Handbook of

LOCAL ANESTHESIA

SIXTH EDITION

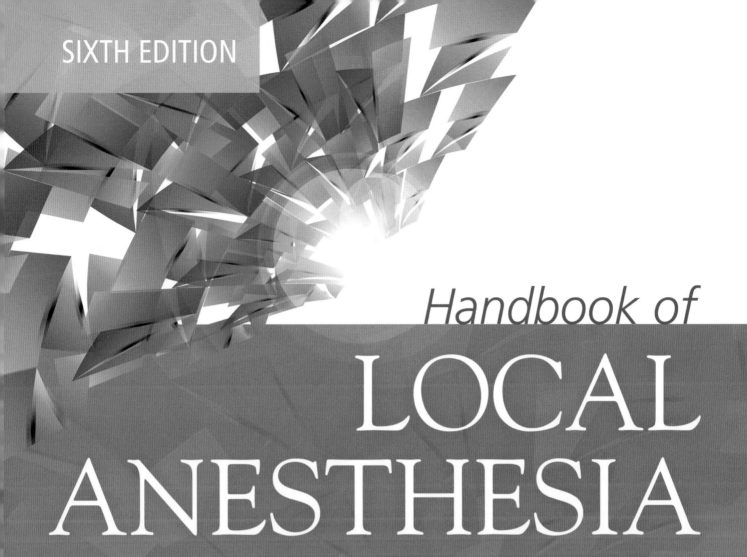

Handbook of LOCAL ANESTHESIA

Stanley F. Malamed, DDS
Professor of Anesthesia and Medicine
School of Dentistry
University of Southern California
Los Angeles, California

with 441 illustrations

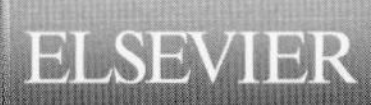

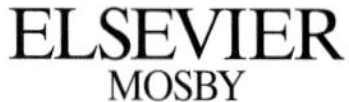

ELSEVIER
MOSBY

3251 Riverport Lane
St. Louis, Missouri 63043

HANDBOOK OF LOCAL ANESTHESIA ISBN: 978-0-323-07413-1

Copyright © 2013 by Mosby, an imprint of Elsevier Inc.
Copyright © 2004 by Mosby, Inc., an affiliate of Elsevier Inc.

No part of this publication may be reproduced or transmitted in any form or by any means, electronic or mechanical, including photocopying, recording, or any information storage and retrieval system, without permission in writing from the publisher. Details on how to seek permission, further information about the Publisher's permissions policies and our arrangements with organizations such as the Copyright Clearance Center and the Copyright Licensing Agency, can be found at our website: www.elsevier.com/permissions.
This book and the individual contributions contained in it are protected under copyright by the Publisher (other than as may be noted herein).

Notices

Knowledge and best practice in this field are constantly changing. As new research and experience broaden our understanding, changes in research methods, professional practices, or medical treatment may become necessary.

Practitioners and researchers must always rely on their own experience and knowledge in evaluating and using any information, methods, compounds, or experiments described herein. In using such information or methods they should be mindful of their own safety and the safety of others, including parties for whom they have a professional responsibility.

With respect to any drug or pharmaceutical products identified, readers are advised to check the most current information provided (i) on procedures featured or (ii) by the manufacturer of each product to be administered, to verify the recommended dose or formula, the method and duration of administration, and contraindications. It is the responsibility of practitioners, relying on their own experience and knowledge of their patients, to make diagnoses, to determine dosages and the best treatment for each individual patient, and to take all appropriate safety precautions.

To the fullest extent of the law, neither the Publisher nor the authors, contributors, or editors, assume any liability for any injury and/or damage to persons or property as a matter of products liability, negligence or otherwise, or from any use or operation of any methods, products, instructions, or ideas contained in the material herein.

Library of Congress Cataloging-in-Publication Data
Malamed, Stanley F., 1944-
Handbook of local anesthesia / Stanley F. Malamed.—6th ed.
p. ; cm.
Includes bibliographical references and index.
ISBN 978-0-323-07413-1 (hardcover : alk. paper)
I. Title.
[DNLM: 1. Anesthesia, Dental. 2. Anesthesia, Local. 3. Injections. WO 460]
617.9'67–dc23
2011051243

Vice President and Publishing Director: Linda Duncan
Executive Content Strategist: John J. Dolan
Senior Content Development Specialist: Brian S. Loehr
Publishing Services Manager: Catherine Jackson
Senior Project Manager: Rachel E. McMullen
Design Direction: Maggie Reid

Printed in China

Last digit is the print number: 9 8 7 6 5 4 3

Working together to grow
libraries in developing countries
www.elsevier.com | www.bookaid.org | www.sabre.org
ELSEVIER BOOK AID International Sabre Foundation

To Beverly, Heather, Jennifer, and Jeremy,
and the next generation: Matthew, Rachel, Gabriella,
Ashley, Rebecca, Elijah, and Ethan

Contributors

Daniel L. Orr II, BS, DDS, MS (Anesthesiology), PhD, JD, MD
Professor and Director
Oral and Maxillofacial Surgery and Advanced Pain Control
University of Nevada Las Vegas School of Dental Medicine
Las Vegas, Nevada
Clinical Professor
Oral and Maxillofacial Surgery
University of Nevada School of Medicine
Las Vegas, Nevada

Mark N. Hochman, DDS
Private Practice Limited to Periodontics
Orthodontics and Implant Dentistry
Specialized Dentistry of New York
New York City, New York
Clinical Associate Professor
New York University
College of Dentistry
New York City, New York
Clinical Consultant
Milestone Scientific, Inc.
Livingston, New Jersey

Preface

The sixth edition of Handbook of Local Anesthesia!

As happened with previous editions, I truly find it hard to comprehend how many years have transpired since the 1st edition was published in 1978. It has been 8 years since the fifth edition and in this time there have been a significant number of changes, many of them advances, in the art and science of pain control in dentistry.

Though the drugs remain the same—articaine HCl, bupivacaine HCl, lidocaine HCl, mepivacaine HCl, and prilocaine HCl—the years since the fifth edition have seen the introduction and refinement of drugs and devices which work to help the dental profession come ever closer to the twin goals of truly pain free dentistry and truly pain free local anesthetic injections.

As I have stated repeatedly in previous editions, "Local anesthetics are the safest and the most effective drugs available in all of medicine for the prevention and the management of pain. Indeed, there are no other drugs that truly prevent pain; no other drugs which actually prevent a propagated nociceptive nerve impulse from reaching the patient's brain, where it would be interpreted as pain. Deposit a local anesthetic drug in close proximity to a sensory nerve and clinically adequate pain control will result in essentially all clinical situations."

Find the nerve with a local anesthetic drug and pain control is virtually assured. Yet in certain clinical situations "finding the nerve" remains a vexing problem. This is especially so in the mandible, primarily permanent mandibular molars. Over my 39 years as a teacher of anesthesia in dentistry I and my dentist anesthesiologist colleagues have worked at "fixing" this problem.

Have we succeeded? Not yet.

Are we getting close to a solution? Yes.

This sixth edition of Local Anesthesia includes new and/or expanded discussions of the periodontal ligament (PDL) injection—including the use of computer-controlled local anesthetic delivery (C-CLAD) systems for PDL (and other injections); the administration of the local anesthetic articaine HCl by mandibular infiltration in the adult mandible; buffering of local anesthetic solutions (the local anesthetic "ON" switch) to increase patient comfort during injection, decrease onset time of anesthesia, and, perhaps, increase the depth of anesthesia; phentolamine mesylate (the local anesthetic "OFF" switch) giving the doctor the opportunity to significantly minimize the duration of a patients residual soft tissue anesthesia, thereby minimizing the risk of self-inflicted soft tissue injury.

I have asked Dr. Mark Hochman to rewrite the discussions in this edition on C-CLAD devices (Chapter 5—The Syringe) and the local anesthetic techniques associated with it (Chapter 15—Supplemental Injections and Chapter 20—Future Considerations). Dr. Hochman has been intimately involved with the development of C-CLAD since the mid-1990s and is the author of a number of refereed papers on the subject including two injection techniques—AMSA (anterior middle superior alveolar nerve block) and P-ASA (palatal—anterior superior alvelar nerve block) that were developed as a result of his research into computer delivery of local anesthetics.

A DVD accompanied the fifth edition of Local Anesthesia. It followed the structure of the textbook, providing clinical demonstrations of the techniques and concepts presented in the text. The DVD has proven to be a highly effective teaching device and is used, both legally and (sadly) illegally, by students, dentists and dental hygienists throughout the world.

A supplemental disk has been incuded with the original 2-disk set which accompanies this sixth edition. The disk presents clinical updates on a number of the newer additions to the local anesthetic armamentarium. It is my feeling, as an educator that the combination of the written text plus the visual impact of the DVD provides a more optimal learning experience for all who come to study this critically important subject.

Feedback from readers of this textbook is always appreciated. Should errors be noted, or suggestions for improvement be made, contact me at malamed@usc.edu.

Stanley F. Malamed

October 2011
Los Angeles, California, USA

Acknowledgments

The people involved with the video production of the new supplemental DVD cannot receive enough thanks: Dr. Joseph Massad and his excellent team at Millennium Productions.

Thanks, too, to the manufacturers of local anesthetic drugs and devices in North America, including Beutlich Pharmaceuticals; Dentsply; Kodak (Cook-Waite); Midwest; Milestone Scientific; Novocol; Septodont, Inc; and Sultan Safety, LLC, for their assistance in supplying photographs and graphics for use in this edition.

I also want to thank Brian S. Loehr, Senior Content Development Specialist; Rachel E. McMullen, Senior Project Manager; and John J. Dolan, Executive Content Strategist, from Mosby (an affiliate of Elsevier) who had the unenviable task of dealing with a frequently lazy, usually hard-to-reach author. Their perseverance—once again—has paid off with this sixth edition.

Finally, I wish to thank the many members of our profession, the dentists and dental hygienists, who have provided me with written and verbal input regarding prior editions of this textbook. Many of their suggestions for additions, deletions, and corrections have been incorporated into this new text. Thanks to you all!

Stanley F. Malamed
December 2011
Los Angeles, California

Contents

New to this Edition

DVD SUPPLEMENT

A supplemental disk has been added to the original 2-disk set. The new DVD supplement presents clinical updates on a number of the newer additions to the local anesthetic armamentarium, including the local anesthesia "ON" and "OFF" switches, and Computer-Controlled Local Anesthetic Delivery (C-CLAD).

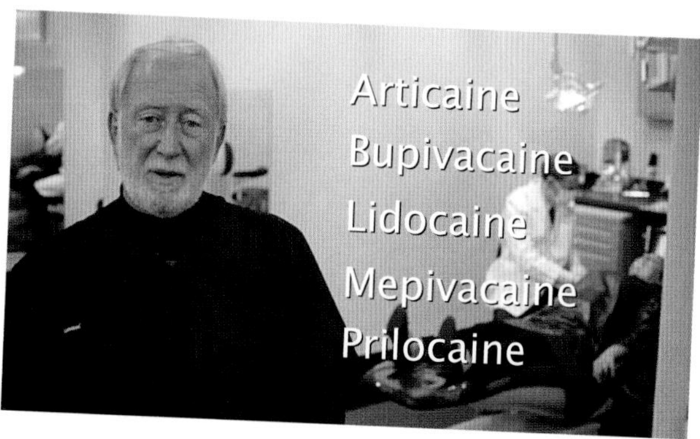

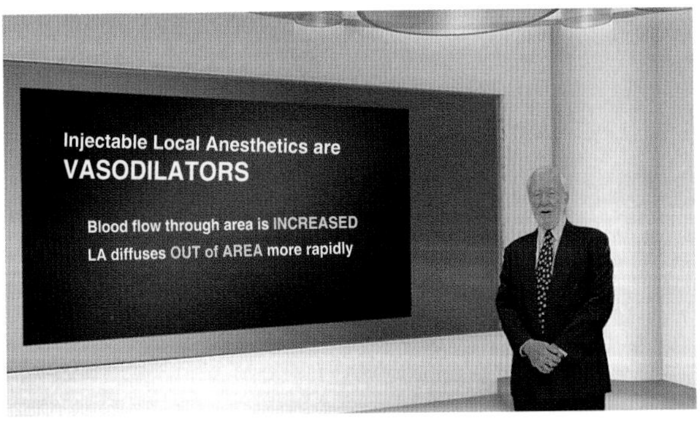

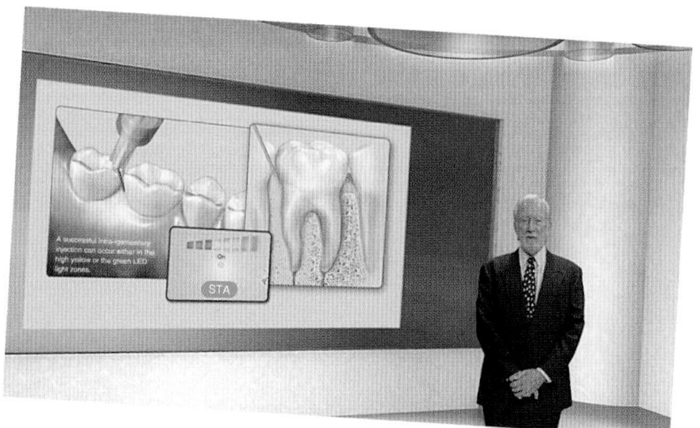

NEW INFORMATION

Updated discussions of the armamentarium needed to succeed in local anesthesia delivery

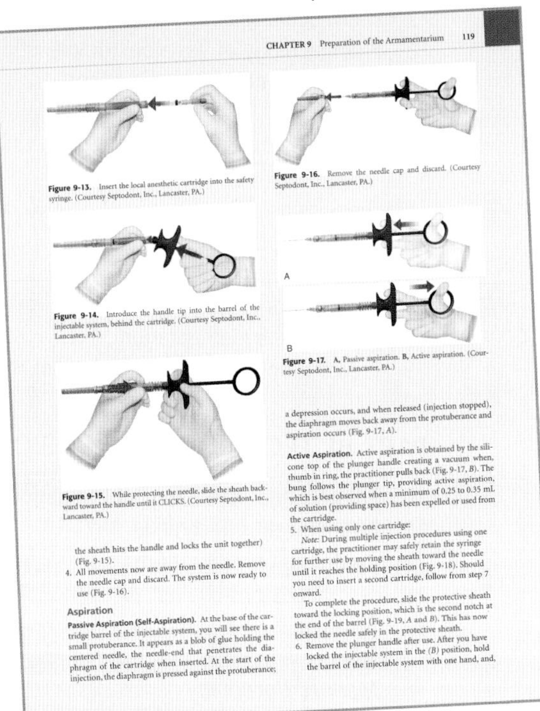

CHAPTER 9 Preparation of the Armamentarium 119

Figure 9-13. Insert the local anesthetic cartridge into the safety syringe. (Courtesy Septodont, Inc., Lancaster, PA.)

Figure 9-14. Introduce the handle tip into the barrel of the injectable system, behind the cartridge. (Courtesy Septodont, Inc., Lancaster, PA.)

Figure 9-15. While protecting the needle, slide the sheath backward toward the handle until it CLICKS. (Courtesy Septodont, Inc., Lancaster, PA.)

the sheath hits the handle and locks the unit together) (Fig. 9-15).

4. All movements now are away from the needle. Remove the needle cap and discard. The system is now ready to use (Fig. 9-16).

Aspiration

Passive Aspiration (Self-Aspiration). At the base of the cartridge barrel of the injectable system, you will see there is a small protuberance. It appears as a blob of glue holding the centered needle, the needle-end that penetrates the diaphragm of the cartridge when inserted. At the start of the injection, the diaphragm is pressed against the protuberance;

Figure 9-16. Remove the needle cap and discard. (Courtesy Septodont, Inc., Lancaster, PA.)

A

B

Figure 9-17. A, Passive aspiration. B, Active aspiration. (Courtesy Septodont, Inc., Lancaster, PA.)

a depression occurs, and when released (injection stopped), the diaphragm moves back away from the protuberance and aspiration occurs (Fig. 9-17, *A*).

Active Aspiration. Active aspiration is obtained by the silicone top of the plunger handle creating a vacuum when, thumb in ring, the practitioner pulls back (Fig. 9-17, *B*). The bung follows the plunger tip, providing active aspiration, which is best observed when a minimum of 0.25 to 0.35 mL of solution (providing space) has been expelled or used from the cartridge.

5. When using only one cartridge:

Note: During multiple injection procedures using one cartridge, the practitioner may safely retain the syringe for further use by moving the sheath toward the needle until it reaches the holding position (Fig. 9-18). Should you need to insert a second cartridge, follow from step 7 onward.

To complete the procedure, slide the protective sheath toward the locking position, which is the second notch at the end of the barrel (Fig. 9-19, *A* and *B*). This has now locked the needle safely in the protective sheath.

6. Remove the plunger handle after use. After you have locked the injectable system in the (*B*) position, hold the barrel of the injectable system with one hand, and,

Computer-controlled local anesthetic delivery (C-CLAD) systems

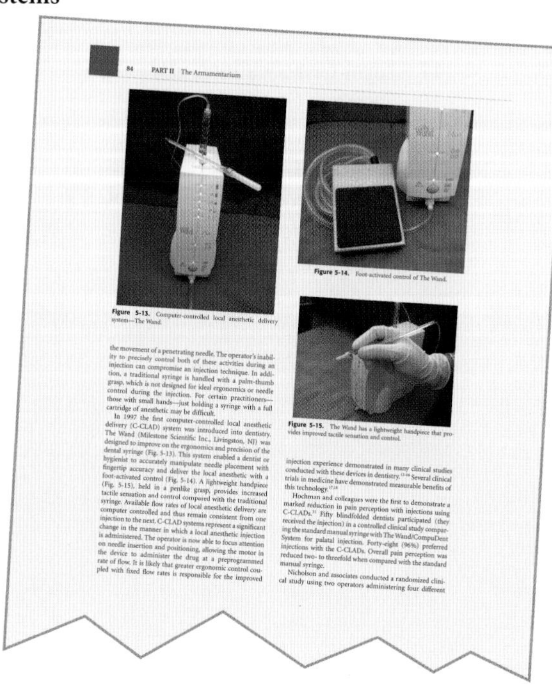

84 PART II The Armamentarium

Figure 5-13. Computer-controlled local anesthetic delivery system—The Wand.

Figure 5-14. Foot-activated control of The Wand.

Figure 5-15. The Wand has a lightweight handpiece that provides improved tactile sensation and control.

the movement of a penetrating needle. The operator's inability to precisely control both of these activities during an injection can compromise an injection technique. In addition, a traditional syringe is handled with a palm-thumb grasp, which is not designed for ideal ergonomics or needle control during the injection. For certain practitioners—those with small hands—just holding a syringe with a full cartridge of anesthetic may be difficult.

In 1997 the first computer-controlled local anesthetic delivery (C-CLAD) system was introduced into dentistry. The Wand (Milestone Scientific Inc., Livingston, NJ) was designed to improve on the ergonomics and precision of the dental syringe (Fig. 5-13). This system enabled a dentist or hygienist to accurately manipulate needle placement with fingertip accuracy and deliver the local anesthetic with a foot-activated control (Fig. 5-14). A lightweight handpiece (Fig. 5-15), held in a penlike grasp, provides increased tactile sensation and control compared with the traditional syringe. Available flow rates of local anesthetic delivery are computer controlled and thus remain consistent from one injection to the next. C-CLAD systems represent a significant change in the manner in which a local anesthetic injection is administered. The operator is now able to focus attention on needle insertion and positioning, allowing the motor in the device to administer the drug at a preprogrammed rate of flow. It is likely that greater ergonomic control coupled with fixed flow rates is responsible for the improved injection experience demonstrated in many clinical studies conducted with these devices in dentistry.[12-16] Several clinical trials in medicine have demonstrated measurable benefits of this technology.[17,18]

Hochman and colleagues were the first to demonstrate a marked reduction in pain perception with injections using C-CLADs.[11] Fifty blindfolded dentists participated (they received the injection) in a controlled clinical study comparing the standard manual syringe with The Wand/CompuDent System for palatal injection. Forty-eight (96%) preferred injections with the C-CLADs. Overall pain perception was reduced two- to threefold when compared with the standard manual syringe.

Nicholson and associates conducted a randomized clinical study using two operators administering four different

NEW ILLUSTRATIONS IDENTIFY CLINICALLY IMPORTANT ANATOMY

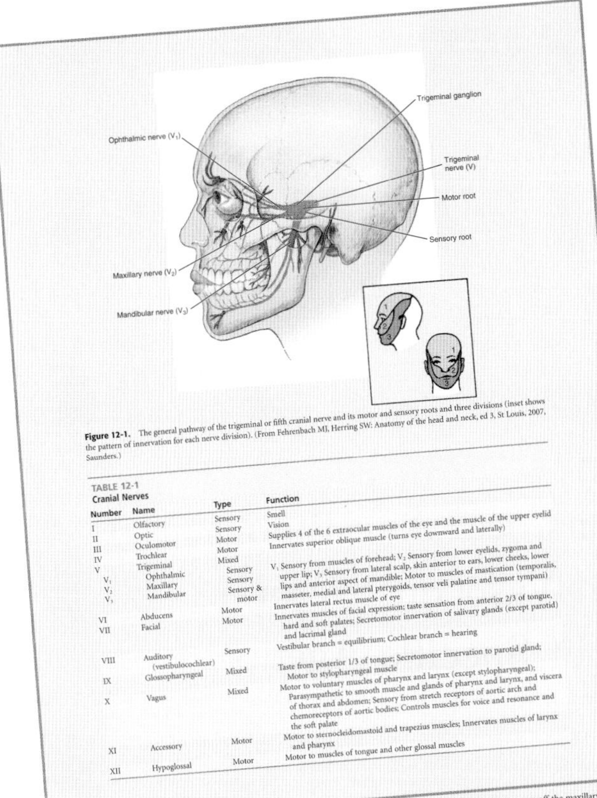

Figure 12-1. The general pathway of the trigeminal or fifth cranial nerve and its motor and sensory roots and three divisions (inset shows the pattern of innervation for each nerve division). (From Fehrenbach MJ, Herring SW: Anatomy of the head and neck, ed 3, St Louis, 2007, Saunders.)

TABLE 12-1
Cranial Nerves

Number	Name	Type	Function
I	Olfactory	Sensory	Smell
II	Optic	Sensory	Vision
III	Oculomotor	Motor	Supplies 4 of the 6 extraocular muscles of the eye and the muscle of the upper eyelid
IV	Trochlear	Motor	Innervates superior oblique muscle (turns eye downward and laterally)
V	Trigeminal	Mixed	
V_1	Ophthalmic	Sensory	V_1 Sensory from muscles of forehead; V_2 Sensory from lower eyelids, zygoma and upper lip; V_3 Sensory from lateral scalp, skin anterior to ears, lower cheeks, lower lips and anterior aspect of mandible; Motor to muscles of mastication (temporalis, masseter, medial and lateral pterygoids, tensor veli palatine and tensor tympani)
V_2	Maxillary	Sensory	
V_3	Mandibular	Sensory & motor	
VI	Abducens	Motor	Innervates lateral rectus muscle of eye
VII	Facial	Motor	Innervates muscles of facial expression; taste sensation from anterior 2/3 of tongue, hard and soft palates; Secretomotor innervation of salivary glands (except parotid) and lacrimal gland
VIII	Auditory (vestibulocochlear)	Sensory	Vestibular branch = equilibrium; Cochlear branch = hearing
IX	Glossopharyngeal	Mixed	Taste from posterior 1/3 of tongue; Secretomotor innervation to parotid gland; Motor to stylopharyngeal muscle
X	Vagus	Mixed	Motor to voluntary muscles of pharynx and larynx (except stylopharyngeal); Parasympathetic to smooth muscle and glands of pharynx and larynx, and viscera of thorax and abdomen; Sensory from stretch receptors of aortic arch and chemoreceptors of aortic bodies; Controls muscles for voice and resonance and the soft palate
XI	Accessory	Motor	Motor to sternocleidomastoid and trapezius muscles; Innervates muscles of larynx and pharynx
XII	Hypoglossal	Motor	Motor to muscles of tongue and other glossal muscles

CHAPTER 12 Anatomic Considerations 171

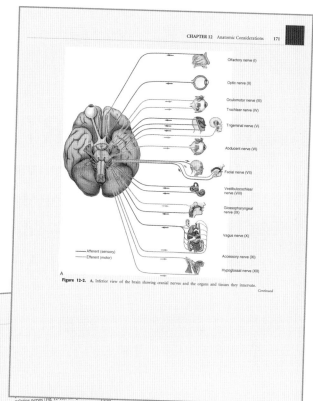

Olfactory nerve (I)
Optic nerve (II)
Oculomotor nerve (III)
Trochlear nerve (IV)
Trigeminal nerve (V)
Abducent nerve (VI)
Facial nerve (VII)
Vestibulocochlear nerve (VIII)
Glossopharyngeal nerve (IX)
Vagus nerve (X)
Accessory nerve (XI)
Hypoglossal nerve (XII)
Afferent (sensory)
Efferent (motor)
A

Figure 12-2. A, Inferior view of the brain showing cranial nerves and the organs and tissues they innervate.

Continued

The zygomatic nerve comes off the maxillary division in the pterygopalatine fossa and travels anteriorly, entering the orbit through the inferior orbital fissure, where it divides into the zygomaticotemporal and zygomaticofacial nerves: the zygomaticotemporal supplying sensory innervation to the skin on the side of the forehead, and the zygomaticofacial supplying the skin on the prominence of the cheek. Just before leaving the orbit, the zygomatic nerve sends a branch that communicates with the lacrimal nerve of the ophthalmic division. This branch carries secretory fibers from the sphenopalatine ganglion to the lacrimal gland.

The pterygopalatine nerves are two short trunks that unite in the pterygopalatine ganglion and are then redistributed into several branches. They also serve as a communication between the pterygopalatine ganglion and the maxillary nerve (V_2). Postganglionic secretomotor fibers from the pterygopalatine ganglion pass through these nerves and back along V_2 to the zygomatic nerve, through which they are routed to the lacrimal nerve and the lacrimal gland.

Branches of the pterygopalatine nerves include those that supply four areas: orbit, nose, palate, and pharynx.

1. The orbital branches supply the periosteum of the orbit.
2. The nasal branches supply the mucous membranes of the superior and middle conchae, the lining of the posterior ethmoidal sinuses, and the posterior portion of the nasal septum. One branch is significant in dentistry, the nasopalatine nerve, which passes across the roof of the nasal cavity downward and forward, where it lies between the mucous membrane and the periosteum of the nasal septum. The nasopalatine nerve

palatine nerves (Fig. 12-10)... palatine nerve descends through the pterygopalatine canal, emerging on the hard palate through the greater palatine foramen (which is usually located about 1 cm toward the palatal midline, just distal to the second molar). Sicher and DuBrul have stated that the greater palatine foramen may be located 3 to 4 mm in front of the posterior border of the hard palate.[1] The nerve courses anteriorly between the mucoperiosteum and the osseous hard palate, supplying sensory innervation to the palatal soft tissues and bone as far anterior as the first premolar, where it communicates with terminal fibers of the nasopalatine nerve (see Fig. 12-10). It also provides sensory innervation to some parts of the soft palate. The middle palatine nerve emerges from the lesser palatine foramen, along with the posterior palatine nerve. The middle palatine nerve provides sensory innervation to the mucous membrane of

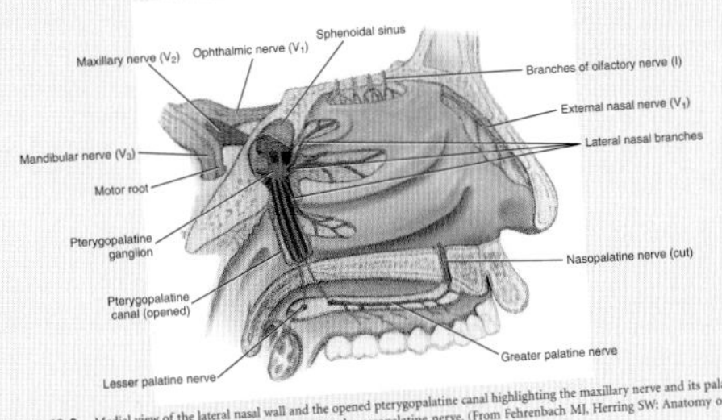

Figure 12-9. Medial view of the lateral nasal wall and the opened pterygopalatine canal highlighting the maxillary nerve and its palatine branches. The nasal septum has been removed, thus severing the nasopalatine nerve. (From Fehrenbach MJ, Herring SW: Anatomy of the head and neck, ed 3, St Louis, 2007, Saunders.)

IN THIS PART

PART I

The Drugs

In the first section of this book, the pharmacologic and clinical properties of the classes of drugs known as local anesthetics (Chapter 2) and vasoconstrictors (Chapter 3) are discussed. Knowledge of both the pharmacologic and clinical properties of these drugs, by all persons permitted to administer them, is absolutely essential for their safe use and for a better understanding of those potentially life-threatening systemic reactions associated with their administration. Emphasis is placed on local anesthetic drug combinations currently used in anesthesia in dentistry in North America (Chapter 4).

Chapter 1 provides a background for understanding how local anesthetics work to transiently block nerve conduction, thus preventing pain from being experienced. The anatomy and physiology of normal neurons and nerve conduction are reviewed as a background for the discussion, which, in subsequent chapters, takes up the pharmacology and clinical actions of various specific agents.

CHAPTER 1

Neurophysiology

DESIRABLE PROPERTIES OF LOCAL ANESTHETICS

Local anesthesia has been defined as loss of sensation in a circumscribed area of the body caused by depression of excitation in nerve endings or inhibition of the conduction process in peripheral nerves.[1] An important feature of local anesthesia is that it produces this loss of sensation without inducing loss of consciousness. In this one major area, local anesthesia differs dramatically from general anesthesia.

Many methods are used to induce local anesthesia:

1. Mechanical trauma (compression of tissues)
2. Low temperature
3. Anoxia
4. Chemical irritants
5. Neurolytic agents such as alcohol and phenol
6. Chemical agents such as local anesthetics

However, only those methods or substances that induce a transient and completely reversible state of anesthesia have application in clinical practice. Following are those properties deemed most desirable for a local anesthetic:

1. It should not be irritating to the tissue to which it is applied.
2. It should not cause any permanent alteration of nerve structure.
3. Its systemic toxicity should be low.
4. It must be effective regardless of whether it is injected into the tissue or is applied locally to mucous membranes.
5. The time of onset of anesthesia should be as short as possible.
6. The duration of action must be long enough to permit completion of the procedure yet not so long as to require an extended recovery.

Most local anesthetics discussed in this section meet the first two criteria: They are (relatively) nonirritating to tissues and are completely reversible. Of paramount importance is systemic toxicity, because all injectable and most topical local anesthetics are eventually absorbed from their site of administration into the cardiovascular system. The potential toxicity of a drug is an important factor in its consideration for use as a local anesthetic. Toxicity varies greatly among the local anesthetics currently in use. Toxicity is discussed more thoroughly in Chapter 2. Although it is a desirable characteristic, not all local anesthetics in clinical use today meet the criterion of being effective, regardless of whether the drug is injected or applied topically. Several of the more potent injectable local anesthetics (e.g., procaine, mepivacaine) prove to be relatively ineffective when applied topically to mucous membranes. To be effective as topical anesthetics, these drugs must be applied in concentrations that prove to be locally irritating to tissues while increasing the risk of systemic toxicity. Dyclonine, a potent topical anesthetic, is not administered by injection because of its tissue-irritating properties. Lidocaine and tetracaine, on the other hand, are effective anesthetics when administered by injection or topical application in clinically acceptable concentrations. The last factors—rapid onset of action and adequate duration of clinical action—are met satisfactorily by most of the clinically effective local anesthetics in use today. Clinical duration of action does vary considerably among drugs and also among different preparations of the same drug, as well as by the type of injection administered (e.g., nerve block vs. supraperiosteal). The duration of anesthesia necessary to complete a procedure is a major consideration in the selection of a local anesthetic.

In addition to these qualities, Bennett[2] lists other desirable properties of an ideal local anesthetic:

7. It should have potency sufficient to give complete anesthesia without the use of harmful concentrated solutions.
8. It should be relatively free from producing allergic reactions.
9. It should be stable in solution and should readily undergo biotransformation in the body.
10. It should be sterile or capable of being sterilized by heat without deterioration.

No local anesthetic in use today satisfies all of these criteria; however, all anesthetics do meet a majority of them. Research is continuing in an effort to produce newer drugs that possess a maximum of desirable factors and a minimum of negative ones.

FUNDAMENTALS OF IMPULSE GENERATION AND TRANSMISSION

The discovery in the late 1800s of a group of chemicals with the ability to prevent pain without inducing loss of consciousness was one of the major steps in the advancement of the medical and dental professions. For the first time, medical and dental procedures, could be carried out easily and in the absence of pain, a fact that is virtually taken for granted by contemporary medical and dental professionals and their patients.

The concept behind the actions of local anesthetics is simple: They prevent both the generation and the conduction of a nerve impulse. In effect, local anesthetics set up a chemical roadblock between the source of the impulse (e.g., the scalpel incision in soft tissues) and the brain. Therefore the aborted impulse, prevented from reaching the brain, cannot be interpreted by the patient as pain.

This is similar to the effect of lighting the fuse on a stick of dynamite. The fuse is the "nerve," whereas the dynamite is the "brain." If the fuse is lit and the flame reaches the dynamite, an explosion occurs (Fig. 1-1). When a nerve is stimulated, an impulse is propagated that will be interpreted as pain when it reaches the brain. If the fuse is lit, but "water" (e.g., local anesthetic) is placed somewhere between the end of the fuse and the dynamite stick, the fuse will burn up to the point of water application and then die out. The dynamite does not explode. When a local anesthetic is placed at some point between the pain stimulus (e.g., the drill) and the brain, the nerve impulse is still propagated and travels up to the point of local anesthetic application and then "dies," never reaching the brain, and pain does not occur (Fig. 1-2).

How, in fact, do local anesthetics, the most used drugs in dentistry, function to abolish or prevent pain? Following is a discussion of current theories seeking to explain the mode of action of local anesthetic drugs. To understand their action better, however, the reader must have an acquaintance with the fundamentals of nerve conduction. A review of the relevant characteristics and properties of nerve anatomy and physiology follows.

The Neuron

The neuron, or nerve cell, is the structural unit of the nervous system. It is able to transmit messages between the central nervous system (CNS) and all parts of the body. There are two basic types of neuron: sensory (afferent) and motor (efferent). The basic structure of these two neuronal types differs significantly (Fig. 1-3).

Sensory neurons that are capable of transmitting the sensation of pain consist of three major portions.[3] The *peripheral process* (also known as the *dendritic zone*), which is composed of an arborization of free nerve endings, is the most distal segment of the sensory neuron. These free nerve

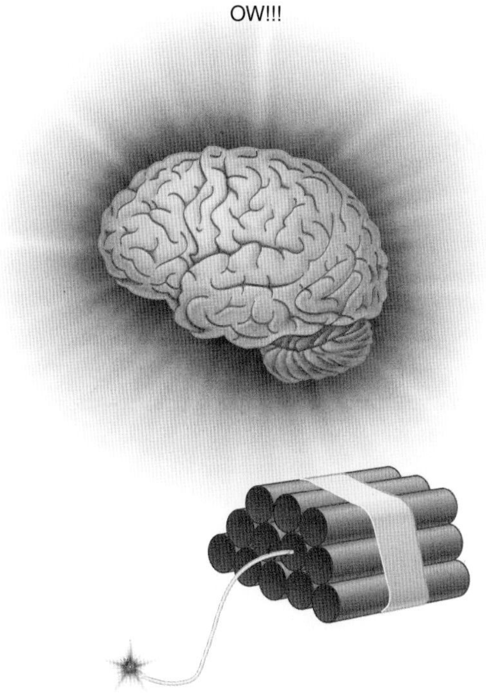

Figure 1-1. The fuse is lit and the flame reaches the dynamite; an explosion occurs, and the patient experiences pain.

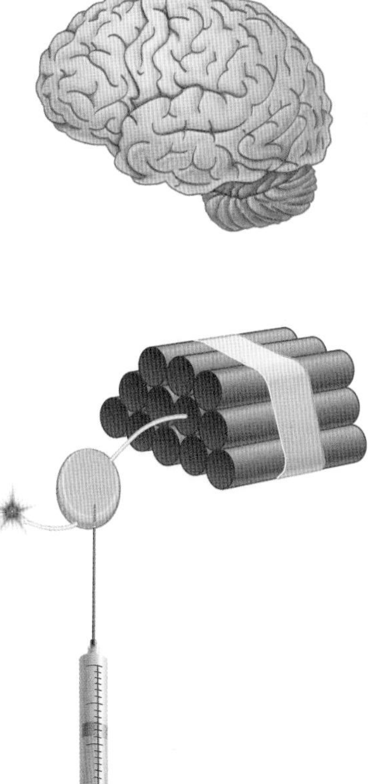

Figure 1-2. Local anesthetic is placed at some point between the pain stimulus and the brain (dynamite). The nerve impulse travels up to the point of local anesthetic application and then "dies," never reaching the brain, and pain does not occur.

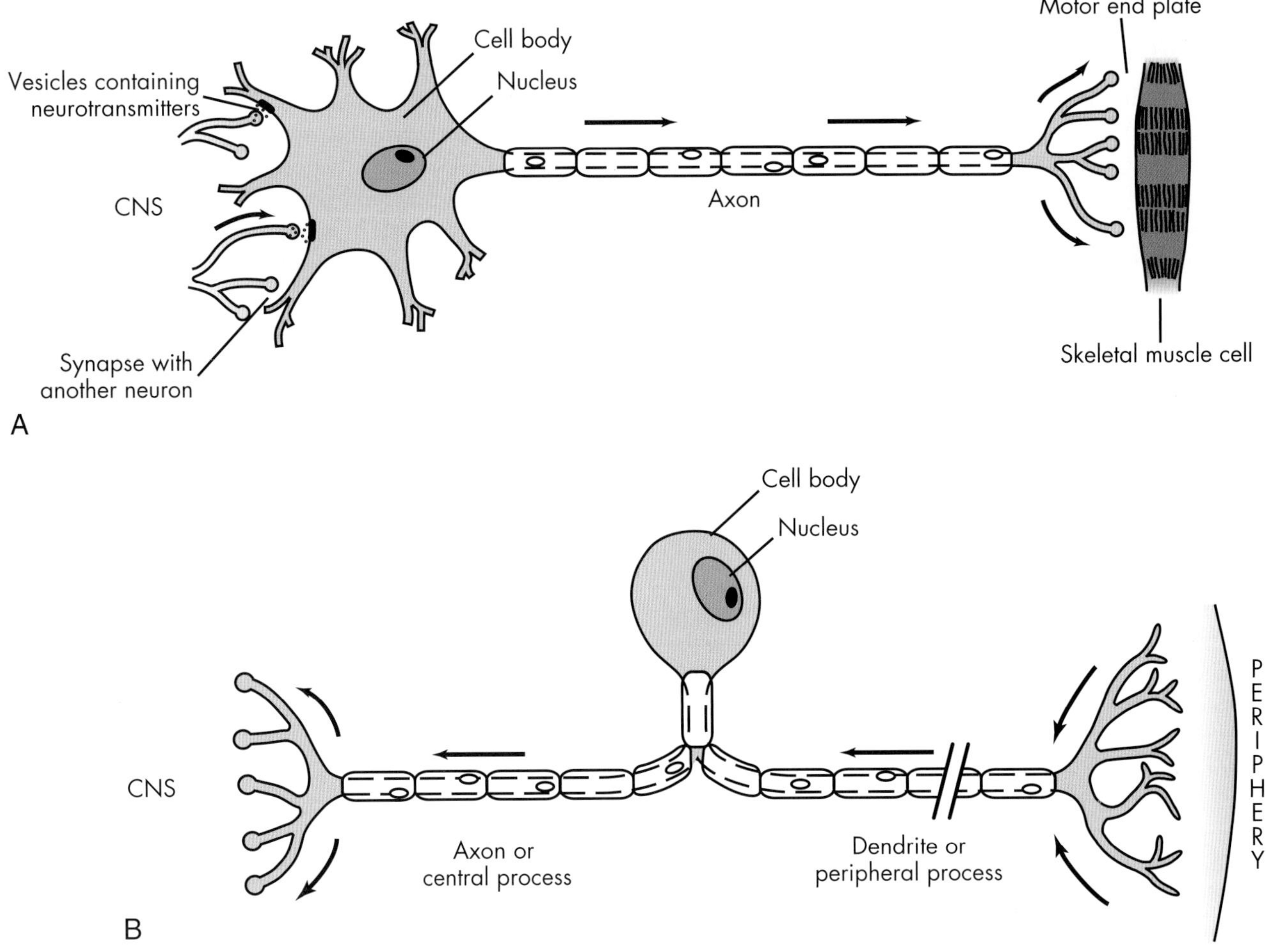

Figure 1-3. **A,** Multipolar motor neuron. **B,** Unipolar sensory neuron. (From Liebgott B: Anatomical basis of dentistry, ed 2, St Louis, 2001, Mosby.)

endings respond to stimulation produced in the tissues in which they lie, provoking an impulse that is transmitted centrally along the axon. The *axon* is a thin cable-like structure that may be quite long (the giant squid axon has been measured at 100 to 200 cm). At its mesial (or central) end is an arborization similar to that seen in the peripheral process. However, in this case the arborization forms synapses with various nuclei in the CNS to distribute incoming (sensory) impulses to their appropriate sites within the CNS for interpretation. The *cell body* is the third part of the neuron. In the sensory neuron described here, the cell body is located at a distance from the axon, the main pathway of impulse transmission in this nerve. The cell body of the sensory nerve therefore is not involved in the process of impulse transmission, its primary function being to provide vital metabolic support for the entire neuron (Fig. 1-3, *B*).

Nerve cells that conduct impulses from the CNS toward the periphery are termed *motor neurons* and are structurally different from the sensory neurons just described in that their cell body is interposed between the axon and dendrites. In motor neurons, the cell body not only is an integral component of the impulse transmission system but also provides metabolic support for the cell. Near its termination, the axon branches with each branch, ending as a bulbous axon terminal (or bouton). Axon terminals synapse with muscle cells (Fig. 1-3, *A*).

The Axon

The single nerve fiber, the axon, is a long cylinder of neural cytoplasm (axoplasm) encased in a thin sheath, the nerve membrane, or axolemma. Neurons have a cell body and a nucleus, as do all other cells; however, neurons differ from other cells in that they have an axonal process from which the cell body may be at a considerable distance. The axoplasm, a gelatinous substance, is separated from extracellular fluids by a continuous nerve membrane. In some nerves, this membrane is itself covered by an insulating lipid-rich layer of myelin.

Current thinking holds that both sensory nerve excitability and conduction are attributable to changes developing within the nerve membrane. The cell body and the axoplasm are not essential for nerve conduction. They are important, however. The metabolic support of the membrane is probably derived from the axoplasm.

The nerve (cell) membrane itself is approximately 70 to 80 Å thick. (An angstrom unit is 1/10,000 of a micrometer.) Figure 1-4 represents a currently acceptable configuration. All biological membranes are organized to block the diffusion of water-soluble molecules; to be selectively permeable to certain molecules via specialized pores or channels; and to transduce information through protein receptors responsive to chemical or physical stimulation by neurotransmitters or hormones (chemical) or light, vibration, or pressure (physical).[4] The membrane is described as a flexible nonstretchable structure consisting of two layers of lipid molecules (bilipid layer of phospholipids) and associated proteins, lipids, and carbohydrates. The lipids are oriented with their hydrophilic (polar) ends facing the outer surface and their hydrophobic (nonpolar) ends projecting to the middle of the membrane (Fig. 1-4, *A*). Proteins are visualized as the primary organizational elements of membranes (Fig. 1-4, *B*).[5] Proteins are classified as transport proteins (channels, carriers, or pumps) and receptor sites. Channel proteins are thought to be continuous pores through the membrane, allowing some ions (Na^+, K^+, Ca^{++}) to flow passively, whereas other channels are gated, permitting ion flow only when the gate is open.[4] The nerve membrane lies at the interface between extracellular fluid and axoplasm. It separates highly diverse ionic concentrations within the axon from those outside. The resting nerve membrane has an electrical resistance about 50 times greater than that of the intracellular and extracellular fluids, thus preventing the passage of sodium, potassium, and chloride ions down their concentration gradients. However, when a nerve impulse passes, electrical conductivity of the nerve membrane increases approximately 100-fold. This increase in conductivity permits the passage of sodium and potassium ions along their concentration gradients through the nerve membrane. It is the movement of these ions that provides an immediate source of energy for impulse conduction along the nerve.

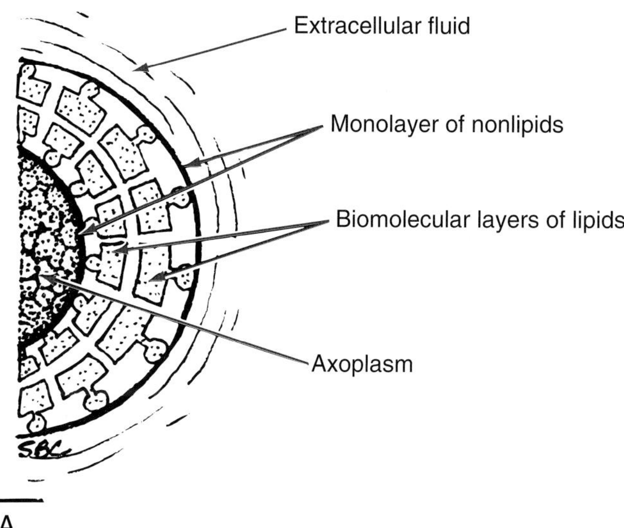

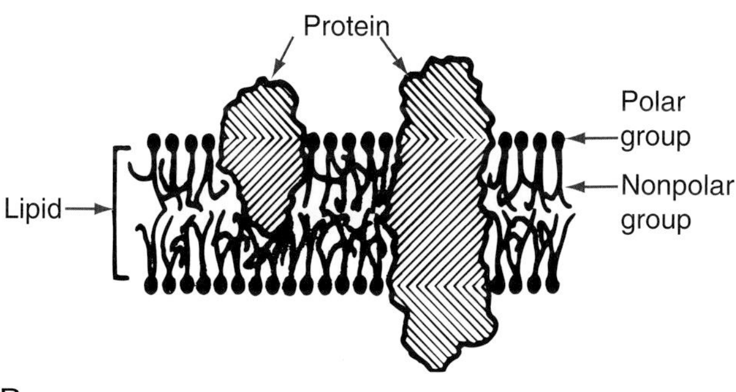

Figure 1-4. **A,** Configuration of a biological membrane. **B,** Heterogeneous lipoprotein membrane as suggested by Singer and Nicholson. (Redrawn from Covino BG, Vassalo HG: Local anesthetics: mechanisms of action and clinical use, New York, 1976, Grune & Stratton.)

Some nerve fibers are covered by an insulating lipid layer of myelin. In vertebrates, myelinated nerve fibers include all but the smallest of axons (Table 1-1).[6] Myelinated nerve fibers (Fig. 1-5) are enclosed in spirally wrapped layers of lipoprotein myelin sheaths, which are actually a specialized form of Schwann cell. Although primarily lipid (75%), the myelin sheath also contains some protein (20%) and carbohydrate (5%).[7] Each myelinated nerve fiber is enclosed in its own myelin sheath. The outermost layer of myelin consists of the Schwann cell cytoplasm and its nucleus. Constrictions are located at regular intervals (approximately every 0.5 to 3 mm) along the myelinated nerve fiber. These are nodes of Ranvier, and they form a gap between two adjoining Schwann cells and their myelin spirals.[8] At these

TABLE 1-1
Classification of Peripheral Nerves According to Fiber Size and Physiologic Properties

Fiber Class	Subclass	Myelin	Diameter, μ	Conduction Velocity, m/s	Location	Function
A	alpha	+	6-22	30-120	Afferent to and efferent from muscles and joints	Motor, proprioception
	beta	+	6-22	30-120	Afferent to and efferent from muscles and joints	Motor, proprioception
	gamma	+	3-6	15-35	Efferent to muscle spindles	Muscle tone
	delta	+	1-4	5-25	Afferent sensory nerves	Pain, temperature, touch
B		+	<3	3-15	Preganglionic sympathetic	Various autonomic functions
C	sC	–	0.3-1.3	0.7-1.3	Postganglionic sympathetic	Various autonomic functions
	d gammaC	–	0.4-1.2	0.1-2.0	Afferent sensory nerves	Various autonomic functions; pain, temperature, touch

From Berde CB, Strichartz GR: Local anesthetics. In Miller RD, editor: Anesthesia, ed 5, Philadelphia, 2000, Churchill Livingstone, pp 491–521.

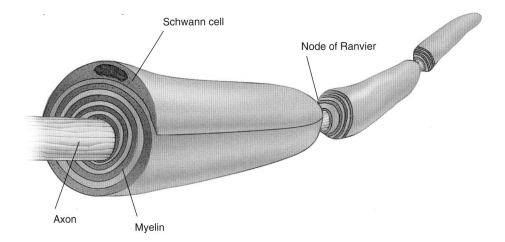

Figure 1-5. Structure of a myelinated nerve fiber. (Redrawn from de Jong RH: Local anesthetics, St Louis, 1994, Mosby.)

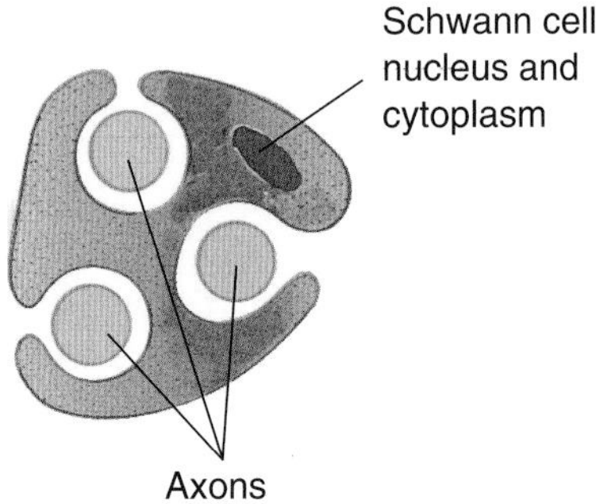

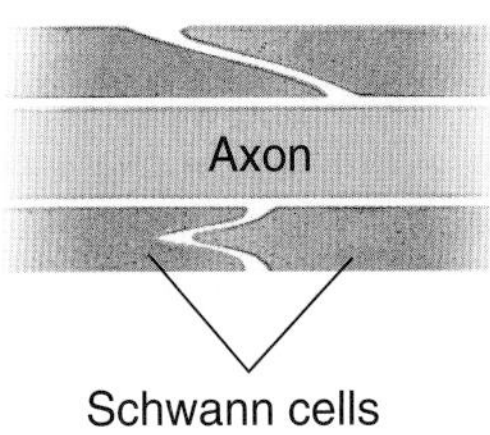

Figure 1-6. Types of Schwann cell sheaths. (Redrawn from Wildsmith JAW: Peripheral nerve and anaesthetic drugs, Br J Anaesth 58:692-700, 1986.)

nodes, the nerve membrane is exposed directly to the extracellular medium.

Unmyelinated nerve fibers (Fig. 1-6) are also surrounded by a Schwann cell sheath. Groups of unmyelinated nerve fibers share the same sheath. The insulating properties of the myelin sheath enable a myelinated nerve to conduct impulses at a much faster rate than an unmyelinated nerve of equal size.

Physiology of the Peripheral Nerves

The function of a nerve is to carry messages from one part of the body to another. These messages, in the form of electrical action potentials, are called *impulses.* Action potentials are transient depolarizations of the membrane that result from a brief increase in the permeability of the membrane to sodium, and usually also from a delayed increase in its permeability to potassium.[9] Impulses are initiated by chemical, thermal, mechanical, or electrical stimuli.

Once an impulse is initiated by a stimulus in any particular nerve fiber, the amplitude and shape of that impulse remain constant, regardless of changes in the quality of the stimulus or in its strength. The impulse remains constant without losing strength as it passes along the nerve because the energy used for its propagation is derived from energy that is released by the nerve fiber along its length and not solely from the initial stimulus. de Jong has described impulse conduction as being like the active progress of a spark along a fuse of gunpowder.[10] Once lit, the fuse burns steadily along its length, with one burning segment providing the energy necessary to ignite its neighbor. Such is the situation with impulse propagation along a nerve.

Electrophysiology of Nerve Conduction

Following is a description of electrical events that occur within a nerve during the conduction of an impulse. Subsequent sections describe the precise mechanisms for each of these steps.

A nerve possesses a resting potential (Fig. 1-7, Step 1). This is a negative electrical potential of –70 mV that exists across the nerve membrane, produced by differing concentrations of ions on either side of the membrane (Table 1-2). The interior of the nerve is negative relative to the exterior.

Step 1. A stimulus excites the nerve, leading to the following sequence of events:

A. An initial phase of slow depolarization. The electrical potential within the nerve becomes slightly less negative (see Fig. 1-7, *Step 1A*).
B. When the falling electrical potential reaches a critical level, an extremely rapid phase of depolarization results. This is termed *threshold potential,* or *firing threshold* (see Fig. 1-7, *Step 1B*).
C. This phase of rapid depolarization results in a reversal of the electrical potential across the nerve membrane

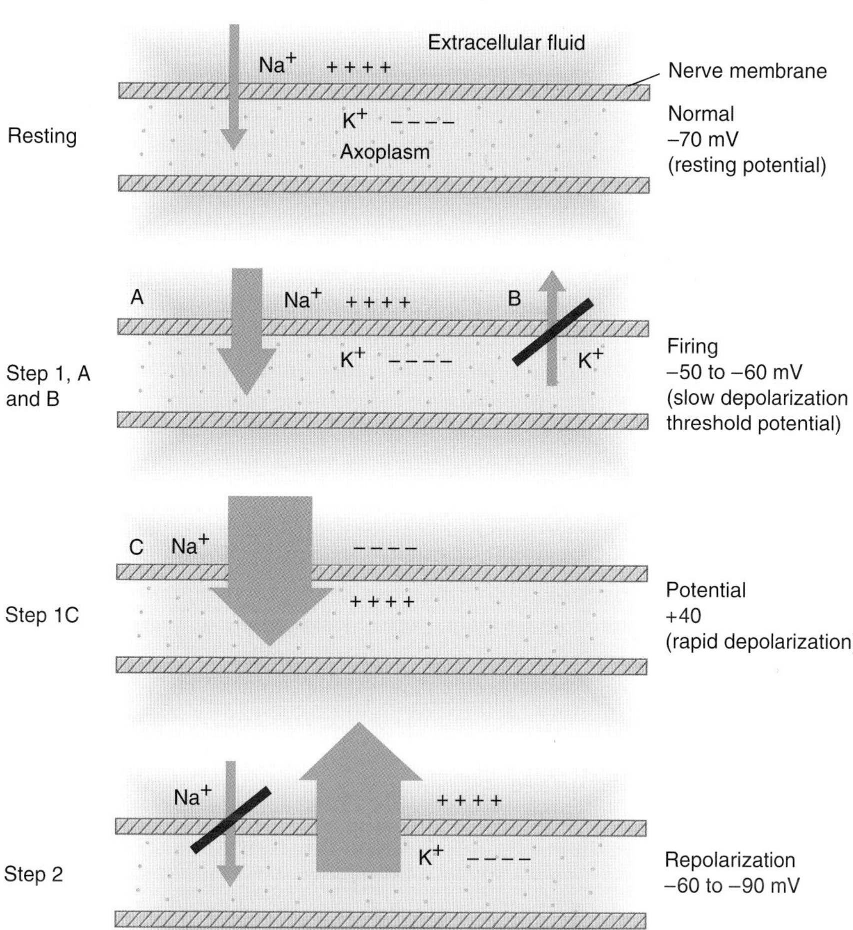

Figure 1-7. *Top,* Resting potential. Step 1, **A** and **B,** Slow depolarization to threshold. Step 1, **C,** Rapid depolarization. Step 2, Repolarization.

TABLE 1-2
Intracellular and Extracellular Ionic Concentrations

Ion	Intracellular, mEq/L	Extracellular, mEq/L	Ratio (approximate)
Potassium (K^+)	110-170	3-5	27:1
Sodium (Na^+)	5-10	140	1:14
Chloride (Cl^-)	5-10	110	1:11

(see Fig. 1-7, *Step 1C*). The interior of the nerve is now electrically positive in relation to the exterior. An electrical potential of +40 mV exists on the interior of the nerve cell.[11]

Step 2. After these steps of depolarization, repolarization occurs (Fig. 1-7, *Step 2*). The electrical potential gradually becomes more negative inside the nerve cell relative to outside until the original resting potential of −70 mV is again achieved.

The entire process (Steps 1 and 2) requires 1 millisecond (msec); depolarization (Step 1) takes 0.3 msec; repolarization (Step 2) takes 0.7 msec.

Electrochemistry of Nerve Conduction

The preceding sequence of events depends on two important factors: the concentrations of electrolytes in the axoplasm (interior of the nerve cell) and extracellular fluids, and the permeability of the nerve membrane to sodium and potassium ions.

Table 1-2 shows the differing concentrations of ions found within neurons and in the extracellular fluids. Significant differences exist for ions between their intracellular and extracellular concentrations. These ionic gradients differ because the nerve membrane exhibits selective permeability.

Resting State. In its resting state, the nerve membrane is

- Slightly permeable to sodium ions (Na^+)
- Freely permeable to potassium ions (K^+)
- Freely permeable to chloride ions (Cl^-)

Potassium remains within the axoplasm, despite its ability to diffuse freely through the nerve membrane and its concentration gradient (passive diffusion usually occurs from a region of greater concentration to one of lesser concentration), because the negative charge of the nerve membrane restrains the positively charged ions by electrostatic attraction.

Chloride remains outside the nerve membrane instead of moving along its concentration gradient into the nerve cell, because the opposing, nearly equal, electrostatic influence (electrostatic gradient from inside to outside) forces outward migration. The net result is no diffusion of chloride through the membrane.

Sodium migrates inwardly because both the concentration (greater outside) and the electrostatic gradient (positive ion attracted by negative intracellular potential) favor such migration. Only the fact that the resting nerve membrane is relatively impermeable to sodium prevents a massive influx of this ion.

Membrane Excitation

Depolarization. Excitation of a nerve segment leads to an increase in permeability of the cell membrane to sodium ions. This is accomplished by a transient widening of transmembrane ion channels sufficient to permit the unhindered passage of hydrated sodium ions. The rapid influx of sodium ions to the interior of the nerve cell causes depolarization of the nerve membrane from its resting level to its firing threshold of approximately −50 to −60 mV (see Fig. 1-7, Steps 1A and 1B).[12] The firing threshold is actually the magnitude of the decrease in negative transmembrane potential that is necessary to initiate an action potential (impulse).

A decrease in negative transmembrane potential of 15 mV (e.g., from −70 to −55 mV) is necessary to reach the firing threshold; a voltage difference of less than 15 mV will not initiate an impulse. In a normal nerve, the firing threshold remains constant. Exposure of the nerve to a local anesthetic raises its firing threshold. Elevating the firing threshold means that more sodium must pass through the membrane to decrease the negative transmembrane potential to a level where depolarization occurs.

When the firing threshold is reached, membrane permeability to sodium increases dramatically and sodium ions rapidly enter the axoplasm. At the end of depolarization (the peak of the action potential), the electrical potential of the nerve is actually reversed; an electrical potential of +40 mV exists (see Fig. 1-7, *Step 1C*). The entire depolarization process requires approximately 0.3 msec.

Repolarization. The action potential is terminated when the membrane repolarizes. This is caused by the extinction *(inactivation)* of increased permeability to sodium. In many cells, permeability to potassium also increases, resulting in the efflux of K^+, and leading to more rapid membrane repolarization and return to its resting potential (see Fig. 1-7, *Step 2*).

Movement of sodium ions into the cell during depolarization and subsequent movement of potassium ions out of the cell during repolarization are passive (not requiring the expenditure of energy), because each ion moves along its concentration gradient (higher → lower). After the return of the membrane potential to its original level (−70 mV), a slight excess of sodium exists within the nerve cell, along with a slight excess of potassium extracellularly. A period of metabolic activity then begins in which active transfer of sodium ions out of the cell occurs via the sodium pump. An expenditure of energy is necessary to move sodium ions out of the nerve cell against their concentration gradient; this energy comes from the oxidative metabolism of adenosine triphosphate (ATP). The same pumping mechanism is thought to be responsible for the active transport of potassium ions into the cell against their concentration gradient. The process of repolarization requires 0.7 msec.

Immediately after a stimulus has initiated an action potential, a nerve is unable, for a time, to respond to another stimulus regardless of its strength. This is termed the *absolute refractory period,* and it lasts for about the duration of the main part of the action potential. The absolute refractory period is followed by a *relative refractory period,* during which a new impulse can be initiated but only by a stronger than normal stimulus. The relative refractory period continues to decrease until the normal level of excitability returns, at which point the nerve is said to be repolarized.

During depolarization, a major proportion of ionic sodium channels are found in their open (O) state (thus permitting the rapid influx of Na^+). This is followed by a slower decline into a state of inactivation (I) of the channels to a nonconducting state. Inactivation temporarily converts the channels to a state from which they cannot open in response to depolarization (absolute refractory period). This inactivated state is slowly converted back, so that most channels are found in their closed (C) resting form when the membrane is repolarized (−70 mV). Upon depolarization, the channels change configuration, first to an open ion-conducting (O) state and then to an inactive nonconducting (I) state. Although both C and I states correspond to nonconducting channels, they differ in that depolarization can recruit channels to the conducting O state from C but not from I. Figure 1-8 describes the sodium channel transition stages.[13]

Membrane Channels. Discrete aqueous pores through the excitable nerve membrane, called *sodium* (or *ion*) *channels,* are molecular structures that mediate its sodium permeability. A channel appears to be a lipoglycoprotein firmly situated in the membrane (see Fig. 1-4). It consists of an aqueous pore spanning the membrane that is narrow enough at least at one point to discriminate between sodium ions and others; Na^+ passes through 12 times more easily than K^+. The channel also includes a portion that changes configuration in response to changes in membrane potential, thereby gating the passage of ions through the pore (C, O, and I states are described). The presence of these channels helps explain membrane permeability or impermeability to certain ions. Sodium channels have an internal diameter of approximately 0.3 × 0.5 nm.[14]

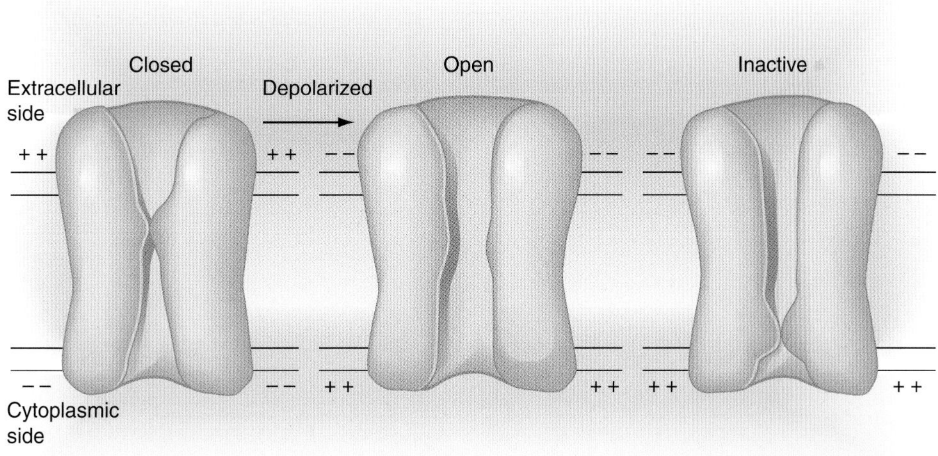

Figure 1-8. Sodium channel transition stages. Depolarization reverses resting membrane potential from interior negative *(left)* to interior positive *(center)*. The channel proteins undergo corresponding conformational changes from resting state *(closed)* to ion-conducting stage *(open)*. State changes continue from open *(center)* to inactive *(right)*, where channel configuration assumes a different, but still impermeable, state. With repolarization, the inactivated refractory channel reverts to the initial resting configuration *(left)*, ready for the next sequence. (Redrawn from Siegelbaum SA, Koester F: Ion channels. In Kandel ER, editor: Principles of neural science, ed 3, Norwalk, Conn, 1991, Appleton-Lange.)

A sodium ion is thinner than a potassium or chloride ion and therefore should diffuse freely down its concentration gradient through membrane channels into the nerve cell. However, this does not occur, because all these ions attract water molecules and thus become hydrated. Hydrated sodium ions have a radius of 3.4 Å, which is approximately 50% greater than the 2.2 Å radius of potassium and chloride ions. Sodium ions therefore are too large to pass through narrow channels when a nerve is at rest (Fig. 1-9). Potassium and chloride ions can pass through these channels. During depolarization, sodium ions readily pass through the nerve membrane because configurational changes that develop within the membrane produce transient widening of these transmembrane channels to a size adequate to allow the unhindered passage of sodium ions down their concentration gradient into the axoplasm (transformation from the C to the O configuration). This concept can be visualized as the opening of a gate during depolarization that is partially occluding the channel in the resting membrane (C) (Fig. 1-10).

Evidence indicates that channel specificity exists in that sodium channels differ from potassium channels.[15] The gates on the sodium channel are located near the external surface of the nerve membrane, whereas those on the potassium channel are located near the internal surface of the nerve membrane.

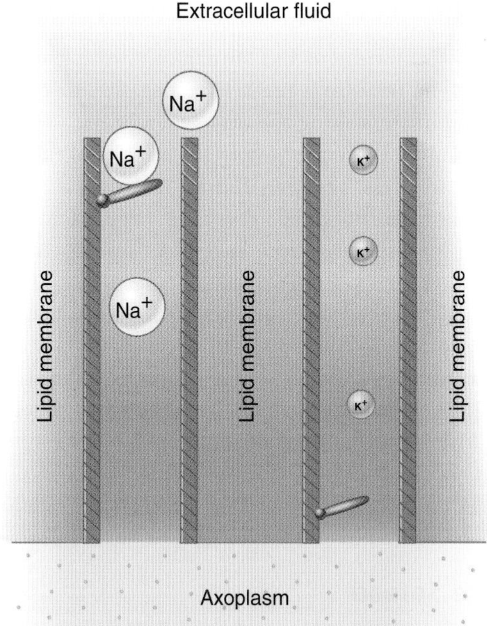

Figure 1-9. Membrane channels are partially occluded; the nerve is at rest. Hydrated sodium ions (Na^+) are too large to pass through channels, although potassium ions (K^+) can pass through unimpeded.

Impulse Propagation

After initiation of an action potential by a stimulus, the impulse must move along the surface of the axon. Energy for impulse propagation is derived from the nerve membrane in the following manner.

The stimulus disrupts the resting equilibrium of the nerve membrane; the transmembrane potential is reversed momentarily, with the interior of the cell changing from negative to positive, and the exterior changing from positive to negative. This new electrical equilibrium in this segment of nerve produces local currents that begin to flow between

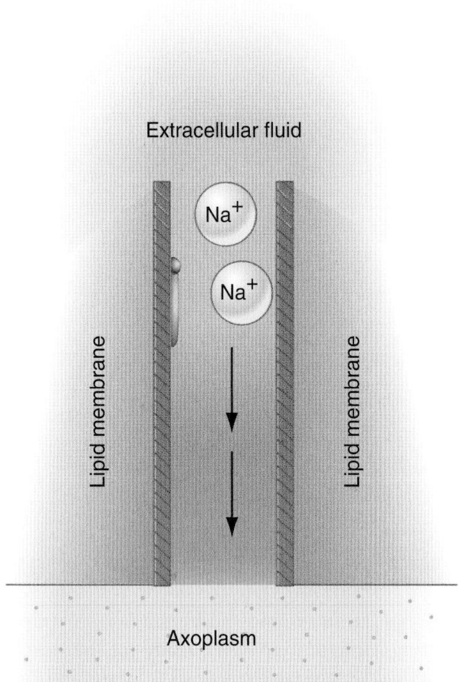

Figure 1-10. Membrane channels are open; depolarization occurs. Hydrated sodium ions (Na^+) now pass unimpeded through the sodium channel.

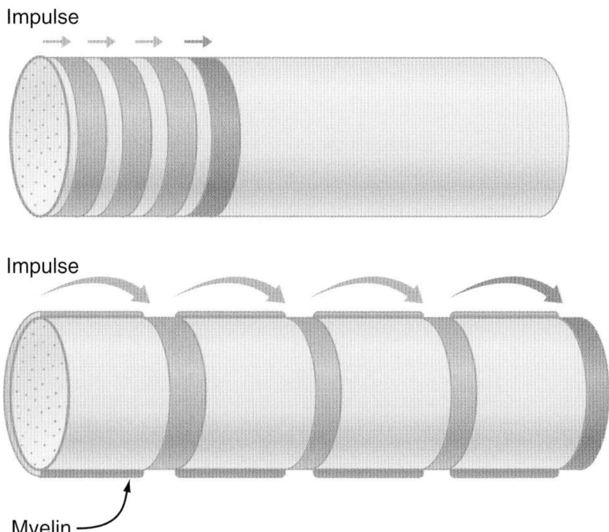

Figure 1-11. Saltatory propagation. Comparison of impulse propagation in nonmyelinated *(upper)* and myelinated *(lower)* axons. In nonmyelinated axons, the impulse moves forward by sequential depolarization of short adjoining membrane segments. Depolarization in myelinated axons, on the other hand, is discontinuous; the impulse leaps forward from node to node. Note how much farther ahead the impulse is in the myelinated axon after four depolarization sequences. (Redrawn from de Jong RH: Local anesthetics, St Louis, 1994, Mosby.)

the depolarized segment and the adjacent resting area. These local currents flow from positive to negative, extending for several millimeters along the nerve membrane.

As a result of this current flow, the interior of the adjacent area becomes less negative and its exterior less positive. Transmembrane potential decreases, approaching firing threshold for depolarization. When transmembrane potential is decreased by 15 mV from resting potential, a firing threshold is reached and rapid depolarization occurs. The newly depolarized segment sets up local currents in adjacent resting membrane, and the entire process starts anew.

Conditions in the segment that has just depolarized return to normal after the absolute and relative refractory periods. Because of this, the wave of depolarization can spread in only one direction. Backward (retrograde) movement is prevented by the inexcitable, refractory segment.

Impulse Spread

The propagated impulse travels along the nerve membrane toward the CNS. The spread of this impulse differs depending on whether or not a nerve is myelinated.

Unmyelinated Nerves. An unmyelinated nerve fiber is basically a long cylinder with a high–electrical resistance cell membrane surrounding a low-resistance conducting core of axoplasm, all of which is bathed in low-resistance extracellular fluid.

The high-resistance cell membrane and low-resistance intracellular and extracellular media produce a rapid decrease in the density of current within a short distance of the depolarized segment. In areas immediately adjacent to this depolarized segment, local current flow may be adequate to initiate depolarization in the resting membrane. Farther away it will prove to be inadequate to achieve a firing threshold.

The spread of an impulse in an unmyelinated nerve fiber therefore is characterized as a relatively slow forward-creeping process (Fig. 1-11). The conduction rate in unmyelinated C fibers is 1.2 m/sec compared with 14.8 to 120 m/sec in myelinated A-alpha and A-delta fibers.[16]

Myelinated Nerves. Impulse spread within myelinated nerves differs from that in unmyelinated nerves because of the layer of insulating material separating the intracellular and extracellular charges. The farther apart are the charges, the smaller is the current necessary to charge the membrane. Local currents thus can travel much farther in a myelinated nerve than in an unmyelinated nerve before becoming incapable of depolarizing the nerve membrane ahead of it.

Impulse conduction in myelinated nerves occurs by means of current leaps from node to node, a process termed *saltatory conduction* (see Fig. 1-11) (*saltare* is the Latin verb "to leap"). This form of impulse conduction proves to be much faster and more energy efficient than that employed in unmyelinated nerves. The thickness of the myelin sheath increases with increasing diameter of the axon. In addition, the distance between adjacent nodes of Ranvier increases with greater axonal diameter. Because of these two factors, saltatory conduction is more rapid in a thicker axon.

Saltatory conduction usually progresses from one node to the next in a stepwise manner. However, it can be demonstrated that the current flow at the next node still exceeds that necessary to reach the firing threshold of the nodal membrane. If conduction of an impulse is blocked at one node, the local current skips over that node and proves adequate to raise the membrane potential at the next node to its firing potential, producing depolarization. A minimum of perhaps 8 to 10 mm of nerve must be covered by anesthetic solution to ensure thorough blockade.[17]

MODE AND SITE OF ACTION OF LOCAL ANESTHETICS

How and where local anesthetics alter the processes of impulse generation and transmission needs to be discussed. It is possible for local anesthetics to interfere with the excitation process in a nerve membrane in one or more of the following ways:

1. Altering the basic resting potential of the nerve membrane
2. Altering the threshold potential (firing level)
3. Decreasing the rate of depolarization
4. Prolonging the rate of repolarization

It has been established that the primary effects of local anesthetics occur during the depolarization phase of the action potential.[18] These effects include a decrease in the rate of depolarization, particularly in the phase of slow depolarization. Because of this, cellular depolarization is not sufficient to reduce the membrane potential of a nerve fiber to its firing level, and a propagated action potential does not develop. There is no accompanying change in the rate of repolarization.

Where Do Local Anesthetics Work?

The nerve membrane is the site at which local anesthetics exert their pharmacologic actions. Many theories have been promulgated over the years to explain the mechanism of action of local anesthetics, including the acetylcholine, calcium displacement, and surface charge theories. The *acetylcholine theory* stated that acetylcholine was involved in nerve conduction, in addition to its role as a neurotransmitter at nerve synapses.[19] No evidence indicates that acetylcholine is involved in neural transmission along the body of the neuron. The *calcium displacement theory,* once popular, maintained that local anesthetic nerve block was produced by the displacement of calcium from some membrane site that controlled permeability to sodium.[20] Evidence that varying the concentration of calcium ions bathing a nerve does not affect local anesthetic potency has diminished the credibility of this theory. The *surface charge (repulsion) theory* proposed that local anesthetics act by binding to the nerve membrane and changing the electrical potential at the membrane surface.[21] Cationic (RNH^+) (p. 16) drug molecules were aligned at the membrane–water interface, and because some of the local anesthetic molecules carried a net positive charge, they made the electrical potential at the membrane surface more positive, thus decreasing the excitability of the nerve by increasing the threshold potential. Current evidence indicates that the resting potential of the nerve membrane is unaltered by local anesthetics (they do not become hyperpolarized), and that conventional local anesthetics act within membrane channels rather than at the membrane surface. Also, the surface charge theory cannot explain the activity of uncharged anesthetic molecules in blocking nerve impulses (e.g., benzocaine).

Two other theories, membrane expansion and specific receptor, are given credence today. Of the two, the specific receptor theory is more widely held.

The *membrane expansion theory* states that local anesthetic molecules diffuse to hydrophobic regions of excitable membranes, producing a general disturbance of the bulk membrane structure, expanding some critical region(s) in the membrane, and preventing an increase in permeability to sodium ions.[22,23] Local anesthetics that are highly lipid soluble can easily penetrate the lipid portion of the cell membrane, producing a change in configuration of the lipoprotein matrix of the nerve membrane. This results in a decreased diameter of sodium channels, which leads to inhibition of both sodium conductance and neural excitation (Fig. 1-12). The membrane expansion theory serves as a possible explanation for the local anesthetic activity of a drug such as benzocaine, which does not exist in cationic form yet still exhibits potent topical anesthetic activity. It has been demonstrated that nerve membranes, in fact, do expand and become more fluid when exposed to local anesthetics. However, no direct evidence suggests that nerve conduction is entirely blocked by membrane expansion per se.

The *specific receptor theory,* the most favored today, proposes that local anesthetics act by binding to specific receptors on the sodium channel (Fig. 1-13).[24] The action of the drug is direct, not mediated by some change in the general properties of the cell membrane. Both biochemical and electrophysiologic studies have indicated that a specific receptor site for local anesthetics exists in the sodium channel either on its external surface or on the internal axoplasmic surface.[25,26] Once the local anesthetic has gained access to the receptors, permeability to sodium ions is decreased or eliminated, and nerve conduction is interrupted.

Local anesthetics are classified by their ability to react with specific receptor sites in the sodium channel. It appears that drugs can alter nerve conduction in at least four sites within the sodium channel (see Fig. 1-13):

1. Within the sodium channel (tertiary amine local anesthetics)
2. At the outer surface of the sodium channel (tetrodotoxin, saxitoxin)

3 and 4. At the activation or the inactivation gate (scorpion venom)

Table 1-3 is a biological classification of local anesthetics based on their site of action and the active form of the compound. Drugs in Class C exist only in the uncharged

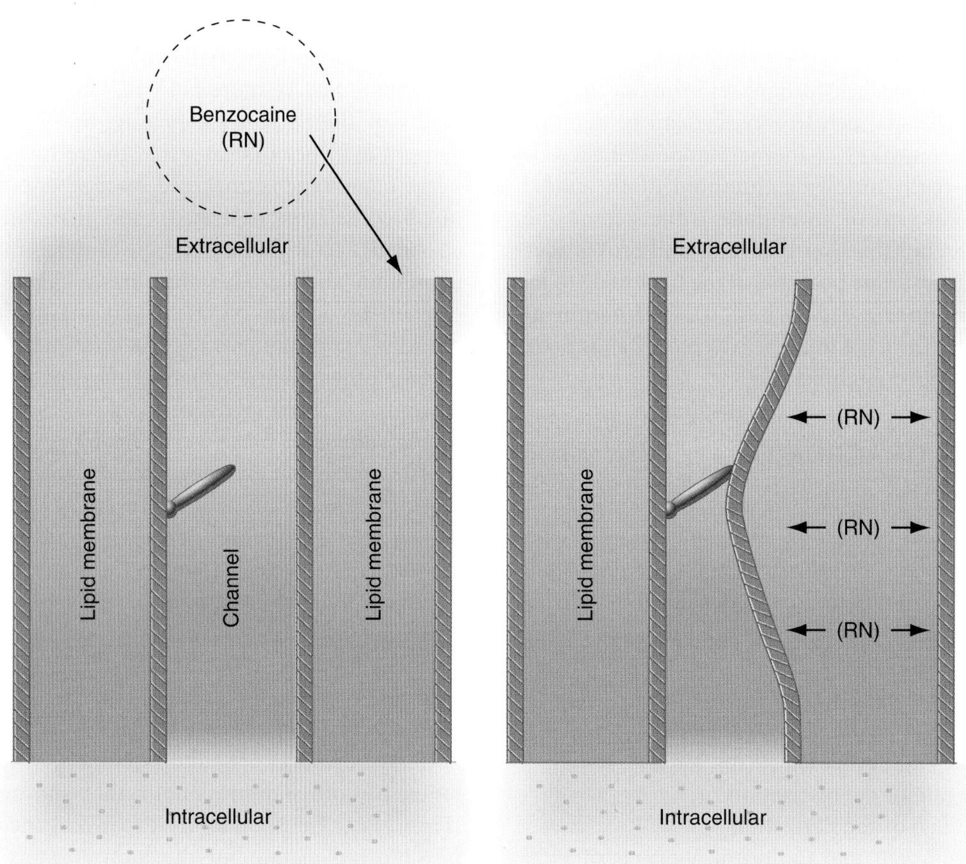

Figure 1-12. Membrane expansion theory.

TABLE 1-3
Classification of Local Anesthetic Substances According to Biological Site and Mode of Action

Classification	Definition	Chemical Substance
Class A	Agents acting at receptor site on external surface of nerve membrane	Biotoxins (e.g., tetrodotoxin, saxitoxin)
Class B	Agents acting at receptor site on internal surface of nerve membrane	Quaternary ammonium analogs of lidocaine Scorpion venom
Class C	Agents acting by a receptor-independent physico-chemical mechanism	Benzocaine
Class D	Agents acting by combination of receptor and receptor-independent mechanisms	Most clinically useful local anesthetic agents (e.g., articaine, lidocaine, mepivacaine, prilocaine)

Modified from Covino BG, Vassallo HG: Local anesthetics: mechanisms of action and clinical use, New York, 1976, Grune & Stratton. Used by permission.

form (RN), whereas Class D drugs exist in both charged and uncharged forms. Approximately 90% of the blocking effects of Class D drugs are caused by the cationic form of the drug; only 10% of blocking action is produced by the base (Fig. 1-14).

Myelinated Nerve Fibers. One additional factor should be considered with regard to the site of action of local anesthetics in myelinated nerves. The myelin sheath insulates the axon both electrically and pharmacologically. The only site at which molecules of local anesthetic have access to the nerve membrane is at the nodes of Ranvier, where sodium channels are found in abundance. Ionic changes that develop during impulse conduction arise only at the nodes.

Because an impulse may skip over or bypass one or two blocked nodes and continue on its way, it is necessary for at least two or three nodes immediately adjacent to the anesthetic solution to be blocked to ensure effective anesthesia—a length of approximately 8 to 10 mm.

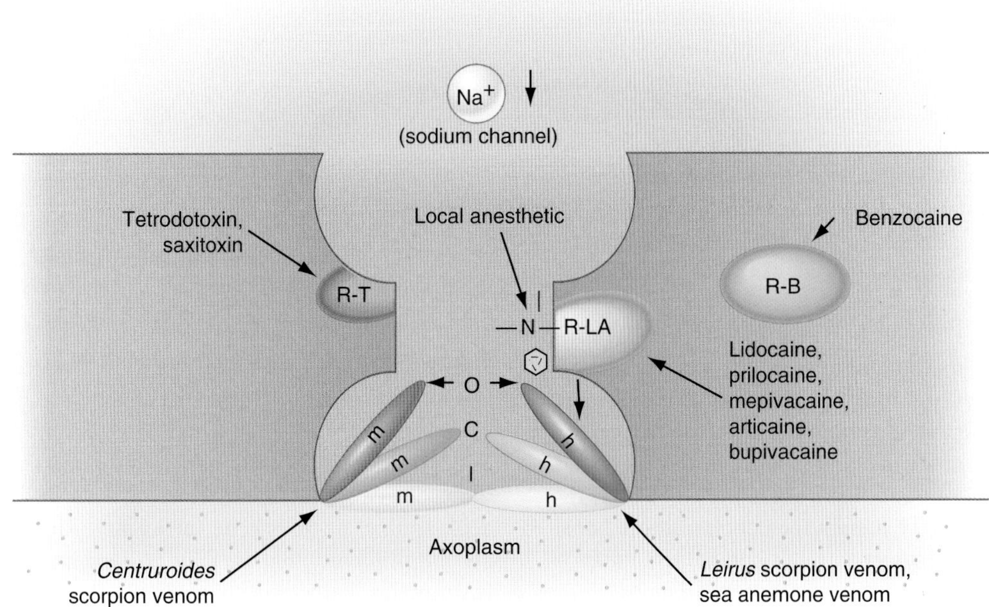

Figure 1-13. **A,** Tertiary amine local anesthetics inhibit the influx of sodium during nerve conduction by binding to a receptor within the sodium channel (R-LA). This blocks the normal activation mechanism (O gate configuration, depolarization) and also promotes movement of the activation and inactivation gates (m and h) to a position resembling that in the inactivated state (I). **B,** Biotoxins (R-T) block the influx of sodium at an outer surface receptor; various venoms do it by altering the activity of the activation and inactivation gates; and benzocaine (R-B) does it by expanding the membrane. **C,** Channel in the closed configuration. (Redrawn from Pallasch TJ: Dent Drug Serv Newsletter 4:25, 1983.)

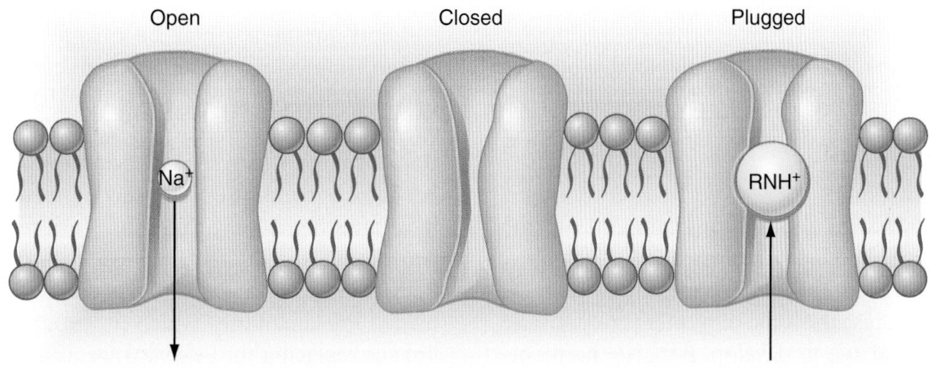

Figure 1-14. Channel entry. On the left is an open channel, inward permeant to sodium ion. The center channel is in the resting closed configuration; although impermeant to sodium ion here, the channel remains voltage responsive. The channel on the right, although in open configuration, is impermeant because it has local anesthetic cation bound to the gating receptor site. Note that local anesthetic enters the channel from the axoplasmic *(lower)* side; the channel filter precludes direct entry via the external mouth. Local anesthetic renders the membrane impermeant to sodium ion, hence inexcitable by local action currents. (Redrawn from de Jong RH: Local anesthetics, St Louis, 1994, Mosby.)

Sodium channel densities differ in myelinated and unmyelinated nerves. In small unmyelinated nerves, the density of sodium channels is about 35/μm, whereas at the nodes of Ranvier in myelinated fibers, it may be as high as 20,000/μm. On an average nerve length basis, relatively few sodium channels are present in unmyelinated nerve membranes. For example, in the garfish olfactory nerve, the ratio of sodium channels to phospholipid molecules is 1:60,000, corresponding to a mean distance between channels of 0.2 μm, whereas at densely packed nodes of Ranvier, the channels are separated by only 70 Å.[27,28]

How Local Anesthetics Work

The primary action of local anesthetics in producing a conduction block is to decrease the permeability of ion channels to sodium ions (Na^+). Local anesthetics selectively inhibit the peak permeability of sodium, whose value is normally about five to six times greater than the minimum necessary for impulse conduction (e.g., there is a safety factor for conduction of 5× to 6×).[29] Local anesthetics reduce this safety factor, decreasing both the rate of rise of the action potential and its conduction velocity. When the safety factor falls below unity,[10] conduction fails and nerve block occurs.

Local anesthetics produce a very slight, virtually insignificant decrease in potassium (K^+) conductance through the nerve membrane.

Calcium ions (Ca^{++}), which exist in bound form within the cell membrane, are thought to exert a regulatory role on the movement of sodium ions across the nerve membrane. Release of bound calcium ions from the ion channel receptor site may be the primary factor responsible for increased sodium permeability of the nerve membrane. This represents the first step in nerve membrane depolarization. Local anesthetic molecules may act through competitive antagonism with calcium for some site on the nerve membrane.

The following sequence is a proposed mechanism of action of local anesthetics[1]:

1. Displacement of calcium ions from the sodium channel receptor site, which permits …
2. Binding of the local anesthetic molecule to this receptor site, which produces …
3. Blockade of the sodium channel, and a …
4. Decrease in sodium conductance, which leads to …
5. Depression of the rate of electrical depolarization, and …
6. Failure to achieve the threshold potential level, along with …
7. Lack of development of propagated action potentials, which is called …
8. Conduction blockade.

The mechanism whereby sodium ions gain entry to the axoplasm of the nerve, thereby initiating an action potential, is altered by local anesthetics. The nerve membrane remains in a polarized state because the ionic movements responsible for the action potential fail to develop. Because the membrane's electrical potential remains unchanged, local currents do not develop, and the self-perpetuating mechanism of impulse propagation is stalled. An impulse that arrives at a blocked nerve segment is stopped because it is unable to release the energy necessary for its continued propagation. Nerve block produced by local anesthetics is called a *nondepolarizing nerve block.*

ACTIVE FORMS OF LOCAL ANESTHETICS

Local Anesthetic Molecules

Most injectable local anesthetics are tertiary amines. Only a few (e.g., prilocaine, hexylcaine) are secondary amines. The typical local anesthetic structure is shown in Figures 1-15 and 1-16. The lipophilic part is the largest portion of the molecule. Aromatic in structure, it is derived from benzoic acid, aniline, or thiophene (articaine). All local anesthetics are amphipathic, that is, they possess both lipophilic and hydrophilic characteristics, generally at opposite ends of the molecule. The hydrophilic part is an amino derivative of ethyl alcohol or acetic acid. Local anesthetics without a hydrophilic part are not suited for injection but are good topical anesthetics (e.g., benzocaine). The anesthetic structure is completed by an intermediate hydrocarbon chain containing an ester or an amide linkage. Other chemicals, especially histamine blockers and anticholinergics, share this basic structure with local anesthetics and commonly exhibit weak local anesthetic properties.

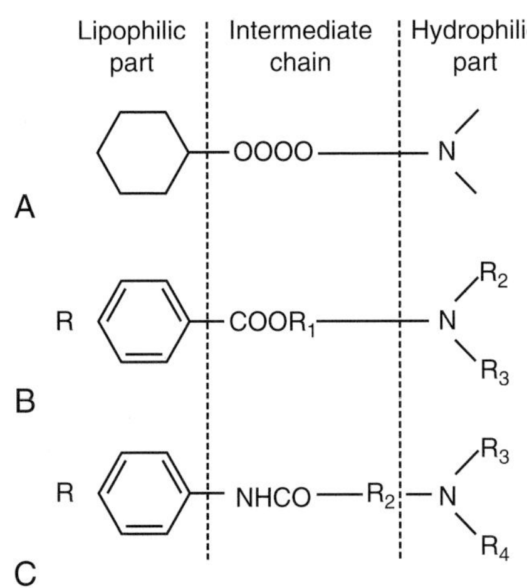

Figure 1-15. **A,** Typical local anesthetic. **B,** Ester type. **C,** Amide type.

Local anesthetics may be classified as amino esters or amino amides according to their chemical linkages. The nature of the linkage is important in defining several properties of the local anesthetic, including the basic mode of biotransformation. Ester-linked local anesthetics (e.g., procaine) are readily hydrolyzed in aqueous solution. Amide-linked local anesthetics (e.g., lidocaine) are relatively resistant to hydrolysis. A greater percentage of an amide-linked drug than of an ester-linked drug is excreted unchanged in the urine. Procainamide, which is procaine with an amide linkage replacing the ester linkage, is as potent a local anesthetic as procaine, yet because of its amide linkage, it is hydrolyzed much more slowly. Procaine is hydrolyzed in plasma in only a few minutes, but just approximately 10% of procainamide is hydrolyzed in 1 day.

As prepared in the laboratory, local anesthetics are basic compounds that are poorly soluble in water and unstable on exposure to air.[30] Their pK_a values range from 7.5 to 10. In this form, they have little or no clinical value. However, because they are weakly basic, they combine readily with acids to form local anesthetic salts, in which form they are quite soluble in water and comparatively stable. Thus local anesthetics used for injection are dispensed as acid salts, most commonly the hydrochloride salt (e.g., lidocaine HCl, articaine HCl), dissolved in sterile water or saline.

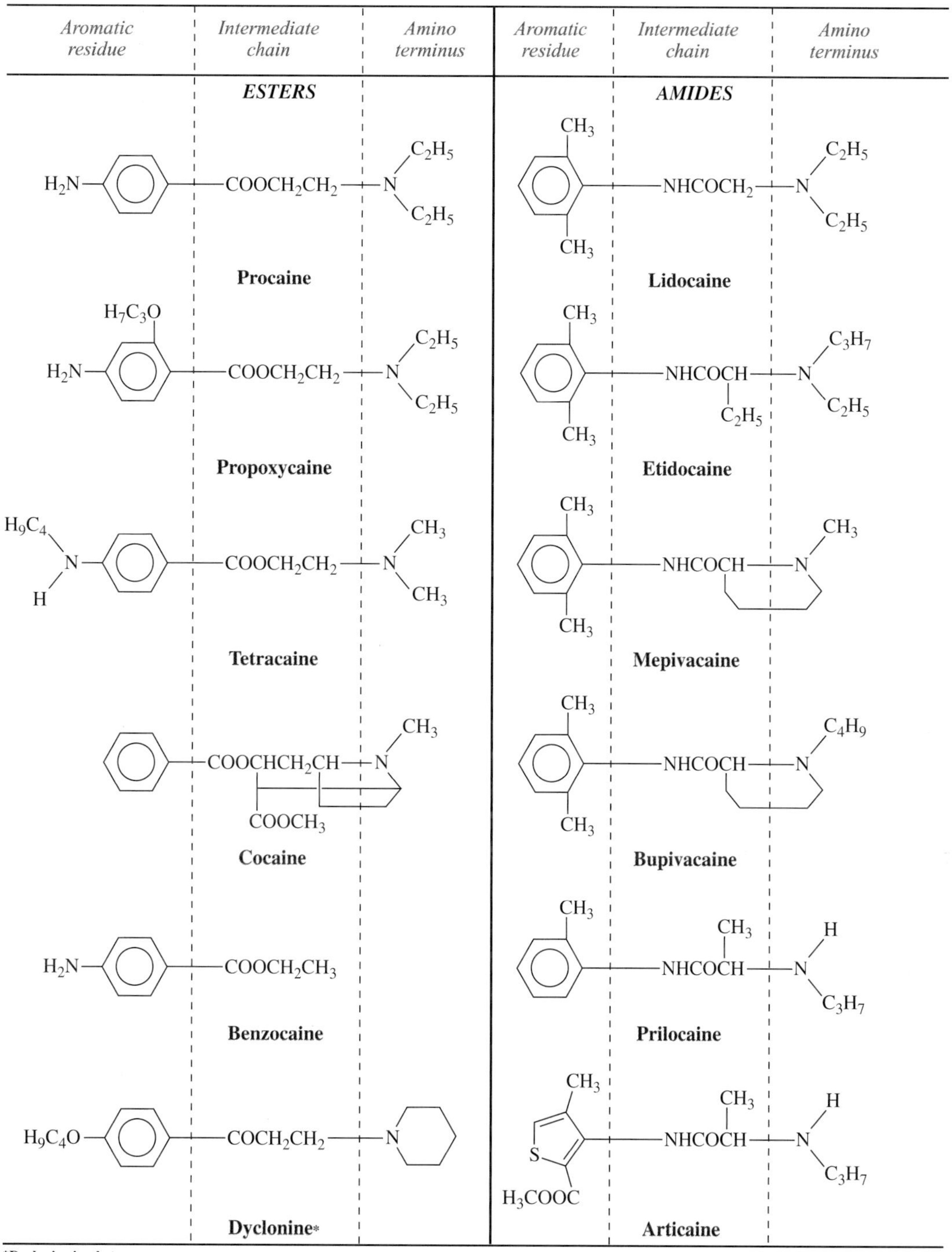

Aromatic residue	Intermediate chain	Amino terminus	Aromatic residue	Intermediate chain	Amino terminus
	ESTERS			*AMIDES*	
H_2N– (ring)	$COOCH_2CH_2$	N (C_2H_5, C_2H_5)	(ring) CH_3, CH_3	$NHCOCH_2$	N (C_2H_5, C_2H_5)
	Procaine			**Lidocaine**	
H_7C_3O, H_2N– (ring)	$COOCH_2CH_2$	N (C_2H_5, C_2H_5)	(ring) CH_3, CH_3	$NHCOCH$ (C_2H_5)	N (C_3H_7, C_2H_5)
	Propoxycaine			**Etidocaine**	
H_9C_4, H, N– (ring)	$COOCH_2CH_2$	N (CH_3, CH_3)	(ring) CH_3, CH_3	$NHCOCH$	N (CH_3)
	Tetracaine			**Mepivacaine**	
	$COOCHCH_2CH$ ($COOCH_3$)	N (CH_3)	CH_3, CH_3	$NHCOCH$	N (C_4H_9)
	Cocaine			**Bupivacaine**	
H_2N– (ring)	$COOCH_2CH_3$		(ring) CH_3	$NHCOCH$ (CH_3)	N (H, C_3H_7)
	Benzocaine			**Prilocaine**	
H_9C_4O– (ring)	$COCH_2CH_2$	N (ring)	CH_3, S, H_3COOC (ring)	$NHCOCH$ (CH_3)	N (H, C_3H_7)
	Dyclonine*			**Articaine**	

*Dyclonine is a ketone.

Figure 1-16. Chemical configuration of local anesthetics. (From Yagiela JA, Neidle EA, Dowd FJ: Pharmacology and therapeutics for dentistry, ed 6, St Louis, 2010, Mosby.)

It is well known that the pH of a local anesthetic solution (as well as the pH of the tissue into which it is injected) greatly influences its nerve-blocking action. Acidification of tissue decreases local anesthetic effectiveness. Inadequate anesthesia results when local anesthetics are injected into inflamed or infected areas. The inflammatory process produces acidic products: The pH of normal tissue is 7.4; the pH of an inflamed area is 5 to 6. Local anesthetics containing epinephrine or other vasopressors are acidified by the manufacturer to inhibit oxidation of the vasopressor (p. 18). The pH of solutions without epinephrine is about 6.5; epinephrine-containing solutions have a pH of about 3.5. Clinically, this lower pH is more likely to produce a burning sensation on injection, as well as a slightly slower onset of anesthesia.

Elevating the pH (alkalinization) of a local anesthetic solution speeds its onset of action, increases its clinical effectiveness, and makes its injection more comfortable. However, the local anesthetic base, because it is unstable, precipitates out of alkalinized solutions, making these preparations ill-suited for clinical use. Buffered (e.g., carbonated) local anesthetics have received much attention in recent years both in medicine and, more recently, in dentistry.[31] Sodium bicarbonate or carbon dioxide (CO_2) added to the anesthetic solution immediately before injection provides greater comfort and more rapid onset of anesthesia (see Chapter 19).[32,33] The use of buffered local anesthetics in dentistry is reviewed in depth in Chapter 20.

Despite potentially wide pH variation in extracellular fluids, the pH at the interior of a nerve remains stable. Normal functioning of a nerve therefore is affected very little by changes in the extracellular environment. However, the ability of a local anesthetic to block nerve impulses is profoundly altered by changes in extracellular pH.

Dissociation of Local Anesthetics

As discussed, local anesthetics are available as acid salts (usually hydrochloride) for clinical use. The local anesthetic salt, both water soluble and stable, is dissolved in sterile water or saline. In this solution, it exists simultaneously as uncharged molecules (RN), also called the *base,* and as positively charged molecules (RNH^+), called the *cation.*

$$RNH^+ \rightleftharpoons RN + H^+$$

The relative proportion of each ionic form in the solution varies with the pH of the solution or surrounding tissues. In the presence of a high concentration of hydrogen ions (low pH), the equilibrium shifts to the left, and most of the anesthetic solution exists in cationic form:

$$RNH^+ > RN + H^+$$

As hydrogen ion concentration decreases (higher pH), the equilibrium shifts toward the free base form:

$$RNH^+ < RN + H^+$$

The relative proportion of ionic forms also depends on the pK_a, or dissociation constant, of the specific local anesthetic. The pK_a is a measure of the affinity of a molecule for hydrogen ions (H^+). When the pH of the solution has the same value as the pK_a of the local anesthetic, exactly 50% of the drug exists in the RNH^+ form and 50% in the RN form. The percentage of drug existing in either form can be determined from the Henderson-Hasselbalch equation.

Table 1-4 lists the pK_a values for commonly used local anesthetics.

Actions on Nerve Membranes

The two factors involved in the action of a local anesthetic are (1) diffusion of the drug through the nerve sheath, and (2) binding at the receptor site in the ion channel. The uncharged, lipid-soluble, free base form (RN) of the anesthetic is responsible for diffusion through the nerve sheath. This process is explained in the following example:

TABLE 1-4
Dissociation Constants (pK_a) of Local Anesthetics

Agent	pK_a	% Base (RN) at pH 7.4	Approximate Onset of Action, min
Benzocaine	3.5	100	—
Mepivacaine	7.7	33	2-4
Lidocaine	7.7	29	2-4
Prilocaine	7.7	25	2-4
Articaine	7.8	29	2-4
Etidocaine	7.9	25	2-4
Ropivacaine	8.1	17	2-4
Bupivacaine	8.1	17	5-8
Tetracaine	8.6	7	10-15
Cocaine	8.6	7	—
Chloroprocaine	8.7	6	6-12
Propoxycaine	8.9	4	9-14
Procaine	9.1	2	14-18
Procainamide	9.3	1	—

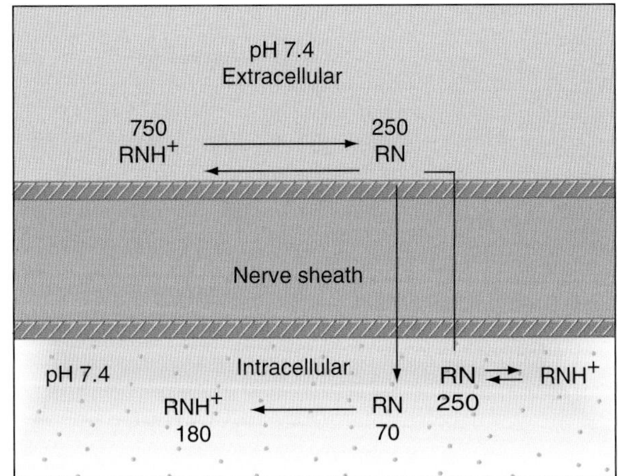

Figure 1-17. Mechanism of action of the local anesthetic molecule. Anesthetic pK_a of 7.9; tissue pH of 7.4.

1. One thousand molecules of a local anesthetic with a pK_a of 7.9 are injected into the tissues outside a nerve. The tissue pH is normal (7.4) (Fig. 1-17).
2. From Table 1-4 and the Henderson-Hasselbalch equation, it can be determined that at normal tissue pH, 75% of local anesthetic molecules are present in the cationic form (RNH^+) and 25% in the free base form (RN).
3. In theory then, all 250 lipophilic RN molecules will diffuse through the nerve sheath to reach the interior (axoplasm) of the neuron.
4. When this happens, the extracellular equilibrium between $RNH^+ \rightleftharpoons RN$ has been disrupted by passage of the free base forms into the neuron. The remaining 750 extracellular RNH^+ molecules will now reequilibrate according to the tissue pH and the pK_a of the drugs:

$$RNH^+(570) \rightleftharpoons RN(180) + H^+$$

5. The 180 newly created lipophilic RN molecules diffuse into the cell, starting the entire process (Step 4) again. Theoretically, this will continue until all local anesthetic molecules diffuse into the axoplasm.

   The reality, however, is somewhat different. Not all the local anesthetic molecules will eventually reach the interior of the nerve, because of the process of diffusion (drugs will diffuse in all possible directions, not just toward the nerve), and because some will be absorbed into blood vessels and extracellular soft tissues at the injection site.
6. The inside of the nerve should be viewed next. After penetration of the nerve sheath and entry into the axoplasm by the lipophilic RN form of the anesthetic, reequilibration takes place inside the nerve, because a local anesthetic cannot exist in only the RN form at an intracellular pH of 7.4. Seventy-five percent of those RN molecules present within the axoplasm revert into the RNH^+ form; the remaining 25% of molecules remain in the uncharged RN form.
7. From the axoplasmic side, the RNH^+ ions enter into the sodium channels, bind to the channel receptor site, and ultimately are responsible for the conduction blockade that results (see Figs. 1-13 and 1-14).

Of the two factors—diffusibility and binding—responsible for local anesthetic effectiveness, the former is extremely important in actual practice. The ability of a local anesthetic to diffuse through the tissues surrounding a nerve is of critical significance, because in clinical situations the local anesthetic cannot be applied directly to the nerve membrane, as it can in a laboratory setting. Local anesthetic solutions better able to diffuse through soft tissue provide an advantage in clinical practice.

A local anesthetic with a high pK_a value has very few molecules available in the RN form at a tissue pH of 7.4. The onset of anesthetic action of this drug is slow because too few base molecules are available to diffuse through the nerve membrane (e.g., procaine, with a pK_a of 9.1). The rate of onset of anesthetic action is related to the pK_a of the local anesthetic (see Table 1-4).

A local anesthetic with a lower pK_a (<7.5) has a greater number of lipophilic free base molecules available to diffuse through the nerve sheath; however, the anesthetic action of this drug is inadequate because at an intracellular pH of 7.4, only a very small number of base molecules dissociate back to the cationic form necessary for binding at the receptor site.

In actual clinical situations with the local anesthetics currently available, the pH of the extracellular fluid determines the ease with which a local anesthetic moves from the site of its administration into the axoplasm of the nerve cell. The intracellular pH remains stable and independent of the extracellular pH, because hydrogen ions (H^+), such as the local anesthetic cations (RNH^+), do not readily diffuse through tissues. The pH of extracellular fluid therefore may differ from that of the nerve membrane. The ratio of anesthetic cations to uncharged base molecules (RNH^+/RN) also may vary greatly at these sites. Differences in extracellular

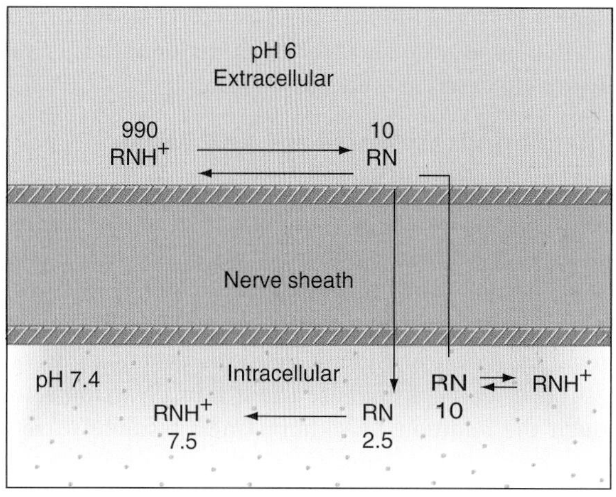

Figure 1-18. Effect of decreased tissue pH on the actions of a local anesthetic.

and intracellular pH are highly significant in pain control when inflammation or infection is present.[34] The effect of a decrease in tissue pH on the actions of a local anesthetic is described in Figure 1-18. This can be compared with the example in Figure 1-17, involving normal tissue pH:

1. Approximately 1000 molecules of a local anesthetic with a pK_a of 7.9 are deposited outside a nerve. The tissue is inflamed and infected and has a pH of 6.
2. At this tissue pH, approximately 99% of local anesthetic molecules are present in the charged cationic (RNH^+) form, with approximately 1% in the lipophilic free base (RN) form.
3. Approximately 10 RN molecules diffuse across the nerve sheath to reach the interior of the cell (contrasting with 250 RN molecules in the healthy example). The pH of the interior of the nerve cell remains normal (e.g., 7.4).
4. Extracellularly, the equilibrium between $RNH^+ \rightleftharpoons RN$, which has been disrupted, is reestablished. The relatively few newly created RN molecules diffuse into the cell, starting the entire process again. However, a sum total of fewer RN molecules succeed in eventually crossing the nerve sheath than would succeed at a normal pH because of greatly increased absorption of anesthetic molecules into the blood vessels in the region (increased vascularity is noted in the area of inflammation and infection).
5. After penetration of the nerve sheath by the base form, reequilibrium occurs inside the nerve. Approximately 75% of the molecules present intracellularly revert to the cationic form (RNH^+), 25% remaining in the uncharged free base form (RN).
6. The cationic molecules bind to receptor sites within the sodium channel, resulting in conduction blockade.

Adequate blockade of the nerve is more difficult to achieve in inflamed or infected tissues because of the relatively small number of molecules able to cross the nerve sheath (RN) and the increased absorption of remaining anesthetic molecules into dilated blood vessels in this region. Although it presents a potential problem in all aspects of dental practice, this situation is seen most often in endodontics. Possible remedies are described in Chapter 16.

Clinical Implications of pH and Local Anesthetic Activity

Most commercially prepared solutions of local anesthetics without a vasoconstrictor have a pH between 5.5 and 7. When injected into tissue, the vast buffering capacity of tissue fluids returns the pH at the injection site to a normal 7.4. Local anesthetic solutions containing a vasopressor (e.g., epinephrine) are acidified by the manufacturer through the addition of sodium (meta)bisulfite to retard oxidation of the vasoconstrictor, thereby prolonging the period of effectiveness of the drug. (See Chapter 3 for a discussion of the appropriate use of vasoconstrictors in local anesthetics.)

Epinephrine may be added to a local anesthetic solution immediately before its administration without the addition of antioxidants; however, if the solution is not used in a short time, it will oxidize, slowly turning yellow then brown (much like a sliced apple oxidizing).

Rapid oxidation of the vasopressor may be delayed, thereby increasing the shelf life of the product, through the addition of antioxidants. Sodium bisulfite in a concentration between 0.05% and 0.1% is commonly used. A 2% solution of lidocaine HCl, with a pH of 6.8, is acidified to 4.2 by the addition of sodium bisulfite.

Even in this situation, the enormous buffering capacity of the tissues tends to maintain a normal tissue pH; however, it does require a longer time to do so after injection of a pH 4.2 solution than with a pH 6.8 solution. During this time, the local anesthetic is not able to function at its full effectiveness, resulting in a slower onset of clinical action for local anesthetics with vasoconstrictors compared with their plain counterparts.

Local anesthetics are clinically effective on both axons and free nerve endings. Free nerve endings lying below intact skin may be reached only by injection of anesthetic beneath the skin. Intact skin forms an impenetrable barrier to the diffusion of local anesthetics. EMLA (eutectic mixture of local anesthetics lidocaine and prilocaine) enables local anesthetics to penetrate intact skin, albeit slowly.[35]

Mucous membranes and injured skin (e.g., burns, abrasions) lack the protection afforded by intact skin, permitting topically applied local anesthetics to diffuse through to reach free nerve endings. Topical anesthetics can be employed effectively wherever skin is no longer intact because of injury, as well as on mucous membranes (e.g., cornea, gingiva, pharynx, trachea, larynx, esophagus, rectum, vagina, bladder).[36]

The buffering capacity of mucous membrane is poor; thus topical application of a local anesthetic with a pH between 5.5 and 6.5 lowers the regional pH to below normal, and less local anesthetic base is formed. Diffusion of the drug across the mucous membrane to free nerve endings is limited, and nerve block is ineffective. Increasing the pH of the drug provides more RN form, thereby increasing the potency of the topical anesthetic; however, the drug in this form is more rapidly oxidized. The effective shelf life of the local anesthetic is decreased as the pH of the drug is increased.[30]

To enhance the clinical efficacy of topical anesthetics, a more concentrated form of the drug is commonly used (5% or 10% lidocaine) than for injection (2% lidocaine). Although only a small percentage of the drug is available in the base form, raising the concentration provides additional RN molecules for diffusion and dissociation to the active cation form at free nerve endings.

Some topical anesthetics (e.g., benzocaine) are not ionized in solution; thus their anesthetic effectiveness is unaffected by pH. Because of the poor water solubility of benzocaine, its absorption from the site of application is minimal, and systemic reactions (e.g., overdose) are rarely encountered.

KINETICS OF LOCAL ANESTHETIC ONSET AND DURATION OF ACTION

Barriers to Diffusion of the Solution

A peripheral nerve is composed of hundreds to thousands of tightly packed axons. These axons are protected, supported, and nourished by several layers of fibrous and elastic tissues. Nutrient blood vessels and lymphatics course throughout the layers.

Individual nerve fibers (axons) are covered with, and are separated from each other by, the endoneurium. The perineurium then binds these nerve fibers together into bundles called *fasciculi.* The radial nerve, located in the wrist, contains between 5 and 10 fasciculi. Each fasciculus contains between 500 and 1000 individual nerve fibers. Five thousand nerve fibers occupy approximately 1 mm^2 of space.

The thickness of the perineurium varies with the diameter of the fasciculus it surrounds. The thicker the perineurium, the slower the rate of local anesthetic diffusion across it.[37] The innermost layer of perineurium is the *perilemma.* It is covered with a smooth mesothelial membrane. The perilemma represents the main barrier to diffusion into a nerve.

Fasciculi are contained within a loose network of areolar connective tissue called the *epineurium.* The epineurium constitutes between 30% and 75% of the total cross-section of a nerve. Local anesthetics are readily able to diffuse through the epineurium because of its loose consistency. Nutrient blood vessels and lymphatics traverse the epineurium. These vessels absorb local anesthetic molecules, removing them from the site of injection.

The outer layer of the epineurium surrounding the nerve is denser and is thickened, forming what is termed the *epineural sheath* or *nerve sheath.* The epineural sheath does not constitute a barrier to diffusion of local anesthetic into a nerve.

Table 1-5 summarizes the layers of a typical peripheral nerve.

Induction of Local Anesthesia

Following administration of a local anesthetic into the soft tissues near a nerve, molecules of the local anesthetic traverse the distance from one site to another according to their concentration gradient. During the induction phase of anesthesia, the local anesthetic moves from its extraneural site of deposition toward the nerve (as well as in all other possible directions). This process is termed *diffusion.* It is the unhindered migration of molecules or ions through a fluid medium under the influence of the concentration gradient. Penetration of an anatomic barrier to diffusion occurs when a drug passes through a tissue that tends to restrict free molecular movement. The perineurium is the greatest barrier to penetration of local anesthetics.

Diffusion. The rate of diffusion is governed by several factors, the most significant of which is the concentration gradient. The greater the initial concentration of the local anesthetic, the faster the diffusion of its molecules and the more rapid its onset of action.

TABLE 1-5
Organization of a Peripheral Nerve

Structure	Description
Nerve fiber	Single nerve cell
Endoneurium	Covers each nerve fiber
Fasciculi	Bundles of 500 to 1000 nerve fibers
Perineurium*	Covers fasciculi
Perilemma*	Innermost layer of perineurium
Epineurium	Alveolar connective tissue supporting fasciculi and carrying nutrient vessels
Epineural sheath	Outer layer of epineurium

*The perineurium and perilemma constitute the greatest anatomic barriers to diffusion in a peripheral nerve.

Fasciculi that are located near the surface of the nerve are termed *mantle bundles* (Fig. 1-19, *A*). Mantle bundles are the first ones reached by the local anesthetic and are exposed to a higher concentration of it. Mantle bundles usually are blocked completely shortly after injection of a local anesthetic (Fig. 1-19, *B*).

Fasciculi found closer to the center of the nerve are called *core bundles.* Core bundles are contacted by a local anesthetic only after much delay and by a lower anesthetic concentration because of the greater distance that the solution must traverse and the greater number of barriers it must cross.

As the local anesthetic diffuses into the nerve, it becomes increasingly diluted by tissue fluids with some being absorbed by capillaries and lymphatics. Ester anesthetics undergo almost immediate enzymatic hydrolysis. Thus core fibers are exposed to a decreased concentration of local anesthetic, a fact that may explain the clinical situation of inadequate pulpal anesthesia developing in the presence of subjective symptoms of adequate soft tissue anesthesia. Complete conduction blockade of all nerve fibers in a peripheral nerve requires that an adequate volume, as well as an adequate concentration, of the local anesthetic be deposited. In no clinical situation are 100% of the fibers within a peripheral nerve blocked, even in cases of clinically excellent pain control.[38] Fibers near the surface of the nerve (mantle fibers) tend to innervate more proximal regions (e.g., the molar area with an inferior alveolar nerve block), whereas fibers in the core bundles innervate the more distal points of nerve distribution (e.g., the incisors and canine with an inferior alveolar block).

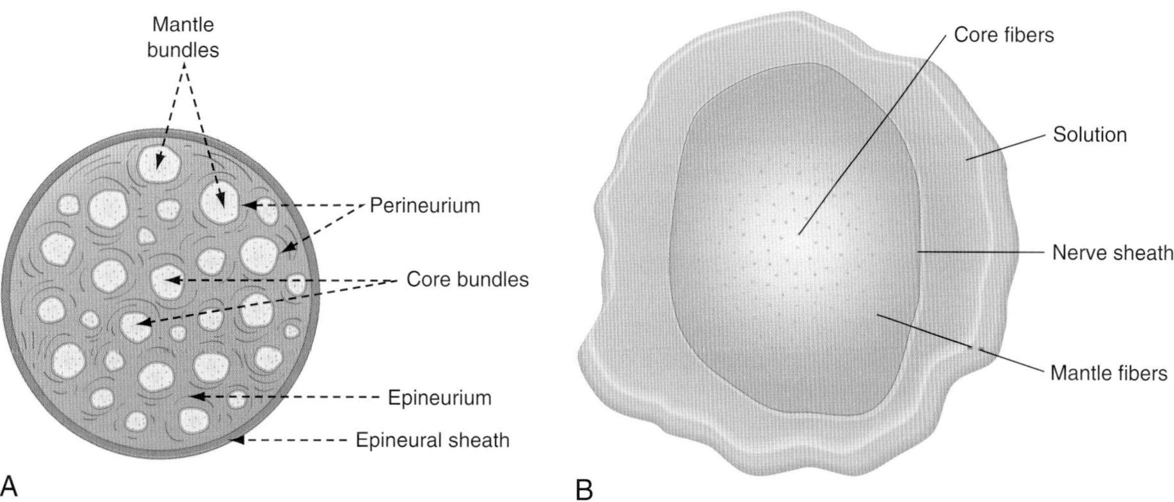

Figure 1-19. **A,** Composition of nerve fibers and bundles within a peripheral nerve. **B,** In a large peripheral nerve (containing hundreds or thousands of axons), local anesthetic solution must diffuse inward toward the nerve core from the extraneural site of injection. Local anesthetic molecules are removed by tissue uptake while tissue fluid mixes with the carrier solvent. This results in gradual dilution of the local anesthetic solution as it penetrates the nerve toward the core. A concentration gradient occurs during induction so that the outer mantle fibers are solidly blocked, whereas the inner core fibers are not yet blocked. Not only are core fibers exposed to a lower local anesthetic concentration, but the drug arrives later. Delay depends on the tissue mass to be penetrated and the diffusivity of the local anesthetic. (Redrawn from **B,** de Jong RH: Local anesthetics, St Louis, 1994, Mosby.)

Blocking Process. After deposition of local anesthetic as close to the nerve as possible, the solution diffuses in all directions according to prevailing concentration gradients. A portion of the injected local anesthetic diffuses toward the nerve and into the nerve. However, a significant portion of the injected drug also diffuses away from the nerve. The following reactions then occur:

1. Some of the drug is absorbed by nonneural tissues (e.g., muscle, fat).
2. Some is diluted by interstitial fluid.
3. Some is removed by capillaries and lymphatics from the injection site.
4. Ester-type anesthetics are hydrolyzed.

The sum total effect of these factors is to decrease the local anesthetic concentration outside the nerve; however, the concentration of local anesthetic within the nerve continues to rise as diffusion progresses. These processes continue until an equilibrium results between intraneural and extraneural concentrations of anesthetic solution.

Induction Time. *Induction time* is defined as the period from deposition of the anesthetic solution to complete conduction blockade. Several factors control the induction time of a given drug. Those under the operator's control are the concentration of the drug and the pH of the local anesthetic solution. Factors not under the clinician's control include the diffusion constant of the anesthetic drug and the anatomic diffusion barriers of the nerve.

Physical Properties and Clinical Actions. Other physicochemical factors of a local anesthetic may influence its clinical characteristics.

The effect of the *dissociation constant* (pK_a) on the rate of onset of anesthesia has been described. Although both molecular forms of the anesthetic are important in neural blockade, drugs with a lower pK_a possess a more rapid onset of action than those with a higher pK_a.[39]

Lipid solubility of a local anesthetic appears to be related to its intrinsic potency. The estimated lipid solubilities of various local anesthetics are presented in Table 1-6. Greater lipid solubility permits the anesthetic to penetrate the nerve membrane (which itself is 90% lipid) more easily. This is reflected biologically in increased potency of the anesthetic. Local anesthetics with greater lipid solubility produce more effective conduction blockade at lower concentrations (lower percentage solutions or smaller volumes deposited) than is produced by less lipid-soluble local anesthetics.

The degree of *protein binding* of the local anesthetic molecule is responsible for the duration of anesthetic activity. After penetration of the nerve sheath, a reequilibrium occurs between the base and cationic forms of the local anesthetic according to the Henderson-Hasselbach equation. Now, in the sodium channel itself, RNH^+ ions bind at the receptor site. Proteins constitute approximately 10% of the nerve membrane, and local anesthetics (e.g., etidocaine, ropivacaine, bupivacaine) possessing a greater degree of protein binding (see Table 1-6) than others (e.g., procaine) appear to attach more securely to the protein receptor sites and to possess a longer duration of clinical activity.[40]

Vasoactivity affects both the anesthetic potency and the duration of anesthesia provided by a drug. Injection of local anesthetics, such as procaine, with greater vasodilating properties increases perfusion of the local site with blood. The injected local anesthetic is absorbed into the cardiovascular compartment more rapidly and is carried away from the injection site and from the nerve, thus providing for a shortened duration of anesthesia, as well as decreased potency of the drug. Table 1-7 summarizes the influence of various factors on local anesthetic action.

Recovery from Local Anesthetic Block

Emergence from a local anesthetic nerve block follows the same diffusion patterns as induction; however, it does so in the reverse order.

The extraneural concentration of local anesthetic is continually depleted by diffusion, dispersion, and uptake of the drug, whereas the intraneural concentration of local anesthetic remains relatively stable. The concentration gradient is reversed, the intraneural concentration exceeds the extraneural concentration, and anesthetic molecules begin to diffuse out of the nerve.

Fasciculi in the mantle begin to lose the local anesthetic much sooner than do the core bundles. Local anesthetic within the core then diffuses into the mantle, so that the first nerve fibers to entirely lose anesthesia are those centermost in the nerve. Mantle fibers remain anesthetized the longest, and core fibers the shortest, time. Recovery from anesthesia is a slower process than induction because the local anesthetic is bound to the drug receptor site in the sodium channel and therefore is released more slowly than it is absorbed.

Readministration of Local Anesthetic

Occasionally a dental procedure outlasts the duration of clinically effective pain control, and a repeat injection of local anesthetic is necessary. Usually this repeat injection immediately results in a return of profound anesthesia. On some occasions, however, the clinician may encounter greater difficulty in reestablishing adequate pain control with subsequent injections.

Recurrence of Immediate Profound Anesthesia. At the time of reinjection, the concentration of local anesthetic in the core fibers is less than that in the mantle fibers. Partially recovered core fibers still contain some local anesthetic, although not enough to provide complete anesthesia. After deposition of a new high concentration of anesthetic near the nerve, the mantle fibers are once again exposed to a concentration gradient directed inward toward the nerve; this eventually leads to an increased concentration in the core fibers. This combination of residual local anesthetic (in the nerve) and the newly deposited supply results in rapid onset of profound anesthesia and administration of a smaller volume of local anesthetic drug.

TABLE 1-6
Chemical Structure, Physicochemical Properties, and Pharmacologic Properties of Local Anesthetic Agents

Agent	CHEMICAL CONFIGURATION			PHYSICOCHEMICAL PROPERTIES			PHARMACOLOGIC PROPERTIES			
	Aromatic (lipophilic)	Intermediate Chain	Amine (hydrophilic)	Molecular Weight (base)	pKa (36° C)	Onset	Approx Lipid Solubility	Usual Effective Concentration, %	Protein Binding	Duration
Esters										
Procaine	$H-N(H)-C_6H_4-$	$-COOCH_2CH_2-$	$N(C_2H_5)_2$	236	9.1	Slow	1.0	2-4	5	Short
Chloroprocaine	$H-N(H)-C_6H_3(Cl)-$	$-COOCH_2CH_2-$	$N(C_2H_5)_2$	271	8.7	Fast	NA	2	NA	Short
Tetracaine	$H_9C_4N(H)-C_6H_4-$	$-COOCH_2CH_2-$	$N(CH_3)_2$	264	8.4	Slow	80	0.15	85	Long
Amides										
Mepivacaine	$C_6H_3(CH_3)_2-$	$-NHCO-$	N-CH_3 piperidine ring	246	7.9	Fast	1.0	2-3	75	Moderate
Prilocaine	$C_6H_4(CH_3)-$	$-NHCOCH(CH_3)-$	$N(H)(C_3H_7)$	220	7.7	Fast	1.5	4	55	Moderate
Lidocaine	$C_6H_3(CH_3)_2-$	$-NHCOCH_2-$	$N(C_2H_5)_2$	234	7.7	Fast	4.0	2	65	Moderate

Modified from Rogers MC, et al, editors: Principles and practice of anesthesiology, St Louis, 1993, Mosby.
NA, Not available.

Continued

TABLE 1-6
Chemical Structure, Physicochemical Properties, and Pharmacologic Properties of Local Anesthetic Agents—cont'd

	CHEMICAL CONFIGURATION			PHYSICOCHEMICAL PROPERTIES			PHARMACOLOGIC PROPERTIES			
Agent	Aromatic (lipophilic)	Intermediate Chain	Amine (hydrophilic)	Molecular Weight (base)	pKa (36° C)	Onset	Approx Lipid Solubility	Usual Effective Concentration, %	Protein Binding	Duration
Ropivacaine	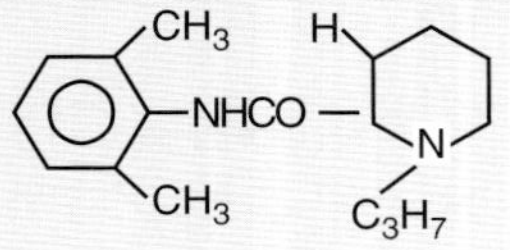 CH_3, CH_3	—NHCO—, H, N, C_3H_7		274	8.1	Moderate	2.8	0.2-0.5	94	Long
Bupivacaine	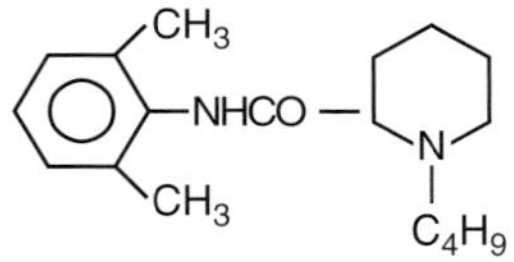 CH_3, CH_3	—NHCO—, N, C_4H_9		288	8.1	Moderate	NA	0.5-0.75	95	Long
Etidocaine	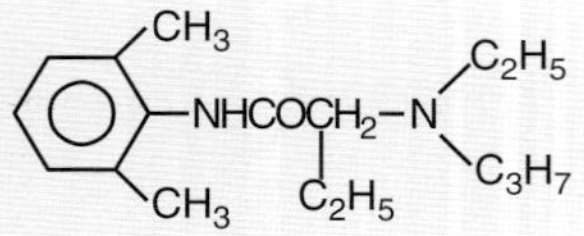 CH_3, CH_3	—NHCOCH—N, C_2H_5, C_2H_5, C_3H_7		276	7.9	Fast	140	0.5-1.5	94	Long
Articaine	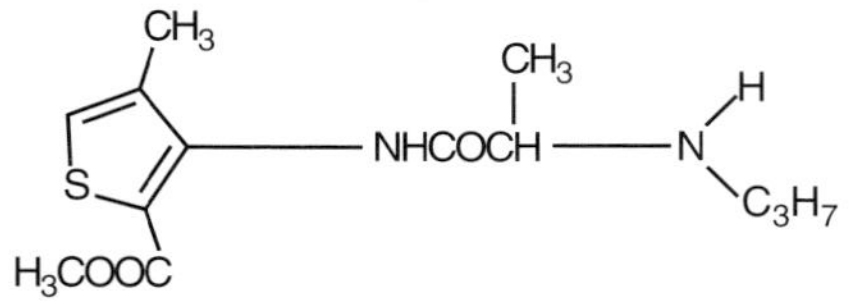 CH_3, S, H_3COOC	NHCOCH, CH_3	N, H, C_3H_7	320	7.8	Fast	17	4	95	Moderate

TABLE 1-7
Factors Affecting Local Anesthetic Action

Factor	Action Affected	Description
pK_a	Onset	Lower pK_a = More rapid onset of action, more RN molecules present to diffuse through nerve sheath; thus onset time is decreased
Lipid solubility	Anesthetic potency	Increased lipid solubility = Increased potency (e.g., procaine = 1; etidocaine = 140) Etidocaine produces conduction blockade at very low concentrations, whereas procaine poorly suppresses nerve conduction, even at higher concentrations
Protein binding	Duration	Increased protein binding allows anesthetic cations (RNH^+) to be more firmly attached to proteins located at receptor sites; thus duration of action is increased
Nonnervous tissue diffusibility	Onset	Increased diffusibility = Decreased time of onset
Vasodilator activity	Anesthetic potency and duration	Greater vasodilator activity = Increased blood flow to region = Rapid removal of anesthetic molecules from injection site; thus anesthetic potency and duration are decreased

From Cohen S, Burns RC: Pathways of the pulp, ed 6, St Louis, 1994, Mosby.

Difficulty Reachieving Profound Anesthesia. In this second situation, as in the first, the dental procedure has outlasted the clinical effectiveness of the local anesthetic drug, and the patient is experiencing pain. The doctor readministers a volume of local anesthetic, but unlike in the first scenario, effective control of pain does not occur.

Tachyphylaxis. In this second clinical situation, a process known as *tachyphylaxis* occurs. Tachyphylaxis is defined as increasing tolerance to a drug that is administered repeatedly. It is much more likely to develop if nerve function is allowed to return before reinjection (e.g., if the patient complains of pain). The duration, intensity, and spread of anesthesia with reinjection are greatly reduced.[41]

Although difficult to explain, tachyphylaxis is probably brought about by some or all of the following factors: edema, localized hemorrhage, clot formation, transudation, hypernatremia, and decreased pH of tissues. The first four factors isolate the nerve from contact with the local anesthetic solution. The fifth, hypernatremia, raises the sodium ion gradient, thus counteracting the decrease in sodium ion conduction brought about by the local anesthetic. The last factor, a decrease in pH of the tissues, is brought about by the first injection of the acidic local anesthetic. The ambient pH in the area of injection may be somewhat lower, so that fewer local anesthetic molecules are transformed into the free base (RN) on reinjection.

Duration of Anesthesia

As the local anesthetic is removed from the nerve, the function of the nerve returns rapidly at first, but then it gradually slows. Compared with onset of the nerve block, which is rapid, recovery from the nerve block is much slower because the local anesthetic is bound to the nerve membrane. Longer-acting local anesthetics (e.g., bupivacaine, etidocaine, ropivacaine, tetracaine) are more firmly bound in the nerve membrane (increased protein binding) than are shorter-acting drugs (e.g., procaine, lidocaine) and therefore are released more slowly from receptor sites in the sodium channels. The rate at which an anesthetic is removed from a nerve has an effect on the duration of neural blockade; in addition to increased protein binding, other factors that influence the rate of removal of a drug from the injection site are the vascularity of the injection site and the presence or absence of a vasoactive substance. Anesthetic duration is increased in areas of decreased vascularity (e.g., Gow-Gates mandibular nerve block vs. inferior alveolar nerve block), and the addition of a vasopressor decreases tissue perfusion to a local area, thus increasing the duration of the block.

References

1. Covino BG, Vassallo HG: Local anesthetics: mechanisms of action and clinical use, New York, 1976, Grune & Stratton.
2. Bennett CR: Monheim's local anesthesia and pain control in dental practice, ed 5, St Louis, 1974, Mosby.
3. Fitzgerald MJT: Neuroanatomy: basic and clinical, London, 1992, Baillière Tyndall.
4. Noback CR, Strominger NL, Demarest RJ: The human nervous system: introduction and review, ed 4, Philadelphia, 1991, Lea & Febiger.
5. Singer SJ, Nicholson GL: The fluid mosaic model of the structure of cell membranes, Science 175:720–731, 1972.
6. Guyton AC: Basic neuroscience: anatomy and physiology, ed 2, Philadelphia, 1991, WB Saunders.
7. Guidotti G: The composition of biological membranes, Arch Intern Med 129:194–201, 1972.
8. Denson DD, Maziot JX: Physiology, pharmacology, and toxicity of local anesthetics: adult and pediatric considerations. In Raj PP, editor: Clinical practice of regional anesthesia, New York, 1991, Churchill Livingstone.
9. Heavner JE: Molecular action of local anesthetics. In Raj PP, editor: Clinical practice of regional anesthesia, New York, 1991, Churchill Livingstone.
10. de Jong RH: Local anesthetics, ed 2, Springfield, Ill, 1977, Charles C Thomas.
11. Hodgkin AL, Huxley AF: A quantitative description of membrane current and its application to conduction and excitation in nerve, J Physiol (London) 117:500–544, 1954.
12. Noback CR, Demarest RJ: The human nervous system: basic principles of neurobiology, ed 3, New York, 1981, McGraw-Hill, pp 44–45.
13. Keynes RD: Ion channels in the nerve-cell membrane, Sci Am 240:326–335, 1979.

14. Cattarall WA: Structure and function of voltage-sensitive ion channels, Science 242:50–61, 1988.
15. Hille B: Ionic selectivity, saturation, and block in sodium channels: a four-barrier model, J Gen Physiol 66:535–560, 1975.
16. Ritchie JM: Physiological basis for conduction in myelinated nerve fibers. In Morell P, editor: Myelin, ed 2, New York, 1984, Plenum Press, pp 117–145.
17. Franz DN, Perry RS: Mechanisms for differential block among single myelinated and non-myelinated axons by procaine, J Physiol 235:193–210, 1974.
18. de Jong RH, Wagman IH: Physiological mechanisms of peripheral nerve block by local anesthetics, Anesthesiology 24:684–727, 1963.
19. Dettbarn WD: The acetylcholine system in peripheral nerve, Ann N Y Acad Sci 144:483–503, 1967.
20. Goldman DE, Blaustein MP: Ions, drugs and the axon membrane, Ann N Y Acad Sci 137:967–981, 1966.
21. Wei LY: Role of surface dipoles on axon membrane, Science 163:280–282, 1969.
22. Lee AG: Model for action of local anesthetics, Nature 262:545–548, 1976.
23. Seeman P: The membrane actions of anesthetics and tranquilizers, Pharmacol Rev 24:583–655, 1972.
24. Strichartz GR, Ritchie JM: The action of local anesthetics on ion channels of excitable tissues. In Strichartz GR, editor: Local anesthetics, New York, 1987, Springer-Verlag.
25. Butterworth JF IV, Strichartz GR: Molecular mechanisms of local anesthesia: a review, Anesthesiology 72:711–734, 1990.
26. Ritchie JM: Mechanisms of action of local anesthetic agents and biotoxins, Br J Anaesth 47:191–198, 1975.
27. Rasminsky M: Conduction in normal and pathological nerve fibers. In Swash M, Kennard C, editors: Scientific basis of clinical neurology, Edinburgh, 1985, Churchill Livingstone.
28. Ritchie JM: The distribution of sodium and potassium channels in mammalian myelinated nerve. In Ritchie JM, Keyes RD, Bolis L, editors: Ion channels in neural membranes, New York, 1986, Alan R Liss.
29. Hille B, Courtney K, Dum R: Rate and site of action of local anesthetics in myelinated nerve fibers. In Fink BR, editor: Molecular mechanisms of anesthesia, New York, 1975, Raven Press, pp 13–20.
30. Setnikar I: Ionization of bases with limited solubility: investigation of substances with local anesthetic activity, J Pharm Sci 55:1190–1195, 1990.
31. Malamed SF: Buffering local anesthetics in dentistry, ADSA Pulse 44(3):8–9, 2011.
32. Stewart JH, Chinn SE, Cole GW, Klein JA: Neutralized lidocaine with epinephrine for local anesthesia-II, J Dermatol Surg Oncol 16:942–945, 1990.
33. Bokesch PM, Raymond SA, Strichartz GR: Dependence of lidocaine potency on pH and pCO_2. Anesth Analg 66:9–17, 1987.
34. Bieter RN: Applied pharmacology of local anesthetics, Am J Surg 34:500–510, 1936.
35. Buckley MM, Benfield P: Eutectic lidocaine/prilocaine cream: a review of the topical anesthetic/analgesic efficacy of a eutectic mixture of local anesthetics (EMLA), Drugs 46:126–151, 1993.
36. Campbell AH, Stasse JA, Lord GH, Willson JE: In vivo evaluation of local anesthetics applied topically, J Pharm Sci 57:2045–2048, 1968.
37. Noback CR, Demarest RJ: The human nervous system: basic principles of neurobiology, ed 3, New York, 1981, McGraw-Hill.
38. de Jong RH: Local anesthetics, ed 2, Springfield, Ill, 1977, Charles C Thomas, pp 66–68.
39. Ritchie JM, Ritchie B, Greengard P: The active structure of local anesthetics, J Pharmacol Exp Ther 150:152, 1965.
40. Tucker GT: Plasma binding and disposition of local anesthetics, Int Anesthesiol Clin 13:33, 1975.
41. Cohen EN, Levine DA, Colliss JE, Gunther RE: The role of pH in the development of tachyphylaxis to local anesthetic agents, Anesthesiology 29:994–1001, 1968.

CHAPTER 2

Pharmacology of Local Anesthetics

Local anesthetics, when used for the management of pain, differ from most other drugs commonly used in medicine and dentistry in one important manner. Virtually all other drugs, regardless of the route through which they are administered, must ultimately enter into the circulatory system in sufficiently high concentrations (e.g., attain therapeutic blood levels in their target organ[s]) before they can begin to exert a clinical action. Local anesthetics, however, when used for pain control, *cease* to provide a clinical effect when they are absorbed from the site of administration into the circulation. One prime factor involved in the termination of action of local anesthetics used for pain control is their redistribution from the nerve fiber into the cardiovascular system.

The presence of a local anesthetic in the circulatory system means that the drug will be transported to every part of the body. Local anesthetics have the ability to alter the functioning of some of these cells. In this chapter, the actions of local anesthetics, other than their ability to block conduction in nerve axons of the peripheral nervous system, are reviewed. A classification of local anesthetics is shown in Box 2-1.

PHARMACOKINETICS OF LOCAL ANESTHETICS

Uptake

When injected into soft tissues, local anesthetics exert pharmacologic action on blood vessels in the area. All local anesthetics possess a degree of vasoactivity, most producing dilation of the vascular bed into which they are deposited, although the degree of vasodilation may vary, and some may produce vasoconstriction. To some degree, these effects may be concentration dependent.[1] Relative vasodilating values of amide local anesthetics are shown in Table 2-1.

Ester local anesthetics are also potent vasodilating drugs. Procaine, the most potent vasodilator among local anesthetics, is occasionally injected clinically to induce vasodilation when peripheral blood flow has been compromised because of (accidental) intra-arterial (IA) injection of a drug (e.g., thiopental)[2] or injection of epinephrine or norepinephrine into a fingertip or toe.[3] IA administration of an irritating drug such as thiopental may produce arteriospasm with an attendant decrease in tissue perfusion that if prolonged could lead to tissue death, gangrene, and loss of the affected limb. In this situation, procaine is administered IA in an attempt to break the arteriospasm and reestablish blood flow to the affected limb. Tetracaine, chloroprocaine, and propoxycaine also possess vasodilating properties to varying degrees but not to the degree of procaine.

Cocaine is the only local anesthetic that consistently produces vasoconstriction.[4] The initial action of cocaine is vasodilation followed by an intense and prolonged vasoconstriction. It is produced by inhibition of the uptake of catecholamines (especially norepinephrine) into tissue binding sites. This results in an excess of free norepinephrine, leading to a prolonged and intense state of vasoconstriction. This inhibition of the reuptake of norepinephrine has not been demonstrated with other local anesthetics, such as lidocaine and bupivacaine.

A significant clinical effect of vasodilation is an increase in the rate of absorption of the local anesthetic into the blood, thus decreasing the duration and quality (e.g., depth) of pain control, while increasing the anesthetic blood (or plasma) concentration and its potential for overdose (toxic reaction). The rates at which local anesthetics are absorbed into the bloodstream and reach their peak blood level vary according to the route of administration (Table 2-2).

Oral Route. With the exception of cocaine, local anesthetics are absorbed poorly, if at all, from the gastrointestinal tract after oral administration. In addition, most local anesthetics (especially lidocaine) undergo a significant hepatic first-pass effect after oral administration. After absorption of lidocaine from the gastrointestinal tract into the enterohepatic circulation, a fraction of the drug dose is carried to the liver, where approximately 72% of the dose is biotransformed into inactive metabolites.[5] This has seriously hampered the use of lidocaine as an oral antidysrhythmic drug. In 1984, Astra Pharmaceuticals and Merck Sharp & Dohme introduced an analog of lidocaine, tocainide hydrochloride, which is effective orally.[6] The chemical structures of tocainide and lidocaine are presented in Figure 2-1.

BOX 2-1 Classification of Local Anesthetics

Esters

Esters of benzoic acid

Butacaine
Cocaine
Ethyl aminobenzoate (benzocaine)
Hexylcaine
Piperocaine
Tetracaine

Esters of para-aminobenzoic acid

Chloroprocaine
Procaine
Propoxycaine

Amides

Articaine
Bupivacaine
Dibucaine
Etidocaine
Lidocaine
Mepivacaine
Prilocaine
Ropivacaine

Quinoline

Centbucridine

TABLE 2-2
Time to Achieve Peak Blood Level

Route	Time, min
Intravenous	1
Topical	5 (approximately)
Intramuscular	5-10
Subcutaneous	30-90

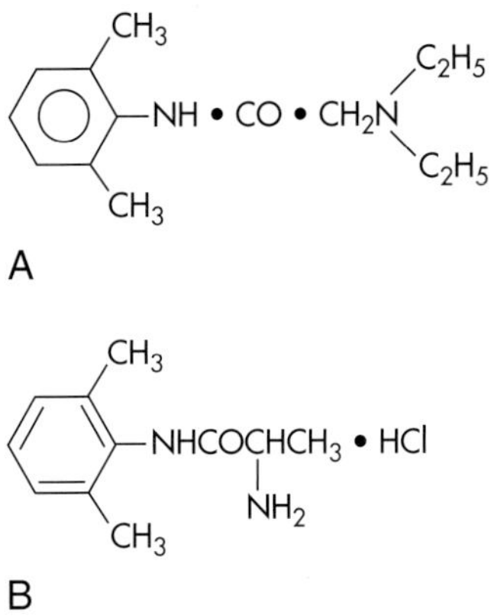

A: CH_3, CH_3 — NH • CO • $CH_2N(C_2H_5)_2$

B: CH_3, CH_3 — NHCOCHCH$_3$ • HCl, NH_2

Figure 2-1. Tocainide. **A,** Represents a modification of lidocaine (**B**) that is able to pass through the liver after oral administration with minimal hepatic first-pass effect.

TABLE 2-1
Relative Vasodilating Values of Amide-Type Local Anesthetics

	Vasodilating Activity	MEAN % INCREASE IN FEMORAL ARTERY BLOOD FLOW IN DOGS AFTER INTRA-ARTERIAL INJECTION* 1 min	5 min
Articaine	1 (approx)	NA	NA
Bupivacaine	2.5	45.4	30
Etidocaine	2.5	44.3	26.6
Lidocaine	1	25.8	7.5
Mepivacaine	0.8	35.7	9.5
Prilocaine	0.5	42.1	6.3
Tetracaine	NA	37.6	14

Modified from Blair MR: Cardiovascular pharmacology of local anaesthetics, Br J Anaesth 47(suppl):247-252, 1975.
NA, Not available.
*Each agent injected rapidly at a dose of 1 mg/0.1 mL saline.

Topical Route. Local anesthetics are absorbed at differing rates after application to mucous membrane: In the tracheal mucosa, absorption is almost as rapid as with intravenous (IV) administration (indeed, intratracheal drug administration [epinephrine, lidocaine, atropine, naloxone, and flumazenil] is used in certain emergency situations); in the pharyngeal mucosa, absorption is slower; and in the esophageal or bladder mucosa, uptake is even slower than occurs through the pharynx. Wherever no layer of intact skin is present, topically applied local anesthetics can produce an anesthetic effect. Sunburn remedies (e.g., Solarcaine, Schering-Plough HealthCare Products, Inc., Memphis, Tenn) usually contain lidocaine, benzocaine, or other anesthetics in an ointment formulation. Applied to intact skin, they do not provide an anesthetic action, but with skin damaged by sunburn, they bring rapid relief of pain. A eutectic mixture of local anesthetics lidocaine and prilocaine (EMLA) has been developed that is able to provide surface anesthesia of intact skin.[7]

Injection. The rate of uptake (absorption) of local anesthetics after parenteral administration (subcutaneous, intramuscular, or IV) is related to both the vascularity of the injection site and the vasoactivity of the drug.

IV administration of local anesthetics provides the most rapid elevation of blood levels and is used clinically in the primary management of ventricular dysrhythmias.[8] Rapid IV administration can lead to significantly high local anesthetic blood levels, which can induce serious toxic reactions. The benefits to be accrued from IV drug administration must always be carefully weighed against any risks associated with IV administration. Only when the benefits clearly outweigh the risks should the drug be administered, as is the case with pre-fatal ventricular dysrhythmias such as premature ventricular contractions (PVCs).[9]

Distribution

Once absorbed into the blood, local anesthetics are distributed throughout the body to all tissues (Fig. 2-2). Highly perfused organs (and areas), such as the brain, head, liver, kidneys, lungs, and spleen, initially will have higher anesthetic blood levels than less highly perfused organs. Skeletal muscle, although not as highly perfused as these areas, contains the greatest percentage of local anesthetic of any tissue or organ in the body because it constitutes the largest mass of tissue in the body (Table 2-3).

The plasma concentration of a local anesthetic in certain target organs has a significant bearing on the potential toxicity of the drug. The blood level of the local anesthetic is influenced by the following factors:

1. Rate at which the drug is absorbed into the cardiovascular system
2. Rate of distribution of the drug from the vascular compartment to the tissues (more rapid in healthy patients than in those who are medically compromised [e.g., congestive heart failure], thus leading to lower blood levels in healthier patients)
3. Elimination of the drug through metabolic or excretory pathways

The latter two factors serve to decrease the blood level of the local anesthetic.

The rate at which a local anesthetic is removed from the blood is described as its *elimination half-life.* Simply stated, the elimination half-life is the time necessary for a 50% reduction in the blood level (one half-life = 50% reduction; two half-lives = 75% reduction; three half-lives = 87.5% reduction; four half-lives = 94% reduction; five half-lives = 97% reduction; six half-lives = 98.5% reduction) (Table 2-4).

All local anesthetics readily cross the blood–brain barrier. They also readily cross the placenta and enter the circulatory system of the developing fetus.

Metabolism (Biotransformation, Detoxification)

A significant difference between the two major groups of local anesthetics, the esters and the amides, is the means by which the body biologically transforms the active drug into one that is pharmacologically inactive. Metabolism (or biotransformation or detoxification) of local anesthetics is important because the overall toxicity of a drug depends on a balance between its rate of absorption into the bloodstream at the site of injection and its rate of removal from

TABLE 2-3
Percentages of Cardiac Output Distributed to Different Organ Systems

Region	Percent of Cardiac Output Received
Kidney	22
Gastrointestinal system, spleen	21
Skeletal muscle	15
Brain	14
Skin	6
Liver	6
Bone	5
Heart muscle	3
Other	8

Adapted from Mohrman DE, Heller LJ: Cardiovascular physiology, ed 7, New York, 2010, Lange Medical Books/McGraw-Hill.

TABLE 2-4
Half-Life of Local Anesthetics

Drug	Half-life, hours
Chloroprocaine*	0.1
Procaine*	0.1
Tetracaine*	0.3
Articaine†	0.5
Cocaine*	0.7
Prilocaine†	1.6
Lidocaine†	1.6
Mepivacaine†	1.9
Ropivacaine†	1.9
Etidocaine†	2.6
Bupivacaine†	3.5
Propoxycaine*	NA

NA, Not available.
*Ester.
†Amide.

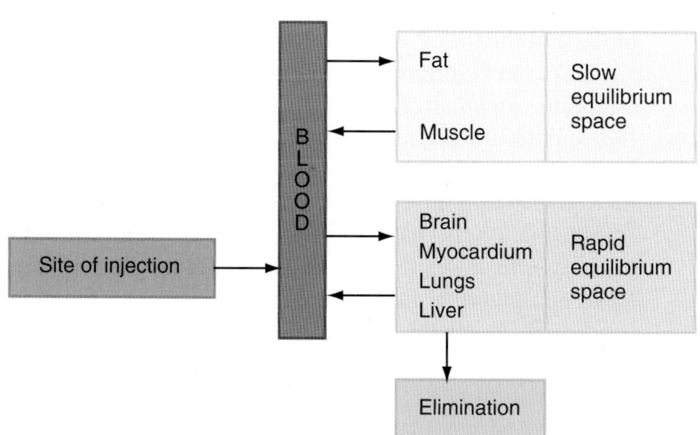

Figure 2-2. Pattern of distribution of local anesthetics after absorption. (Redrawn from Wildsmith JAW, Armitage EN, McClure JH: Principles and practice of regional anesthesia, ed 3, Edinburgh, 2003, Churchill Livingstone.)

TABLE 2-5
Hydrolysis Rate of Esters

Drug	Rate of Hydrolysis, μmol/mL/hr
Chloroprocaine	4.7
Procaine	1.1
Tetracaine	0.3

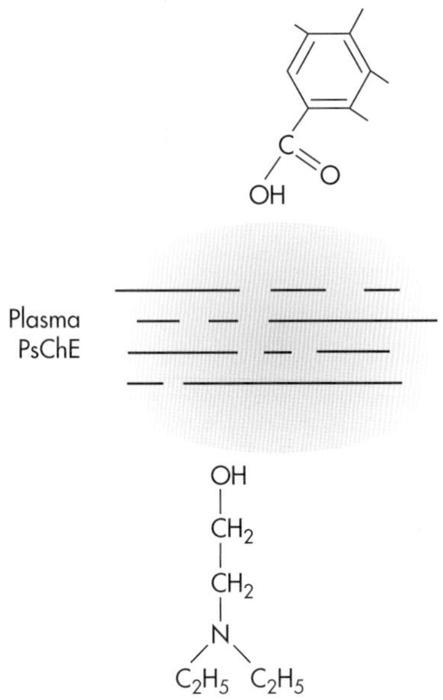

Figure 2-3. Metabolic hydrolysis of procaine. *PsChE,* Pseudocholinesterase. (From Tucker GT: Biotransformation and toxicity of local anesthetics, Acta Anaesthesiol Belg 26[Suppl]: 123, 1975.)

the blood through the processes of tissue uptake and metabolism.

Ester Local Anesthetics. Ester local anesthetics are hydrolyzed in the plasma by the enzyme pseudocholinesterase.[10] The rate at which hydrolysis of different esters occurs varies considerably (Table 2-5).

The rate of hydrolysis has an impact on the potential toxicity* of a local anesthetic. Chloroprocaine, the most rapidly hydrolyzed, is the least toxic, whereas tetracaine, hydrolyzed 16 times more slowly than chloroprocaine, has the greatest potential toxicity. Procaine undergoes hydrolysis to para-aminobenzoic acid (PABA), which is excreted unchanged in the urine, and to diethylamine alcohol, which undergoes further biotransformation before excretion (Fig. 2-3). Allergic reactions that occur in response to ester local anesthetics usually are not related to the parent compound (e.g., procaine) but rather to PABA, which is a major metabolic product of many ester local anesthetics.

*ALL chemicals (drugs) have the potential to be poisons, also called *toxins.* When the resulting blood level is too high, drugs exert negative actions, which we call a *toxic reaction* or *overdose.*

Approximately 1 of every 2800 persons has an atypical form of pseudocholinesterase, which causes an inability to hydrolyze ester local anesthetics and other chemically related drugs (e.g., succinylcholine).[11] Its presence leads to prolongation of higher local anesthetic blood levels and increased potential for toxicity.

Succinylcholine is a short-acting muscle relaxant commonly employed during the induction phase of general anesthesia. It produces respiratory arrest (apnea) for a period of approximately 2 to 3 minutes. Then plasma pseudocholinesterase hydrolyzes succinylcholine, blood levels fall, and spontaneous respiration resumes. Persons with atypical pseudocholinesterase are unable to hydrolyze succinylcholine at a normal rate; therefore the duration of apnea is prolonged. Atypical pseudocholinesterase is a hereditary trait. Any familial history of difficulty during general anesthesia should be carefully evaluated by the doctor before dental care commences. A confirmed or strongly suspected history, in the patient or biological family, of atypical pseudocholinesterase represents a relative contraindication to administration of ester-type local anesthetics.

There are absolute and relative contraindications to the administration of drugs. An *absolute contraindication* implies that under no circumstance should the drug in question be administered to this patient because the possibility of potentially toxic or lethal reactions is increased, whereas a *relative contraindication* means that the drug in question may be administered to the patient after careful weighing of the risk associated with use of the drug versus the potential benefit to be gained, and if an acceptable alternative drug is not available. However, the smallest clinically effective dose always should be used because the likelihood of adverse reaction to this drug is increased in this patient.

Amide Local Anesthetics. The biotransformation of amide local anesthetics is more complex than that of the esters. The primary site of biotransformation of amide local anesthetics is the liver. Virtually the entire metabolic process occurs in the liver for lidocaine, mepivacaine, etidocaine, and bupivacaine. Prilocaine undergoes primary metabolism in the liver, with some also possibly occurring in the lung.[12,13] Articaine, a hybrid molecule containing both ester and amide components, undergoes metabolism in both the blood and the liver.[14]

The rates of biotransformation of lidocaine, mepivacaine, etidocaine, and bupivacaine are similar. Therefore liver function and hepatic perfusion significantly influence the rate of biotransformation of an amide local anesthetic. Approximately 70% of a dose of injected lidocaine undergoes biotransformation in patients with normal liver function.[5] Patients with lower than usual hepatic blood flow (hypotension, congestive heart failure) or poor liver function (cirrhosis) are unable to biotransform amide local anesthetics at a normal rate.[15,16] This slower than normal biotransformation rate results in higher anesthetic blood levels and increased risk of toxicity. Significant liver dysfunction

(American Society of Anesthesiologists Physical Status classification system [ASA] 4 to 5) or heart failure (ASA 4 to 5) represents a relative contraindication to the administration of amide local anesthetic drugs (Table 2-6). Articaine has a shorter half-life than other amides (27 minutes vs. 90 minutes) because a portion of its biotransformation occurs in the blood by the enzyme plasma cholinesterase.[17]

The biotransformation products of certain local anesthetics can possess significant clinical activity if they are permitted to accumulate in the blood. This may be seen in renal or cardiac failure and during periods of prolonged drug administration. A clinical example is the production of methemoglobinemia in patients receiving large doses of prilocaine.[18,19] Prilocaine, the parent compound, does not produce methemoglobinemia, but orthotoluidine, a primary metabolite of prilocaine, does induce the formation of methemoglobin, which is responsible for methemoglobinemia. When methemoglobin blood levels become elevated, clinical signs and symptoms are observed. Methemoglobinemia is discussed more fully in Chapter 10. Another example of pharmacologically active metabolites is the sedative effect occasionally observed after lidocaine administration. Lidocaine does not produce sedation; however, two metabolites—monoethylglycinexylidide and glycine xylidide—are thought to be responsible for this clinical action.[20]

The metabolic pathways of lidocaine and prilocaine are shown in Figures 2-4 and 2-5.

TABLE 2-6
Lidocaine Disposition in Various Groups of Patients

Group	Lidocaine Half-Life, hr	Mean Total Body Clearance, mL/kg/min
Normal	1.8	10
Heart failure	1.9	6.3
Hepatic disease	4.9	6
Renal disease	1.3	13.7

Data from Thomson PD, et al: Lidocaine pharmacokinetics in advanced heart failure, liver disease, and renal failure in humans, Ann Intern Med 78:499–513, 1973.

Excretion

The kidneys are the primary excretory organ for both the local anesthetic and its metabolites. A percentage of a given dose of local anesthetic is excreted unchanged in the urine. This percentage varies according to the drug. Esters appear only in very small concentrations as the parent compound in the urine because they are hydrolyzed almost completely in the plasma. Procaine appears in the urine as PABA (90%) with 2% unchanged. Ten percent of a cocaine dose is found in the urine unchanged. Amides usually are present in the urine as the parent compound in a greater percentage than the esters, primarily because of their more complex process of biotransformation. Although the percentages of parent drug found in urine vary from study to study, less than 3% lidocaine, 1% mepivacaine, and 1% etidocaine is found unchanged in the urine.

Patients with significant renal impairment may be unable to eliminate the parent local anesthetic compound or its major metabolites from the blood, resulting in slightly elevated blood levels and therefore increased potential for toxicity. This may occur with the esters or amides and is especially likely with cocaine. Thus significant renal disease (ASA 4 to 5) represents a relative contraindication to the administration of local anesthetics. This includes patients undergoing renal dialysis and those with chronic glomerulonephritis or pyelonephritis.

SYSTEMIC ACTIONS OF LOCAL ANESTHETICS

Local anesthetics are chemicals that reversibly block action potentials in all excitable membranes. The central nervous system (CNS) and the cardiovascular system (CVS) therefore are especially susceptible to their actions. Most of the systemic actions of local anesthetics are related to their blood or plasma level in the target organ (CNS, CVS). The higher the level, the greater will be the clinical action.

Centbucridine (a quinoline derivative) has proved to be five to eight times as potent a local anesthetic as lidocaine, with an equally rapid onset of action and an equivalent duration.[21,22] Of potentially great importance is the finding that it does not adversely affect the CNS or CVS, except in very high doses.

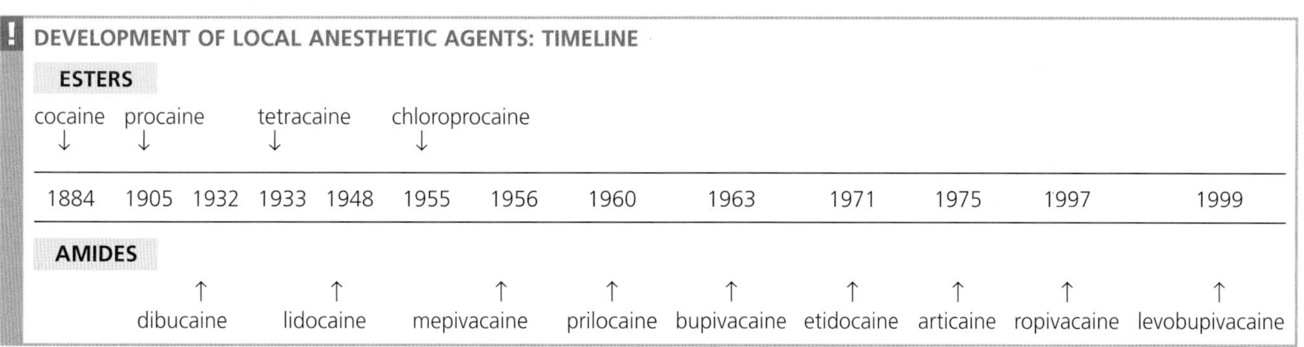

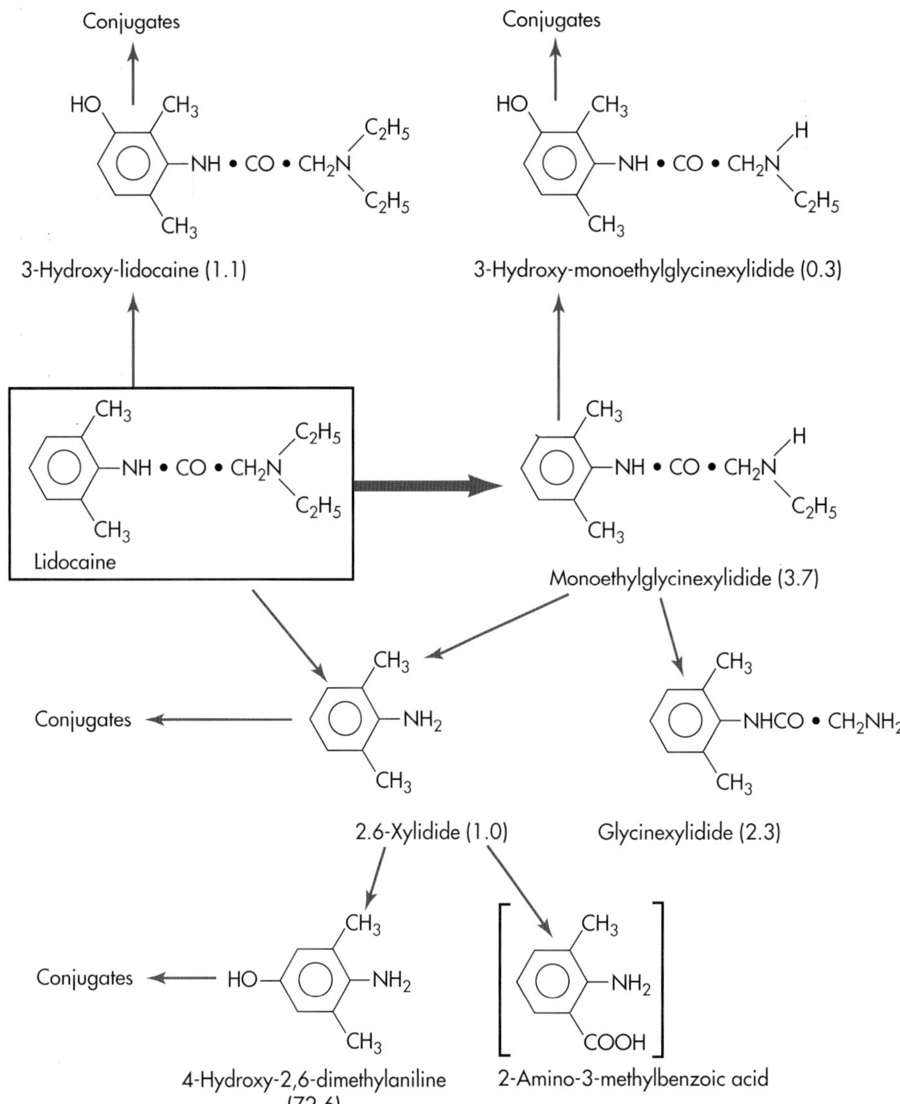

Figure 2-4. Metabolic pathways of lidocaine. Percentages of dose found in urine are indicated in parentheses. (From Kennaghan JB, Boyes RN: The tissue distribution, metabolism, and excretion of lidocaine in rats, guinea pigs, dogs and man, J Pharmacol Exp Ther Feb 180(2):454–463, 1972.)

Local anesthetics are absorbed from their site of administration into the circulatory system, which effectively dilutes them and carries them to all cells of the body. The ensuing blood level of the local anesthetic depends on its rate of uptake from the site of administration into the circulatory system (increasing the blood level), and on the rates of distribution in tissue and biotransformation (in the liver), processes that remove the drug from the blood (decreasing the blood level) (see Fig. 2-2).

Central Nervous System

Local anesthetics readily cross the blood–brain barrier. Their pharmacologic action on the CNS is seen as depression. At low (therapeutic, nontoxic) blood levels, no CNS effects of any clinical significance have been noted. At higher (toxic, overdose) levels, the primary clinical manifestation is a generalized tonic–clonic convulsion. Between these two extremes exists a spectrum of other clinical signs and symptoms. (See Box 2-2, "Preconvulsive Signs and Symptoms of Central Nervous Toxicity.")

Anticonvulsant Properties. Some local anesthetics (e.g., procaine, lidocaine, mepivacaine, prilocaine, even cocaine) have demonstrated anticonvulsant properties.[23,24] These occur at a blood level considerably below that at which the same drugs produce seizure activity. Values for anticonvulsive blood levels of lidocaine are shown in Table 2-7.[25]

Procaine, mepivacaine, and lidocaine have been used intravenously to terminate or decrease the duration of both grand mal and petit mal seizures.[23,26] The anticonvulsant blood level of lidocaine (about 0.5 to 4 μg/mL) is very close to its cardiotherapeutic range (see following). It has been demonstrated to be effective in temporarily arresting seizure activity in a majority of human epileptic patients.[27] It was especially effective in interrupting status epilepticus

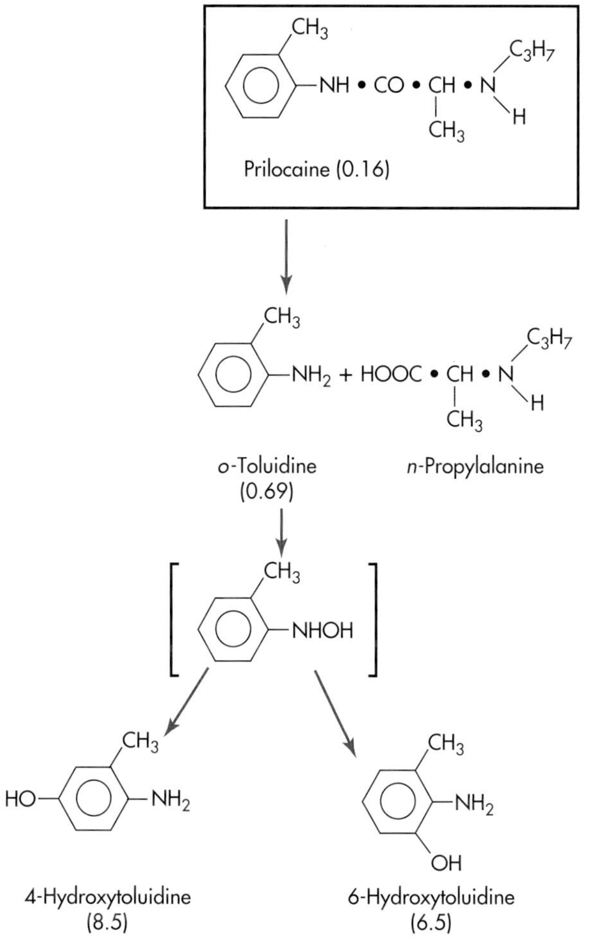

Prilocaine (0.16)

o-Toluidine (0.69) + n-Propylalanine

4-Hydroxytoluidine (8.5)

6-Hydroxytoluidine (6.5)

Figure 2-5. Metabolic pathways of prilocaine. Percentages of dose found in urine are indicated in parentheses.

BOX 2-2 Preconvulsive Signs and Symptoms of Central Nervous System Toxicity

Signs (objectively observable)	Symptoms (subjectively felt)
Slurred speech	Numbness of tongue and circumoral region
Shivering	Warm, flushed feeling of skin
Muscular twitching	Pleasant dreamlike state
Tremor of muscles of face and distal extremities	
Generalized lightheadedness	
Dizziness	
Visual disturbances (inability to focus)	
Auditory disturbance (tinnitus)	
Drowsiness	
Disorientation	

TABLE 2-7
Anticonvulsive Blood Levels of Lidocaine

Clinical Situation	Lidocaine Blood Level, μg/mL
Anticonvulsive level	0.5-4
Preseizure signs and symptoms	4.5-7
Tonic–clonic seizure	>7.5

at therapeutic doses of 2 to 3 mg/kg when given at a rate of 40 to 50 mg/min.

Mechanism of Anticonvulsant Properties. Epileptic patients possess hyperexcitable cortical neurons at a site within the brain where the convulsive episode originates (called the *epileptic focus*). Local anesthetics, by virtue of their depressant actions on the CNS, raise the seizure threshold by decreasing the excitability of these neurons, thereby preventing or terminating seizures.

Preconvulsive Signs and Symptoms. With a further increase in the blood level of the local anesthetic to above its therapeutic level, adverse reactions may be observed. Because the CNS is much more susceptible than other systems to the actions of local anesthetics, it is not surprising that the initial clinical signs and symptoms of overdose (toxicity) are CNS in origin. With lidocaine, this second phase is observed at a level between 4.5 and 7 μg/mL in the average normal healthy patient.* Initial clinical signs and symptoms of CNS toxicity are usually excitatory in nature (see Box 2-2).

All of these signs and symptoms, except for the sensation of circumoral and lingual numbness, are related to the direct depressant action of the local anesthetic on the CNS. Numbness of the tongue and circumoral regions is not caused by CNS effects of the local anesthetic.[28] Rather it is the result of a direct anesthetic action of the local anesthetic, which is present in high concentrations in these highly vascular tissues, on free nerve endings. The anesthetic has been transported to these tissues by the CVS. A dentist treating a patient might have difficulty conceptualizing why anesthesia of the tongue is considered to be a sign of a toxic reaction when lingual anesthesia is commonly produced after mandibular nerve blocks. Consider for a moment a physician administering a local anesthetic into the patient's foot. Overly high blood levels would produce bilateral numbing of the tongue, as contrasted with the usual unilateral anesthesia seen after dental nerve blocks.

Lidocaine and procaine differ somewhat from other local anesthetics in that the usual progression of signs and symptoms just noted may not be seen. Lidocaine and procaine frequently produce an initial mild sedation or drowsiness (more common with lidocaine).[29] Because of this potential,

*Individual variation in response to drugs, as depicted in the normal distribution curve, may produce clinical symptoms at levels lower than these (in hyperresponders) or may fail to produce them at higher levels (in hyporesponders).

the U.S. Air Force and the U.S. Navy ground airplane pilots for 24 hours after receipt of a local anesthetic.[30]

Sedation may develop in place of the excitatory signs. If excitation or sedation is observed during the first 5 to 10 minutes after intraoral administration of a local anesthetic, it should serve as a warning to the clinician of a rising local anesthetic blood level and the possibility (if the blood level continues to rise) of a more serious reaction, including a generalized convulsive episode.

TABLE 2-8
Effects of pCO_2 on the Convulsive Threshold (CD_{100}) of Various Local Anesthetics in Cats

	CD_{100}, mg/kg		Percent
Agent	**pCO_2 (25-40 torr)**	**pCO_2 (6581 torr)**	**Change in CD_{100}**
Procaine	35	17	51
Mepivacaine	18	10	44
Prilocaine	22	12	45
Lidocaine	15	7	53
Bupivacaine	5	2.5	50

Data from Englesson S, Grevsten S, Olin A: Some numerical methods of estimating acid-base variables in normal human blood with a haemoglobin concentration of 5 g/100 cm^3, Scand J Lab Clin Invest 32:289–295, 1973.

TABLE 2-9
Convulsant Dose (CD_{100}) and Acid-Base Status*

	pH 7.10	pH 7.20	pH 7.30	pH 7.40
pCO_2 30	—	—	27.5	26.6
pCO_2 40	—	20.6	21.4	22.0
pCO_2 60	13.1	15.4	17.5	—
pCO_2 80	11.3	14.3	—	—

From Englesson S: The influence of acid-base changes on central nervous toxicity of local anaesthetic agents, Acta Anaesthesiol Scand 18:88–103, 1974.

*Intravenous lidocaine 5 mg/kg/min, cats; doses in mg/kg.

Convulsive Phase. Further elevation of the local anesthetic blood level leads to signs and symptoms consistent with a generalized tonic–clonic convulsive episode. The duration of seizure activity is related to the local anesthetic blood level and is inversely related to the arterial partial pressure of carbon dioxide (pCO_2) level.[31] At a normal pCO_2, a lidocaine blood level between 7.5 and 10 μg/mL usually results in a convulsive episode. When carbon dioxide (CO_2) levels are increased, the blood level of local anesthetic necessary for seizures decreases while the duration of the seizure increases.[31] Seizure activity generally is self-limiting, because cardiovascular activity usually is not significantly impaired, and redistribution and biotransformation of the local anesthetic continue throughout the episode. This results in a decrease in anesthetic blood level and termination of seizure activity, usually within 1 minute.

However, several other mechanisms also at work unfortunately act to prolong the convulsive episode. Both cerebral blood flow and cerebral metabolism are increased during local anesthetic-induced convulsions. Increased blood flow to the brain leads to an increase in the volume of local anesthetic being delivered to the brain, tending to prolong the seizure. Increased cerebral metabolism leads to a progressive metabolic acidosis as the seizure continues, and this tends to prolong the seizure activity (by lowering the blood level of anesthetic necessary to provoke a seizure), even in the presence of a declining local anesthetic level in the blood. As noted in Tables 2-8 and 2-9, the dose of local anesthetic necessary to induce seizures is markedly diminished in the presence of hypercarbia (see Table 2-8) or acidosis (see Table 2-9).[31,32]

Further increases in local anesthetic blood level result in cessation of seizure activity as electroencephalographic (EEG) tracings become flattened, indicative of a generalized CNS depression. Respiratory depression occurs at this time, eventually leading to respiratory arrest if anesthetic blood levels continue to rise. Respiratory effects are a result of the depressant action of the local anesthetic drug on the CNS.

Mechanism of Preconvulsant and Convulsant Actions. It is known that local anesthetics exert a depressant action on excitable membranes, yet the primary clinical manifestation associated with high local anesthetic blood levels is related to varying degrees of stimulation. How can a drug that depresses the CNS be responsible for the production of varying degrees of stimulation, including tonic–clonic seizure activity? It is thought that local anesthetics produce clinical signs and symptoms of CNS excitation (including convulsions) through selective blockade of inhibitory pathways in the cerebral cortex.[32-35] de Jong states that "inhibition of inhibition thus is a presynaptic event that follows local anesthetic blockade of impulses traveling along inhibitory pathways."[36]

The cerebral cortex has pathways of neurons that are essentially inhibitory and others that are facilitatory (excitatory). A state of balance normally is maintained between the degrees of effect exerted by these neuronal paths (Fig. 2-6). At preconvulsant local anesthetic blood levels, observed clinical signs and symptoms are produced because the local anesthetic selectively depresses the action of inhibitory neurons (Fig. 2-7). Balance then is tipped slightly in favor of excessive facilitatory (excitatory) input, leading to symptoms of tremor and slight agitation.

At higher (convulsive) blood levels, inhibitory neuron function is completely depressed, allowing unopposed function of facilitatory neurons (Fig. 2-8). Pure facilitatory input without inhibition produces the tonic–clonic activity observed at these levels.

Further increases in anesthetic blood level lead to depression of the facilitatory and inhibitory pathways, producing generalized CNS depression (Fig. 2-9). The precise site of action of the local anesthetic within the CNS is not known but is thought to be at the inhibitory cortical synapses or directly on the inhibitory cortical neurons.

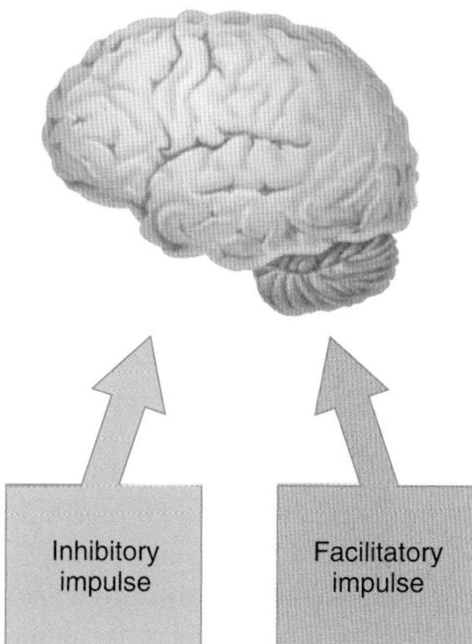

Figure 2-6. Balance between inhibitory and facilitatory impulses in a normal cerebral cortex.

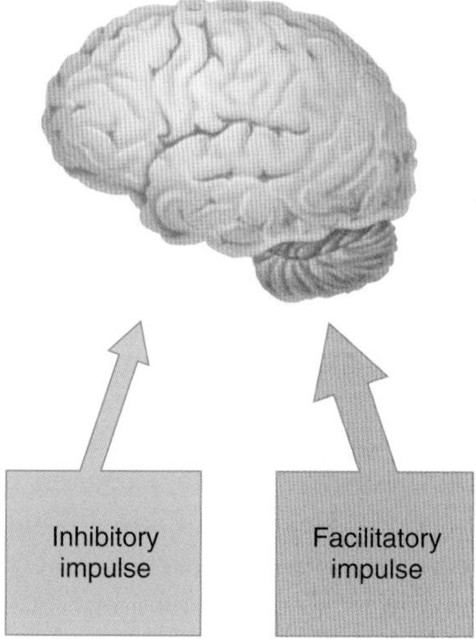

Figure 2-7. In the preconvulsive stage of local anesthetic action, the inhibitory impulse is more profoundly depressed than the facilitatory impulse.

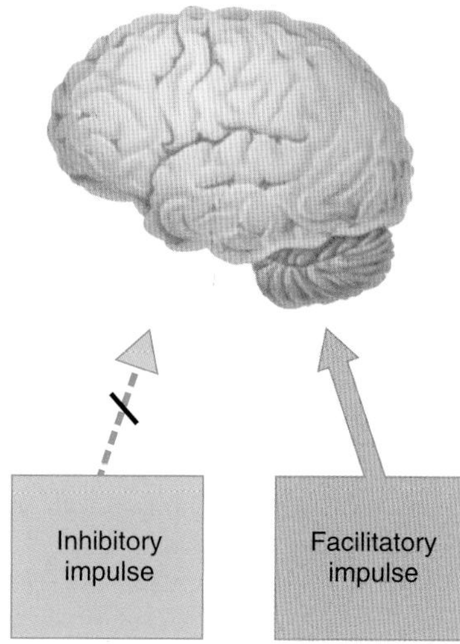

Figure 2-8. In the convulsive stage of local anesthetic action, the inhibitory impulse is totally depressed, permitting unopposed facilitatory impulse activity.

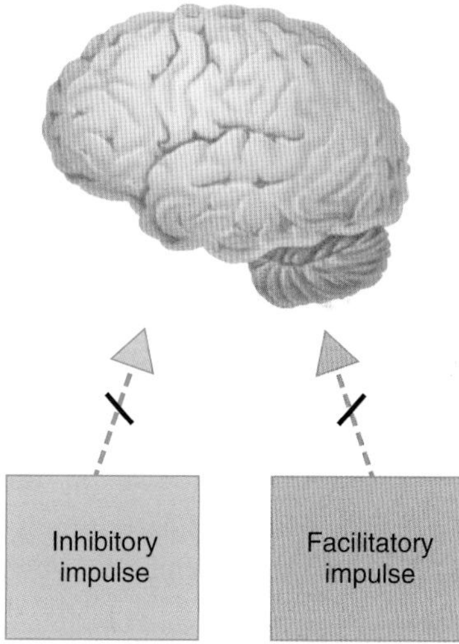

Figure 2-9. In the final stage of local anesthetic action, both inhibitory and facilitatory impulses are totally depressed, producing generalized central nervous system depression.

Analgesia. Local anesthetics possess a second action in relation to the CNS. Administered intravenously, they increase the pain reaction threshold and also produce a degree of analgesia.

In the 1940s and 1950s, procaine was administered intravenously for the management of chronic pain and arthritis.[37] The "procaine unit" was commonly used for this purpose; it consisted of 4 mg/kg of body weight administered over 20 minutes. The technique was ineffective for acute pain. Because of the relatively narrow safety margin between the analgesic actions of procaine and the occurrence of signs and symptoms of overdose, this technique is no longer in use today.

Mood Elevation. The use of local anesthetic drugs for mood elevation and rejuvenation has persisted for centuries, despite documentation of both catastrophic events (mood elevation) and lack of effect (rejuvenation).

Cocaine has long been used for its euphoria-inducing and fatigue-lessening actions, dating back to the chewing of coca leaves by Incas and other South American natives.[38,39] Unfortunately, as is well documented today, prolonged use of cocaine leads to habituation. William Stewart Halsted (1852-1922), the father of American surgery, cocaine researcher, and the first person to administer a local anesthetic by injection, suffered greatly because of an addiction to cocaine.[40] In more recent times, the sudden, unexpected deaths of several prominent professional athletes caused by cocaine and the addiction of many others clearly demonstrate the dangers involved in the casual use of potent drugs.[41,42]

More benign, but totally unsubstantiated, is the use of procaine (Novocain) as a rejuvenating drug. Clinics

TABLE 2-10
Intravenous Dose of Local Anesthetic Agents Required for Convulsive Activity (CD_{100}) and Irreversible Cardiovascular Collapse (LD_{100}) in Dogs

Agent	CD_{100}, mg/kg	LD_{100}, mg/kg	LD_{100}/CD_{100} Agent Ratio
Lidocaine	22	76	3.5
Etidocaine	8	40	5.0
Bupivacaine	4	20	5.0
Tetracaine	5	27	5.4

Data from Liu P, et al: Acute cardiovascular toxicity of intravenous amide local anesthetics in anesthetized ventilated dogs, Anesth Analg 61:317–322, 1982.

professing to "restore youthful vigor" claim that procaine is a literal Fountain of Youth. These clinics operate primarily in central Europe and Mexico, where procaine is used under the proprietary name Gerovital. de Jong states that "whatever the retarding effect on aging, it probably is relegated most charitably to mood elevation."[43]

Cardiovascular System

Local anesthetics have a direct action on the myocardium and peripheral vasculature. In general, however, the cardiovascular system appears to be more resistant than the CNS to the effects of local anesthetic drugs (Table 2-10).[44]

Direct Action on the Myocardium. Local anesthetics modify electrophysiologic events in the myocardium in a manner similar to their actions on peripheral nerves. As the local anesthetic blood level increases, the rate of rise of various phases of myocardial depolarization is reduced. No significant change in resting membrane potential occurs, and no significant prolongation of the phases of repolarization is seen.[45]

Local anesthetics produce a myocardial depression that is related to the local anesthetic blood level. Local anesthetics decrease the electrical excitability of the myocardium, decrease the conduction rate, and decrease the force of contraction.[46-48]

Therapeutic advantage is taken of this depressant action in managing the hyperexcitable myocardium, which manifests as various cardiac dysrhythmias. Although many local anesthetics have demonstrated antidysrhythmic actions in animals, only procaine and lidocaine have gained significant clinical reliability in humans. Lidocaine is the most widely used and intensively studied local anesthetic in this regard.[9,29,49,50] Procainamide is the procaine molecule with an amide linkage replacing the ester linkage. Because of this, it is hydrolyzed much more slowly than procaine.[51] Tocainide, a chemical analog of lidocaine, was introduced in 1984 as an oral antidysrhythmic drug, because lidocaine is ineffective after oral administration.[52] Tocainide also is effective in managing ventricular dysrhythmias but is associated with a 40% incidence of adverse effects, including nausea, vomiting, tremor, paresthesias, agranulocytosis, and pulmonary fibrosis.[53,54] Tocainide worsens symptoms of congestive heart failure in about 5% of patients and may provoke dysrhythmias (i.e., is prodysrhythmic) in 1% to 8%.[55]

Blood levels of lidocaine usually noted after intraoral injection of one or two dental cartridges, 0.5 to 2 μg/mL, are not associated with cardiodepressant activity. Increasing lidocaine blood levels slightly is nontoxic and is associated with antidysrhythmic actions. Therapeutic blood levels of lidocaine for antidysrhythmic activity range from 1.8 to 6 μg/mL.[48,56]

Lidocaine usually is administered intravenously in a bolus of 50 to 100 mg at a rate of 25 to 50 mg/min. This dose is based on 1 to 1.5 mg/kg of body weight every 3 to 5 minutes and is frequently followed by a continuous IV infusion of 1 to 4 mg/min. Signs and symptoms of local anesthetic overdose will be noted if the blood level rises beyond 6 μg/mL of blood.[56]

Lidocaine is used clinically primarily in the management of PVCs and ventricular tachycardia. It also is used as a (class-indeterminate) drug in advanced cardiovascular life support and in management of cardiac arrest caused by ventricular fibrillation.[57]

Direct cardiac actions of local anesthetics at blood levels greater than the therapeutic (antidysrhythmic) level include a decrease in myocardial contractility and decreased cardiac output, both of which lead to circulatory collapse (see Table 2-10).

Box 2-3 summarizes the CNS and cardiovascular effects of increasing local anesthetic blood levels.

Direct Action on the Peripheral Vasculature. Cocaine is the only local anesthetic drug that consistently produces vasoconstriction at commonly employed dosages.[4] Ropivacaine causes cutaneous vasoconstriction, whereas its congener bupivacaine produces vasodilation.[58] All other local anesthetics produce a peripheral vasodilation through relaxation of smooth muscle in the walls of blood vessels. This leads to increased blood flow to and from the site of local anesthetic deposition (see Table 2-1). Increased local blood flow increases the rate of drug absorption, in turn leading to decreased depth and duration of local anesthetic action, increased bleeding in the treatment area, and increased local anesthetic blood levels.

Table 2-11 provides examples of peak blood levels achieved after local anesthetic injection with and without the presence of a vasopressor.[58-60]

The primary effect of local anesthetics on blood pressure is hypotension. Procaine produces hypotension more frequently and significantly than does lidocaine: 50% of patients in one study receiving procaine became hypotensive, compared with 6% of those receiving lidocaine.[61] This action is produced by direct depression of the myocardium and smooth muscle relaxation in the vessel walls by the local anesthetic.

In summary, negative effects on the cardiovascular system are not noted until significantly elevated local anesthetic

BOX 2-3 Minimal to Moderate Overdose Levels

Signs
Talkativeness
Apprehension
Excitability
Slurred speech
Generalized stutter, leading to muscular twitching and tremor in the face and distal extremities
Euphoria
Dysarthria
Nystagmus
Sweating
Vomiting
Failure to follow commands or be reasoned with
Elevated blood pressure
Elevated heart rate
Elevated respiratory rate

Symptoms (progressive with increasing blood levels)
Lightheadedness and dizziness
Restlessness
Nervousness
Sensation of twitching before actual twitching is observed (see "Generalized stutter" under "SIGNS")
Metallic taste
Visual disturbances (inability to focus)
Auditory disturbances (tinnitus)
Drowsiness and disorientation
Loss of consciousness

Moderate to High Overdose Levels
Tonic–clonic seizure activity followed by
Generalized central nervous system depression
Depressed blood pressure, heart rate, and respiratory rate

From Malamed SF: Medical emergencies in the dental office, ed 6, St Louis, 2007, Mosby.

TABLE 2-11
Peak Plasma Levels Following Local Anesthetic Administration With and Without Vasopressor

Injection Site	Anesthetic	Dose, mg	Epinephrine Dilution	Peak Level, µg/mL
Infiltration	Lidocaine	400	None	2.0
Infiltration	Lidocaine	400	1:200,000	1.0
Intercostal	Lidocaine	400	None	6.5
Intercostal	Lidocaine	400	1:200,000	5.3
Intercostal	Lidocaine	400	1:80,000	4.9
Infiltration	Mepivacaine	5 mg/kg	None	1.2
Infiltration	Mepivacaine	5 mg/kg	1:200,000	0.7

Data from Kopacz DJ, Carpenter RL, Mackay DL: Effect of ropivacaine on cutaneous capillary flow in pigs, Anesthesiology 71:69, 1989; Scott DB, et al: Factors affecting plasma levels of lignocaine and prilocaine, Br J Anaesth 44:1040-1049, 1972; Duhner KG, et al: Blood levels of mepivacaine after regional anaesthesia, Br J Anaesth 37:746–752, 1965.

blood levels are reached. The usual sequence of local anesthetic–induced actions on the cardiovascular system is as follows:

1. At nonoverdose levels, a slight increase or no change in blood pressure occurs because of increased cardiac output and heart rate as a result of enhanced sympathetic activity; direct vasoconstriction of certain peripheral vascular beds is also noted.
2. At levels approaching yet still below overdose, a mild degree of hypotension is noted; this is produced by a direct relaxant action on the vascular smooth muscle.
3. At overdose levels, profound hypotension is caused by decreased myocardial contractility, cardiac output, and peripheral resistance.
4. At lethal levels, cardiovascular collapse is noted. This is caused by massive peripheral vasodilation and decreased myocardial contractility and heart rate (sinus bradycardia).
5. Certain local anesthetics such as bupivacaine (and to a lesser degree ropivacaine and etidocaine) may precipitate potentially fatal ventricular fibrillation.[62,63]

Local Tissue Toxicity

Skeletal muscle appears to be more sensitive than other tissues to the local irritant properties of local anesthetics. Intramuscular and intraoral injection of articaine, lidocaine, mepivacaine, prilocaine, bupivacaine, and etidocaine can produce skeletal muscle alterations.[64-67] It appears that longer-acting local anesthetics cause more localized skeletal muscle damage than shorter-acting drugs. The changes that occur in skeletal muscle are reversible, with muscle regeneration being complete within 2 weeks after local anesthetic administration. These muscle changes have not been associated with any overt clinical signs of local irritation.

Respiratory System

Local anesthetics exert a dual effect on respiration. At nonoverdose levels, they have a direct relaxant action on bronchial smooth muscle, whereas at overdose levels, they may produce respiratory arrest as a result of generalized CNS depression. In general, respiratory function is unaffected by local anesthetics until near-overdose levels are achieved.

Miscellaneous Actions

Neuromuscular Blockade. Many local anesthetics have been demonstrated to block neuromuscular transmission in humans. This is a result of the inhibition of sodium diffusion through a blockade of sodium channels in the cell membrane. This action normally is slight and usually is clinically insignificant. On occasion, however, it can be additive to that produced by both depolarizing (e.g., succinylcholine) and nondepolarizing (e.g., atracurium, vecuronium) muscle relaxants; this may lead to abnormally prolonged periods of muscle paralysis. Such actions are unlikely to occur in the dental outpatient.

Drug Interactions. In general, CNS depressants (e.g., opioids, antianxiety drugs, phenothiazines, barbiturates), when administered in conjunction with local anesthetics, lead to potentiation of the CNS-depressant actions of the local anesthetic. The conjoint use of local anesthetics and drugs that share a common metabolic pathway can produce adverse reactions. Both ester local anesthetics and the depolarizing muscle relaxant succinylcholine require plasma pseudocholinesterase for hydrolysis. Prolonged apnea may result from concomitant use of these drugs.

Drugs that induce the production of hepatic microsomal enzymes (e.g., barbiturates) may alter the rate at which amide local anesthetics are metabolized. Increased hepatic microsomal enzyme induction increases the rate of metabolism of the local anesthetic.

Specific drug–drug interactions related to the administration of local anesthetics are reviewed in Chapter 10.

Malignant Hyperthermia. Malignant hyperthermia (MH; hyperpyrexia) is a pharmacogenic disorder in which a genetic variant in an individual alters that person's response to certain drugs. Acute clinical manifestations of MH include tachycardia, tachypnea, unstable blood pressure, cyanosis, respiratory and metabolic acidosis, fever (as high as 42° C [108° F] or more), muscle rigidity, and death. Mortality ranges from 63% to 73%. Many commonly used anesthetic drugs can trigger MH in certain individuals.

Until recently, the amide local anesthetics were thought to be capable of provoking MH and were considered to be absolutely contraindicated in MH-susceptible patients.[68] The Malignant Hyperthermia Association of the United States (MHAUS), after evaluating recent clinical research, concluded that in fact no documented cases in the medical or dental literature (over the past 30 years) support the concept of amide anesthetics triggering malignant hyperthermia.[69-73]

MHAUS maintains a Website with information for both health care providers and patients: www.mhaus.org.

References

1. Aps C, Reynolds F: The effect of concentration in vasoactivity of bupivacaine and lignocaine, Br J Anaesth 48:1171–1174, 1976.
2. Covino BG: Pharmacology of local anaesthetic agents, Br J Anaesth 58:701–716, 1986.
3. U.S. Food and Drug Administration: Center for Drug Evaluation and Research: Approval letter for phentolamine mesylate, 1998. Available at: www.fda.gov/cder/foi/anda/98/40235ap.pdf. Accessed November 6, 2007.
4. Benowitz NL: Clinical pharmacology and toxicology of cocaine, Pharmacol Toxicol 72:1–12, 1993.
5. Arthur GR: Pharmacokinetics of local anesthetics. In Strichartz GR, editor: Local anesthetics: handbook of experimental pharmacology, vol 81, Berlin, 1987, Springer-Verlag.
6. Hohnloser SH, Lange HW, Raeder E, et al: Short- and long-term therapy with tocainide for malignant ventricular tachyarrhythmias, Circulation 73:143–149, 1986.
7. Soliman IE, Broadman LM, Hannallah RS, McGill WA: Comparison of the analgesic effects of EMLA (eutectic mixture of local anesthetics) to intradermal lidocaine infiltration prior to venous cannulation in unpremedicated children, Anesthesiology 68:804–806, 1988.
8. American Heart Association: ACLS provider manual, Dallas, Tex, 2001, American Heart Association, pp 83–84.
9. Haugh KH: Antidysrhythmic agents at the turn of the twenty-first century: a current review, Crit Care Nursing Clin North Am 14:13–69, 2002.
10. Kalow W: Hydrolysis of local anesthetics by human serum cholinesterase, J Pharmacol Exp Ther 104:122–134, 1952.
11. Watson CB: Respiratory complications associated with anesthesia, Anesth Clin North Am 20:375–399, 2002.
12. Harris WH, Cole DW, Mital M, Laver MB: Methemoglobin formation and oxygen transport following intravenous regional anesthesia using prilocaine, Anesthesiology 29:65, 1968.
13. Arthur GR: Distribution and elimination of local anesthetic agents: the role of the lung, liver, and kidneys, PhD thesis, Edinburgh, 1981, University of Edinburgh.
14. Oertel R, Berndt A, Kirch W: Saturable in vitro metabolism of articaine by serum esterases: does it contribute to the resistance of the local anesthetic effect? Reg Anesth 21:576–581, 1996.
15. Nation RL, Triggs EJ: Lidocaine kinetics in cardiac patients and aged subjects, Br J Clin Pharmacol 4:439–448, 1977.
16. Thomson PD, Melmon KL, Richardson JA, et al: Lidocaine pharmacokinetics in advanced heart failure, liver disease, and renal failure in humans, Ann Intern Med 78:499–508, 1973.
17. Oertel R, Rahn R, Kirch W: Clinical pharmacokinetics of articaine, Clin Pharmacokinet 33:617–625, 1997.
18. Prilocaine-induced methemoglobinemia—Wisconsin, 1993, MMWR Morb Mortal Wkly Rep 43:3555–3557, 1994.

19. Wilburn-Goo D, Lloyd LM: When patients become cyanotic: acquired methemoglobinemia, J Am Dent Assoc 130:626–631, 1999.
20. Strong JM, Parker M, Atkinson AJ Jr: Identification of glycinexylidide in patients treated with intravenous lidocaine, Clin Pharmacol Ther 14:67–72, 1973.
21. Gupta PP, Tangri AN, Saxena RC, Dhawan BN: Clinical pharmacology studies on 4-N-butylamino-1,2,3,4,-tetrahydroacridine hydrochloride (Centbucridine), a new local anaesthetic agent, Indian J Exp Biol 20:344–346, 1982.
22. Vacharajani GN, Parikh N, Paul T, Satoskar RS: A comparative study of Centbucridine and lidocaine in dental extraction, Int J Clin Pharmacol Res 3:251–255, 1983.
23. Bernhard CG, Bohm E: Local anaesthetics as anticonvulsants: a study on experimental and clinical epilepsy, Stockholm, 1965, Almqvist & Wiksell.
24. Bernhard CG, Bohm E, Wiesel T: On the evaluation of the anticonvulsive effect of different local anesthetics, Arch Int Pharmacodyn Ther 108:392–407, 1956.
25. Julien RM: Lidocaine in experimental epilepsy: correlation of anticonvulsant effect with blood concentrations, Electroencephalogr Clin Neurophysiol 34:639–645, 1973.
26. Berry CA, Sanner JH, Keasling HH: A comparison of the anticonvulsant activity of mepivacaine and lidocaine, J Pharmacol Exp Ther 133:357–363, 1961.
27. Walker IA, Slovis CM: Lidocaine in the treatment of status epilepticus, Acad Emerg Med 4:918–922, 1997.
28. Chen AH: Toxicity and allergy to local anesthesia, J Calif Dent Assoc 26:983–992, 1998.
29. Katz J, Feldman MA, Bass EB, et al: Injectable versus topical anesthesia for cataract surgery: patient perceptions of pain and side effects: the Study of Medical Testing for Cataract Surgery Study Team, Ophthalmology 107:2054–2060, 2000.
30. Bureau of Medicine and Surgery. Available at: http://navymedicine.med.navy.mil/. Accessed October 28, 2011.
31. Englesson S: The influence of acid-base changes on central nervous system toxicity of local anesthetic agents. I. An experimental study in cats, Acta Anaesthesiol Scand 18:79, 1974.
32. Englesson S, Grevsten S, Olin A: Some numerical methods of estimating acid-base variables in normal human blood with a haemoglobin concentration of 5 g-100 cm^3, Scand J Lab Clin Invest 32:289–295, 1973.
33. de Jong RH, Robles R, Corbin RW: Central actions of lidocaine-synaptic transmission, Anesthesiology 30:19, 1969.
34. Huffman RD, Yim GKW: Effects of diphenylaminoethanol and lidocaine on central inhibition, Int J Neuropharmacol 8:217, 1969.
35. Tanaka K, Yamasaki M: Blocking of cortical inhibitory synapses by intravenous lidocaine, Nature 209:207, 1966.
36. de Jong RH: Local anesthetics, St Louis, 1994, Mosby.
37. Graubard DJ, Peterson MC: Clinical uses of intravenous procaine, Springfield, Ill, 1950, Charles C Thomas.
38. Garcilasso de la Vega: Commentarios reales de los Incas (1609–1617). In Freud S, editor: Uber coca, Wien, 1884, Verlag von Moritz Perles.
39. Disertacion sobre el aspecto, cultivo, comercio y virtudes de la famosa planta del Peru nombrado coca: Lima, 1794. In Freud S, editor: Uber coca, Wien, 1884, Verlag von Moritz Perles.
40. Olch PD, William S: Halsted and local anesthesia: contributions and complications, Anesthesiology 42:479–486, 1975.
41. Preboth M: Cocaine abuse among athletes, Am Fam Physician 62:1850–2000, 1915.
42. Harriston K, Jenkins S: Maryland basketball star Len Bias is dead at 22. Washington Post, 20 June 1986.
43. de Jong RH: Local anesthetics, ed 2, Springfield, Ill, 1977, Charles C Thomas, p 89.
44. Scott DB: Toxicity caused by local anaesthetic drugs, Br J Anaesth 53:553–554, 1981.
45. Pinter A, Dorian P: Intravenous antiarrhythmic agents, Curr Opin Cardiol 16:17–22, 2001.
46. Sugi K: Pharmacological restoration and maintenance of sinus rhythm by antiarrhythmic agents, J Cardiol 33(Suppl 1):59–64, 1999.
47. Alexander JH, Granger CB, Sadowski Z, et al: Prophylactic lidocaine use in acute myocardial infarction: incidence and outcomes from two international trials. The GUSTO-I and GUSTO-IIb Investigators, Am Heart J 137:599–805, 1999.
48. Cannom DS, Prystowsky EN: Management of ventricular arrhythmias: detection, drugs, and devices, JAMA 281:272–279, 1999.
49. Tan HL, Lie KI: Prophylactic lidocaine use in acute myocardial infarction revisited in the thrombolytic era, Am Heart J 137:570–573, 1999.
50. Kowey PR: An overview of antiarrhythmic drug management of electrical storm, Can J Cardiol 12(Suppl B):3B–8B; discussion 27B–28B, 1996.
51. Slavik RS, Tisdale JE, Borzak S: Pharmacologic conversion of atrial fibrillation: a systematic review of available evidence, Prog Cardiovasc Dis 44:221–252, 2001.
52. Lalka D, Meyer MB, Duce BR, Elvin AT: Kinetics of the oral antiarrhythmic lidocaine congener, tocainide, Clin Pharmacol Ther 19:757–766, 1976.
53. Perlow GM, Jain BP, Pauker SC, et al: Tocainide-associated interstitial pneumonitis, Ann Intern Med 94(4 Pt 1):489–490, 1981.
54. Volosin K, Greenberg RM, Greenspon AJ: Tocainide associated agranulocytosis, Am Heart J 109:1392, 1985.
55. Bronheim D, Thys DM: Cardiovascular drugs. In Longnecker DE, Tinker JH, Morgan GE Jr, editors: Principles and practice of anesthesiology, ed 2, St Louis, 1998, Mosby.
56. Kudenchuk PJ: Advanced cardiac life support antiarrhythmic drugs, Cardiol Clin 20:19–87, 2002.
57. American Heart Association: Guidelines 2000 for cardiopulmonary resuscitation and emergency cardiovascular care, Circulation 102:8–149, 2000.
58. Kopacz DJ, Carpenter RL, MacKay DL: Effect of ropivacaine on cutaneous capillary flow in pigs, Anesthesiology 71:69, 1989.
59. Scott DB, Jebson PJR, Braid DP, et al: Factors affecting plasma levels of lignocaine and prilocaine, Br J Anaesth 44:1040–1049, 1972.
60. Duhner KG, Harthon JGL, Hebring BG, Lie T: Blood levels of mepivacaine after regional anaesthesia, Br J Anaesth 37:746–752, 1965.
61. Kimmey JR, Steinhaus JE: Cardiovascular effects of procaine and lidocaine (Xylocaine) during general anesthesia, Acta Anaesthesiol Scand 3:9–15, 1959.
62. de Jong RH, Ronfeld R, DeRosa R: Cardiovascular effects of convulsant and supraconvulsant doses of amide local anesthetics, Anesth Analg 61:3, 1982.
63. Feldman HS, Arthur GR, Covino BG: Comparative systemic toxicity of convulsant and supraconvulsant doses of intravenous ropivacaine, bupivacaine and lidocaine in the conscious dog, Anesth Analg 69:794, 1989.

64. Zink W, Graf BM, Sinner B, et al: Differential effects of bupivacaine on intracellular Ca^{2+} regulation: potential mechanisms of its myotoxicity, Anesthesiology 97:710–716, 2002.
65. Irwin W, Fontaine E, Agnolucci L, et al: Bupivacaine myotoxicity is mediated by mitochondria, J Biol Chem 277:12221–12227, 2002.
66. Benoit PW, Yagiela JA, Fort NF: Pharmacologic correlation between local anesthetic-induced myotoxicity and disturbances of intracellular calcium distribution, Toxicol Appl Pharmacol 52:187–198, 1980.
67. Hinton RJ, Dechow PC, Carlson DS: Recovery of jaw muscle function following injection of a myotoxic agent (lidocaine-epinephrine), Oral Surg Oral Med Oral Pathol 59:247–251, 1986.
68. Denborough MA, Forster JF, Lovell RR, et al: Anaesthetic deaths in a family, Br J Anaesth 34:395–396, 1962.
69. Gielen M, Viering W: 3-in-1 lumbar plexus block for muscle biopsy in malignant hyperthermia patients: amide local anaesthetics may be used safely, Acta Anaesthesiol Scand 30:581–583, 1986.
70. Ording H: Incidence of malignant hyperthermia in Denmark, Anesth Analg 64:700–704, 1985.
71. Paasuke PT, Brownell AKW: Amine local anaesthetics and malignant hyperthermia (editorial), Can Anaesth Soc J 33:126–129, 1986.
72. Jastak JT, Yagiela JA, Donaldson D: Local anesthesia of the oral cavity, Philadelphia, 1995, WB Saunders, pp 141–142.
73. Malignant Hyperthermia Association of the United States. Available at: www.mhaus.org. Accessed October 28, 2011.

CHAPTER 3

Pharmacology of Vasoconstrictors

All clinically effective injectable local anesthetics are vasodilators, the degree of vasodilation varying from significant (procaine) to minimal (prilocaine, mepivacaine) and also possibly with both the injection site and individual patient response. After local anesthetic injection into tissues, blood vessels (arterioles and capillaries primarily) in the area dilate, resulting in increased perfusion at the site, leading to the following reactions:

1. An increased rate of absorption of the local anesthetic into the cardiovascular system, which in turn removes it from the injection site (redistribution)
2. Higher plasma levels of the local anesthetic, with an attendant increase in the risk of local anesthetic toxicity (overdose)
3. Decrease in both the depth and duration of anesthesia because the local anesthetic diffuses away from the injection site more rapidly
4. Increased bleeding at the site of treatment as a result of increased perfusion

Vasoconstrictors are drugs that constrict blood vessels and thereby control tissue perfusion. They are added to local anesthetic solutions to oppose the inherent vasodilatory actions of the local anesthetics. Vasoconstrictors are important additions to a local anesthetic solution for the following reasons:

1. By constricting blood vessels, vasoconstrictors decrease blood flow (perfusion) to the site of drug administration.
2. Absorption of the local anesthetic into the cardiovascular system is slowed, resulting in lower anesthetic blood levels.[1,2] Table 3-1 illustrates levels of local anesthetic in the blood with and without a vasoconstrictor.[1]
3. Local anesthetic blood levels are lowered, thereby decreasing the risk of local anesthetic toxicity.
4. More local anesthetic enters into the nerve, where it remains for longer periods, thereby increasing (in some cases significantly,[3] in others minimally[4]) the duration of action of most local anesthetics.
5. Vasoconstrictors decrease bleeding at the site of administration; therefore they are useful when increased bleeding is anticipated (e.g., during a surgical procedure).[5,6]

The vasoconstrictors commonly used in conjunction with injected local anesthetics are chemically identical or similar to the sympathetic nervous system mediators epinephrine and norepinephrine. The actions of the vasoconstrictors so resemble the response of adrenergic nerves to stimulation that they are classified as sympathomimetic, or adrenergic, drugs. These drugs have many clinical actions besides vasoconstriction.

Sympathomimetic drugs also may be classified according to their chemical structure and mode of action.

CHEMICAL STRUCTURE

Classification of sympathomimetic drugs by chemical structure is related to the presence or absence of a catechol nucleus. Catechol is orthodihydroxybenzene. Sympathomimetic drugs that have hydroxyl (OH) substitutions in the third and fourth positions of the aromatic ring are termed *catechols.*

HO–(ring)(HO)–CH(OH)–CH(①)–NH(②)

	①	②
Epinephrine	H	CH_3
Levonordefrin	CH_3	H
Norepinephrine	H	H

If they also contain an amine group (NH_2) attached to the aliphatic side chain, they are then called *catecholamines.* Epinephrine, norepinephrine, and dopamine are the naturally occurring catecholamines of the sympathetic nervous system. Isoproterenol and levonordefrin are synthetic catecholamines.

TABLE 3-1
Effects of Vasoconstrictor (Epinephrine 1:200,000) on Peak Local Anesthetic Levels in Blood

		PEAK LEVEL, μg/mL	
Local Anesthetic	Dose, mg	Without Vasoconstrictor	With Vasoconstrictor
Mepivacaine	500	4.7	3
Lidocaine	400	4.3	3
Prilocaine	400	2.8	2.6
Etidocaine	300	1.4	1.3

Data from Cannall H, Walters H, Beckett AH, Saunders A: Circulating blood levels of lignocaine after peri-oral injections, Br Dent J 138:87–93, 1975.

BOX 3-1 Categories of Sympathomimetic Amines

Direct-Acting	Indirect-Acting	Mixed-Acting
Epinephrine	Tyramine	Metaraminol
Norepinephrine	Amphetamine	Ephedrine
Levonordefrin	Methamphetamine	
Isoproterenol	Hydroxyamphetamine	
Dopamine		
Methoxamine		
Phenylephrine		

Vasoconstrictors that do not possess OH groups in the third and fourth positions of the aromatic molecule are not catechols but are amines because they have an NH_2 group attached to the aliphatic side chain.

Catecholamines	Noncatecholamines
Epinephrine	Amphetamine
Norepinephrine	Methamphetamine
Levonordefrin	Ephedrine
Isoproterenol	Mephentermine
Dopamine	Hydroxyamphetamine
	Metaraminol
	Methoxamine
	Phenylephrine

Felypressin, a synthetic analog of the polypeptide vasopressin (antidiuretic hormone), is available in many countries as a vasoconstrictor. As of the time of this writing (November 2011), felypressin is not available in the United States.

MODES OF ACTION

Three categories of sympathomimetic amines are known: direct-acting drugs, which exert their action directly on adrenergic receptors; indirect-acting drugs, which act by releasing norepinephrine from adrenergic nerve terminals; and mixed-acting drugs, with both direct and indirect actions (Box 3-1).[1-3]

Adrenergic Receptors

Adrenergic receptors are found in most tissues of the body. The concept of adrenergic receptors was proposed by Ahlquist in 1948 and is well accepted today.[7] Ahlquist recognized two types of adrenergic receptor, termed alpha (α) and beta (β), based on inhibitory or excitatory actions of catecholamines on smooth muscle.

Activation of α receptors by a sympathomimetic drug usually produces a response that includes contraction of smooth muscle in blood vessels (vasoconstriction). Based on differences in their function and location, α receptors have since been subcategorized. Whereas α_1 receptors are excitatory-postsynaptic, α_2 receptors are inhibitory-postsynaptic.[8]

Activation of β receptors produces smooth muscle relaxation (vasodilation and bronchodilation) and cardiac stimulation (increased heart rate and strength of contraction).

Beta receptors are further divided into β_1, and β_2:β_1 are found in the heart and small intestines and are responsible for cardiac stimulation and lipolysis; β_2, found in the bronchi, vascular beds, and uterus, produce bronchodilation and vasodilation.[9]

Table 3-2 illustrates the differences in varying degrees of α and β receptor activity of three commonly used vasoconstrictors.

Table 3-3 lists the systemic effects, based on α and β receptor activity, of epinephrine and norepinephrine.

TABLE 3-2
Adrenergic Receptor Activity of Vasoconstrictors

Drug	α_1	α_2	β_1	β_2
Epinephrine	+++	+++	+++	+++
Norepinephrine	++	++	++	+
Levonordefrin	+	++	++	+

Relative potency of drugs is indicated as follows: +++, high, ++, intermediate, and +, low.
From Jastak JT, Yagiela JA, Donaldson D: Local anesthesia of the oral cavity, Philadelphia, 1995, WB Saunders.

Release of Catecholamines

Other sympathomimetic drugs, such as tyramine and amphetamine, act indirectly by causing the release of the catecholamine norepinephrine from storage sites in adrenergic nerve terminals. In addition, these drugs may exert direct action on α and β receptors.

The clinical actions of this group of drugs therefore are quite similar to the actions of norepinephrine. Successively repeated doses of these drugs will prove to be less effective than those given previously because of depletion of norepinephrine from storage sites. This phenomenon is termed *tachyphylaxis* and is not seen with drugs that act directly on adrenergic receptors.

DILUTIONS OF VASOCONSTRICTORS

The dilution of vasoconstrictors is commonly referred to as a *ratio* (e.g., 1 to 1000 [written 1:1000]). Because maximum doses of vasoconstrictors are presented in milligrams, or more commonly today as micrograms (μg), the following interpretations should enable the reader to convert these terms readily:

- A concentration of 1:1000 means that 1 g (1000 mg) of solute (drug) is contained in 1000 mL of solution.
- Therefore, a 1:1000 dilution contains 1000 mg in 1000 mL or 1.0 mg/mL of solution (1000 μg/mL).

Vasoconstrictors, as used in dental local anesthetic solutions, are much less concentrated than the 1:1000 dilution described in the preceding paragraph. To produce these more dilute, clinically safer, yet effective concentrations, the 1:1000 dilution must be diluted further. This process is described here:

- To produce a 1:10,000 concentration, 1 mL of a 1:1000 solution is added to 9 mL of solvent (e.g., sterile water); therefore 1:10,000 = 0.1 mg/mL (100 μg/mL).
- To produce a 1:100,000 concentration, 1 mL of a 1:10,000 concentration is added to 9 mL of solvent; therefore 1:100,000 = 0.01 mg/mL (10 μg/mL).

The milligram per milliliter and μg per milliliter values of the various vasoconstrictor dilutions used in medicine and dentistry are shown in Table 3-4.

The genesis of vasoconstrictor dilutions in local anesthetics began with the discovery of adrenalin in 1897 by Abel. In 1903, Braun suggested using adrenalin as a chemical tourniquet to prolong the duration of local anesthetics.[10] Braun recommended the use of a 1:10,000 dilution of epinephrine, ranging to as dilute as 1:100,000, with cocaine in nasal surgery (a highly vascular area). It appears at present that an epinephrine concentration of 1:200,000 provides comparable results, with fewer systemic side effects. The 1:200,000 dilution, which contains 5 μg/mL (or 0.005 mg/mL), has become widely used in both medicine and dentistry and is currently found in articaine, prilocaine, lidocaine (though not in North America), etidocaine, and bupivacaine. In several European and Asian countries, lidocaine with epinephrine concentrations of 1:300,000 and 1:400,000 is available in dental cartridges.

Although it is the most used vasoconstrictor in local anesthetics in both medicine and dentistry, epinephrine is *not* an

TABLE 3-3
Systemic Effects of Sympathomimetic Amines

Effector Organ or Function	Epinephrine	Norepinephrine
Cardiovascular System		
Heart rate	+	–
Stroke volume	++	++
Cardiac output	+++	0, –
Arrhythmias	++++	++++
Coronary blood flow	++	++
Blood Pressure		
Systolic arterial	+++	+++
Mean arterial	+	++
Diastolic arterial	+, 0, –	++
Peripheral Circulation		
Total peripheral resistance	–	++
Cerebral blood flow	+	0, –
Cutaneous blood flow	–	–
Splanchnic blood flow	+++	0, +
Respiratory System		
Bronchodilation	+++	0
Genitourinary System		
Renal blood flow	–	–
Skeletal Muscle		
Muscle blood flow	+++	0, –
Metabolic Effects		
Oxygen consumption	++	0, +
Blood glucose	+++	0, +
Blood lactic acid	+++	0, +

Data from Goldenberg M, Aranow H Jr, Smith AA, Faber M: Pheochromocytoma and essential hypertensive vascular disease, Arch Intern Med 86:823–836, 1950.

+, Increase; –, decrease; *0*, no effect.

TABLE 3-4
Concentrations of Clinically Used Vasoconstrictors

Concentration (Dilution)	Milligrams per Milliliter (mg/mL)	Micrograms per Milliliter (μg/mL)	μg per Cartridge (1.8 mL)	Therapeutic Use
1:1000	1.0	1000		Epinephrine—Emergency medicine (IM/SC anaphylaxis)
1:2500	0.4	400		Phenylephrine
1:10,000	0.1	100		Epinephrine—Emergency medicine (IV/ET cardiac arrest)
1:20,000	0.05	50	90	Levonordefrin—Local anesthetic
1:30,000	0.033	33.3	73 (2.2-mL cartridge)	Norepinephrine—Local anesthetic
1:50,000	0.02	20	36	Epinephrine—Local anesthetic
1:80,000	0.0125	12.5	27.5 (2.2-mL cartridge)	Epinephrine—Local anesthetic (United Kingdom)
1:100,000	0.01	10	18	Epinephrine—Local anesthetic
1:200,000	0.005	5	9	Epinephrine—Local anesthetic
1:400,000	0.0025	2.5	4.5	Epinephrine—Local anesthetic

ideal drug. The benefits to be gained from adding epinephrine (or any vasoconstrictor, for that matter) to a local anesthetic solution must be weighed against any risks that might be present. Epinephrine is absorbed from the site of injection, just as is the local anesthetic. Measurable epinephrine blood levels are obtained, and these influence the heart and blood vessels. Resting plasma epinephrine levels (39 pg/mL) are doubled after administration of one cartridge of lidocaine with 1 : 100,000 epinephrine.[11] Elevation of epinephrine plasma levels is linearly dose dependent and persists from several minutes to a half-hour.[12] Contrary to a previously held position that intraoral administration of usual volumes of epinephrine produced no cardiovascular response, and that patients were more at risk from endogenously released epinephrine than they were from exogenously administered epinephrine,[13,14] recent evidence demonstrates that epinephrine plasma levels equivalent to those achieved during moderate to heavy exercise may occur after intraoral injection.[15,16] These are associated with moderate increases in cardiac output and stroke volume (see the following section). Blood pressure and heart rate, however, are minimally affected at these dosages.[17]

In patients with preexisting cardiovascular or thyroid disease, the side effects of absorbed epinephrine must be weighed against those of elevated local anesthetic blood levels. It is currently thought that the cardiovascular effects of conventional epinephrine doses are of little practical concern, even in patients with heart disease.[12] However, even following usual precautions (e.g., aspiration, slow injection), sufficient epinephrine can be absorbed to cause sympathomimetic reactions such as apprehension, tachycardia, sweating, and pounding in the chest (palpitation)—the so-called epinephrine reaction.[18]

Intravascular administration of vasoconstrictors and their administration to sensitive individuals (hyperresponders), or the occurrence of unanticipated drug–drug interactions, can however produce significant clinical manifestations. Intravenous administration of 0.015 mg of epinephrine with lidocaine results in an increase in the heart rate ranging from 25 to 70 beats per minute, with elevations in systolic blood from 20 to 70 mm Hg.[12,19,20] Occasional rhythm disturbances may be observed, and premature ventricular contractions (PVCs) are most often noted.

Other vasoconstrictors used in medicine and dentistry include norepinephrine, phenylephrine, levonordefrin, and felypressin. Norepinephrine, lacking significant β_2 actions, produces intense peripheral vasoconstriction with possible dramatic elevation of blood pressure, and is associated with a side effect ratio nine times higher than that of epinephrine.[21] Although it is currently available in some countries in local anesthetic solutions, the use of norepinephrine as a vasopressor in dentistry is diminishing and cannot be recommended. The use of a mixture of epinephrine and norepinephrine is to be absolutely avoided.[22] Phenylephrine, a pure α-adrenergic agonist, theoretically possesses advantages over other vasoconstrictors. However, in clinical trials, peak blood levels of lidocaine were actually higher with phenylephrine 1 : 20,000 (lidocaine blood level = 2.4 μg/mL) than with epinephrine 1 : 200,000 (1.4 μg/mL).[23] The cardiovascular effects of levonordefrin most closely resemble those of norepinephrine.[24] Felypressin was shown to be about as effective as epinephrine in reducing cutaneous blood flow.[5]

Epinephrine remains the most effective and the most used vasoconstrictor in medicine and dentistry.

PHARMACOLOGY OF SPECIFIC AGENTS

The pharmacologic properties of the sympathomimetic amines commonly used as vasoconstrictors in local anesthetics are reviewed. Epinephrine is the most useful and represents the best example of a drug mimicking the activity of sympathetic discharge. Its clinical actions are reviewed in depth. The actions of other drugs are compared with those of epinephrine.

Epinephrine

Proprietary Name. Adrenalin.

Chemical Structure. Epinephrine as the acid salt is highly soluble in water. Slightly acid solutions are relatively stable if they are protected from air. Deterioration (through oxidation) is hastened by heat and the presence of heavy metal ions. Sodium bisulfite is commonly added to epinephrine solutions to delay this deterioration. The shelf life of a local anesthetic cartridge containing a vasoconstrictor is somewhat shorter (18 months) than that of a cartridge containing no vasoconstrictor (36 months).

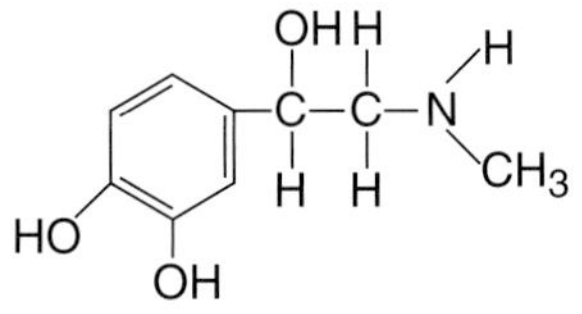

Source. Epinephrine is available as a synthetic and is also obtained from the adrenal medulla of animals (epinephrine constitutes approximately 80% of adrenal medullary secretions). It exists in both levorotatory and dextrorotatory forms; the levorotatory form is approximately 15 times as potent as the dextrorotatory form.

Mode of Action. Epinephrine acts directly on both α- and β-adrenergic receptors; β effects predominate.

Systemic Actions

Myocardium. Epinephrine stimulates β_1 receptors of the myocardium. There is a positive inotropic (force of contraction) and a positive chronotropic (rate of contraction) effect. Both cardiac output and heart rate are increased.

Pacemaker Cells. Epinephrine stimulates β_1 receptors and increases the irritability of pacemaker cells, leading to an increased incidence of dysrhythmias. Ventricular tachycardia (VT) and premature ventricular contractions (PVCs) are common.

Coronary Arteries. Epinephrine produces dilation of the coronary arteries, increasing coronary artery blood flow.

Blood Pressure. Systolic blood pressure is increased. Diastolic pressure is decreased when small doses are administered because of the greater sensitivity to epinephrine of β_2 receptors compared with α receptors in vessels supplying the skeletal muscles. Diastolic pressure is increased with larger epinephrine doses because of constriction of blood vessels supplying the skeletal muscles caused by α receptor stimulation.

Cardiovascular Dynamics. The overall action of epinephrine on the heart and cardiovascular system is direct stimulation:

- Increased systolic and diastolic pressures
- Increased cardiac output
- Increased stroke volume
- Increased heart rate
- Increased strength of contraction
- Increased myocardial oxygen consumption

These actions lead to an overall *decrease* in cardiac efficiency.

The cardiovascular responses of increased systolic blood pressure and increased heart rate develop with the administration of one to two dental cartridges of a 1:100,000 epinephrine dilution.[25] Administration of four cartridges of 1:100,000 epinephrine will bring about a slight decrease in diastolic blood pressure.

Vasculature. The primary action of epinephrine is on smaller arterioles and precapillary sphincters. Blood vessels supplying the skin, mucous membranes, and kidneys primarily contain α receptors. Epinephrine produces constriction in these vessels. Vessels supplying the skeletal muscles contain both α and β_2 receptors, with β_2 predominating. Small doses of epinephrine produce dilation of these vessels as a result of β_2 actions. β_2 receptors are more sensitive to epinephrine than are α receptors. Larger doses produce vasoconstriction because α receptors are stimulated.

Hemostasis. Clinically, epinephrine is used frequently as a vasoconstrictor for hemostasis during surgical procedures. Injection of epinephrine directly into surgical sites rapidly produces high tissue concentrations, predominant α receptor stimulation, and hemostasis. As epinephrine tissue levels decrease over time, its primary action on blood vessels reverts to vasodilation because β_2 actions predominate; therefore it is common for some bleeding to be noted at about 6 hours after a surgical procedure. In a clinical trial involving extraction of third molars, postsurgical bleeding occurred in 13 of 16 patients receiving epinephrine with their local anesthetic for hemostasis, whereas 0 of 16 patients receiving local anesthetic without vasoconstrictor (mepivacaine plain) had bleeding 6 hours post surgery.[26] Additional findings of increased postsurgical pain and delayed wound healing were noted in the epinephrine-receiving group.[26]

Respiratory System. Epinephrine is a potent dilator (β_2 effect) of bronchiole smooth muscle. It is an important drug for management of more refractory episodes of bronchospasm (e.g., status asthmaticus).

Central Nervous System. In usual therapeutic dosages, epinephrine is not a potent central nervous system (CNS) stimulant. Its CNS-stimulating actions become prominent when an excessive dose is administered.

Metabolism. Epinephrine increases oxygen consumption in all tissues. Through β action, it stimulates glycogenolysis in the liver and skeletal muscle, elevating blood sugar levels at plasma epinephrine concentrations of 150 to 200 pg/mL.[25] The equivalent of four dental local anesthetic cartridges of 1:100,000 epinephrine must be administered to elicit this response.[27]

Termination of Action and Elimination. The action of epinephrine is terminated primarily by its reuptake by adrenergic nerves. Epinephrine that escapes reuptake is rapidly inactivated in the blood by the enzymes catechol-*O*-methyltransferase (COMT) and monoamine oxidase (MAO), both of which are present in the liver.[28] Only small amounts (approximately 1%) of epinephrine are excreted unchanged in the urine.

Side Effects and Overdose. The clinical manifestations of epinephrine overdose relate to CNS stimulation and include increasing fear and anxiety, tension, restlessness, throbbing headache, tremor, weakness, dizziness, pallor, respiratory difficulty, and palpitation.

With increasing levels of epinephrine in the blood, cardiac dysrhythmias (especially ventricular) become more common; ventricular fibrillation is a rare but possible consequence. Dramatic increases in both systolic (>300 mm Hg) and diastolic (>200 mm Hg) pressures may be noted and have led to cerebral hemorrhage.[29] Anginal episodes may be precipitated in patients with coronary artery insufficiency. Because of the rapid inactivation of epinephrine, the stimulatory phase of the overdose (toxic) reaction usually is brief. Vasoconstrictor overdose is discussed in greater depth in Chapter 18.

Clinical Applications

- Management of acute allergic reactions
- Management of refractory bronchospasm (status asthmaticus)
- Management of cardiac arrest
- As a vasoconstrictor, for hemostasis
- As a vasoconstrictor in local anesthetics, to decrease absorption into the cardiovascular system
- As a vasoconstrictor in local anesthetics, to increase depth of anesthesia
- As a vasoconstrictor in local anesthetics, to increase duration of anesthesia
- To produce mydriasis

Availability in Dentistry. Epinephrine is the most potent and widely used vasoconstrictor in dentistry. It is available in the following dilutions and drugs:

Epinephrine Dilution	Local Anesthetic (generic)
1:50,000	Lidocaine
1:80,000	Lidocaine (lignocaine) (United Kingdom)
1:100,000	Articaine Lidocaine
1:200,000	Articaine Bupivacaine Etidocaine† Lidocaine Mepivacaine* Prilocaine
1:300,000	Lidocaine*
1:400,000	Articaine*

*Not available in the United States (August 2011).
†No longer marketed in the United State (2002).

Maximum Doses. The least concentrated solution that produces effective pain control should be used. Lidocaine is available with two dilutions of epinephrine—1:50,000 and 1:100,000—in the United States and Canada, and with 1:80,000, 1:200,000, and 1:300,000 dilutions in other countries. The duration of effective pulpal and soft tissue anesthesia is equivalent with all forms. Therefore it is recommended (in North America) that the 1:100,000 epinephrine concentration be used with lidocaine when extended pain control is necessary. Where 1:200,000 or 1:300,000 epinephrine is available with lidocaine, these concentrations are preferred for pain control.[30]

The dosages in Table 3-5 represent recommended maximums as suggested by this author and others.[31] They are conservative figures but still provide the dental practitioner with adequate volumes to produce clinically acceptable anesthesia. The American Heart Association as far back as 1964 stated that "the typical concentrations of vasoconstrictors contained in local anesthetics are not contraindicated in patients with cardiovascular disease so long as preliminary aspiration is practiced, the agent is injected slowly, and the smallest effective dose is administered."[32] In 1954 the New York Heart Association recommended that maximal epinephrine doses be limited to 0.2 mg per appointment.[33] In the following years, the American Heart Association recommended the restriction of epinephrine in local anesthetics when administered to patients with ischemic heart disease.[34]

More recently, the Agency for Healthcare Research and Quality (AHRQ) reviewed the published literature on the subject of the effects of epinephrine in dental patients with high blood pressure.[35] The report reviewed six studies that evaluated the effects of dental treatment (extraction of teeth) in hypertensive patients when they received local anesthetics with and without epinephrine. Results suggest that hypertensive subjects undergoing an extraction experience small increases in systolic blood pressure and heart rate associated with the use of a local anesthetic containing epinephrine. These increases associated with the use of epinephrine occur in addition to increases in systolic and diastolic blood pressures and heart rate associated with undergoing the procedure without epinephrine that are larger for hypertensive than for normotensive patients. No adverse outcomes were reported among any of the subjects in the studies included in the review, and only one report of an adverse event associated with the use of epinephrine in local anesthetic in a hypertensive patient was identified in the literature (Table 3-6).[35]

In cardiovascularly compromised patients, it seems prudent to limit or avoid exposure to vasoconstrictors, if possible. These include poorly controlled American Society of Anesthesiologists Physical Status classification system (ASA) 3 and all ASA 4 and greater cardiovascular risk patients. However, as stated, the risk of epinephrine administration must be weighed against the benefits to be gained

TABLE 3-5
Recommended Maximum Dosages of Epinephrine

	CARTRIDGES (ROUNDED OFF)	
Epinephrine Concentration (μg/Cartridge)	Normal, Healthy Patient (ASA I)*	Patient With Clinically Significant Cardiovascular Disease (ASA III or IV)†
1:50,000 (36)	5.5	1
1:100,000 (18)	11‡	2
1:200,000 (9)	22‡	4

*Maximum epinephrine dose of 0.2 mg or 200 μg per appointment.
†Maximum recommended dose of 0.04 or 40 μg per appointment.
‡Actual maximum volume of administration is limited by the dosage of local anesthetic drug.

TABLE 3-6
Means of Maximum Changes from Baseline for Blood Pressure and Heart Rate*

	max Δ SBP, mm	max Δ DBP, mm	max Δ HR, bpm
Hypertensives			
Anesthesia with epinephrine	15.3	2.3	9.3
Anesthesia without epinephrine	11.7	3.3	4.7
Normotensives			
Anesthesia with epinephrine	5.0	−0.7	6.3
Anesthesia without epinephrine*	5.0	4.0	0.7

Data from Cardiovascular effects of epinephrine in hypertensive dental patients: summary, evidence report/technology assessment number 48. AHRQ Publication Number 02-E005, Rockville, Md. March 2002, Agency for Healthcare Research and Quality. Available at: http://www.ahrq.gov/clinic/epcsums/ephypsum.htm
DBP, Diastolic blood pressure; *HR*, heart rate; *SBP*, systolic blood pressure.
*Unweighted mean of subject means reported in three studies.

from its inclusion in the local anesthetic solution. Can clinically adequate pain control be provided for this patient without a vasoconstrictor in the solution? What is the potential negative effect of poor anesthesia on endogenous release of catecholamines in response to sudden, unexpected pain?

The use of vasoconstrictors for cardiovascularly compromised patients is reviewed in greater depth in Chapter 20.

Hemostasis. Epinephrine-containing local anesthetic solutions are used, via infiltration into the surgical site, to prevent or to minimize hemorrhage during surgical and other procedures. The 1:50,000 dilution of epinephrine is more effective in this regard than less concentrated 1:100,000 or 1:200,000 solutions.[36] Epinephrine dilutions of 1:50,000 and 1:100,000 are considerably more effective in restricting surgical blood loss than are local anesthetics without vasoconstrictor additives.[26]

Clinical experience has shown that effective hemostasis can be obtained with concentrations of 1:100,000 epinephrine. Although the small volume of 1:50,000 epinephrine required for hemostasis does not increase a patient's risk, consideration always should be given to use of the 1:100,000 dilution, especially in patients known to be more sensitive to catecholamines. These include hyperresponders on the Bell-shaped curve, as well as ASA 3 or 4 risk cardiovascularly compromised individuals and geriatric patients.

Norepinephrine (Levarterenol)

Proprietary Names. Levophed, Noradrenalin; levarterenol is the official name of norepinephrine.

Chemical Structure. Norepinephrine (as the bitartrate) in dental cartridges is relatively stable in acid solutions, deteriorating on exposure to light and air. The shelf life of a cartridge containing norepinephrine bitartrate is 18 months. Acetone-sodium bisulfite is added to the cartridge to retard deterioration.

OH H
C–C–NH_2
H H
HO
OH

Source. Norepinephrine is available in both synthetic and natural forms. The natural form constitutes approximately 20% of the catecholamine production of the adrenal medulla. In patients with pheochromocytoma, a tumor of the adrenal medulla, norepinephrine may account for up to 80% of adrenal medullary secretions. It exists in both levorotatory and dextrorotatory forms; the levorotatory form is 40 times as potent as the dextrorotatory form. Norepinephrine is synthesized and is stored at postganglionic adrenergic nerve terminals.

Mode of Action. The actions of norepinephrine are almost exclusively on α receptors (90%). It also stimulates β actions in the heart (10%). Norepinephrine is one fourth as potent as epinephrine.

Systemic Actions

Myocardium. Norepinephrine has a positive inotropic action on the myocardium through β_1 stimulation.

Pacemaker Cells. Norepinephrine stimulates pacemaker cells and increases their irritability, leading to a greater incidence of cardiac dysrhythmias (β_1 action).

Coronary Arteries. Norepinephrine produces an increase in coronary artery blood flow through a vasodilatory effect.

Heart Rate. Norepinephrine produces a decrease in heart rate caused by reflex actions of the carotid and aortic baroreceptors and the vagus nerve after a marked increase in both systolic and diastolic pressures.

Blood Pressure. Both systolic and diastolic pressures are increased, systolic to a greater extent. This effect is produced through the α-stimulating actions of norepinephrine, which lead to peripheral vasoconstriction and a concomitant increase in peripheral vascular resistance.

Cardiovascular Dynamics. The overall action of norepinephrine on the heart and cardiovascular system is as follows:

- Increased systolic pressure
- Increased diastolic pressure
- Decreased heart rate
- Unchanged or slightly decreased cardiac output
- Increased stroke volume
- Increased total peripheral resistance

Vasculature. Norepinephrine, through α stimulation, produces constriction of cutaneous blood vessels. This leads to increased total peripheral resistance and increased systolic and diastolic blood pressures.

The degree and duration of ischemia noted after norepinephrine infiltration into the palate have led to soft tissue necrosis (Fig. 3-1).

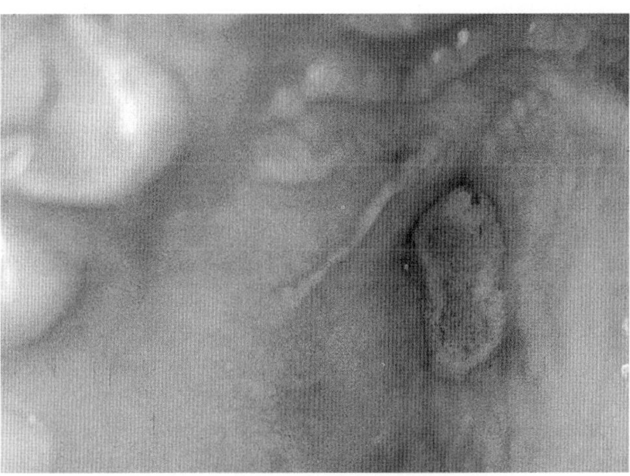

Figure 3-1. Sterile abscess on the palate produced by excessive use of a vasoconstrictor (norepinephrine).

Respiratory System. Norepinephrine does not relax bronchial smooth muscle, as does epinephrine. It does, however, produce α-induced constriction of lung arterioles, which reduces airway resistance to a small degree. Norepinephrine is not clinically effective in the management of bronchospasm.

Central Nervous System. Similar to epinephrine, norepinephrine does not exhibit CNS-stimulating actions at usual therapeutic doses; its CNS-stimulating properties are most prominent after overdose. Clinical manifestations are similar to those of epinephrine overdose (p. 43) but are less frequent and usually are not as severe.

Metabolism. Norepinephrine increases the basal metabolic rate. Tissue oxygen consumption is also increased in the area of injection. Norepinephrine produces an elevation in the blood sugar level in the same manner as epinephrine, but to a lesser degree.

Termination of Action and Elimination. The action of norepinephrine is terminated through its reuptake at adrenergic nerve terminals and its oxidation by MAO. Exogenous norepinephrine is inactivated by COMT.

Side Effects and Overdose. Clinical manifestations of norepinephrine overdose are similar to but less frequent and less severe than those of epinephrine. They normally involve CNS stimulation. Excessive levels of norepinephrine in the blood produce markedly elevated systolic and diastolic pressures with increased risk of hemorrhagic stroke, headache, anginal episodes in susceptible patients, and cardiac dysrhythmias.

Extravascular injection of norepinephrine into tissues may produce necrosis and sloughing because of intense α stimulation. In the oral cavity, the most likely site to encounter this phenomenon is the hard palate (see Fig. 3-1). Norepinephrine should be avoided for vasoconstricting purposes (e.g., hemostasis), especially on the palate. An increasing number of authorities have stated that norepinephrine should not be used at all with local anesthetics.[30,37]

Clinical Applications. Norepinephrine is used as a vasoconstrictor in local anesthetics and for the management of hypotension.

Availability in Dentistry. In the United States, norepinephrine is no longer available in local anesthetic solutions used in dentistry. In the past, it was included with the local anesthetics propoxycaine and procaine in a 1:30,000 concentration. In other countries, norepinephrine is included with lidocaine (Germany) and mepivacaine (Germany) or as the combination of norepinephrine and epinephrine with lidocaine (Germany) or tolycaine (Japan).[21]

Maximum Doses. When given, norepinephrine should be used for pain control only, there being no justification for its use in obtaining hemostasis. It is approximately 25% as potent a vasopressor as epinephrine and therefore is used clinically as a 1:30,000 dilution.

Recommendations of the International Federation of Dental Anesthesiology Societies (IFDAS) suggest that norepinephrine be eliminated as a vasoconstrictor in dental local anesthetics, a statement with which this author wholeheartedly agrees.[30]

Normal healthy patient: 0.34 mg per appointment; 10 mL of a 1:30,000 solution

Patient with clinically significant cardiovascular disease (ASA 3 or 4): 0.14 mg per appointment; approximately 4 mL of a 1:30,000 solution

Levonordefrin

Proprietary Name. Neo-Cobefrin.

Chemical Structure. Levonordefrin is freely soluble in dilute acidic solutions. Sodium bisulfite is added to the solution to delay its deterioration. The shelf life of a cartridge containing levonordefrin-sodium bisulfite is 18 months.

Source. Levonordefrin, a synthetic vasoconstrictor, is prepared by the resolution of nordefrin into its optically active isomers. The dextrorotatory form of nordefrin is virtually inert.

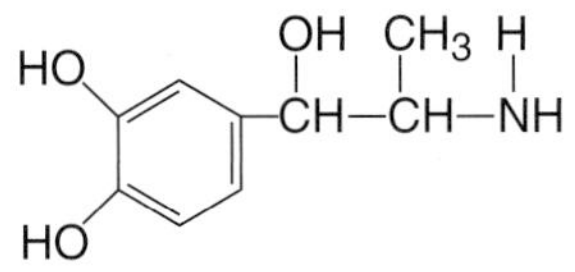

HO, HO — OH CH_3 H — CH—CH—NH

Mode of Action. It appears to act through direct α receptor stimulation (75%) with some β activity (25%), but to a lesser degree than epinephrine. Levonordefrin is 15% as potent a vasopressor as epinephrine.

Systemic Actions. Levonordefrin produces less cardiac and CNS stimulation than is produced by epinephrine.

Myocardium. The same action as epinephrine is seen, but to a lesser degree.

Pacemaker Cells. The same action as epinephrine is seen, but to a lesser degree.

Coronary Arteries. The same action as epinephrine is seen, but to a lesser degree.

Heart Rate. The same action as epinephrine is seen, but to a lesser degree.

Vasculature. The same action as epinephrine is seen, but to a lesser degree.

Respiratory System. Some bronchodilation occurs, but to a much smaller degree than with epinephrine.

Central Nervous System. The same action as epinephrine is seen, but to a lesser degree.

Metabolism. The same action as epinephrine is seen, but to a lesser degree.

Termination of Action and Elimination. Levonordefrin is eliminated through the actions of COMT and MAO.

Side Effects and Overdose. These are the same as with epinephrine, but to a lesser extent. With higher doses, additional side effects include hypertension, ventricular tachycardia, and anginal episodes in patients with coronary artery insufficiency.

Clinical Applications. Levonordefrin is used as a vasoconstrictor in local anesthetics.

Availability in Dentistry. It can be obtained with mepivacaine in a 1:20,000 dilution.

Maximum Doses. Levonordefrin is considered one sixth (15%) as effective a vasopressor as epinephrine; therefore it is used in a higher concentration (1:20,000).

For all patients, the maximum dose should be 1 mg per appointment; 20 mL of a 1:20,000 dilution (11 cartridges).*

In the concentration at which it is available, levonordefrin has the same effect on the clinical activity of local anesthetics as does epinephrine in 1:50,000 or 1:100,000 concentration.

Phenylephrine Hydrochloride

Proprietary Name. Neo-Synephrine.

Chemical Structure. Phenylephrine is quite soluble in water. It is the most stable and the weakest vasoconstrictor employed in dentistry.

HO–(benzene ring)–CH(OH)–CH_2–N(H)–CH_3

Source. Phenylephrine is a synthetic sympathomimetic amine.

Mode of Action. Direct α receptor stimulation occurs (95%). Although the effect is less than with epinephrine, duration is longer. Phenylephrine exerts little or no β action on the heart. Only a small portion of its activity results from its ability to release norepinephrine. Phenylephrine is only 5% as potent as epinephrine.

Systemic Actions

Myocardium. It has little chronotropic or inotropic effect on the heart.

Pacemaker Cells. Little effect is noted.

Coronary Arteries. Increased blood flow occurs as the result of dilation.

Blood Pressure. α action produces increases in both systolic and diastolic pressures.

Heart Rate. Bradycardia is produced by reflex actions of the carotid–aortic baroreceptors and the vagus nerve. Cardiac dysrhythmias are rarely noted, even after large doses of phenylephrine.

Cardiovascular Dynamics. Overall, the cardiovascular actions of phenylephrine are as follows:

- Increased systolic and diastolic pressures
- Reflex bradycardia
- Slightly decreased cardiac output (resulting from increased blood pressure and bradycardia)
- Powerful vasoconstriction (most vascular beds constricted, peripheral resistance increased significantly) but without marked venous congestion
- Rarely associated with provoking cardiac dysrhythmias

Respiratory System. Bronchi are dilated but to a lesser degree than with epinephrine. Phenylephrine is not effective in treating bronchospasm.

Central Nervous System. A minimum effect on CNS activity is noted.

Metabolism. Some increase in the metabolic rate is noted. Other actions (e.g., glycogenolysis) are similar to those produced by epinephrine.

Termination of Action and Elimination. Phenylephrine undergoes hydroxylation to epinephrine, then oxidation to metanephrine, after which it is eliminated in the same manner as epinephrine.

Side Effects and Overdose. CNS effects are minimal with phenylephrine. Headache and ventricular dysrhythmias have been noted after overdose. Tachyphylaxis is observed with long-term use.

Clinical Applications. Phenylephrine is used as a vasoconstrictor in local anesthetics, for the management of hypotension, as a nasal decongestant, and in ophthalmic solutions to produce mydriasis.

Availability in Dentistry. Phenylephrine was used with 4% procaine in a 1:2500 dilution (no longer available in dental cartridges).

Maximum Doses. Phenylephrine is considered only one twentieth as potent as epinephrine, hence its use in a 1:2500 dilution (equivalent to a 1:50,000 epinephrine concentration). It is an excellent vasoconstrictor, with few significant side effects.

Normal healthy patient: 4 mg per appointment; 10 mL of a 1:2500 solution

Patient with clinically significant cardiovascular impairment (ASA 3 or 4): 1.6 mg per appointment, equivalent to 4 mL of a 1:2500 solution

Felypressin

Proprietary Name. Octapressin.

Chemical Structure

Cys-Phe-Phe-Gly-Asn-Cys-Pro-Lys-$GlyNH_2$

*Maximum volume for administration may be limited by the dose of the local anesthetic.

Source. Felypressin is a synthetic analog of the antidiuretic hormone vasopressin. It is a nonsympathomimetic amine, categorized as a vasoconstrictor.

Mode of Action. Felypressin acts as a direct stimulant of vascular smooth muscle. Its actions appear to be more pronounced on the venous than on the arteriolar microcirculation.[38]

Systemic Actions

Myocardium. No direct effects are noted.

Pacemaker Cells. Felypressin is nondysrhythmogenic, in contrast to the sympathomimetic amines (e.g., epinephrine, norepinephrine).

Coronary Arteries. When administered in high doses (greater than therapeutic), it may impair blood flow through the coronary arteries.

Vasculature. In high doses (greater than therapeutic), felypressin-induced constriction of cutaneous blood vessels may produce facial pallor.

Central Nervous System. Felypressin has no effect on adrenergic nerve transmission; thus it may be safely administered to hyperthyroid patients and to anyone receiving MAO inhibitors or tricyclic antidepressants.

Uterus. It has both antidiuretic and oxytocic actions, the latter contraindicating its use in pregnant patients.

Side Effects and Overdose. Laboratory and clinical studies with felypressin in animals and humans have demonstrated a wide margin of safety.[39] The drug is well tolerated by the tissues into which it is deposited, with little irritation developing. The incidence of systemic reactions to felypressin is minimal.

Clinical Applications. Felypressin is used as a vasoconstrictor in local anesthetics to decrease their absorption and increase their duration of action.

Availability in Dentistry. Felypressin is employed in a dilution of 0.03 IU/mL (International Units) with 3% prilocaine in Japan, Germany, and other countries. It is not available as a vasoconstrictor in local anesthetics in North America.

Maximum Doses. Felypressin-containing solutions are not recommended for use where hemostasis is necessary because of its predominant effect on the venous rather than the arterial circulation.[40]

For patients with clinically significant cardiovascular impairment (ASA 3 or 4), the maximum recommended dose is 0.27 IU; 9 mL of 0.03 IU/mL.

SELECTION OF A VASOCONSTRICTOR

Two vasoconstrictors are available in local anesthetic solutions in North America: epinephrine and levonordefrin.

In the selection of an appropriate vasoconstrictor, if any, for use with a local anesthetic, several factors must be considered: the length of the dental procedure, the need for hemostasis during and after the procedure, the requirement for postoperative pain control, and the medical status of the patient.

Length of the Dental Procedure

The addition of any vasoactive drug to a local anesthetic prolongs the duration (and depth) of pulpal and soft tissue anesthesia of most local anesthetics. For example, pulpal and hard tissue anesthesia with 2% lidocaine lasts approximately 10 minutes; the addition of 1:50,000, 1:80,000, 1:100,000, or 1:200,000 epinephrine increases this to approximately 60 minutes. The addition of a vasoconstrictor to prilocaine, on the other hand, does not significantly increase the duration of clinically effective pain control. Prilocaine 4%, after nerve block injection, provides pulpal anesthesia of about 40 to 60 minutes' duration. (Infiltration injection with prilocaine 4% provides approximately 10 to 15 minutes of pulpal anesthesia.) The addition of a 1:200,000 epinephrine concentration to prilocaine increases this slightly (to about 60 to 90 minutes).[41]

Average durations of pulpal and hard tissue anesthesia expected from commonly used local anesthetics with and without vasoconstrictors are shown in Table 3-7.

The typical dental patient is scheduled for a 1-hour appointment. The duration of actual treatment (and the desirable duration of profound pulpal anesthesia) is 47.9 minutes (standard deviation [SD] 14.7 minutes) in a general dentistry office, whereas in the offices of dental specialists, treatment time is 39.1 minutes (SD 19.4 minutes).[42]

For routine restorative procedures, it might be estimated that pulpal anesthesia will be required for approximately 40 to 50 minutes. As can be seen in Table 3-7, it is difficult to achieve consistently reliable pulpal anesthesia without inclusion of a vasoconstrictor (see minutes marked with asterisks in Table 3-7).

TABLE 3-7
Average Durations of Pulpal and Hard Tissue Anesthesia

Local Anesthetic	Infiltration, minutes	Nerve Block, minutes
Lidocaine HCL		
2% – no vasoconstrictor	5-10*	≈10-20*
2% + epinephrine 1:50,000	≈60	≥60
2% + epinephrine 1:100,000	≈60	≥60
2% + epinephrine 1:200,000	≈60	≥60
Mepivacaine HCL		
3% – no vasoconstrictor	5-10*	20-40*
2% + levonordefrin 1:20,000	≤60	≥60
2% + epinephrine 1:100,000	≤60	>60
Prilocaine HCL		
4% – no vasoconstrictor	10-15*	40-60*
4% + epinephrine 1:200,000	≤60	60-90
Articaine HCL		
4% + epinephrine 1:100,000	≤60	≥60

*Indicates duration of pulpal anesthesia usually inadequate to provide pain control for a typical 48-minute procedure.

Requirement for Hemostasis

Epinephrine is effective in preventing or minimizing blood loss during surgical procedures. However, epinephrine also produces a rebound vasodilatory effect as the tissue level of epinephrine declines. This leads to possible bleeding postoperatively, which potentially interferes with wound healing.[26]

Epinephrine, which possesses both α and β actions, produces vasoconstriction through its α effects. Used in a 1:50,000 concentration, and even at 1:100,000 (but to a lesser extent), epinephrine produces a definite rebound β effect once α-induced vasoconstriction has ceased. This leads to increased postoperative blood loss, which, if significant (not usually the case in dentistry), could compromise a patient's cardiovascular status.

Phenylephrine, a longer-acting, almost pure α-stimulating vasoconstrictor, does not produce a rebound β effect because its β actions are minimal. Therefore because it is not as potent a vasoconstrictor as epinephrine, hemostasis during the procedure is not as effective; however, because of the long duration of action of phenylephrine compared with that of epinephrine, the postoperative period passes with less bleeding. Total blood loss is usually lower when phenylephrine is used. Phenylephrine is not included in any dental local anesthetic formulation.

Norepinephrine is a potent α stimulator and vasoconstrictor that has produced documented cases of tissue necrosis and sloughing. Norepinephrine cannot be recommended as a vasoconstrictor in dentistry because its disadvantages outweigh its advantages. Other more or equally effective vasoconstrictors are available that do not possess the disadvantages of norepinephrine.[43,44]

Felypressin constricts the venous circulation more than the arteriolar circulation and therefore is of minimal value for hemostasis.

Vasoconstrictors must be deposited locally into the surgical site (area of bleeding) to provide hemostasis. They act directly on α receptors in the vascular smooth muscle. Only small volumes of local anesthetic solutions with vasoconstrictor are required to achieve hemostasis (i.e., just enough to produce ischemia at the site).

Medical Status of the Patient

Few contraindications are known to vasoconstrictor administration in the concentrations in which they are found in dental local anesthetics. For all patients, and for some in particular, the benefits and risks of including the vasopressor in the local anesthetic solution must be weighed against the benefits and risks of using a plain anesthetic solution.[45-47] In general, these groups consist of the following:

- Patients with more significant cardiovascular disease (ASA 3 and 4)*
- Patients with certain noncardiovascular diseases (e.g., thyroid dysfunction, diabetes, sulfite sensitivity)
- Patients receiving MAO inhibitors, tricyclic antidepressants, and phenothiazines

In each of these situations, it is necessary to determine the degree of severity of the underlying disorder to determine whether a vasoconstrictor may be safely included or should be excluded from the local anesthetic solution. It is not uncommon for medical consultation to be sought to aid in determining this information.

Management of these patients is discussed in depth in Chapters 10 and 20. Briefly, however, it may be stated that local anesthetics with vasoconstrictors are not absolutely contraindicated for the patient whose medical condition has been diagnosed and is under control through medical or surgical means (ASA 2 or 3 risk), and if the vasoconstrictor is administered slowly, in minimal doses, after negative aspiration has been ensured.

Patients with a resting blood pressure (minimum 5-minute rest) of greater than 200 mm Hg systolic or greater than 115 mm Hg diastolic should not receive elective dental care until their more significant medical problem of high blood pressure is corrected. Patients with severe cardiovascular disease (ASA 3 or 4 risk) may be at too great a risk for elective dental therapy, for example, a patient who has had a recent (within the past 6 months) acute myocardial infarction with significant myocardial damage; a patient who has been experiencing anginal episodes at rest on a daily basis, or whose signs and symptoms are increasing in severity (preinfarction or unstable angina); or a patient whose cardiac dysrhythmias are refractory to antiarrhythmic drug therapy.[45] Epinephrine and other vasoconstrictors can be administered, within limits, to patients with mild to moderate cardiovascular disease (ASA 2 or 3). Because felypressin has minimum cardiovascular stimulatory action and is nondysrhythmogenic, it is the recommended drug for the ASA 3 or 4 cardiovascular risk patient. Epinephrine also is contraindicated in patients exhibiting clinical evidence of the hyperthyroid state.[46] Signs and symptoms include exophthalmos, hyperhidrosis, tremor, irritability and nervousness, increased body temperature, inability to tolerate heat, increased heart rate, and increased blood pressure. Minimal dosages of epinephrine are recommended as a vasoconstrictor during general anesthesia when a patient (in any ASA category) is receiving a halogenated anesthetic (halothane, isoflurane, sevoflurane, or enflurane). These inhalation (general) anesthetics sensitize the myocardium such that epinephrine administration is frequently associated with the occurrence of ventricular dysrhythmias (PVCs or ventricular fibrillation). Felypressin is recommended in these situations; however, because of its potential oxytocic actions, felypressin is not recommended for pregnant patients. Once the impaired medical status of the patient is improved (e.g., ASA 4 becomes ASA 3), routine dental care involving the administration of local anesthetics with vasoconstrictors is indicated.

*The ASA Physical Status Classification System is discussed in depth in Chapter 10.

Patients being treated with MAO inhibitors may receive vasoconstrictors within the usual dental dosage parameters without increased risk.[47,48] Patients receiving tricyclic antidepressants are at greater risk for the development of dysrhythmias with epinephrine administration. It is recommended that when epinephrine is administered to these patients, its dose be minimal. Administration of levonordefrin or norepinephrine is absolutely contraindicated in patients receiving tricyclic antidepressants.[49] Large doses of vasoconstrictor may induce severe (exaggerated) responses.

Local anesthetic formulations with vasoconstrictors also contain an antioxidant (to delay oxidation of the vasoconstrictor). Sodium bisulfite is the most frequently used antioxidant in dental cartridges. It prolongs the shelf life of the anesthetic solution with vasoconstrictor to approximately 18 months. However, sodium bisulfite renders the local anesthetic considerably more acidic than the same solution without a vasoconstrictor. Acidic solutions of local anesthetics contain a greater proportion of charged cation molecules (RNH^+) than of uncharged base molecules (RN). Because of this, diffusion of the local anesthetic solution into the axoplasm is slower, resulting in (slightly) delayed onset of anesthesia when local anesthetics containing sodium bisulfite (and vasoconstrictors) are injected.

Vasoconstrictors are important additions to local anesthetic solutions. Numerous studies have demonstrated conclusively that epinephrine, when added to short- or medium-duration local anesthetic solutions, slows the rate of absorption, lowers the systemic blood level, delays cresting of the peak blood level, prolongs the duration of anesthesia, intensifies the depth of anesthesia, and reduces the incidence of systemic reactions.[18] In modern dentistry, adequate pain control of sufficient clinical duration and depth is difficult to achieve without inclusion of vasoconstrictors in the local anesthetic solution. Unless specifically contraindicated by a patient's medical status (ASA 4 or above) or by the required duration of treatment (short), inclusion of a vasoconstrictor should be considered routinely. When these drugs are used, however, care always must be taken to avoid unintended intravascular administration of the vasoconstrictor (as well as the local anesthetic) through multiple aspirations and slow administration of minimum concentrations of both the vasoconstrictor and the local anesthetic.

References

1. Moore PA, Hersh EV: Local anesthetics: pharmacology and toxicity, Dent Clin North Am 54:587–599, 2010.
2. Finder RL, Moore PA: Adverse drug reactions to local anesthesia, Dent Clin North Am 46:447–457, 2002.
3. Brown G: The influence of adrenaline, noradrenaline vasoconstrictors on the efficacy of lidocaine, J Oral Ther Pharmacol 4:398–405, 1968.
4. Cowan A: Further clinical evaluation of prilocaine (Citanest), with and without epinephrine, Oral Surg Oral Med Oral Pathol 26:304–311, 1968.
5. Carpenter RL, Kopacz DJ, Mackey DC: Accuracy of Doppler capillary flow measurements for predicting blood loss from skin incisions in pigs, Anesth Analg 68:308–311, 1989.
6. Myers RR, Heckman HM: Effects of local anesthesia on nerve blood flow: studies using lidocaine with and without epinephrine, Anesthesiology 71:757–762, 1989.
7. Ahlquist RP: A study of adrenotropic receptors, Am J Physiol 153:586–600, 1948.
8. Hieble JP: Adrenoceptor subclassification: an approach to improved cardiovascular therapeutics, Pharmaceut Acta Helvet 74:63–71, 2000.
9. Smiley RM, Kwatra MM, Schwinn DA: New developments in cardiovascular adrenergic receptor pharmacology: molecular mechanisms and clinical relevance, J Cardiothorac Vasc Anesth 12:10–95, 1998.
10. Braun H: Uber den Einfluss der Vitalitat der Gewebe auf die ortlichen und allgemeinen Giftwirkungen localabaesthesierender Mittel, und uber die Bedeutung des Adrerenalins fur die Lokalanasthesie, Arch Klin Chir 69:541–591, 1903.
11. Tolas AG, Pflug AE, Halter JB: Arterial plasma epinephrine concentrations and hemodynamic responses after dental injection of local anesthetic with epinephrine, J Am Dent Assoc 104:41–43, 1982.
12. Jastak JT, Yagiela JA, Donaldson D, editors: Local anesthesia of the oral cavity, Philadelphia, 1995, WB Saunders.
13. Holroyd SV, Requa-Clark B: Local anesthetics. In Holroyd SV, Wynn RL, editors: Clinical pharmacology in dental practice, ed 3, St Louis, 1983, Mosby.
14. Malamed SF: Handbook of local anesthesia, ed 5, St Louis, 2004, Mosby.
15. Cryer PE: Physiology and pathophysiology of the human sympathoadrenal neuroendocrine system, N Engl J Med 303:436–444, 1980.
16. Yagiela JA: Epinephrine and the compromised heart, Orofac Pain Manage 1:5–8, 1991.
17. Kaneko Y, Ichinohe T, Sakurai M, et al: Relationship between changes in circulation due to epinephrine oral injection and its plasma concentration, Anesth Prog 36:188–190, 1989.
18. de Jong RH: Uptake, distribution, and elimination. In de Jong RH, editor: Local anesthetics, St Louis, 1994, Mosby.
19. Huang KC: Effect of intravenous epinephrine on heart rate as monitored with a computerized tachometer, Anesthesiology 73:A762, 1990.
20. Narchi P, Mazoit J-X, Cohen S, Samii K: Heart rate response to an IV test dose of adrenaline and lignocaine with and without atropine pretreatment, Br J Anaesth 66:583–586, 1991.
21. Malamed SF, Sykes P, Kubota Y, et al: Local anesthesia: a review, Anesth Pain Control Dent 1:11–24, 1992.
22. Lipp M, Dick W, Daublander M: Examination of the central venous epinephrine level during local dental infiltration and block anesthesia using tritium marked epinephrine as vasoconstrictor, Anesthesiology 69:371, 1988.
23. Stanton-Hicks M, Berges PU, Bonica JJ: Circulatory effects of peridural block. IV. Comparison of the effects of epinephrine and phenylephrine, Anesthesiology 39:308–314, 1973.
24. Robertson VJ, Taylor SE, Gage TW: Quantitative and qualitative analysis of the pressor effects of levonordefrin, J Cardiovasc Pharmacol 6:529–935, 1984.
25. Clutter WE, Bier DM, Shah SD, Cryer PE: Epinephrine plasma metabolic clearance rates and physiologic thresholds for metabolic and hemodynamic actions in man, J Clin Invest 66:94–101, 1980.
26. Sveen K: Effect of the addition of a vasoconstrictor to local anesthetic solution on operative and postoperative bleeding, analgesia, and wound healing, Int J Oral Surg 8:301–306, 1979.

27. Meechan JG: The effects of dental local anaesthetics on blood glucose concentration in healthy volunteers and in patients having third molar surgery, Br Dent J 170:373–376, 1991.
28. Lefkowitz RJ, Hoffman BB, Taylor P: Neurohumoral transmission: the autonomic and somatic motor nervous system. In Brunton LL, Lazo JS, Parker KL editors: Goodman and Gilman's the pharmacological basis of therapeutics, ed 11, New York, 2006, McGraw-Hill Companies.
29. Campbell RL: Cardiovascular effects of epinephrine overdose: case report, Anesth Prog 24:190–193, 1977.
30. Jakob W: Local anaesthesia and vasoconstrictive additional components, Newslett Int Fed Dent Anesthesiol Soc 2:1, 1989.
31. Bennett CR: Monheim's local anesthesia and pain control in dental practice, ed 7, St Louis, 1983, Mosby.
32. Management of dental problems in patients with cardiovascular disease: report of a working conference jointly sponsored by the American Dental Association and American Heart Association, J Am Dent Assoc 68:333–342, 1964.
33. Use of epinephrine in connection with procaine in dental procedures: report of the Special Committee of the New York Heart Association, Inc., on the use of epinephrine in connection with procaine in dental procedures, J Am Dent Assoc 50:108, 1955.
34. Kaplan EL, editor: Cardiovascular disease in dental practice, Dallas, 1986, American Heart Association.
35. Cardiovascular effects of epinephrine in hypertensive dental patients: summary, evidence report/technology assessment number 48. AHRQ Publication Number 02-E005, March 2002, Agency for Healthcare Research and Quality, Rockville, Md. Availableat:http://www.ahrq.gov/clinic/epcsums/ephypsum.htm
36. Buckley JA, Ciancio SG, McMullen JA: Efficacy of epinephrine concentration in local anesthesia during periodontal surgery, J Periodontol 55:653–657, 1984.
37. Kaufman E, Garfunkel A, Findler M, et al: Emergencies evolving from local anesthesia, Refuat Hapeh Vehashinayim 19:13–18, 98, 2002.
38. Altura BM, Hershey SG, Zweifach BW: Effects of a synthetic analogue of vasopressin on vascular smooth muscle, Proc Soc Exp Biol Med 119:258–261, 1965.
39. Sunada K, Nakamura K, Yamashiro M, et al: Clinically safe dosage of felypressin for patients with essential hypertension, Anesth Prog 43:408–415, 1996.
40. Newcomb GM, Waite IM: The effectiveness of local analgesic preparations in reducing haemorrhage during periodontal surgery, J Dent 1:37–42, 1972.
41. Epstein S: Clinical study of prilocaine with varying concentrations of epinephrine, J Am Dent Assoc 78:85–90, 1969.
42. American Dental Association: 2009 survey of dental practice, Chicago, February 2010, American Dental Association.
43. van der Bijl P, Victor AM: Adverse reactions associated with norepinephrine in dental local anesthesia, Anesth Prog 39:37–89, 1992.
44. Hirota Y, Hori T, Kay K, Matsuura H: Effects of epinephrine and norepinephrine contained in 2% lidocaine on hemodynamics of the carotid and cerebral circulation in older and younger adults, Anesth Pain Control Dent 1:343–351, 1992.
45. Goulet JP, Perusse R, Turcotte JY: Contraindications to vasoconstrictors in dentistry. Part I. Cardiovascular diseases, Oral Surg Oral Med Oral Pathol 74:579–686, 1992.
46. Goulet JP, Perusse R, Turcotte JY: Contraindications to vasoconstrictors in dentistry. Part II. Hyperthyroidism, diabetes, sulfite sensitivity, cortico-dependent asthma, and pheochromocytoma, Oral Surg Oral Med Oral Pathol 74:587–691, 1992.
47. Goulet JP, Perusse R, Turcotte JY: Contraindications to vasoconstrictors in dentistry. Part III. Pharmacologic interactions, Oral Surg Oral Med Oral Pathol 74:592–697, 1992.
48. Verrill PJ: Adverse reactions to local anaesthetics and vasoconstrictor drugs, Practitioner 214:380–387, 1975.
49. Jastak JT, Yagiela JA, Donaldson D, editors: Local anesthesia of the oral cavity, Philadelphia, 1995, WB Saunders.

CHAPTER 4

Clinical Action of Specific Agents

SELECTION OF A LOCAL ANESTHETIC

Although many drugs are classified as local anesthetics and find use within the health professions, only a handful are currently used in dentistry. In 1980, when the first edition of this text was published, five local anesthetics were available in dental cartridge form in the United States: lidocaine, mepivacaine, prilocaine, and the combination of procaine and propoxycaine.[1] In the years since that first edition, increased demand for longer-acting local anesthetics led to the introduction, in dental cartridges, of bupivacaine (1982 Canada, 1983 United States) and etidocaine (1985). In 1975 articaine became available in Germany, and later throughout Europe. Articaine came to North America in 1983 (Canada) and to the United States in 2000. Articaine is classified as an intermediate-duration local anesthetic.

The combination of procaine and propoxycaine was withdrawn from the U.S. market in January 1996.

As this sixth edition of *Handbook of Local Anesthesia* goes to press, the local anesthetic armamentarium in North American dentistry includes articaine, bupivacaine, lidocaine, mepivacaine, and prilocaine.

With the availability of these local anesthetics, in various combinations with and without vasoconstrictors, it is possible for a doctor to select a local anesthetic solution that possesses the specific pain controlling properties necessary for the patient for any given dental procedure. Table 4-1 lists local anesthetics and the various combinations in which they are currently available in the United States and Canada. Box 4-1 lists these combinations by their expected duration of clinical action (durations of pulpal and soft tissue anesthesia).

In this chapter, each of the available local anesthetics in its various combinations is described. In addition, the rationale for selection of an appropriate local anesthetic for a given patient at a given appointment is presented. It is strongly suggested that the reader—the potential administrator of these drugs—become familiar with this material, including contraindications to the administration of certain local anesthetic combinations (Table 4-2).

In the following discussion of the clinical properties of specific local anesthetic combinations, several concepts are presented that require some explanation. These include the duration of action of the drug and determination of the maximum recommended dose.

DURATION

The duration of pulpal (hard tissue) and soft tissue (total) anesthesia cited for each drug is an approximation. Many factors affect both the depth and the duration of a drug's anesthetic action, prolonging or (much more commonly) decreasing it. These factors include but are not limited to the following:

1. Individual response to the drug (the "bell-shaped" curve)
2. Accuracy in deposition of the local anesthetic
3. Status of tissues at the site of drug deposition (vascularity, pH)
4. Anatomic variation
5. Type of injection administered (supraperiosteal ["infiltration"] or nerve block)

In the subsequent discussion of individual local anesthetics, the durations of anesthesia (pulpal and soft tissue) are presented as a range (e.g., 40 to 60 minutes). This approach attempts to take into account the factors mentioned that can influence drug action:

1. **Normal distribution curve (bell-shaped curve):** Variation in individual response to a drug is common and expected and is depicted in the so-called bell or normal distribution curve (Fig. 4-1). Most patients will respond in a predictable manner to a drug's actions (e.g., 40 to 60 minutes). However, some patients (with none of the other factors that influence drug action obviously present) will have a shorter or longer duration of anesthesia. This is to be expected and is entirely normal.

   For example, if 100 persons are administered an appropriate dose of 2% lidocaine HCl with epinephrine 1:100,000 via supraperiosteal injection over a maxillary lateral incisor, and a pulp tester is used to assess the

TABLE 4-1
Local Anesthetics Available in North America (August 2011)

Local Anesthetic (+ Vasoconstrictor)	Duration of Action*
Articaine HCl	
4% + epinephrine 1:100,000	Intermediate
4% + epinephrine 1:200,000	Intermediate
Bupivacaine HCl	
0.5% + epinephrine 1:200,000	Long
Lidocaine HCl	
2% + epinephrine 1:50,000	Intermediate
2% + epinephrine 1:100,000	Intermediate
Mepivacaine HCl	
3%	Short
2% + levonordefrin 1:20,000	Intermediate
Prilocaine HCl	
4%	Short (infiltration); intermediate (nerve block)
4% + epinephrine 1:200,000	Intermediate

*The classification of duration of action is approximate, for extreme variations may be noted among patients. Short-duration drugs provide pulpal or deep anesthesia for less than 30 minutes; intermediate-duration drugs for about 60 minutes; and long-duration drugs for longer than 90 minutes.

BOX 4-1 Approximate Duration of Action of Local Anesthetics

Short Duration (Pulpal Anesthesia Approximately 30 Minutes)
Mepivacaine HCl 3%
Prilocaine HCl 4% (by infiltration)

Intermediate Duration (Pulpal Anesthesia Approximately 60 Minutes)
Articaine HCl 4% + epinephrine 1:100,000
Articaine HCl 4% + epinephrine 1:200,000
Lidocaine HCl 2% + epinephrine 1:50,000
Lidocaine HCl 2% + epinephrine 1:100,000
Mepivacaine HCl 2% + levonordefrin 1:20,000
Prilocaine HCl 4% (via nerve block only)
Prilocaine HCl 4% + epinephrine 1:200,000

Long Duration (Pulpal Anesthesia Approximately 90+ Minutes)
Bupivacaine HCl 0.5% + epinephrine 1:200,000 (by nerve block)

TABLE 4-2
Contraindications for Local Anesthetics

Medical Problem	Drugs to Avoid	Type of Contraindication	Alternative Drug
Local anesthetic allergy, documented	All local anesthetics in same chemical class (e.g., esters)	Absolute	Local anesthetics in different chemical class (e.g., amides)
Bisulfite allergy	Vasoconstrictor-containing local anesthetics	Absolute	Any local anesthetic without vasoconstrictor
Atypical plasma cholinesterase	Esters	Relative	Amides
Methemoglobinemia, idiopathic or congenital	Prilocaine	Relative	Other amides or esters
Significant liver dysfunction (ASA 3–4)	Amides	Relative	Amides or esters, but judiciously
Significant renal dysfunction (ASA 3–4)	Amides or esters	Relative	Amides or esters, but judiciously
Significant cardiovascular disease (ASA 3–4)	High concentrations of vasoconstrictors (as in racemic epinephrine gingival retraction cords)	Relative	Local anesthetics with epinephrine concentration of 1:200,000 or 1:100,000, or mepivacaine 3%, or prilocaine 4% (nerve blocks)
Clinical hyperthyroidism (ASA 3–4)	High concentrations of vasoconstrictors (as in racemic epinephrine gingival retraction cords)	Relative	Local anesthetics with epinephrine concentration of 1:200,000 or 1:100,000, or mepivacaine 3%, or prilocaine 4% (nerve blocks)

duration of anesthesia, approximately 70% (68.26%) will have pulpal anesthesia for approximately 60 minutes. These represent the *normo-responders.* Approximately 15% will have pulpal anesthesia that lasts beyond the expected 60 minutes—perhaps 70 or 80 minutes, and even longer for some. These persons are termed *hyperresponders.* No dentist complains about these patients because their dental treatment proceeds and is completed with no pain or need for repeated injection of local anesthetic. However, it is the final 15%, the *hyporesponders,* who are well remembered by the dentist. These patients, given

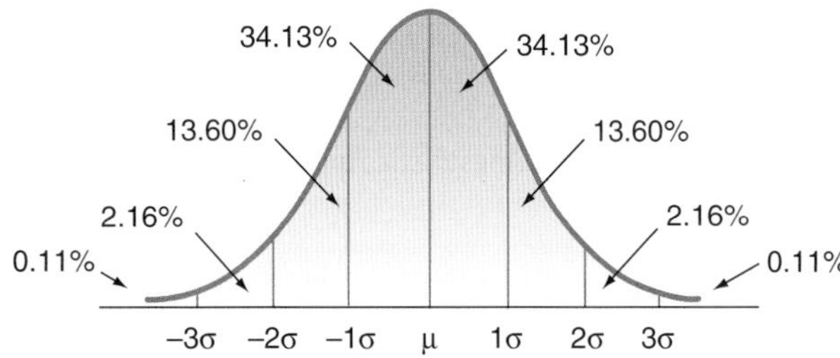

Figure 4-1. "Bell-shaped" curve.

lidocaine with epinephrine, are anesthetized for 45 minutes, 30 minutes, 15 minutes, or even less. These are the patients about whom the doctor states (incorrectly): "They metabolize the drug rapidly." As was mentioned in Chapter 2, metabolism (biotransformation, detoxification) has nothing to do with the clinical effects of a local anesthetic dissipating. The duration of anesthesia is based simply on the way some persons respond to this drug (or group of drugs).

2. **Accuracy in administration of the local anesthetic** is another factor that influences drug action. Although not as significant in certain techniques (e.g., supraperiosteal) or with certain drugs (e.g., articaine), accuracy in deposition is a major factor in many nerve blocks in which a considerable thickness of soft tissue must be penetrated to access the nerve being blocked. Inferior alveolar nerve block (IANB) is the prime example of a technique in which the depth and duration of anesthesia are greatly influenced by the accuracy of injection. Deposition of local anesthetic close to the nerve provides greater depth and duration of anesthesia compared with an anesthetic deposited at a greater distance from the nerve to be blocked.
3. **The status of the tissues into which a local anesthetic is deposited** influences the observed duration of anesthetic action. The presence of normal healthy tissue at the site of drug deposition is assumed. Inflammation, infection, or pain (acute or chronic) usually decreases depth and anticipated duration of anesthesia. Increased vascularity at the site of drug deposition results in more rapid absorption of the local anesthetic and a decreased duration of anesthesia. This is most notable in areas of inflammation and infection but is also a consideration in "normal" anatomy. The recent introduction (February 2011) of buffered local anesthetics promises to help overcome this negative effect of inflammation and infection.[2] The neck of the mandibular condyle, the target for local anesthetic deposition in the Gow-Gates mandibular nerve block, is considerably less vascular than the target area for the IANB. The expected duration of anesthesia for any local anesthetic will be greater in a less vascular region.
4. **Anatomic variation also influences clinical anesthesia.** The normal anatomy of the maxilla and the mandible is described in Chapter 12. The most notable aspect of "normal" anatomy is the presence of extreme variation (e.g., in size and shape of the head or in thickness of bone) from person to person. The techniques presented in subsequent chapters are based on the middle of the bell curve, the so-called normal responders. Anatomic variations away from this "norm" may influence the duration of clinical drug action. Although most obvious in the mandible (height of the mandibular foramen, width of the ramus, thickness of the cortical plate of bone), such variation also may be noted in the maxilla. Supraperiosteal infiltration, usually effective in providing pulpal anesthesia for all maxillary teeth, provides a shorter duration than expected or an inadequate depth of anesthesia when alveolar bone is more dense than usual. Where the zygomatic arch is lower (primarily in children, but occasionally in adults), infiltration anesthesia of the maxillary first and second molars may provide a shorter duration or may even fail to provide adequate depth of pulpal anesthesia. In other cases, the palatal root of maxillary molars may not be adequately anesthetized, even in the presence of normal thickness of the buccal alveolar bone, when that root flares greatly toward the midline of the palate. In the mandible, it is stated that supraperiosteal infiltration is not effective in adults because their cortical plate of bone is too thick; however, according to the bell-shaped curve, 15% of adult patients should have cortical bone that is thinner, perhaps allowing mandibular infiltration to be effective. The use of articaine HCl by mandibular infiltration in adults has been demonstrated to be highly effective (and is discussed in detail in Chapters 15 and 20).[3]
5. **Finally, the duration of clinical anesthesia** is influenced by the type of injection administered. For all drugs presented, administration of a nerve block provides a longer duration of pulpal and soft tissue anesthesia than is provided by supraperiosteal injection (e.g., infiltration). This assumes that the recommended minimum volume of anesthetic is injected. Less than recommended volumes decrease the duration of action. Larger than recommended doses do not provide increased duration. For example, a duration of pulpal anesthesia of 10 to 15 minutes may be expected to follow supraperiosteal injection with prilocaine 4% (no vasoconstrictor), whereas a 40- to 60-minute duration is normal following nerve block (Table 4-3).

TABLE 4-3
Duration of Pulpal Anesthesia by Type of Injection

Local Anesthetic	Infiltration (Minutes)	Nerve Block (Minutes)
Mepivacaine HCl		
3%: no vasoconstrictor	5-10	20-40
Prilocaine HCl		
4%: no vasoconstrictor	10-15	40-60
Bupivacaine HCl		
0.5% + epinephrine 1:200,000	60	Up to 12 hours

MAXIMUM DOSES OF LOCAL ANESTHETICS

Doses of local anesthetic drugs are presented in terms of milligrams of drug per unit of body weight—as milligrams per kilogram (mg/kg) or as milligrams per pound (mg/lb). These numbers, similar to the ones presented for duration, reflect estimated values because there is a wide range (the bell-shaped curve also is seen here) in patient response to blood levels of local anesthetics (or of any drug).

For patients whose responses to anesthetic blood levels lie within the middle of the normal distribution curve, administration of a maximum dose based on body weight produces a local anesthetic blood level below the usual threshold for an overdose (toxic) reaction. The response observed if an overdose reaction occurs at that dose is mild (e.g., tremor of the arms and legs, drowsiness). Patients who are hyporesponders to elevated local anesthetic blood levels may not experience any adverse reaction until their local anesthetic blood level is considerably above this "normal" overdose threshold. These patients represent little increased risk when local anesthetics are administered in "usual" dental doses. However, hyperresponders may demonstrate clinical signs and symptoms of local anesthetic overdose at blood levels that are considerably lower than those normally necessary to produce such reactions. To increase safety for all patients during administration of local anesthetics, but especially in this latter group, one should always minimize drug doses and use the smallest clinically effective dose. Recommended volumes of local anesthetics are presented for each injection technique in Chapters 13, 14, and 15.

The maximum recommended dose (MRD) of local anesthetics has been modified in this 6th edition. In previous editions, both the manufacturer's recommended dose (MRD-m) and the author's recommended dose (MRD-a) were listed. In some instances, these doses differed. Where doses differed, those recommended by this author were more conservative than those recommended by the drug's manufacturer. In this 6th edition of *Local Anesthesia,* only MRDs that have been approved by the U.S. Food and Drug Administration (FDA) are listed (Table 4-4).

Maximum doses are unlikely to be reached in most dental patients, especially adults of normal body weight, for most dental procedures. Two groups of patients, however, represent potentially increased risk from overly high local anesthetic blood levels: the smaller, lighter-weight (and well-behaved) child, and the debilitated elderly individual. Considerable attention must be given to drug administration in these two groups. The maximum recommended dose calculated should always be decreased in medically compromised, debilitated, or elderly persons.

Changes in liver function, plasma protein binding, blood volume, and other important physiologic functions influence the manner in which local anesthetics are distributed and biotransformed in the body.[4] The net result of these changes is increased plasma blood levels of the drug, associated with increased relative risk of overdose reaction. The half-lives of the amide local anesthetics are significantly increased in the presence of decreased liver function or perfusion.[5] Peak plasma local anesthetic blood levels tend to be higher and to remain so longer in these situations. The calculated drug dose (based on body weight) should be decreased in all "at risk" individuals. Unfortunately, there is no magical formula that can aid in determining the degree of dose reduction for a given patient. It is suggested that the doctor evaluate each patient's dental care needs and then devise a treatment plan that takes into account that person's requirement for smaller doses of local anesthetic at every treatment appointment.

A point that has come up in several medicolegal situations related to overdosage (OD) of local anesthetics involves the maximum number of milligrams administered and the effect on the patient. Assume, for example, that the MRD for a local anesthetic in a given patient is 270 mg, and the patient is administered 271 mg. The thinking among laypersons (and, unfortunately, some health care professionals too) is that an overdose will definitely occur. However, this may not be the case. As mentioned, many factors interact to determine how a patient will respond to a given drug. When the

TABLE 4-4
Maximum Recommended Dosages (MRDs) of Local Anesthetics Available in North America

	MANUFACTURER'S AND FDA (MRD)		
Local Anesthetic	**mg/kg**	**mg/lb**	**MRD, mg**
Articaine			
With vasoconstrictor	7.0	3.2	None listed
Bupivacaine			
With vasoconstrictor	None listed	None listed	90
With vasoconstrictor (Canada)	2.0	0.9	90
Lidocaine			
With vasoconstrictor	7.0	3.2	500
Mepivacaine			
No vasoconstrictor	6.6	3.0	400
With vasoconstrictor	6.6	3.0	400
Prilocaine			
No vasoconstrictor	8.0	3.6	600
With vasoconstrictor	8.0	3.6	600

	CALCULATION OF MILLIGRAMS OF LOCAL ANESTHETIC PER DENTAL CARTRIDGE (1.8 mL CARTRIDGE)		
Local Anesthetic	**Percent Concentration**	**mg/mL**	**× 1.8 mL = mg/Cartridge**
Articaine	4	40	72*
Bupivacaine	0.5	5	9
Lidocaine	2	20	36
Mepivacaine	2	20	36
	3	30	54
Prilocaine	4	40	72

MRD, Maximum recommended dose.
*Cartridges of some drugs in the United States read, "1.7 mL. each." The actual volume of all local anesthetic cartridges is approximately 1.76 mL.

BOX 4-2 Calculation of Maximum Dosage and Number of Cartridges (Single Drug)

Patient: 22 Years Old, Healthy, Female, 50 kg
Local Anesthetic: Lidocaine HCl + Epinephrine 1:100,000
Lidocaine 2% = 36 mg/cartridge
Lidocaine: 7.0 mg/kg = 350 mg (MRD)
Number of cartridges: 350/36 = ≈9¾

Patient: 40 Years Old, Healthy, Male, 90 kg
Local Anesthetic: Articaine HCl + Epinephrine 1:200,000
Articaine 4% = 72 mg/cartridge
Articaine: 7.0 mg/kg = 630 mg (MRD)
Number of cartridges: 630/72 = ≈9.0

Patient: 6 Years Old, Healthy, Male, 20 kg
Local Anesthetic: Mepivacaine HCl, No Vasoconstrictor
Mepivacaine 3% = 54 mg/cartridge
Mepivacaine: 6.6 mg/kg = 132 mg (MRD)
Number of cartridges: 130/54 = ≈2.5

MRD, Maximum recommended dose.

BOX 4-3 Calculation of Maximum Dosage and Number of Cartridges (Multiple Drugs)

Patient: 45-kg Female, Healthy
Local Anesthetic: Mepivacaine 2% + Levonordefrin 1:20,000
Mepivacaine 2% = 36 mg/cartridge
Mepivacaine: 6.6 mg/kg = 297 mg (MRD)
Patient receives 2 cartridges = 72 mg, but anesthesia is inadequate.
Doctor wishes to change to articaine 4% + epinephrine 1:100,000.

How Much Articaine Can This Patient Receive?
Articaine 2% = 72 mg/cartridge
Articaine: 7.0 mg/kg = 315 mg (MRD)
Total dose of BOTH local anesthetics should not exceed the lower of the two calculated doses, or 297 mg.
Patient has received 72 mg (lidocaine), thus can still receive 225 mg of articaine.
Therefore, 225 mg/72 mg per cartridge = ≈3.0 cartridges of articaine 4% + epinephrine 1:100,000.

MRD, Maximum recommended dose.

MRD is exceeded, there is no guarantee that an OD will occur, only that there is a greater likelihood of its occurrence. Indeed, in certain individuals, an OD may be seen with dosages below the calculated MRD (hyperresponders to the drug). Another factor in determining whether an OD will occur is the time over which the local anesthetic dose was administered. If all 271 mg is administered within a brief time frame, the resulting local anesthetic blood level will be greater than in a situation in which the same dose is administered a little at a time over several hours. These points are discussed in greater detail in Chapter 18.

Box 4-2 provides examples of how to calculate maximum dosages and numbers of local anesthetic cartridges to be administered to various patients.

A minor point, but one that has led to some confusion primarily among dental and dental hygiene students, and also doctors and hygienists in practice, is that labeling changes on some cartridges of local anesthetics indicate that the volume of solution contained in the cartridge is 1.7 mL, not the "traditional" 1.8 mL. In actual fact, dental cartridges did not always contain 1.8 mL of solution. In the late 1990s, when articaine was undergoing the FDA approval process, the question was asked of its manufacturer: "Can you guarantee that each and every cartridge contains at least 1.8 mL of solution?" The answer was "No." Cartridges are filled mechanically, and very slight variation in volume is noted from one cartridge to the next. When asked if the manufacturer could guarantee that each and every cartridge contains at least 1.7 mL of solution, the answer was "Yes." In actual fact, the average volume of local anesthetic solution in a dental cartridge in the United States is 1.76 mL.[6] When the MRD of a local anesthetic for a given patient is calculated, it is advised that a volume of 1.8 mL should be employed.

A commonly asked question is this: "How do I determine the dose of each local anesthetic administered in clinical situations in which more than one drug is necessary?" The answer is again that no guaranteed formula exists for determining this number. One method is simply to ensure that the total dose of both local anesthetics does not exceed the lower of the two maximum doses for the individual agents.

For example, a 45-kg (100-lb) patient receiving 4% prilocaine with epinephrine may be given 8.0 mg/kg (3.6 mg/lb) (or 360 mg) during a 90-minute procedure (the approximate elimination half-life of prilocaine). She receives two cartridges (144 mg), but anesthesia is inadequate for the treatment to proceed. As is commonly the case, the doctor blames the lack of anesthesia on the anesthetic drug ("I've got a bad batch of local"), not on technique error or unusual patient anatomy, as is more likely. The doctor elects to switch to lidocaine 2% with epinephrine 1:100,000 to provide anesthesia. How does one determine the maximum dose of lidocaine that may be used?

If lidocaine were being administered alone to this patient, its MRD would be 7.0 mg/kg (3.2 mg/lb) or 315 mg. However, she has already received 144 mg of prilocaine within the past few minutes. The amount of lidocaine suggested is the smaller total maximum dose (which in this case is 315 mg [lidocaine] vs. 360 mg [prilocaine]) minus the dose of prilocaine already administered (144 mg), which permits a dose of 171 mg of lidocaine, or about 4.5 cartridges, to be administered to this patient (Box 4-3).

It is extremely unlikely that a "bad batch" of local anesthetic has been distributed to the doctor. The most common causes for failure to achieve adequate pain control are anatomic variation and faulty technique. (However, blaming failure to obtain adequate pain control on the local anesthetic drug serves to soothe the doctor's ego.)

The concept of maximum recommended dose is discussed more fully in Chapter 18.

Clinically available local anesthetics (the amides: articaine, bupivacaine, lidocaine, mepivacaine, and prilocaine) are discussed in detail here. Esters (procaine and propoxycaine) are mentioned in passing, more as a matter of historical interest than of necessity. Agents available for topical application (topical anesthetics) also are discussed.

ESTER-TYPE LOCAL ANESTHETICS

Procaine HCl

Pertinent Information

Classification. Ester.

Chemical Formula. 2-Diethylaminoethyl 4-aminobenzoate hydrochloride.

$$H_2N-C_6H_4-COOCH_2CH_2N(C_2H_5)_2$$

Prepared by. Alfred Einhorn, 1904-1905.

Potency. 1 (procaine = 1)

Toxicity. 1 (procaine = 1)

Metabolism. Hydrolyzed rapidly in plasma by plasma pseudocholinesterase.

Excretion. More than 2% unchanged in the urine (90% as para-aminobenzoic acid [PABA], 8% as diethylaminoethanol).

Vasodilating Properties. Produces the greatest vasodilation of all currently used local anesthetics.

pK_a. 9.1.

pH of Plain Solution. 5.0 to 6.5.

pH of Vasoconstrictor-Containing Solution. 3.5 to 5.5.

Onset of Action. 6 to 10 minutes.

Effective Dental Concentration. 2% to 4%.

Anesthetic Half-Life. 0.1 hour (6 minutes).

Topical Anesthetic Action. Not in clinically acceptable concentrations.

Comments. Procaine HCl, the first synthetic injectable local anesthetic, is no longer available in North America in dental cartridges. However, its proprietary name, Novocain, is synonymous throughout the world with dental local anesthesia. Until 1996, procaine was found in dental cartridges in combination with a second ester anesthetic, propoxycaine.

Used as the sole local anesthetic agent for pain control in dentistry, as it was from its introduction in 1904 until the introduction of the amide local anesthetic lidocaine in the mid-1940s, 2% procaine (plain) provides essentially no pulpal anesthesia and from 15 to 30 minutes of soft tissue anesthesia. This is a result of its profound vasodilating properties. Procaine produces the greatest vasodilation of all clinically used local anesthetics. Thus a clean (e.g., bloodless) surgical field is more difficult to maintain with procaine because of increased bleeding.

Procaine is of importance in the immediate management of inadvertent intra-arterial (IA) injection of a drug; its vasodilating properties are used to aid in breaking arteriospasm.[7]

Although not extremely common, the incidence of allergy to both procaine and other ester local anesthetics is significantly greater than to amide local anesthetics.[8]

Metabolized in the blood by plasma cholinesterase, procaine does not exhibit increased toxicity in patients with hepatic dysfunction.

The maximum recommended dose of procaine, used for peripheral nerve blocks, is 1000 mg.[9]

With a dissociation constant (pK_a) of 9.1, procaine has a slow clinical onset of anesthesia (6 to 10 minutes)—a reason for inclusion of propoxycaine in the anesthetic cartridge.

Propoxycaine HCl

Pertinent Information

Classification. Ester.

Chemical Formula. 2-Diethylaminoethyl-4-amino-2-propoxybenzoate hydrochloride.

$$H_2N-C_6H_3(OC_3H_7)-COOCH_2CH_2-N(C_2H_5)_2$$

Prepared by. Clinton and Laskowski, 1952.

Potency. 7 to 8 (procaine = 1).

Toxicity. 7 to 8 (procaine = 1).

Metabolism. Hydrolyzed in both plasma and the liver.

Excretion. Via the kidneys; almost entirely hydrolyzed.

Vasodilating Properties. Yes, but not as profound as those of procaine.

pK_a. Not available.

pH of Plain Solution. Not available.

Onset of Action. Rapid (2 to 3 minutes).

Effective Dental Concentration. 0.4%.

Anesthetic Half-Life. Not available.

Topical Anesthetic Action. Not in clinically acceptable concentrations.

Comments. Propoxycaine was combined with procaine in solution to provide more rapid onset and a more profound and longer-lasting anesthesia than could be obtained with procaine alone. Propoxycaine was not available alone because its higher toxicity (seven to eight times that of procaine) limited its usefulness as a sole agent.

Procaine HCl + Propoxycaine HCl

Although it is no longer manufactured or available in the United States, the combination of two ester anesthetics, propoxycaine + procaine, was worthy of consideration for inclusion in a dentist's armamentarium of local anesthetics. It was useful when the amides were absolutely contraindicated (e.g., because of documented allergy [although this is an extremely unlikely occurrence]), or when several amide local anesthetics failed to provide clinically adequate anesthesia. Until its removal from the U.S. market in January 1996, the combination of procaine and propoxycaine was the only ester local anesthetic available in dental cartridge form.

A dose of 0.4% propoxycaine/2% procaine with 1:20,000 levonordefrin (United States) or with 1:30,000 norepinephrine (Canada) provided approximately 40 minutes of pulpal anesthesia and 2 to 3 hours of soft tissue anesthesia. The use of norepinephrine in local anesthetic solutions is no longer recommended, especially in areas where prolonged ischemia can lead to tissue necrosis. In the oral cavity, this is most likely to be seen in the palate.

Maximum Recommended Dose. The manufacturer's maximum recommended dose was 3.0 mg/lb or 6.6 mg/kg of body weight for the adult patient.[10] For children, a dose of 3.0 mg/lb was recommended up to a maximum of five cartridges.

AMIDE-TYPE LOCAL ANESTHETICS

Lidocaine HCl

Pertinent Information

Classification. Amide.

Chemical Formula. 2-Diethylamino-2′,6-acetoxylidide hydrochloride.

$$CH_3 \text{ (2,6-substituted benzene ring)}-NH \bullet CO \bullet CH_2N(C_2H_5)_2$$

Prepared by. Nils Löfgren, 1943.

FDA Approved. November 1948.

Potency. 2 (compared with procaine) (procaine = 1; lidocaine remains the standard of comparison [lidocaine = 1] for all local anesthetics).

Toxicity. 2 (compared with procaine).

Metabolism. In the liver, by the microsomal fixed-function oxidases, to monoethylglyceine and xylidide; xylidide is a local anesthetic that is potentially toxic[11] (see Fig. 2-3).

Excretion. Via the kidneys; less than 10% unchanged, more than 80% various metabolites.

Vasodilating Properties. Considerably less than those of procaine; however, greater than those of prilocaine or mepivacaine.

pK_a. 7.9.

pH of Plain Solution. 6.5.

pH of Vasoconstrictor-Containing Solution. ≈3.5.

Onset of Action. Rapid (3 to 5 minutes).

Effective Dental Concentration. 2%.

Anesthetic Half-Life. 1.6 hours (≈90 minutes).

Topical Anesthetic Action. Yes (in clinically acceptable concentrations [5%]).

Pregnancy Classification. B.

Safety During Lactation. S.

Maximum Recommended Dose. The maximum recommended dose by the FDA of lidocaine with or without epinephrine is 3.2 mg/lb or 7.0 mg/kg of body weight for the adult and pediatric patient, not to exceed a an absolute maximum dose of 500 mg[12] (Table 4-5).

Comments. Lidocaine HCl was synthesized in 1943 and in 1948 was the first amide local anesthetic to be marketed. Its entry into clinical practice transformed dentistry; it replaced procaine (Novocain) as the drug of choice for pain control. Compared with procaine, lidocaine possesses a significantly more rapid onset of action (3 to 5 minutes vs. 6 to 10 minutes), produces more profound anesthesia, has a longer duration of action, and has greater potency.

Allergy to amide local anesthetics is virtually nonexistent; true, documented, and reproducible allergic reactions are extremely rare, although possible.[13-18] This is a major clinical advantage of lidocaine (and all amides) over ester-type local anesthetics.[8]

Within only a few years of its introduction, lidocaine had replaced procaine as the most widely used local anesthetic in both medicine and dentistry—a position it maintains today in most countries. It represents the "gold standard," the drug against which all new local anesthetics are compared.

TABLE 4-5
Lidocaine Hydrochloride

			DURATION		
Proprietary	**% LA**	**Vasoconstrictor**	**Pulpal**	**Soft Tissue**	**MRD**
Lidocaine HCl					
	2	Epinephrine 1:50,000	60	180-300	7.0 mg/kg 3.6 mg/lb 500 mg absolute maximum
	2	Epinephrine 1:100,000	60	180-300	7.0 mg/kg 3.6 mg/lb 500 mg absolute maximum

MRD, Maximum recommended dose.

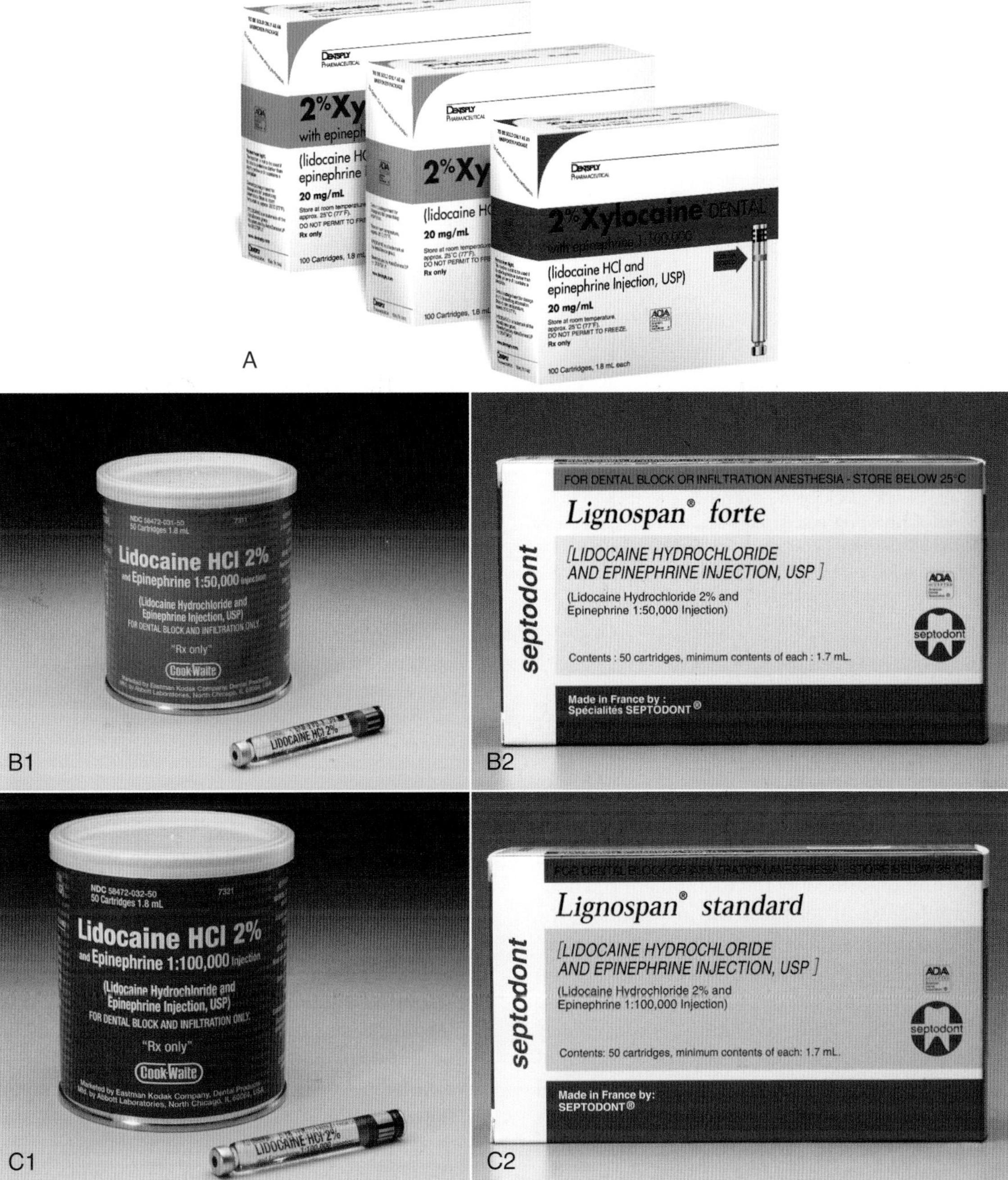

Figure 4-2. **A,** Lidocaine 2%. **B,** Lidocaine 2% with epinephrine 1:50,000. **C,** Lidocaine with epinephrine 1:100,000. (**A,** Courtesy Dentsply, York, Pa. **B** and **C,** Courtesy Eastman Kodak, New York, NY, and Septodont, New Castle, Del.)

Lidocaine HCl is available in North America in two formulations: 2% with epinephrine 1:50,000, and 2% with epinephrine 1:100,000 (Fig. 4-2). A 2% lidocaine with epinephrine 1:300,000 formulation is available in some countries (although not in North America as of August 2011). 2% lidocaine without epinephrine (2% "plain") is no longer available in dental cartridges in North America.

Two Percent Lidocaine HCl Without a Vasoconstrictor (Lidocaine Plain). Its vasodilating properties severely limit the duration and the depth of pulpal anesthesia (5 to 10 minutes). This vasodilatory effect leads to (1) higher blood levels of lidocaine, with an attendant increase in the risk of adverse reactions, along with (2) increased perfusion in the area of drug deposition. Few clinical indications are known for the use of 2% lidocaine without a vasoconstrictor in the typical dental practice. As of August 2011, 2% lidocaine without epinephrine (2% "plain") was no longer available in dental cartridges in North America.

Two Percent Lidocaine With Epinephrine 1:50,000. (Table 4-6)

TABLE 4-6
Lidocaine 2% With Epinephrine 1 : 50,000*†

CONCENTRATION: 2% MRD: 7.0 mg/kg			CARTRIDGE CONTAINS: 36 mg MRD: 3.2 mg/lb		
Weight, kg	mg	Cartridges‡	Weight, lb	mg	Cartridges‡
10	70	2.0	20	72	2.0
20	140	4.0	40	144	4.0
30	210	6.0§	60	216	6.0§
40	280	6.0§	80	288	6.0§
50	350	6.0§	100	360	6.0§
60	420	6.0§	120	432	6.0§
70	490	6.0§	140	500	6.0§
80	500	6.0§	160	500	6.0§
90	500	6.0§	180	500	6.0§
100	500	6.0§	200	500	6.0§

MRD, Maximum recommended dose.
*As with all local anesthetics, the dose varies, depending on the area to be anesthetized, the vascularity of the tissues, individual tolerance, and the technique of anesthesia. The lowest dose needed to provide effective anesthesia should be administered.
†Doses indicated are the maximum suggested for normal healthy individuals (ASA 1); they should be decreased for debilitated or elderly patients.
‡Rounded down to the nearest half-cartridge.
§200 μg of epinephrine is the dose-limiting factor (1:50,000 contains 36 μg/cartridge).

TABLE 4-7
Lidocaine 2% With Epinephrine 1 : 100,000*†‡

CONCENTRATION: 2% MRD: 7.0 mg/kg			CARTRIDGE CONTAINS: 36 mg MRD: 3.2 mg/lb		
Weight, kg	mg	Cartridges*	Weight, lb	mg	Cartridges*
10	70	2.0	20	72	2.0
20	140	4.0	40	144	4.0
30	210	6.0	60	216	6.0
40	280	7.5	80	288	8.0
50	350	9.5	100	360	10.0
60	420	11.0§	120	432	11.0§
70	490	11.0§	140	500	11.0§
80	500	11.0§	160	500	11.0§
90	500	11.0§	180	500	11.0§
100	500	11.0§	200	500	11.0§

MRD, Maximum recommended dose.
*As with all local anesthetics, the dose varies, depending on the area to be anesthetized, the vascularity of the tissues, individual tolerance, and the technique of anesthesia. The lowest dose needed to provide effective anesthesia should be administered.
†Doses indicated are the maximum suggested for normal healthy individuals (ASA 1); they should be decreased for debilitated or elderly patients.
‡Rounded to the nearest half-cartridge.
§200 μg of epinephrine is the dose-limiting factor (1:100,000 contains 18 μg/cartridge).

Inclusion of epinephrine produces a decrease in blood flow (perfusion), leading to decreased bleeding in the area of drug administration caused by the α-stimulating actions of epinephrine. Because of this decrease in perfusion, the local anesthetic is absorbed into the cardiovascular system more slowly (thereby remaining at the site of administration longer, it is hoped near the nerve), leading to an increase in both depth and duration of anesthesia: approximately 60 minutes of pulpal anesthesia and 3 to 5 hours of soft tissue anesthesia. The resultant blood level of local anesthetic is also decreased. The 1:50,000 epinephrine concentration is equal to 20 μg/mL, or 36 μg per cartridge. For patients weighing more than 45 kg (100 lb), the limiting factor in determining the MRD of this local anesthetic combination is the maximum epinephrine dose of 200 μg for the healthy patient. The MRD for epinephrine-sensitive individuals (e.g., certain cardiovascularly compromised patients [American Society of Anesthesiologists Physical Status classification system {ASA} 3] and clinically hyperthyroid patients [ASA 3]) is 40 μg per appointment. This is equivalent to about one cartridge of 1:50,000 epinephrine (see Chapter 20).

The only recommended use of 2% lidocaine with a 1:50,000 epinephrine concentration is for hemostasis (a situation wherein only small volumes are infiltrated directly into the surgical site).

Two Percent Lidocaine With Epinephrine 1:100,000. (Table 4-7)

Administration of 2% lidocaine with epinephrine 1:100,000 decreases blood flow into the area of injection. Duration of action is increased: approximately 60 minutes of pulpal anesthesia and 3 to 5 hours of soft tissue anesthesia. In addition to the lower blood level of lidocaine, less bleeding occurs in the area of drug administration. The epinephrine dilution is 10 μg/mL, or 18 μg per cartridge. Epinephrine-sensitive patients (see earlier discussion for lidocaine with 1:50,000 epineprhine) should be limited to two cartridges of 1:100,000 epinephrine per appointment.

The duration and depth of pulpal anesthesia attained with both lidocaine-epinephrine solutions (1:50,000 and 1:100,000) are equivalent. Each may provide approximately 60 minutes of pulpal anesthesia in ideal circumstances and soft tissue anesthesia of 3 to 5 hours' duration. Indeed, 2% lidocaine with 1:200,000 or 1:300,000 epinephrine provides the same duration of pulpal and soft tissue anesthesia, although not the same level of hemostasis.[19]

In terms of duration and depth of anesthesia for most procedures in a typical dental patient, 2% lidocaine with 1:100,000 epinephrine is preferred to 2% lidocaine with 1:50,000 epinephrine. Both formulations provide equal duration and depth, but the 1:100,000 solution contains only half as much epinephrine as the 1:50,000 solution. Although the dose of epinephrine in the 1:50,000 solution is not dangerous to most patients, ASA-3 and -4 risks with histories of cardiovascular disorders might prove overly sensitive to these concentrations. Also, an elderly patient is likely to be more hyper-responsive to vasoconstrictors. In these individuals, the more dilute formulation (1:100,000 or 1:200,000) should be used.

For hemostasis in procedures in which bleeding is definitely or potentially a problem, 2% lidocaine with 1:50,000 epinephrine is recommended because it decreases bleeding (during periodontal surgery) by 50% compared with a 1:100,000 epinephrine dilution.[20] Vasoconstrictors act directly at the site of administration to decrease tissue perfusion, and the 1:50,000 solution provides excellent hemostatic action. The 1:100,000 dilution also may be used for hemostasis, but it is not as effective. Rebound vasodilation occurs with both 1:50,000 and 1:100,000 epinephrine concentrations as the tissue concentration of epinephrine decreases. Minimum volumes of solution should be administered to provide excellent hemostasis.

Signs and symptoms of lidocaine toxicity (overdose) may be the same (central nervous system [CNS] stimulation followed by CNS depression) as those described in Chapter 2. However, the stimulatory phase may be brief or may not develop at all.[21] Although muscle tremor and seizures commonly occur with overly high lidocaine blood levels, the first signs and symptoms of lidocaine overdose may include drowsiness, leading to loss of consciousness and respiratory arrest.

Mepivacaine HCl

Pertinent Information

Classification. Amide.

Chemical Formula. 1-methyl 2′,6′-pipecoloxylidide hydrochloride.

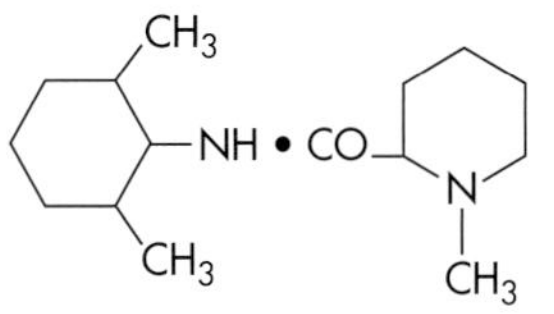

Prepared by. A.F. Ekenstam, 1957; introduced into dentistry in 1960 as a 2% solution containing the synthetic vasopressor levonordefrin, and in 1961 as a 3% solution without a vasoconstrictor.

FDA Approved. April 1960.

Potency. 2 (procaine = 1; lidocaine = 2).

Toxicity. 1.5 to 2 (procaine = 1; lidocaine = 2).

Metabolism. In the liver, by microsomal fixed-function oxidases. Hydroxylation and *N*-demethylation play important roles in the metabolism of mepivacaine.

Excretion. Via the kidneys; approximately 1% to 16% of anesthetic dose is excreted unchanged.

Vasodilating Properties. Mepivacaine produces only slight vasodilation. The duration of pulpal anesthesia with mepivacaine without a vasoconstrictor is 20 to 40 minutes (lidocaine without a vasoconstrictor is but 5 to 10 minutes; procaine without a vasoconstrictor may produce effects up to 2 minutes).

pK_a. 7.6.

pH of Plain Solution. 5.5 to 6.0.

pH of Vasoconstrictor-Containing Solution. 4.0.

Onset of Action. Rapid (3 to 5 minutes).

Effective Dental Concentration. 3% without a vasoconstrictor; 2% with a vasoconstrictor.

Anesthetic Half-Life. 1.9 hours.

Topical Anesthetic Action. Not in clinically acceptable concentrations.

Pregnancy Classification. C.

Safety During Lactation. S?

Maximum Recommended Dose. MRD is 6.6 mg/kg or 3.0 mg/kg of body weight, not to exceed 400 mg[22] (Table 4-8).

Comments. The milder vasodilating property of mepivacaine leads to a longer duration of pulpal anesthesia than is observed with most other local anesthetics when administered without a vasoconstrictor. Mepivacaine 3% plain provides 20 to 40 minutes of pulpal anesthesia (20 minutes via infiltration; 40 minutes via nerve block) and approximately 2 to 3 hours of soft tissue anesthesia.

Three Percent Mepivacaine Without a Vasoconstrictor. (Fig. 4-3 and Table 4-9)

This is recommended for patients in whom a vasoconstrictor is not indicated and for dental procedures requiring

TABLE 4-8
Mepivacaine Hydrochloride

			DURATION		
Proprietary	**% LA**	**Vasoconstrictor**	**Pulpal**	**Soft Tissue**	**MRD**
Mepivacaine HCl	3	None	20—infiltration 40—nerve block	120-180	6.6 mg/kg 3.0 mg/lb 400 mg absolute maximum
Mepivacaine HCl	2	Levonordefrin	60	180-300	6.6 mg/kg 3.0 mg/lb 400 mg absolute maximum

MRD, Maximum recommended dose.

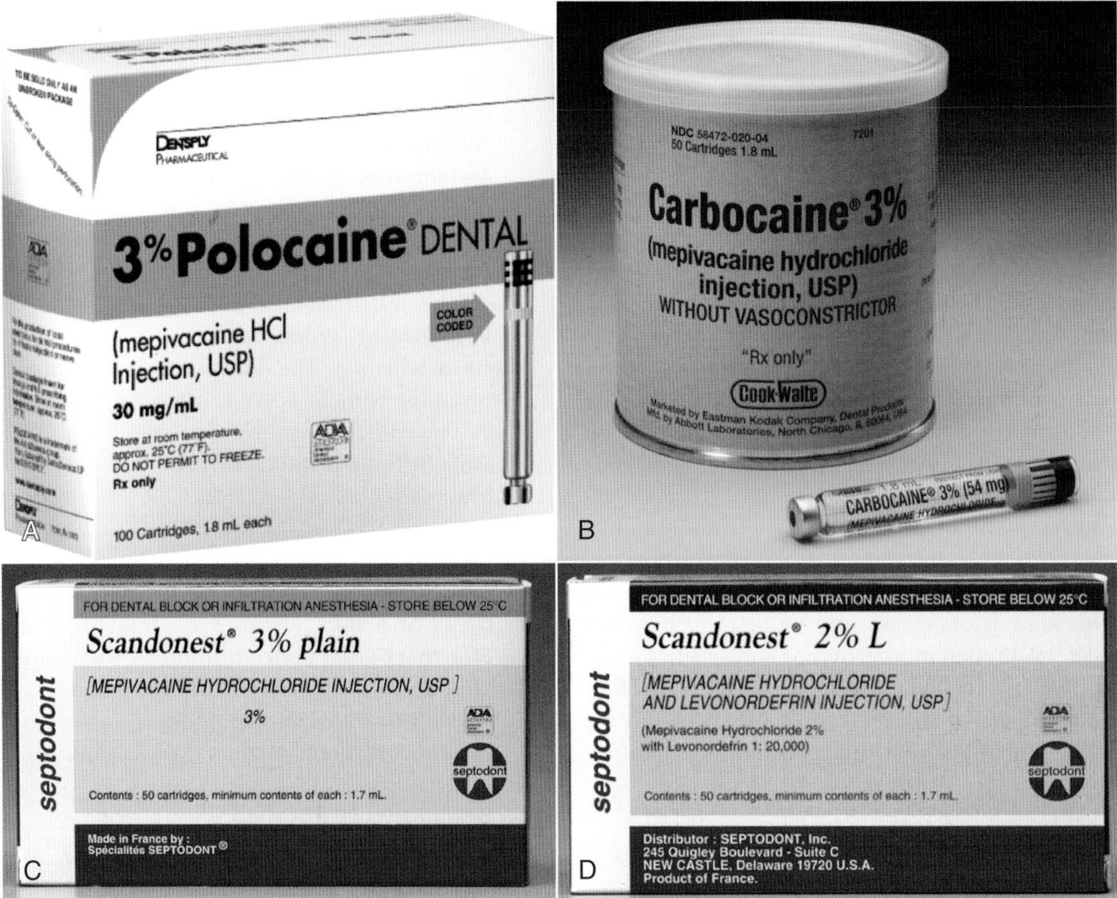

Figure 4-3. A through **C,** Mepivacaine 3%. **D,** Mepivacaine 2% with levonordefrin 1:20,000. (**A,** Courtesy Dentsply, York, Pa. **B,** Courtesy Eastman Kodak, New York, NY. **D,** Courtesy Septodont, New Castle, Del.)

TABLE 4-9
Mepivacaine 3% Without Vasoconstrictor*†

CONCENTRATION: 3% MRD: 6.6 mg/kg			CARTRIDGE CONTAINS: 54 mg MRD: 3.0 mg/lb		
Weight, kg	**mg**	**Cartridges‡**	**Weight, lb**	**mg**	**Cartridges‡**
10	66	1.0	20	60	1.0
20	132	2.5	40	120	2.0
30	198	3.5	60	180	3.0
40	264	4.5	80	240	4.5
50	330	6.0	100	300	5.5
60	396	7.0	120	360	6.5
70	400	7.5	140	400	7.5
80	400	7.5	160	400	7.5
90	400	7.5	180	400	7.5
100	400	7.5	200	400	7.5

MRD, Maximum recommended dose.
*As with all local anesthetics, the dose varies, depending on the area to be anesthetized, the vascularity of the tissues, individual tolerance, and the technique of anesthesia. The lowest dose needed to provide effective anesthesia should be administered.
†Doses indicated are the maximum suggested for normal healthy individuals (ASA 1); they should be decreased for debilitated or elderly patients.
‡Rounded down to the nearest half-cartridge.

neither lengthy nor profound pulpal anesthesia. Mepivacaine plain is the most used local anesthetic in pediatric patients when the treating doctor is not a pediatric dentist (e.g., is a general practitioner) and often is quite appropriate in the management of geriatric patients.

Two Percent Mepivacaine With a Vasoconstrictor, Levonordefrin 1:20,000. (Table 4-10)

This solution provides depth and duration of pulpal (hard tissue) and total (soft tissue) anesthesia similar to those observed with lidocaine-epinephrine solutions. Pulpal anesthesia of approximately 60 minutes' duration and soft tissue anesthesia of 3 to 5 hours are to be expected. Mepivacaine is available in combination with levonordefrin (1:20,000). Where hemostasis is desired , epinephrine is preferred to levonordefrin.

The incidence of true, documented, and reproducible allergy to mepivacaine, an amide local anesthetic, is virtually nonexistent.

Signs and symptoms of mepivacaine overdose usually follow the more typical pattern of CNS stimulation followed by depression. Although possible, absence of stimulation with immediate CNS depression (e.g., drowsiness and unconsciousness, as is seen more commonly with lidocaine) is rare with mepivacaine.

TABLE 4-10
Mepivacaine 2% With Vasoconstrictor*†

CONCENTRATION: 2% MRD: 6.6 mg/kg			CARTRIDGE CONTAINS: 36 mg MRD: 3.0 mg/lb		
Weight, kg	mg	Cartridges‡	Weight, lb	mg	Cartridges‡
10	66	1.5	20	60	1.5
20	132	3.5	40	120	3.0
30	198	5.5	60	180	5.0
40	264	7.0	80	240	6.5
50	330	9.0	100	300	8.0
60	396	11.0	120	360	10.0
70	400	11.0	140	400	11.0
80	400	11.0	160	400	11.0
90	400	11.0	180	400	11.0
100	400	11.0	200	400	11.0

MRD, Maximum recommended dose.
*As with all local anesthetics, the dose varies, depending on the area to be anesthetized, the vascularity of the tissues, individual tolerance, and the technique of anesthesia. The lowest dose needed to provide effective anesthesia should be administered.
†Doses indicated are the maximum suggested for normal healthy individuals (ASA 1); they should be decreased for debilitated or elderly patients.
‡Rounded down to the nearest half-cartridge.

Prilocaine HCl

Pertinent Information

Classification. Amide.

Other Chemical Name. Propitocaine.

Chemical Formula. 2-Propylamino-*o*-propionotoluidide hydrochloride.

$$C_6H_4(CH_3)-NH \cdot CO \cdot CH(CH_3) \cdot N(C_3H_7)H$$

Prepared by. Löfgren and Tegnér, 1953; reported in 1960.

FDA Approved. November 1965.

Potency. 2 (procaine = 1; lidocaine = 2).

Toxicity. 1 (procaine = 1; lidocaine = 2); 40% less toxic than lidocaine.

Metabolism. The metabolism of prilocaine differs significantly from that of lidocaine and mepivacaine. Because it is a secondary amine, prilocaine is hydrolyzed straightforwardly by hepatic amidases into orthotoluidine and *N*-propylalanine. Carbon dioxide is a major end product of prilocaine biotransformation. The efficiency of the body's degradation of prilocaine is demonstrated by the extremely small fraction of intact prilocaine recoverable in the urine.[23] Orthotoluidine can induce the formation of methemoglobin, producing methemoglobinemia if large doses are administered. Minor degrees of methemoglobinemia have been observed following both benzocaine and lidocaine administration,[24,25] but prilocaine consistently reduces the blood's oxygen-carrying capacity, at times sufficiently to cause observable cyanosis.[26,27] Limiting the total prilocaine dose to 600 mg (FDA recommendation) avoids symptomatic cyanosis. Methemoglobin blood levels less than 20% usually do not produce clinical signs or symptoms (which include grayish or slate blue cyanosis of the lips, mucous membranes, and nail beds and [infrequently] respiratory and circulatory distress). Methemoglobinemia may be reversed within 15 minutes with administration of 1 to 2 mg/kg body weight of 1% methylene blue solution intravenously over a 5-minute period.[25] The mechanism of methemoglobin production is discussed in Chapter 10. Prilocaine undergoes biotransformation more rapidly and completely than lidocaine; this takes place not only in the liver but also to a lesser degree in the kidneys and lungs.[27] Plasma levels of prilocaine decrease more rapidly than those of lidocaine.[28] Prilocaine thus is considered to be less toxic systemically than comparably potent local anesthetic amides.[29] Signs of CNS toxicity after prilocaine administration in humans are briefer and less severe than after the same intravenous (IV) dose of lidocaine.[30]

Excretion. Prilocaine and its metabolites are excreted primarily via the kidneys. Renal clearance of prilocaine is faster than for other amides, resulting in its faster removal from the circulation.[31]

Vasodilating Properties. Prilocaine is a vasodilator. It produces greater vasodilation than is produced by mepivacaine but less than lidocaine and significantly less than procaine.

pK_a. 7.9.

pH of Plain Solution. 6.0 to 6.5.

pH of Vasoconstrictor-Containing Solution. 4.0.

Onset of Action. Slightly slower than that of lidocaine (3 to 5 minutes).

Effective Dental Concentration. 4%.

Anesthetic Half-Life. 1.6 hours.

Topical Anesthetic Action. Not in clinically acceptable concentrations.

Prilocaine, in its uncharged base form, is an integral part of EMLA cream (eutectic mixture of the local anesthetics lidocaine and prilocaine), a formulation that permits anesthetics to penetrate the imposing anatomic barrier of intact skin. EMLA cream is used to provide topical anesthesia of skin before venipuncture and other painful cosmetic procedures.[33,34]

Pregnancy Classification. B.

Safety During Lactation. Unknown.

Maximum Recommended Dose. The MRD for prilocaine is 8.0 mg/kg or 3.6 mg/lb of body weight for the adult patient, to a maximum recommended dose of 600 mg (Table 4-11).[31]

TABLE 4-11
Prilocaine Hydrochloride

Proprietary	% LA	Vasoconstrictor	DURATION Pulpal	DURATION Soft Tissue	MRD
Prilocaine HCl	4	None	10-15 infiltration 40-60 nerve block	90-120 infiltration 120-240 nerve block	8.0 mg/kg 3.6 mg/lb 600 mg absolute maximum
Prilocaine HCl	4	Epinephrine 1:200,000	60-90	180-480	8.0 mg/kg 3.6 mg/lb 600 mg absolute maximum

MRD, Maximum recommended dose.

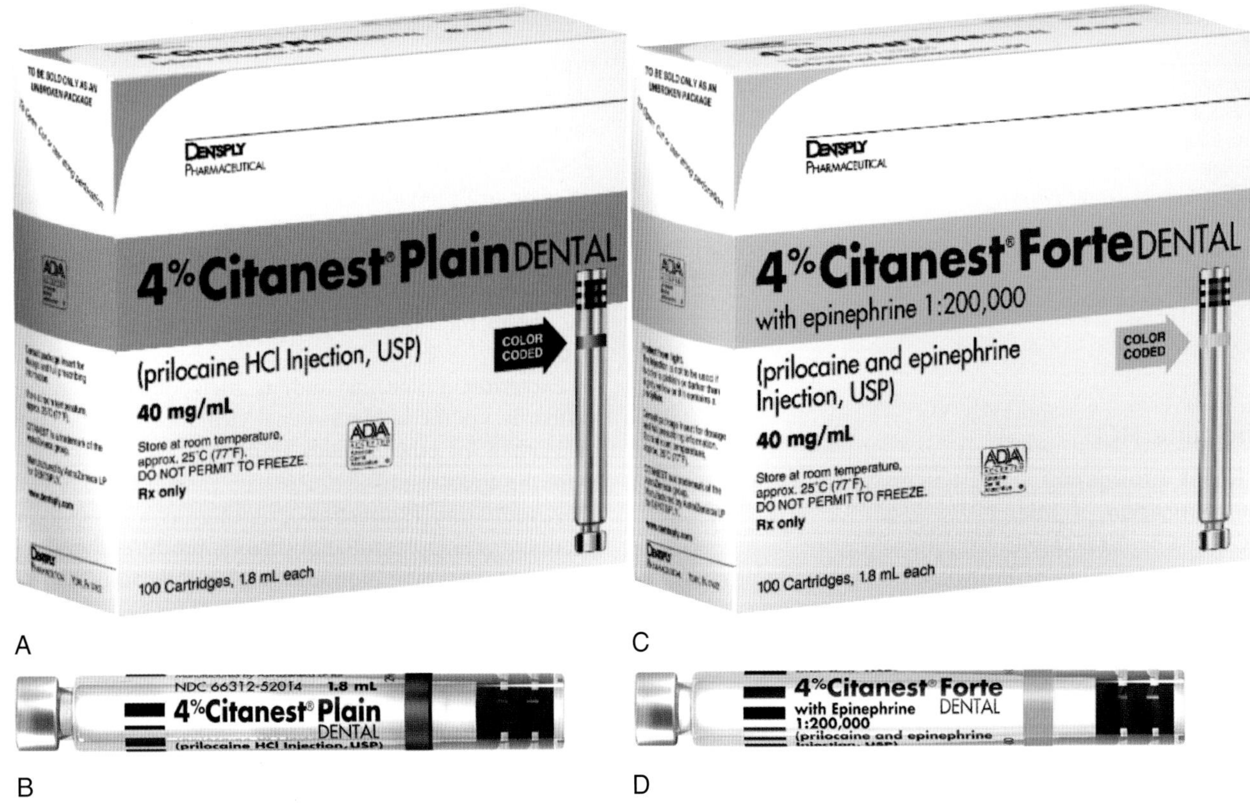

Figure 4-4. **A** and **B**, Prilocaine 4%. **C** and **D**, Prilocaine 4% with epinephrine 1:200,000. (Courtesy Dentsply, York, Pa.)

Comments. Clinical actions of prilocaine plain (Fig. 4-4) vary significantly with the type of injection technique used. Although true for all anesthetics, the variation between supraperiosteal infiltration and nerve block is more pronounced with prilocaine plain (and mepivacaine plain). Infiltration provides short durations of pulpal (10 to 15 minutes) and soft tissue (1½ to 2 hours) anesthesia, whereas regional nerve block (e.g., inferior alveolar nerve block) provides pulpal anesthesia for up to 60 minutes (commonly 40 to 60 minutes) and soft tissue anesthesia for 2 to 4 hours.[32] Thus prilocaine plain frequently is able to provide anesthesia that is equal in duration to that attained with lidocaine or mepivacaine with a vasoconstrictor.

Clinical actions of prilocaine with 1:200,000 epinephrine are not as dependent on anesthetic technique. Prilocaine with epinephrine provides lengthy anesthesia while offering a less concentrated epinephrine dilution: 1:200,000. Pulpal anesthesia of 60 to 90 minutes' duration and soft tissue anesthesia of 3 to 8 hours are common. The cartridge contains 9 μg of epinephrine, therefore epinephrine-sensitive individuals, such as the ASA 3 cardiovascular disease patient, may receive up to four cartridges (36 μg) of prilocaine with epinephrine.

In epinephrine-sensitive patients requiring prolonged pulpal anesthesia (≥60 minutes), prilocaine plain or with 1:200,000 epinephrine is strongly recommended. It is rapidly

TABLE 4-12
Prilocaine 4% With and Without Vasoconstrictor*†

CONCENTRATION: 4% MRD: 8.0 mg/kg			CARTRIDGE CONTAINS: 72 mg MRD: 3.6 mg/lb		
Weight, kg	mg	Cartridges‡	Weight, lb	mg	Cartridges‡
10	80	1.0	20	72	1.0
20	160	2.0	40	144	2.0
30	240	3.0	60	218	3.0
40	320	4.5	80	290	4.0
50	400	5.5	100	362	5.0
60	480	6.5	120	434	6.0
70	560	7.5	140	506	7.0
80	600	8.0	160	578	8.0
90	600	8.0	180	600	8.0
100	600	8.0	200	600	8.0

MRD, Maximum recommended dose.
*As with all local anesthetics, the dose varies, depending on the area to be anesthetized, the vascularity of the tissues, individual tolerance, and the technique of anesthesia. The lowest dose needed to provide effective anesthesia should be administered.
†Doses indicated are the maximum suggested for normal healthy individuals (ASA 1); they should be decreased for debilitated or elderly patients.
‡Rounded to the nearest half-cartridge.

biotransformed and, for this reason, is considered to be a safe local anesthetic (e.g., lower toxicity).[28]

Prilocaine is relatively contraindicated in patients with idiopathic or congenital methemoglobinemia, hemoglobinopathies (sickle cell anemia), anemia, or cardiac or respiratory failure evidenced by hypoxia, because methemoglobin levels are increased, decreasing oxygen-carrying capacity. Prilocaine administration is also relatively contraindicated in patients receiving acetaminophen or phenacetin, both of which produce elevations in methemoglobin levels (Table 4-12).

It has been claimed that prilocaine HCl 4% solution (with or without vasopressor) is associated with a higher risk of paresthesia, primarily of the lingual nerve, than other anesthetic formulations following inferior alveolar nerve block.[34,35] Although the "evidence" remains anecdotal, it appears that this drug, as formulated in North America [as a 4% solution], might be more neurotoxic than other commonly used local anesthetic formulations.[36] This question will be discussed in greater detail in Chapter 17.

Articaine HCl

Pertinent Information

Classification. Hybrid molecule. Classified as an amide; however, it possesses both amide and ester characteristics.

Chemical Formula. 3-*N*-Propylamino-proprionylamino-2-carbomethoxy-4-methylthiophene hydrochloride.

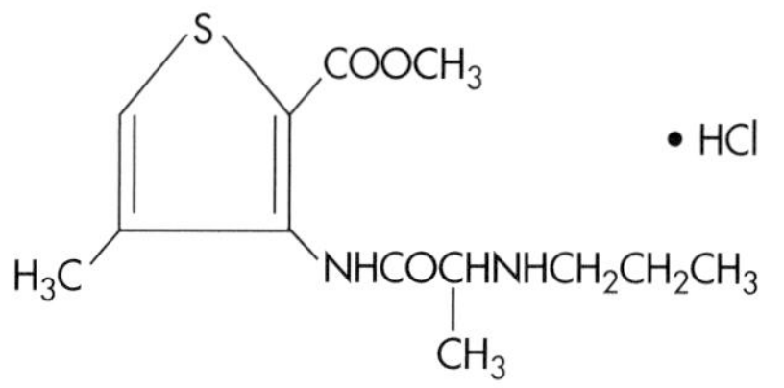

S
$COOCH_3$
• HCl
H_3C
$NHCOCHNHCH_2CH_2CH_3$
CH_3

Prepared by. H. Rusching et al, 1969.

FDA Approved. April 2000 (United States).

Introduced. 1976 in Germany and Switzerland, 1983 in Canada, 2000 in the United States.

Potency. 1.5 times that of lidocaine; 1.9 times that of procaine.

Toxicity. Similar to lidocaine and procaine.

Metabolism. Articaine is the only amide-type local anesthetic that contains a thiophene group. Because articaine HCl is the only widely used amide-type local anesthetic that contains an ester group, biotransformation of articaine HCl occurs in both plasma (hydrolysis by plasma esterase) and liver (hepatic microsomal enzymes). Degradation of articaine HCl is initiated by hydrolysis of the carboxylic acid ester groups to obtain free carboxylic acid.[37] Its primary metabolite, articainic acid, is pharmacologically inactive, undergoing additional biotransformation to form articainic acid glucuronide.[37] Additional metabolites have been detected in animal studies.[38] From this point, the reaction can follow several pathways: cleavage of carboxylic acid, formation of an acid amino group by internal cyclization, and oxidation.

Excretion. Via the kidneys; approximately 5% to 10% unchanged, approximately 90% metabolites (M_1 at 87%, M_2 at 2%).

Vasodilating Properties. Articaine has a vasodilating effect equal to that of lidocaine. Procaine is slightly more vasoactive.

pK_a. 7.8.

pH of Plain Solution. Not available in North America (4% articaine HCl "plain" is available in Germany).

pH of Vasoconstrictor-Containing Solution. 3.5 to 4.0.

Onset of Action. Articaine 1:200,000, infiltration 1 to 2 minutes, mandibular block 2 to 3 minutes; articaine 1:100,000, infiltration 1 to 2 minutes, mandibular block 2 to 2½ minutes.

Effective Dental Concentration. 4% with 1:100,000 or 1:200,000 epinephrine. Articaine HCl is available with epinephrine 1:400,000 in Germany.

Anesthetic Half-Life. 0.5 hours [27 minutes].[39]

Topical Anesthetic Action. Not in clinically acceptable concentrations.

Pregnancy Classification. C.

Safety During Lactation. Unknown (use with caution in females who are breast-feeding because it is not known whether articaine is excreted in milk).

Maximum Recommended Dose. The FDA maximum recommended dose is 7.0 mg/kg or 3.2 mg/lb of body weight for the adult patient (Tables 4-13 and 4-14).[22,40]

TABLE 4-13
Articaine Hydrochloride

Proprietary	% LA	Vasoconstrictor	DURATION Pulpal	DURATION Soft Tissue	MRD
Articaine HCl	4	Epinephrine 1:100,000	60-75	180-360	7.0 mg/kg 3.2 mg/lb No absolute maximum
Articaine HCl	4	Epinephrine 1:200,000	45-60	120-300	7.0 mg/kg 3.2 mg/lb No absolute maximum

MRD, Maximum recommended dose.

TABLE 4-14
Articaine 4% With Epinephrine 1:100,000 or 1:200,000*†

CONCENTRATION: 4% MRD: 7.0 mg/kg			CARTRIDGE CONTAINS: 72 mg MRD: 3.6 mg/lb		
Weight, kg	mg	Cartridges‡	Weight, lb	mg	Cartridges‡
10	70	1.0	20	72	1.0
20	140	2.0	40	144	2.0
30	210	3.0	60	216	3.0
40	280	4.0	80	288	4.0
50	350	5.0	100	360	5.0
60	420	6.0	120	432	6.0
70	490	7.0	140	504	7.0
80	560	8.0	160	576	8.0
90	630	9.0	180	648	9.0
100	700	10.0	200	720	10.0

MRD, Maximum recommended dose.
*As with all local anesthetics, the dose varies, depending on the area to be anesthetized, the vascularity of the tissues, individual tolerance, and the technique of anesthesia. The lowest dose needed to provide effective anesthesia should be administered.
†Doses indicated are the maximum suggested for normal healthy individuals (ASA 1); they should be decreased for debilitated or elderly patients.
‡Rounded to the nearest half-cartridge.

Comments. Originally known as carticaine, the generic nomenclature of this local anesthetic was changed in 1984 to articaine. Literature appearing before 1984 should be reviewed under the original name.

Articaine is the only anesthetic of the amide type to possess a thiophene ring as its lipophilic moiety. It has many of the physicochemical properties of other local anesthetics, with the exception of the aromatic moiety and the degree of protein binding.

Articaine has been available in Europe since 1976 and in Canada since 1984 in two formulations: 4% with 1:100,000 epinephrine and 4% with 1:200,000 epinephrine (Fig. 4-5). In 2000 the FDA approved articaine HCl with epinephrine 1:100,000 for marketing in the United States.[41-43] The formulation with 1:100:000 epinephrine provides between 60 and 75 minutes of pulpal anesthesia; the 1:200,000 formulation, approximately 45 to 60 minutes.[44,45]

Since its introduction into the U.S. dental market in June 2000, articaine has steadily become increasingly popular. As of May 2011 articaine was the second most used dental local anesthetic in the United States (≈40% market share).[46] Articaine, as the newest local anesthetic drug marketed, has been the subject of intense discussion and of many (anecdotal) claims made by dentists, some good (faster onset, increased success rates; "don't miss as often"), some bad (increased risk of paresthesia). It has been claimed that articaine is able to diffuse through soft and hard tissues more reliably than other local anesthetics.[47,48] Clinically, it is claimed that following maxillary buccal infiltration, articaine on occasion may provide palatal soft tissue anesthesia, obviating the need for palatal injection, which, in many hands, is traumatic.[48]

Some initial claims about articaine have been shown to be true, specifically, the significant success of articaine administered by buccal infiltration in the mandible of adult patients. [49-55] This is discussed more fully in Chapter 20.

The success of articaine in the United States mirrors its success elsewhere. In Germany, the first country to have articaine (1976), by 1989 it was used by 71.7% of German dentists,[56] and by 2010 it commanded 95% of the dental local anesthetic market.[57] Articaine has become the leading local anesthetic in Canada, which acquired it in 1983; in the United States, where articaine has been available since June of 2000, it presently (May 2011) commands 40% of the local anesthetic market.[46]

Reports of paresthesia following local anesthetic administration became more frequent after the introduction of articaine into the United States. An overwhelming majority of reported cases occurred following inferior alveolar nerve block and primarily involved the lingual nerve. The question of paresthesia related to local anesthetic drug administration is addressed in depth in Chapter 17.

In previous editions of this textbook, methemoglobinemia was listed as a potential side effect of administration of large doses of articaine.[58] Such reactions had been noted after the IV administration of articaine for regional anesthetic

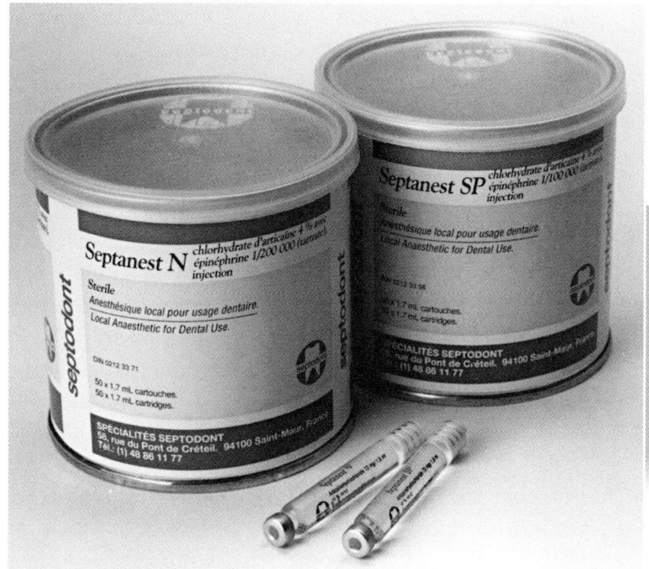

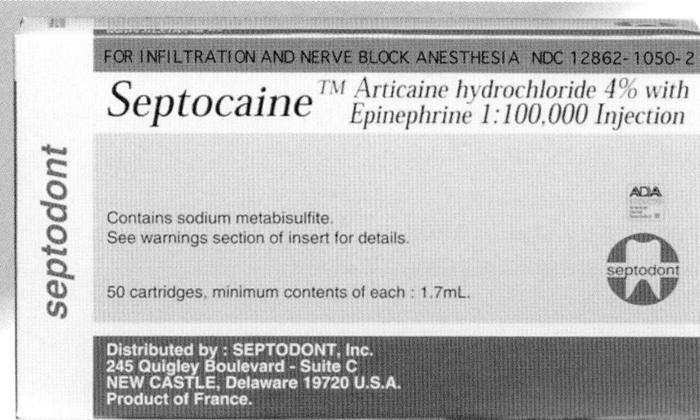

Figure 4-5. Articaine 4% with epinephrine 1:100,000 and 1:200,000. (Courtesy Septodont, New Castle, Del.)

purposes; however, no cases have ever been reported when articaine was administered in the usual manner and volume for dental procedures.

Articaine HCl with epinephrine is contraindicated in persons with known sensitivity to amide-type local anesthetics (few to none) and in persons with sulfite sensitivity (such as some asthmatic patients with allergic-type asthma, as epinephrine-containing LA formulations contain the antioxidant Na metabisulfite). Articaine HCl should be used with caution in persons with hepatic disease and significant impairment in cardiovascular function because amide-type local anesthetics undergo biotransformation in the liver and possess myocardial depressant properties. Articaine is listed by the U.S. FDA as a Class C drug during pregnancy. Use with caution in females who are breast-feeding because it is not known whether articaine is excreted in milk.[59] Administration to children younger than 4 years is not recommended because insufficient data are available to support such usage.

Cartridges of articaine marketed in the United States are listed as containing "1.7 mL" (Fig. 4-6), in contrast to other local anesthetic cartridges, which are labeled as "1.8 mL." Some might interpret this to mean that the cartridge consists of 68 mg. This is incorrect. Articaine HCl cartridges are identical in all ways to other dental cartridges. However, as discussed earlier in this chapter, a change was made to labeling, not to content.

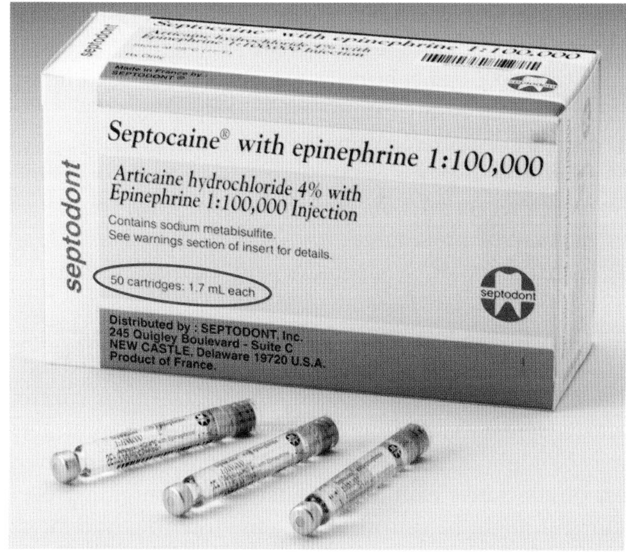

Figure 4-6. Articaine box showing "1.7 mL each."

CH_3
NH • CO
N
CH_3
C_4H_9

Bupivacaine HCl

Pertinent Information

Classification. Amide.

Chemical Formula. 1-Butyl-2′,6′-pipecoloxylidide hydrochloride; structurally related to mepivacaine except for a butyl group replacing a methyl group.

Prepared by. A.F. Ekenstam, 1957.

FDA Approved. October 1972.

Potency. Four times that of lidocaine, mepivacaine, and prilocaine.

Toxicity. Less than four times that of lidocaine and mepivacaine.

Metabolism. Metabolized in the liver by amidases.

Excretion. Via the kidney; 16% unchanged bupivacaine has been recovered from human urine.

Vasodilating Properties. Relatively significant: greater than those of lidocaine, prilocaine, and mepivacaine, yet considerably less than those of procaine.

pK_a. 8.1.

pH of Plain Solution. 4.5 to 6.0.

pH of Vasoconstrictor-Containing Solution. 3.0 to 4.5.

Onset of Action. Slower onset time than other commonly used local anesthetics (e.g., 6 to 10 minutes).

Effective Dental Concentration. 0.5%.

Anesthetic Half-Life. 2.7 hours.

Topical Anesthetic Action. Not in clinically acceptable concentrations.

Pregnancy Classification. C.

Safety During Lactation. S?

Maximum Recommended Dose. The FDA maximum recommended dose of bupivacaine is 90 mg. There is no recommended dosage for bupivacaine based on body weight in the United States (Table 4-15).[60] In Canada, the maximum dose is based on 2.0 mg/kg (0.9 mg/lb).

Comments. Bupivacaine has been available in cartridge form since February 1982 in Canada and July 1983 in the United States. Bupivacaine is available as a 0.5% solution with 1:200,000 epinephrine (Fig. 4-7); there are two primary indications for its utilization in dentistry:

1. Lengthy dental procedures for which pulpal (deep) anesthesia in excess of 90 minutes is necessary (e.g., full mouth reconstruction, implant surgery, extensive periodontal procedures)
2. Management of postoperative pain (e.g., endodontic, periodontal, postimplant, surgical)

The patient's requirement for postoperative opioid analgesics is considerably lessened when bupivacaine is administered for pain control.[61] For postoperative pain control after a short surgical procedure (<30 minutes), bupivacaine may be administered at the start of the procedure; however, for postoperative pain control after lengthy surgical procedures, it might be reasonable to administer bupivacaine at the conclusion of the procedure, shortly before the patient's discharge from the office.

A regimen for management of postsurgical pain has been developed that is clinically quite effective.[62-64] It suggests the pretreatment administration of one oral dose of a nonsteroidal anti-inflammatory drug (NSAID), followed by administration of any suitable (e.g., intermediate-duration) local anesthetic to manage periprocedural pain. A long-duration local anesthetic (bupivacaine) is administered immediately before patient discharge (if deemed necessary), with the patient continuing to take the oral dose of NSAID every "x" hours as indicated (not "prn pain") for "y" number of days. The requirement for opioid agonist analgesics is significantly diminished with this protocol. Hargreaves demonstrated that the preoperative oral dose of NSAID is not necessary as long as the initial oral dose can be ingested within 1 hour of the start of the surgical procedure.[65]

Onset of anesthesia with bupivacaine is commonly delayed for from 6 to 10 minutes, a fact that is understandable in view of its pK_a of 8.1. If this occurs, it may be advisable, at subsequent appointments, to initiate procedural pain control with a more rapid-acting amide (e.g., articaine, mepivacaine, lidocaine, prilocaine), which provides clinically acceptable pain control within a few moments, allowing the procedure to commence more promptly. Follow this with an injection of bupivacaine for long-duration anesthesia.

Bupivacaine is not recommended in younger patients or in those for whom the risk of postoperative soft tissue injury produced by self-mutilation is increased, such as physically and mentally disabled persons. Bupivacaine is

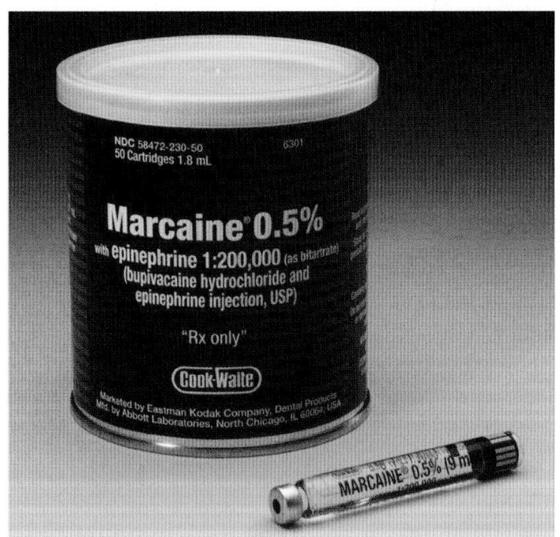

Figure 4-7. Bupivacaine 0.5% with epinephrine 1:200,000. (Courtesy Eastman Kodak, New York, NY.)

TABLE 4-15
Bupivacaine Hydrochloride

Proprietary	% LA	Vasoconstrictor	DURATION Pulpal	DURATION Soft Tissue	MRD
Bupivacaine HCl	0.5	Epinephrine 1:200,000	90-180	240-540 (reports up to 720)	United States: no mg/kg or mg/lb listed Canada: 2.0 mg/kg, 0.9 mg/lb, 90 mg absolute maximum

MRD, Maximum recommended dose.

rarely indicated in children because pediatric dental procedures are usually of short duration.

Etidocaine HCl

Pertinent Information

Classification. Amide.

Chemical Formula. 2-(*N*-Ethylpropylamino) butyro-2,6-xylidide hydrochloride; structurally similar to lidocaine.

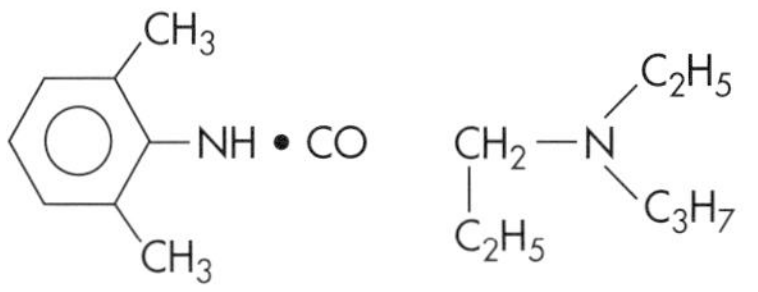

CH_3 / CH_3 (2,6-dimethylphenyl)—NH • CO — $CH(C_2H_5)$ — $N(C_2H_5)(C_3H_7)$

Prepared by. Takman, 1971.

FDA Approved. August 1976.

Dental cartridges of etidocaine HCl with epinephrine 1:200,000 were withdrawn from the North American market in 2002. For a detailed description of etidocaine HCl, the reader is referred to the 5th edition of this textbook.[66]

ANESTHETICS FOR TOPICAL APPLICATION

Use of topically applied local anesthetics is an important component of the atraumatic administration of intraoral local anesthesia (see Chapter 11). Conventional topical anesthetics are unable to penetrate intact skin but do diffuse through abraded skin (e.g., sunburn) and any mucous membranes.

The concentration of a local anesthetic applied topically is typically greater than that of the same local anesthetic administered by injection. The higher concentration facilitates diffusion of the drug through the mucous membrane. Higher concentration also increases the risk of toxicity, both locally to tissues and systemically if the drug is efficiently absorbed.[67] Because topical anesthetic formulations do not contain vasoconstrictors and local anesthetics have vasodilatory properties, vascular absorption of some topical formulations is rapid, and blood levels may quickly reach those achieved by direct IV administration.[67]

Many local anesthetics used effectively via injection prove ineffective when applied topically (e.g., articaine HCl, mepivacaine HCl, prilocaine HCl, procaine HCl) because the concentrations necessary to produce anesthesia via topical application are high, with significantly increased overdose and local tissue toxicity potential (Table 4-16).

As a general rule, topical anesthetics are effective only on surface tissues (2 to 3 mm). Tissues deep to the area of application are poorly anesthetized, if at all. However, surface anesthesia does allow for atraumatic needle penetration of the mucous membrane.[68,69]

The topical anesthetics benzocaine and lidocaine base (not the HCl form used by injection) are insoluble in water. However, they are soluble in alcohol, propylene glycol, polyethylene glycol, and other vehicles suitable for surface application. The base forms of benzocaine and lidocaine are slowly absorbed into the cardiovascular system and therefore are less likely to produce an overdose reaction following typical dental application.

TABLE 4-16
Effective Concentrations for Injection and Topical Application of Local Anesthetics

	EFFECTIVE CONCENTRATION		
Agent	**Injection, %**	**Topical, %**	**Useful as Topical**
Lidocaine	2	2-5	Yes
Mepivacaine	2-3	12-15	No
Procaine	2-4	10-20	No
Tetracaine	0.25-1	0.2-1	Yes

Some topical anesthetics are marketed in pressurized spray containers. Although they are no more effective than other forms, it is difficult to control the amount of anesthetic expelled and to confine it to the desired site of application. Spray devices that do not deliver measured doses should not be used intraorally.

Benzocaine

Benzocaine (ethyl *p*-aminobenzoate) is an ester local anesthetic:

1. Poor solubility in water

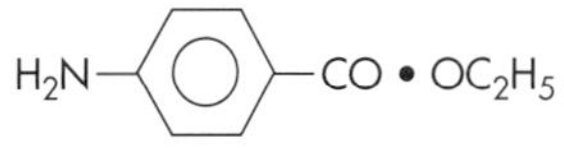

H_2N—(benzene ring)—$CO \bullet OC_2H_5$

2. Poor absorption into the cardiovascular system
3. Systemic toxic (overdose) reactions virtually unknown
4. Remains at the site of application longer, providing a prolonged duration of action
5. Not suitable for injection
6. Localized allergic reactions may occur after prolonged or repeated use. Although allergic reaction to ester anesthetics is rare, ester local anesthetics are more allergenic than amide local anesthetics.[70]
7. Inhibits the antibacterial action of sulfonamides[71]
8. Availability (Fig. 4-8): Benzocaine is available in the following formulations in numerous dosages: aerosol, gel, gel patch, ointment, and solution.

Benzocaine, Butamben, and Tetracaine HCl

Aerosol, gel, ointment, and solution: benzocaine 140 mg/mL; butamben 20 mg/mL; tetracaine HCl, 20 mg/mL.

Cocaine Hydrochloride

Cocaine hydrochloride (benzoylmethylecgonine hydrochloride) occurs naturally as a white crystalline solid that is highly soluble in water:

1. Used exclusively via topical application. Injection of cocaine is contraindicated because of the ready

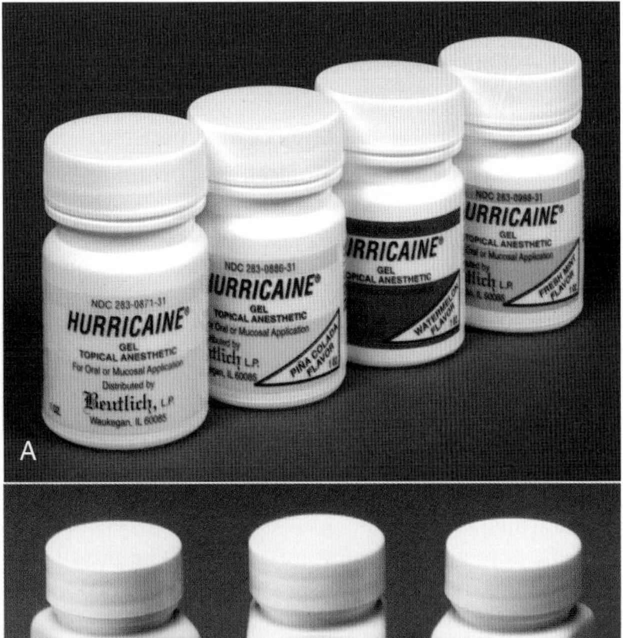

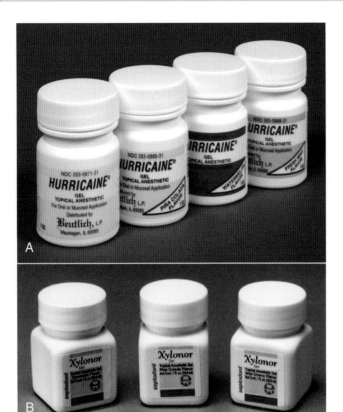

Figure 4-8. **A** and **B**, Topical anesthetics containing benzocaine. (**A**, Courtesy Beautlich Pharmaceuticals, Waukegan, Ill. **B**, Courtesy Septodont, New Castle, Del.)

availability of more effective and much less toxic local anesthetics. Cocaine is an ester local anesthetic.
2. Onset of topical anesthetic action is quite rapid, usually occurring within 1 minute.
3. Duration of anesthetic action may be as long as 2 hours.
4. It is absorbed rapidly but eliminated slowly (elimination half-life = 42 minutes).
5. It undergoes metabolism in the liver and plasma.
6. Unmetabolized cocaine may be found in the urine.
7. Cocaine is the only local anesthetic consistently demonstrated to produce vasoconstriction, which develops as a result of its ability to potentiate the actions of endogenous epinephrine and norepinephrine.[27] Addition of vasoconstrictors to cocaine therefore is unnecessary and is potentially dangerous, increasing the likelihood of dysrhythmias, including ventricular fibrillation.
8. Classified as a Schedule II drug under the Controlled Substances Act. Repeated use results in psychological dependence and tolerance.
9. Overdose of cocaine is not uncommon following illicit use, primarily because the drug is readily absorbed from the nasal mucosa and its dosage is not carefully monitored.
10. Clinical manifestations of mild overdose include euphoria, excitement, restlessness, tremor, hypertension, tachycardia, and tachypnea.
11. Clinical manifestations of acute cocaine overdose include excitement, restlessness, confusion, tremor, hypertension, tachycardia, tachypnea, nausea and vomiting, abdominal pain, exophthalmos, and mydriasis; these are followed by depression (CNS, cardiovascular, respiratory) and death from respiratory arrest.
12. It is available in concentrations ranging from 2% to 10%.
13. It is recommended that the concentration of cocaine not exceed 4% for topical application to oral mucous membranes.
14. Solutions of cocaine are unstable and deteriorate on standing.
15. Because of the extreme abuse potential of cocaine, its use as a topical anesthetic in dentistry is not recommended.
16. Topically applied cocaine is used occasionally before nasal-endotracheal intubation is performed in the operating theater to minimize bleeding from this highly vascular region and pain as the endotracheal tube is passed.

Dyclonine Hydrochloride

Dyclonine hydrochloride (4′-butoxy-3-piperidinopropiophenone hydrochloride) is a ketone derivative without an ester or amide linkage that may be used in patients who are allergic to the common anesthetics. Dyclonine offers advantages over other topical anesthetic agents. Extensive experience with the topical preparation has shown it to be effective and safe.[72] Dyclonine is marketed in 0.5% and 1% solutions:

1. Cross-sensitization with other local anesthetics does not occur; therefore dyclonine may be used in patients with known sensitivities to local anesthetics of other chemical groups.
2. Slightly soluble in water
3. Potency equal to that of cocaine
4. Onset of anesthesia slow, requiring up to 10 minutes
5. Duration of anesthesia may be as long as 1 hour.
6. Systemic toxicity is extremely low, primarily because of the agent's poor water solubility.
7. Not indicated for use by injection; irritating to tissues at the site of application
8. A 0.5% solution is used in dentistry. Maximum recommended dose is 200 mg (40 mL of a 0.5% solution).
9. Dyclonine was available as Dyclone in a 0.5% solution: each 100 mL of solution contained 500 mg of dyclonine HCl, 300 mg of chlorobutanol as a preservative, sodium chloride for isotonicity, and hydrochloric acid, as needed, to adjust pH. The Dyclone brand was withdrawn from the North American market in 2001.

EMLA (Eutectic Mixture of Local Anesthetics)

EMLA cream (composed of lidocaine 2.5% and prilocaine 2.5%) is an emulsion in which the oil phase is a eutectic mixture of lidocaine and prilocaine in a ratio of 1:1 by weight. It was designed as a topical anesthetic able to provide surface anesthesia for intact skin (other topical anesthetics do not produce anesthesia on intact skin, only abraded skin), and as such is used primarily before painful procedures such as venipuncture and other needle insertions. Originally marketed for use in pediatrics, EMLA has gained popularity among needle-phobic adults and persons having other superficial, but painful, procedures performed (e.g., hair removal).

EMLA use has become almost routine during circumcision,[73] during leg ulcer débridement,[74] and in gynecologic procedures.[75] Because intact skin is a barrier to drug diffusion, EMLA must be applied 1 hour before the procedure. Satisfactory numbing of the skin occurs 1 hour after application, reaches a maximum at 2 to 3 hours, and lasts for 1 to 2 hours after removal.

EMLA is supplied in a 5-g or 30-g tube or as an EMLA anesthetic disc. The EMLA disc is a white, round, cellulose disc preloaded with EMLA, packaged in protective laminate foil surrounded by adhesive tape.

EMLA is contraindicated for use in patients with congenital or idiopathic methemoglobinemia, infants younger than 12 months who are receiving treatment with methemoglobin-inducing agents, and patients with known sensitivity to amide-type local anesthetics or any other component of the product.[76]

Because EMLA is effective in penetrating intact skin, its ability to produce effective topical anesthesia in the oral cavity seems obvious. Although the drug package insert[76] stated originally that "EMLA is not recommended for use on mucous membranes," subsequent clinical trials have demonstrated satisfactory results.[77-80]

Bernardi and associates demonstrated statistically significant analgesia in 52 dental patients requiring removal of metal maxillary or mandibular splints used to contain fractures.[77] The authors concluded, "the analgesic effect[s] of EMLA cream on oral mucosa allow the application of contact anesthesia to be broadened to oral surgery and dentistry, limiting it to those procedures that do not involve deep tissues and only require short-term anesthesia."[77]

Munshi and associates reported on the use of EMLA cream in 30 pediatric patients undergoing a variety of clinical procedures, including extraction of mobile primary teeth and root stumps and pulpal therapy procedures in the primary teeth, in which EMLA is used as the sole anesthetic agent.[78] Results show that use of EMLA could eliminate to some extent use of the needle in procedures performed in pediatric dentistry.[79,80]

Lidocaine

Lidocaine is available in two forms for topical application: lidocaine base, which is poorly soluble in water, is used as a 5% concentration, and is indicated for use on ulcerated, abraded, or lacerated tissue; and lidocaine hydrochloride, its water-soluble preparation, which is used as a 2% concentration. The water-soluble form of lidocaine penetrates tissue more efficiently than the base form. However, systemic absorption is also greater, providing greater risk of toxicity than the base form:

1. Lidocaine is an amide local anesthetic with an exceptionally low incidence of allergic reactions.
2. Maximum recommended dose following topical application is 200 mg.
3. Availability: Lidocaine base is available as an aerosol spray, ointment, patch, and solution in various dosage forms (Fig. 4-9).
4. Availability: Lidocaine HCl is available as an oral topical solution in 20 mg/mL (viscous) and 40 mg/mL (solution).

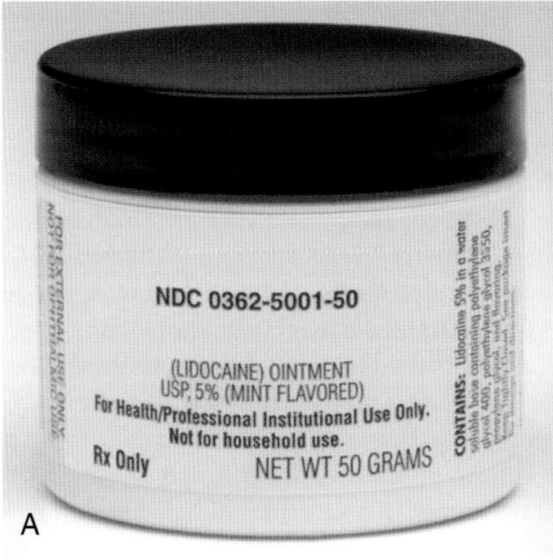

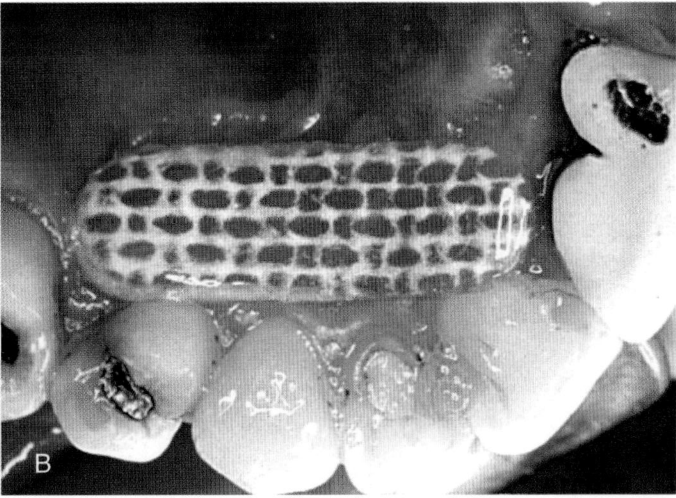

Figure 4-9. Topical anesthetics—Lidocaine. **A,** Octocaine ointment. **B,** Dentipatch. (**A,** Courtesy Septodent, New Castle, DE. **B,** Courtesy Noven Pharmaceuticals Inc., Miami, FL, www.noven.com.)

Tetracaine Hydrochloride

Tetracaine hydrochloride (2-dimethylaminoethyl-4-butylaminobenzoate hydrochloride) is a long-duration ester local anesthetic that can be injected or applied topically.

1. Highly soluble in water
2. Applied topically, five to eight times more potent than cocaine
3. Onset of action after topical application is slow.
4. Duration of action is approximately 45 minutes after topical application.
5. Metabolized in plasma and the liver by plasma pseudocholinesterase at a slower rate than procaine
6. When used by injection, available as a 0.15% concentration
7. 2% concentration is used for topical application.
8. Rapidly absorbed through mucous membranes. Use should be limited to small areas to avoid rapid absorption. Other, more slowly or poorly absorbed agents should be used in lieu of tetracaine when larger areas of topical anesthesia are necessary.
9. Maximum recommended dose of 20 mg when used for topical application. This represents 1 mL of a 2% solution.
10. Caution is urged because of great potential for systemic toxicity.
11. Availability (Canada):
    a. Aerosol: 0.7 mg/metered spray
        1. Supracaine
12. Tetracaine in a 3% concentration, with the vasoconstrictor oxymetazocine, has been shown to provide pulpal anesthesia of maxillary teeth when administered by aerosol spray into a patient's nares.[81] Use of intranasal local anesthesia for dental pain control in discussed in Chapter 20.

SELECTION OF A LOCAL ANESTHETIC

Because of the many local anesthetic combinations available for injection, it sometimes is difficult to select an ideal drug for a given patient. Many dentists simply deal with this by using one local anesthetic for all procedures, regardless of their duration. For example, the dentist may elect to use 2% lidocaine with 1:100,000 epinephrine for procedures lasting 5 to 10 minutes and for procedures involving 90 minutes of treatment time. Although the duration of pulpal anesthesia achievable with this drug, in ideal circumstances, may permit pain-free treatment in both these instances, the patient who requires only 10 minutes of pulpal anesthesia will remain anesthetized unnecessarily for an additional 3 to 5 hours (soft tissues), whereas the patient requiring 90 minutes of pulpal anesthesia will likely experience pain toward the end of the procedure.

A rational approach to selection of an appropriate local anesthetic for a patient includes consideration of several factors: (1) the length of time for which pain control is necessary; (2) the need for posttreatment pain control; (3) the need for hemostasis; and (4) whether any contraindications exist to administration of the selected local anesthetic.[1,22] Table 4-17 lists currently available local anesthetic formulations according to their expected duration of pulpal and soft tissue anesthesia. Again, it must be noted that these numbers are approximations, and the actual duration of clinical anesthesia may be somewhat longer or shorter than indicated.

TABLE 4-17
Duration of Pulpal and Soft Tissue Anesthesia for Available Local Anesthetics

Drug Formulation	DURATION (APPROXIMATE MINUTES) Pulpal	Soft Tissue
Mepivacaine 3% (infiltration)	5-10	90-120
Prilocaine 4% (infiltration)	10-15	60-120
Prilocaine 4% (nerve block)	40-60	120-240
Articaine 4% + epinephrine 1:200,000	45-60	180-240
Lidocaine 2% + epinephrine 1:50,000	60	180-300
Lidocaine 2% + epinephrine 1:100,000	60	180-300
Mepivacaine 2% + levonordefrin 1:20,000	60	180-300
Articaine 4% + epinephrine 1:100,000	60-75	180-300
Prilocaine 4% + epinephrine 1:200,000	60-90	180-480
Bupivacaine 0.5% + epinephrine 1:200,000	>90	240-720

A second consideration in the selection of a local anesthetic must be the requirement for pain control after treatment. A long-duration local anesthetic can be administered when postoperative pain is thought to be a factor. Local anesthetics providing a shorter duration of soft tissue anesthesia can be used for nontraumatic procedures. When postoperative pain is considered likely, 0.5% bupivacaine (for 8 to 12 hours of soft tissue anesthesia [via nerve block]) is suggested.

For patients in whom postoperative anesthesia represents a potential risk, a shorter-duration anesthetic should be considered. These patients include younger children, the older-old patient, and the physically or mentally disabled, who might accidentally bite or chew their lips or tongue, and persons unable to miss a meal (e.g., those with type 1 diabetes) because of residual soft tissue anesthesia. For these patients, 3% mepivacaine is recommended for use in short procedures. However in situations in which these patients require a more profound and/or longer duration of pulpal anesthesia, use of a local anesthetic containing a vasoconstrictor is necessary. The introduction of the local anesthesia reversal agent, phentolamine mesylate (Oraverse), has made it possible to significantly shorten the duration of residual soft tissue anesthesia, thereby minimizing the risk of accidental self-inflicted soft tissue injury (e.g., biting of the lip or tongue).[82-84] Reversal of soft tissue anesthesia in discussed in Chapter 20.

A third factor in choosing a local anesthetic is the requirement for hemostasis during the procedure. Anesthetic solutions containing epinephrine in a 1:50,000 or 1:100,000 concentration are recommended, via local infiltration into the surgical site, when hemostasis is considered necessary. More dilute epinephrine formulations (e.g., 1:200,000, 1:400,000) are not effective for hemostasis, nor is levonordefrin or felypressin.

A fourth factor in the selection of a local anesthetic involves the presence of any contraindications to use of the selected local anesthetic (see Table 4-2).

Absolute contraindications require that the offending drug(s) is not administered to the patient under any condition. The risk that a life-threatening situation will arise is unacceptably elevated. Most absolute contraindications to local anesthetic administration are, in fact, medical contraindications to the delivery of elective dental care (e.g., the patient is too ill to tolerate dentistry). However, one absolute contraindication to local anesthetic administration does exist: true, documented reproducible allergy. Although the incidence of "alleged" local anesthetic allergy is high, true, documented and reproducible allergy is an extremely rare occurrence with amide local anesthetics. Management of alleged and documented allergy to local anesthetics is discussed in Chapter 18.

In cases of a relative contraindication, it is preferable to avoid administration of the drug in question because the risk that an adverse reaction will occur is increased. An alternative drug that is not contraindicated is recommended. However, if an acceptable alternative is not available, the drug in question may be used, but judiciously, with the minimum dose that will provide adequate pain control administered. One example of a relative contraindication is the presence of atypical plasma (pseudo)cholinesterase, which decreases the rate of biotransformation of ester local anesthetics. Amides may be used without increased risk in these patients. Contraindications (both absolute and relative) are reviewed in Chapter 10.

Box 4-4 summarizes the criteria used in selection of a local anesthetic for administration to a given patient at a given dental appointment.

Table 4-18 lists the proprietary names of injectable local anesthetics available in the United States (as of November 2011).

The local anesthetic armamentarium for a dentist or dental hygienist therefore should include drugs of varying durations of action, such as the selection that follows. A minimum of two drugs is recommended for most offices. Amides are preferred to esters whenever possible:

1. Short-duration pulpal anesthetic (≈30 minutes)
2. Intermediate-duration pulpal anesthetic (≈60 minutes)
3. Long-duration pulpal anesthetic (90 or more minutes)
4. Topical anesthetic for tissue preparation before injection of local anesthetic

BOX 4-4 Factors in Selection of a Local Anesthetic for a Patient

1. Length of time pain control is necessary
2. Potential need for posttreatment pain control
3. Possibility of self-mutilation in the postoperative period
4. Requirement for hemostasis
5. Presence of any contraindications (absolute or relative) to the local anesthetic solution selected for administration

TABLE 4-18
Proprietary Names of Injectable Local Anesthetics (United States)

Articaine HCl	Articadent, Orabloc, Septocaine, Zorcaine
Bupivacaine HCl	Marcaine, Vivacaine
Lidocaine HCl	Lignospan, Octocaine, Xylocaine
Mepivacaine HCl	Carbocaine, Isocaine, Polocaine, Scandanest
Prilocaine HCl	Citanest

References

1. Malamed SF: Handbook of local anesthesia, St Louis, 1980, Mosby.
2. Malamed SF: Buffering local anesthetics in dentistry, ADSA Pulse 44:8–9, 2011.
3. Meechan JG: Infiltration anesthesia in the mandible, Dent Clin North Am 54:621–629, 2010.
4. Iwatsubo T, Hirota N, Ooie T, et al: Prediction of in vivo drug metabolism in the human liver from in vitro metabolism data, Pharmacol Ther 73:147–171, 1997.
5. Thompson P, Melmon K, Richardson J, et al: Lidocaine pharmacokinetics in advanced heart failure, liver disease, and renal failure in humans, Ann Intern Med 78:499, 1973.
6. Haase A, Reader A, Nusstein J, Beck M, Drum M. Comparing anesthetic efficacy of articaine versus lidocaine as a supplemental buccal infiltration of the mandibular first molar after an inferior alveolar nerve block, J Amer Dent Assoc 139:1228–1235, 2008.
7. Malamed SF: Sedation: a guide to patient management, ed 4, St Louis, 2003, Mosby.
8. Wilson AW, Deacock S, Downie IP, et al: Allergy to local anesthetic: the importance of thorough investigation, Br Dent J 188:320–322, 2000.
9. Covino BG: Clinical pharmacology of local anesthetic agents. In Cousins MJ, Bridenbaugh PO, editors: Neural blockade in clinical anesthesia and management of pain, ed 2, Philadelphia, 1988, JB Lippincott.
10. Prescribing information: Ravocaine and Novocain with Levophed, New York, 1993, Cook-Waite, Sterling Winthrop.
11. Moore PA, Hersh EV: Local anesthetics: pharmacology and toxicity, Dent Clin North Am 54:587–599, 2010.
12. Prescribing information: 2% Xylocaine Dental, York, Pa, March 2009, Dentsply Pharmaceutical.

13. Brown RS, Paluvoi S, Choksi S, et al: Evaluating a dental patient for local anesthesia allergy, Comp Contin Educ Dent 23:225–228, 131–132, 134, 140, 2002.
14. Jackson D, Chen AH, Bennett CR: Identifying true lidocaine allergy, J Am Dent Assoc 125:1362–1366, 1994.
15. Sindel LJ, deShazo RD: Accidents resulting from local anesthetics: true or false allergy? Clin Rev Allergy 9:379–395, 1991.
16. Ball IA: Allergic reactions to lignocaine, Br Dent J 186:524–526, 1999.
17. Baluga JC: Allergy to local anaesthetics in dentistry: myth or reality? Rev Alerg Mex 50:176–181, 2003.
18. Thyssen JP, Menne T, Elberling J, et al: Hypersensitivity to local anaesthetics—update and proposal of evaluation algorithm, Contact Dermatitis 59:69–78, 2008.
19. Young ER, Mason DR, Saso MA, et al: Some clinical properties of Octocaine 200 (2 percent lidocaine with epinephrine 1:200,000), J Can Dent Assoc 55:987–991, 1989.
20. Buckley JA, Ciancio SG, McMullen JA: Efficacy of epinephrine concentration in local anesthesia during periodontal surgery, J Periodontol 55:653–657, 1984.
21. DeToledo JC: Lidocaine and seizures, Ther Drug Monit 22:320–322, 2000.
22. Malamed SF, Yagiela J: Local anesthetics. In ADA Guide to Dental Therapeutics, Chicago, Ill, 1998, American Dental Association.
23. Geddes IC: Metabolism of local anesthetic agents, Int Anesthesiol Clin 5:525–549, 1967.
24. Severinghaus JW, Xu F-D, Spellman MJ: Benzocaine and methemoglobin: recommended actions, Anesthesiology 74: 385–386, 1991.
25. Schroeder TH, Dieterich HJ, Muhlbauer B: Methemoglobinemia after maxillary block with bupivacaine and additional injection of lidocaine in the operative field, Acta Anaesthesiol Scand 43:480–482, 1999.
26. Wilburn-Goo D, Lloyd LM: When patients become cyanotic: acquired methemoglobinemia, J Am Dent Assoc 130:626–631, 1999.
27. de Jong RH: Local anesthetics, St Louis, 1994, Mosby.
28. Akerman B, Astrom A, Ross S, et al: Studies on the absorption, distribution, and metabolism of labeled prilocaine and lidocaine in some animal species, Acta Pharmacol Toxicol 24:389–403, 1966.
29. Foldes FF, Molloy R, McNall PG, et al: Comparison of toxicity of intravenously given local anesthetic agents in man, JAMA 172:1493–1498, 1960.
30. Englesson S, Eriksson E, Ortengren B: Differences in tolerance to intravenous Xylocaine and Citanest, Acta Anaesthesiol Scand Suppl 16:141–145, 1965.
31. Deriksson E, Granberg PO: Studies on the renal excretion of Citanest and Xylocaine, Acta Anaesthesiol Scand Suppl 16:79–85, 1985.
32. Smith DW, Peterson MR, DeBerard SC: Local anesthesia: topical application, local infiltration, and field block, Postgrad Med 106:27–60, 64–66, 1999.
33. Akinturk S, Eroglu A: A clinical comparison of topical piroxicam and EMLA cream for pain relief and inflammation in laser hair removal, Lasers Med Sci 24:535–538, 2009.
34. Haas DA, Lennon D: A 21 year retrospective study of reports of paresthesia following local anesthetic administration, J Can Dent Assoc 61:319–320, 323–326, 329–330, 1995.
35 Garisto GA, Gaffen AS, Lawrence HP, et al: Occurrence of paresthesia after dental local anesthetic administration in the United States, J Am Dent Assoc 141:836–844, 2010.
36. Pogrel MA: Permanent nerve damage from inferior alveolar nerve blocks—an update to include articaine, J Calif Dent Assoc 35:271–273, 2007.
37. van Oss GE, Vree TB, Baars AM, et al: Pharmacokinetics, metabolism, and renal excretion of articaine and its metabolite articainic acid in patients after epidural administration, Eur J Anaesthesiol 6:19–56, 1989.
38. van Oss GE, Vree TB, Baars AM, et al: Clinical effects and pharmacokinetics of articainic acid in one volunteer after intravenous administration, Pharm Weekbl (Sc) 10:284–286, 1988.
39. Vree TB, Baars AM, van Oss GE, et al: High performance liquid chromatography and preliminary pharmacokinetics of articaine and its 2-carboxy metabolite in human serum and urine, J Chromatogr 424:240–444, 1988.
40. Prescribing information: Septocaine, Louisville, Colo, 2011, Septodont Inc.
41. Malamed SF, Gagnon S, Leblanc D: Safety of articaine: a new amide local anesthetic, J Am Dent Assoc 132:177–185, 2001.
42. Malamed SF, Gagnon S, Leblanc D: Articaine hydrochloride in pediatric dentistry: safety and efficacy of a new amide-type local anesthetic, Pediatr Dent 22:307–311, 2000.
43. Malamed SF, Gagnon S, Leblanc D: Efficacy of articaine: a new amide local anesthetic, J Am Dent Assoc 131:535–642, 2000.
44. Donaldson D, James-Perdok L, Craig BJ, et al: A comparison of Ultracaine DS (articaine HCl) and Citanest Forte (prilocaine HCl) in maxillary infiltration and mandibular nerve block, J Can Dent Assoc 53:38–42, 1987.
45. Knoll-Kohler E, Rupprecht S: Articaine for local anaesthesia in dentistry: a lidocaine controlled double blind cross-over study, Eur J Pain 13:59–63, 1992.
46. Septodont Inc., NA: Personal communications, May 2011.
47. Schulze-Husmann M: Experimental evaluation of the new local anesthetic Ultracaine in dental practice, doctoral dissertation, Bonn, 1974, University of Bonn.
48. Clinicians guide to dental products and techniques, Septocaine. CRA Newsletter June 2001.
49. Kanaa MD, Whitworth JM, Corbett IP, et al: Articaine buccal infiltration enhances the effectiveness of lidocaine inferior alveolar nerve block, Int Endod J 42:238–246, 2009.
50. Meechan JG: Infiltration anesthesia in the mandible, Dent Clin North Am 54:621–629, 2010.
51. Yonchak T, Reader A, Beck M, et al: Anesthetic efficacy of infiltrations in mandibular anterior teeth, Anesth Prog 48:55–60, 2001.
52. Meechan JG, Ledvinka JI: Pulpal anaesthesia for mandibular central incisor teeth: a comparison of infiltration and intraligamentary injections, Int Endod J 35:629–634, 2002.
53. Kanaa MD, Whitworth JM, Corbett IP, et al: Articaine and lidocaine mandibular buccal infiltration anesthesia: a prospective randomized double blind cross-over study, J Endod 32:296–298, 2006.
54. Robertson D, Nusstein J, Reader A, et al: The anesthetic efficacy of articaine in buccal infiltration of mandibular posterior teeth, J Am Dent Assoc 138:1104–1112, 2007.
55. Haase A, Reader A, Nusstein J, et al: Comparing anesthetic efficacy of articaine versus lidocaine as a supplemental buccal infiltration of the mandibular first molar after an inferior alveolar nerve block, J Am Dent Assoc 139:1228–1235, 2008.

56. Jakobs W: Status of dental anesthesia in Germany, Anesth Prog 36:10–212, 1989.
57. Deutscher Dentalmarkt Jahresbericht (DDM) 2010 (German Dental Market Annual Report 2010) GfK HealthCare, Nuremberg, Germany.
58. Malamed SF: Handbook of local anesthesia, ed 4, St Louis, 1997, Mosby, pp 63–64.
59. Articaine, epinephrine: contraindications/precautions, MD Consult. Available at: http://www.mdconsult.com/php/25067 9983–2/homepage. Revised April 21, 2010. Accessed May 24, 2011.
60. Jakobs W: Actual aspects of dental anesthesia in Germany. Presented at the 10th International Dental Congress on Modern Pain Control, IFDAS, Edinburgh, Scotland, UK, June 2003.
61. Prescribing information: Bupivacaine HCl, Lake Forest, Ill, November 2009, Hospira, Inc.
62. Moore PA: Bupivacaine: a long-lasting local anesthetic for dentistry, Oral Surg 58:369, 1984.
63. Acute Pain Management Guideline Panel: Acute pain management: operative or medical procedures and trauma. Clinical practice guideline. AHCPR Publication Number 92-0032, Rockville, Md, 1992, Agency for Health Care Policy and Research, Public Health Service, U.S. Department of Health and Human Services.
64. Oxford League Table of Analgesics in Acute Pain: Bandolier Website. Available at: http://www.medicine.ox.ac.uk/bandolier/booth/painpag/acutrev/analgesics/lftab.html. Accessed May 24, 2011.
65. Hargreaves KM, Keiser K: Development of new pain management strategies, J Dent Educ 66:113–121, 2002.
66. Malamed SF: Handbook of local anesthesia, ed 5, St Louis, 2003, CV Mosby, pp 74–75.
67. Adriani J, Campbell D: Fatalities following topical application of local anesthetics to mucous membranes, JAMA 162:1527, 1956.
68. Jeske AH, Blanton PL: Misconceptions involving dental local anesthesia. Part 2. Pharmacology, Texas Dent J 119:310–314, 2002.
69. Rosivack RG, Koenigsberg SR, Maxwell KC: An analysis of the effectiveness of two topical anesthetics, Anesth Prog 37:290–292, 1990.
70. Patterson RP, Anderson J: Allergic reactions to drugs and biologic agents, JAMA 248:2637–2645, 1982.
71. Alston TA: Antagonism of sulfonamides by benzocaine and chloroprocaine, Anesthesiology 76:375–476, 1992.
72. Adriani J, Zepernick R: Clinical effectiveness of drugs used for topical anesthesia, JAMA 188:93, 1964.
73. Taddio A: Pain management for neonatal circumcision, Paediatr Drugs 3:101–111, 2001.
74. Vanscheidt W, Sadjadi Z, Lillieborg S: EMLA anaesthetic cream for sharp leg ulcer debridement: a review of the clinical evidence for analgesic efficacy and tolerability, Eur J Dermatol 11:20–96, 2001.
75. Wright VC: Vulvar biopsy: techniques for reducing patient discomfort, Adv Nurse Pract 9:17–60, 2001.
76. EMLA, MD Consult. Available at: http://www.mdconsult.com/php/250679983–2/homepage. Revised May 12, 2010. Accessed May 24, 2011.
77. Bernardi M, Secco F, Benech A: Anesthetic efficacy of a eutectic mixture of lidocaine and prilocaine (EMLA) on the oral mucosa: prospective double-blind study with a placebo, Minerva Stomatol 48:9–43, 1999.
78. Munshi AK, Hegde AM, Latha R: Use of EMLA: is it an injection free alternative? J Clin Pediatr Dent 25:215–219, 2001.
79. Franz-Montan M, Ranali J, Ramacciato JC, et al: Ulceration of gingival mucosa after topical application of EMLA: report of four cases, Br Dent J 204:133–134, 2008.
80. Nayak R, Sudha P: Evaluation of three topical anaesthetic agents against pain: a clinical study, Indian J Dent Res 17:155–160, 2006.
81. University of Buffalo, The State University of New York: Nasap spray may end dental needle injections for upper teeth repair. Available at: www.buffalo.edu/news/9911. Accessed February 17, 2009.
82. Moore PA, Hersh EV, Papas AS, et al: Pharmacokinetics of lidocaine with epinephrine following local anesthesia reversal with phentolamine mesylate, Anesth Prog 55:40–48, 2008.
83. Hersh EV, Moore PA, Papas AS, et al, Soft Tissue Anesthesia Recovery Group: Reversal of soft-tissue local anesthesia with phentolamine mesylate in adolescents and adults, J Am Dent Assoc 139:1080–1093, 2008.
84. Tavares M, Goodson JM, Studen-Pavlovich D, et al, Soft Tissue Anesthesia Reversal Group: Reversal of soft-tissue local anesthesia with phentolamine mesylate in pediatric patients, J Am Dent Assoc 139:1095–1104, 2008.

IN THIS PART

PART II

The Armamentarium

The equipment necessary for the administration of local anesthetics is introduced and discussed in this section. This includes the syringe, needle, and local anesthetic cartridge, as well as additional items of equipment. In addition to providing a description of the armamentarium, each chapter reviews the proper care and handling of the equipment and problems that may be encountered with its use. A discussion of the proper technique for assembling and disassembling the equipment follows.

The introduction of computer-controlled local anesthetic delivery (C-CLAD) systems has enhanced the delivery of local anesthetic for many dentists and their patients. These devices have demonstrated great utility in the painless delivery of dental local anesthetics and are described in detail in this section.

CHAPTER 5

The Syringe

The syringe is one of three essential components of the local anesthetic armamentarium (others include the needle and the cartridge). It is the vehicle whereby the contents of the anesthetic cartridge are delivered through the needle to the patient.

TYPES OF SYRINGES

Eight types of syringes for local anesthetic administration are available for use in dentistry today. They represent a considerable improvement over the local anesthetic syringes formerly used. These various types of syringes are listed in Box 5-1.

Syringes that do not permit aspiration (i.e., nonaspirating syringes) are not discussed because their use unacceptably increases the risk of inadvertent intravascular drug administration. Use of aspirating dental syringes (capable of the aspiration of blood) represents the standard of care.

American Dental Association criteria for acceptance of local anesthetic syringes include the following[1,2]:

1. They must be durable and able to withstand repeated sterilization without damage. (If the unit is disposable, it should be packaged in a sterile container.)
2. They should be capable of accepting a wide variety of cartridges and needles of different manufacture, and should permit repeated use.
3. They should be inexpensive, self-contained, lightweight, and simple to use with one hand.
4. They should provide for effective aspiration and be constructed so that blood may be easily observed in the cartridge.

Nondisposable Syringes

Breech-Loading, Metallic, Cartridge-Type, Aspirating. The breech-loading, metallic, cartridge-type syringe (Fig. 5-1) is the most commonly used in dentistry. The term *breech-loading* implies that the cartridge is inserted into the syringe from the side of the barrel of the syringe. The needle is attached to the barrel of the syringe at the needle adaptor. The needle then passes into the barrel, where it penetrates the diaphragm of the local anesthetic cartridge. The needle adaptor (screw hub or convertible tip) is removable and sometimes is discarded inadvertently along with the disposable needle.

The aspirating syringe has a device such as a sharp, hook-shaped end (often called the *harpoon*) attached to the piston that is used to penetrate the thick silicone rubber stopper (bung) at the opposite end of the cartridge (from the needle). Provided the needle is of adequate gauge, when negative pressure is exerted on the thumb ring by the administrator, blood will enter into the needle and will be visible in the cartridge if the needle tip rests within the lumen of a blood vessel. Positive pressure applied to the thumb ring forces local anesthetic into the needle lumen and the tissues wherever the needle tip lies. The thumb ring and finger grips give the administrator added control over the syringe. Almost all syringe manufacturers provide syringes with both "regular" and "small" thumb rings (Fig. 5-2). Most metallic, breech-loading, aspirating syringes are constructed of chrome-plated brass and stainless steel.

Advantages and disadvantages of the metallic, breech-loading, aspirating syringe are listed in Box 5-2.

Breech-Loading, Plastic, Cartridge-Type, Aspirating. A plastic, reusable, dental aspirating syringe is available that is both autoclavable and chemically sterilizable. With proper care and handling, this syringe may be used for multiple anesthetic administrations before it is discarded. Advantages and disadvantages of the plastic, reusable, aspirating syringe are listed in Box 5-3.

Breech-Loading, Metallic, Cartridge-Type, Self-Aspirating. Potential hazards of intravascular administration of local anesthetics are great and are discussed more fully in Chapter 18. The incidence of positive aspiration may be as high as 10% to 15% with some injection techniques.[3] It is accepted by the dental profession that an aspiration test before administration of a local anesthetic drug is of great importance. Unfortunately, it is abundantly clear that in

BOX 5-1 Syringe Types Available in Dentistry

1. Nondisposable syringes:
   a. Breech-loading, metallic, cartridge-type, aspirating
   b. Breech-loading, plastic, cartridge-type, aspirating
   c. Breech-loading, metallic, cartridge-type, self-aspirating
   d. Pressure syringe for periodontal ligament injection
   e. Jet injector ("needle-less" syringe)
2. Disposable syringes
3. "Safety" syringes
4. Computer-controlled local anesthetic delivery systems

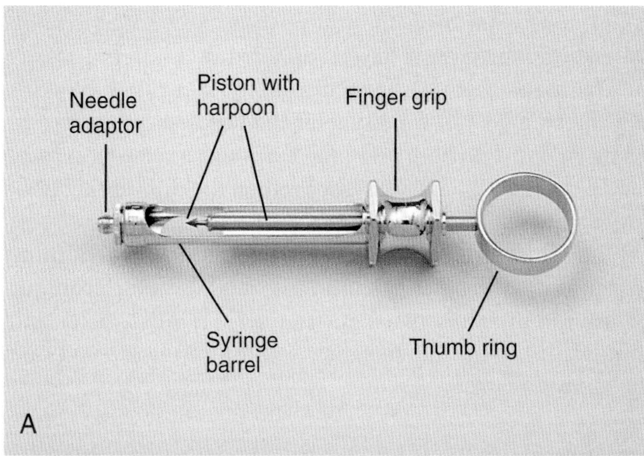

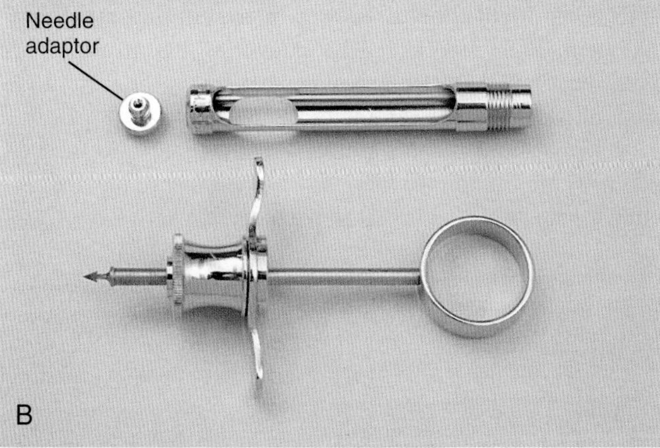

Figure 5-1. **A,** Breech-loading, metallic, cartridge-type syringe; assembled. **B,** Disassembled local anesthetic syringe.

actual clinical practice, too little attention is paid to this procedure (Table 5-1).

With commonly used breech-loading, metallic, cartridge-type syringes, an aspiration test must be carried out purposefully by the administrator before or during drug deposition. The key word here is *purposefully.* However, as demonstrated in Table 5-1, many dentists do not purposefully perform an aspiration test before injection of the anesthetic drug.[4]

BOX 5-2 Advantages and Disadvantages of the Metallic, Breech-Loading, Aspirating Syringe

Advantages	Disadvantages
Visible cartridge	Weight (heavier than plastic syringe)
Aspiration with one hand	Syringe may be too big for small operators
Autoclavable	Possibility of infection with improper care
Rust resistant	
Long lasting with proper maintenance	

BOX 5-3 Advantages and Disadvantages of the Plastic, Reusable, Aspirating Syringe

Advantages	Disadvantages
Plastic eliminates metallic, clinical look	Size (may be too big for small operators)
Lightweight: provides better "feel" during injection	Possibility of infection with improper care
Cartridge is visible	Deterioration of plastic with repeated autoclaving
Aspiration with one hand	
Rust resistant	
Long lasting with proper maintenance	
Lower cost	

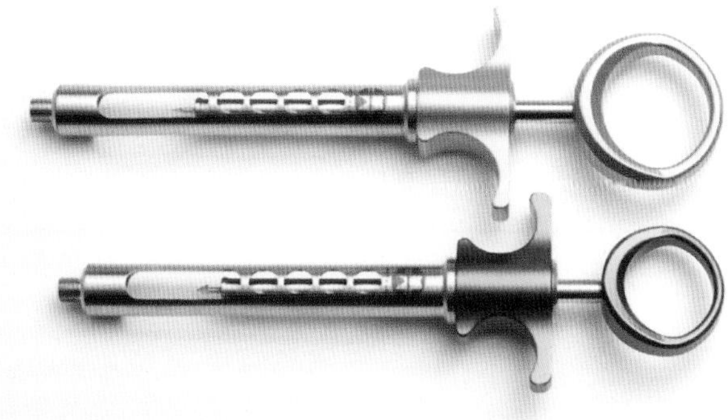

Figure 5-2. Harpoon-type aspirating syringes with small and large thumb rings.

TABLE 5-1
Percentages of Dentists Who Aspirate Before Injection

	INFERIOR ALVEOLAR NERVE BLOCK		MAXILLARY INFILTRATION	
Frequency	**Percent**	**Cumulative**	**Percent**	**Cumulative**
Always	63.2		40.2	
Sometimes	14.7	77.9	24.1	64.3
Rarely	9.2	87.1	18.4	82.7
Never	12.9		17.3	

To increase the ease of aspiration, self-aspirating syringes have been developed (Fig. 5-3). These syringes use the elasticity of the rubber diaphragm in the anesthetic cartridge to obtain the necessary negative pressure for aspiration. The diaphragm rests on a metal projection inside the syringe that directs the needle into the cartridge (Fig. 5-4). Pressure acting directly on the cartridge through the thumb disc (Fig. 5-5) or indirectly through the plunger shaft distorts (stretches) the rubber diaphragm, producing positive pressure within the anesthetic cartridge. When that pressure is released, sufficient negative pressure develops within the cartridge to permit aspiration. The thumb ring produces twice as much negative pressure as the plunger shaft. The use of a self-aspirating dental syringe permits easy performance of multiple aspirations throughout the period of local anesthetic deposition.

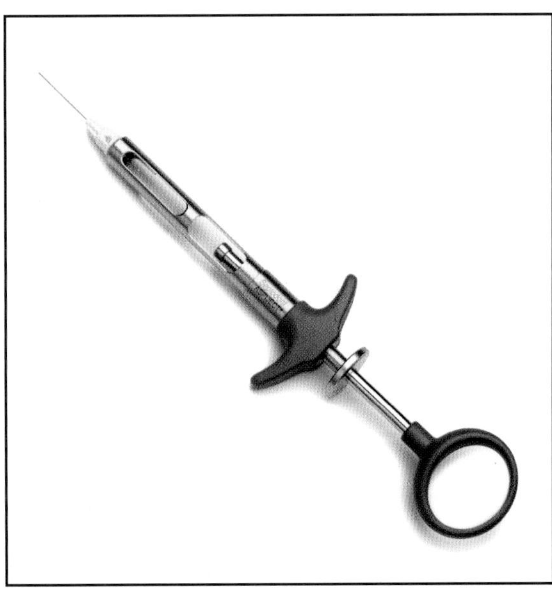

Figure 5-3. Self-aspirating syringe.

The self-aspirating syringe was introduced into the United States in 1981. After an initial period of enthusiasm, the popularity of this syringe decreased. Some dentists believed that the self-aspirating syringe did not provide the same reliable degree of aspiration that was possible with the harpoon-aspirating syringe. It has been demonstrated, however, that this syringe does in fact aspirate as reliably as the harpoon-aspirating syringe.[5-7] The notion can occur that aspiration may not be as reliable with the self-aspirating syringe because the administrator simply has to depress and release the thumb ring to aspirate, rather than pulling back on the thumb ring. Moving the thumb off the thumb ring and onto the thumb disc for aspiration has been mentioned by many dentists as uncomfortable for them. Although this is the preferred means of obtaining a satisfactory aspiration test with these syringes, pressure adequate for aspiration may be obtained by simply releasing the pressure of the thumb on the thumb ring. Second-generation self-aspirating syringes have eliminated the thumb disc.

The major factor influencing ability to aspirate blood is not the syringe, but the gauge of the needle being used.[7] In addition, most doctors using the harpoon-aspirating syringe tend to overaspirate, that is, they retract the thumb ring back too far and with excessive force (and, on occasion, disengage the harpoon from the stopper). These doctors feel more insecure with the self-aspirating syringe. Proper technique of aspiration is discussed in Chapter 11. Advantages and disadvantages of the metallic, self-aspirating syringe are listed in Box 5-4.

Pressure Syringes. Introduced in the late 1970s, pressure syringes brought about a renewed interest in the periodontal ligament (PDL) injection (also known as the intraligamentary injection [ILI]). Discussed in Chapter 16, the PDL injection, although usable for any tooth, helped make it possible to achieve more reliable pulpal anesthesia of one isolated tooth in the mandible where, in the past, nerve block anesthesia (e.g., inferior alveolar nerve block [IANB], Gow-Gates

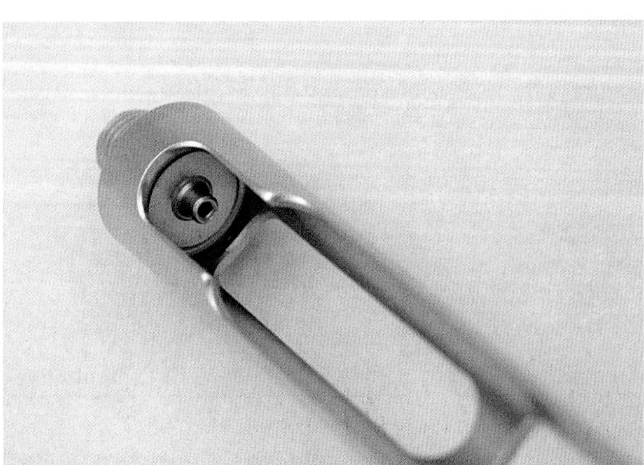

Figure 5-4. A metal projection within the barrel depresses the diaphragm of the local anesthetic cartridge.

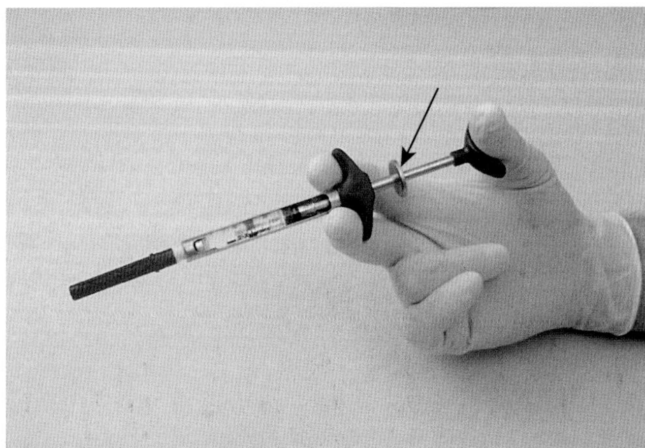

Figure 5-5. Pressure on the thumb disc *(arrow)* increases pressure within the cartridge. Release of pressure on the thumb disc produces the self-aspiration test.

BOX 5-4 Advantages and Disadvantages of the Metallic, Self-Aspirating Syringe

Advantages	Disadvantages
Cartridge visible	Weight
Easier to aspirate with small hands	Feeling of "insecurity" for doctors accustomed to harpoon-type syringe
Autoclavable	Finger must be moved from thumb ring to thumb disc to aspirate
Rust resistant	Possibility of infection with improper care
Long lasting with proper maintenance	
Piston is scored (indicates volume of local anesthetic administered)	

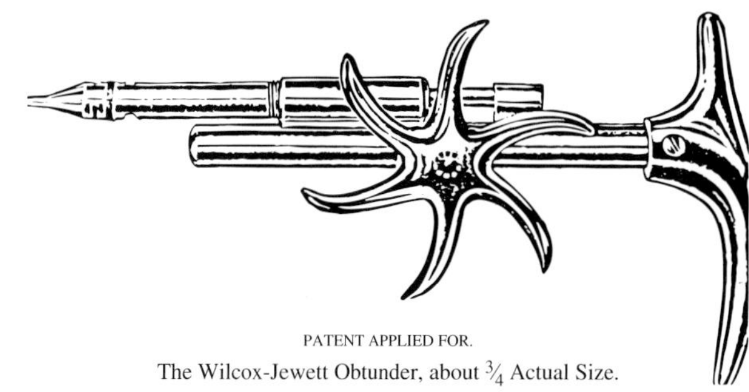

THE WILCOX-JEWETT OBTUNDER.
LEE S. SMITH & SON, PITTSBURG.
PATENT APPLIED FOR.
The Wilcox-Jewett Obtunder, about ¾ Actual Size.

Figure 5-7. Pressure syringe (1905) designed for a periodontal injection.

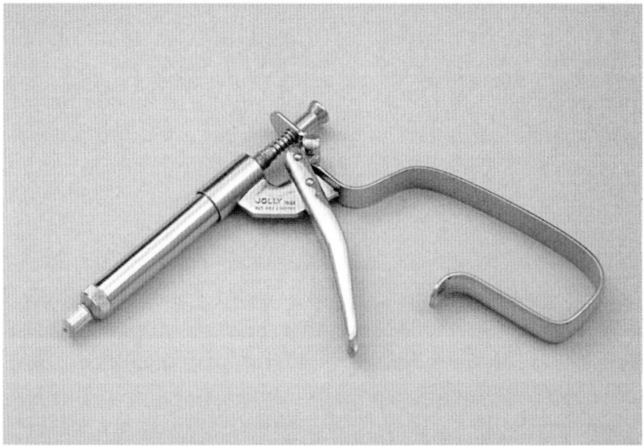

Figure 5-6. Original design of pressure syringe for periodontal ligament (PDL) injection or intraligamentary (ILI) injection.

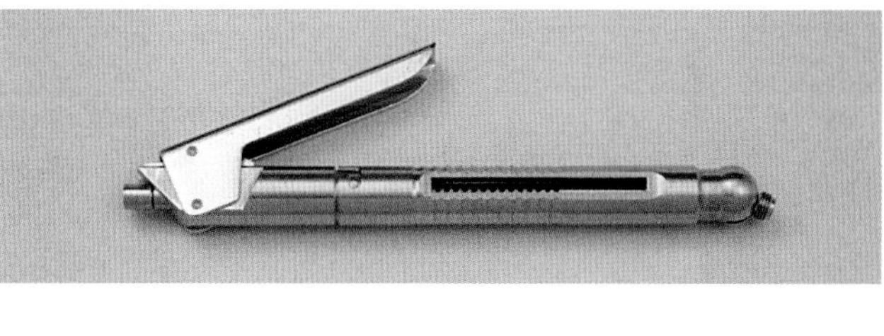

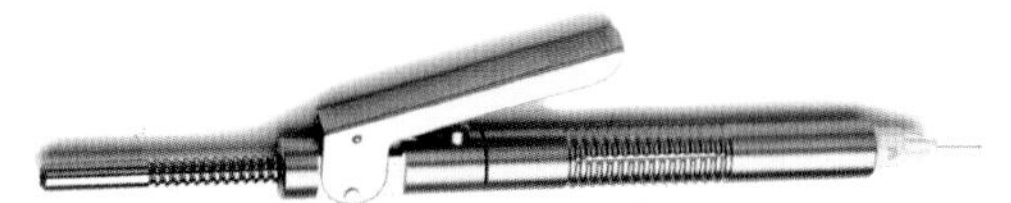

Figure 5-8. Second-generation syringe for periodontal ligament (PDL) injection.

mandibular nerve block), with its attendant prolonged soft tissue (e.g., lingual) anesthesia, was necessary.

The original pressure devices, Peripress (Universal Dental Implements, Edison, NJ) and Ligmaject (IMA Associates, Bloomington, Ind) (Fig. 5-6), were modeled after a device that was available in dentistry in 1905—the Wilcox-Jewett obtunder (Fig. 5-7). These first-generation devices, using a pistol grip, are somewhat larger than the newer, pen-grip devices (Fig. 5-8). Although "special" syringes such as these are not necessary for a successful PDL injection, several advantages are associated with their use, not the least of which is the mechanical advantage they provide the administrator, making the local anesthetic easier to administer. This same mechanical advantage, however, makes the injection somewhat "too easy" to administer, leading to "too rapid" injection of the anesthetic solution and patient discomfort both during the injection and later, when the anesthetic has worn off. However, when used slowly, as recommended by manufacturers, pressure syringes are of some benefit in administration of this valuable technique of anesthesia.

Pressure syringes offer advantages over the conventional syringe when used for PDL injections because their trigger delivers a measured dose of local anesthetic and enables a relatively physically weak administrator to overcome the significant tissue resistance encountered when the technique is administered properly. This mechanical advantage may also prove to be detrimental if the administrator deposits the anesthetic solution too quickly (<20 sec/0.2 mL dose). All pressure syringes completely encase the glass dental cartridge with plastic or metal, thereby protecting the patient in the unlikely event that the glass cartridge cracks or shatters during injection. The original pressure syringes looked somewhat threatening, having the appearance of a gun (see Fig. 5-6). Newer devices are smaller and are much less intimidating.

Probably the greatest disadvantage of using the pressure syringe is its cost; most are priced at considerably more than US $200 (November 2011). For this reason among others, it is recommended that pressure devices be considered for use only after the PDL injection has been found to be ineffective after several attempts with a conventional syringe and needle. Box 5-5 lists the advantages and disadvantages of the pressure syringe.

BOX 5-5 Advantages and Disadvantages of the Pressure Syringe

Advantages	Disadvantages
Measured dose	Cost
Overcomes tissue resistance	Easy to inject too rapidly
Nonthreatening (new devices)	Threatening (original devices)
Cartridges protected	

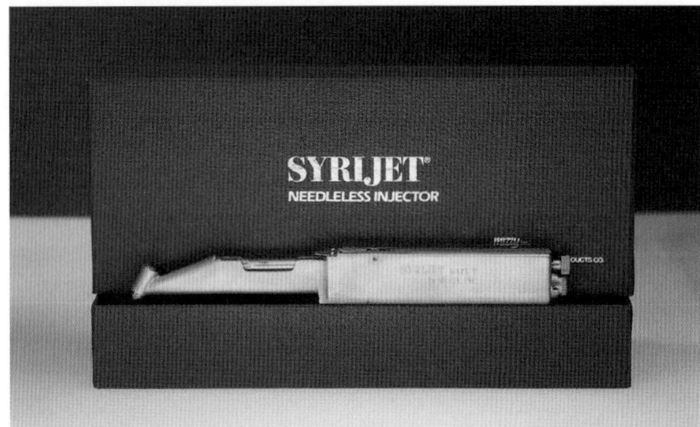

Figure 5-9. SyriJet needleless injector. (Courtesy Mizzy Inc., Cherry Hill, NJ.)

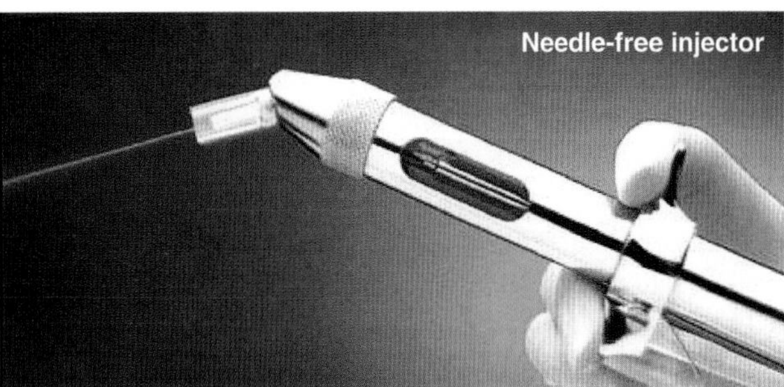

Figure 5-10. MadaJet.

Jet Injector. In 1947 Figge and Scherer introduced a new approach to parenteral injection—the jet or needle-less injection.[8] This represented the first fundamental change in the basic principles of injection since 1853, when Alexander Wood introduced the hypodermic syringe. The first report of the use of jet injections in dentistry was published in 1958 by Margetis and associates.[9] Jet injection is based on the principle that liquids forced through very small openings, called *jets,* at very high pressure can penetrate intact skin or mucous membrane (visualize water flowing through a garden hose that is being crimped). The most frequently used jet injectors in dentistry are the SyriJet Mark II (Mizzy Inc., Cherry Hill, NJ) (Fig. 5-9) and the MadaJet (Mada Medical Products Incorporated, Carlstadt, NJ) (Fig. 5-10). The SyriJet holds any 1.8-mL dental cartridge of local anesthetic. It is calibrated to deliver 0.05 to 0.2 mL of solution at 2000 psi.

BOX 5-6 Advantages and Disadvantages of the Jet Injector

Advantages	Disadvantages
Does not require use of needle (recommended for needle phobics)	Inadequate for pulpal anesthesia or for regional block
Delivers very small volumes of local anesthetic (0.01 to 0.2 mL)	Some patients are disturbed by the jolt of the injection.
Used in lieu of topical anesthetics	Cost
	May damage periodontal tissues

The primary purpose of the jet injector is to obtain topical anesthesia before insertion of a needle. In addition, it may be used to obtain mucosal anesthesia of the palate. Regional nerve blocks or supraperiosteal injections are still necessary for complete anesthesia. The jet injector is not an adequate substitute for the more traditional needle and syringe in obtaining pulpal or regional block anesthesia. Additionally, many patients dislike the feeling that accompanies use of the jet injector, as well as the possible postinjection soreness of soft tissue that may develop even with proper use of the device. Topical anesthetics, applied properly, serve the same purpose as jet injectors at a fraction of the cost (SyriJet Mark II, US $1950 [November 2011]*; MadaJet XL Dental, US $600 [November 2011]) and with minimum risk. Advantages and disadvantages of jet injectors are listed in Box 5-6.

Disposable Syringes

Plastic disposable syringes are available in a variety of sizes with an assortment of needle gauges. Most often they are used for intramuscular or intravenous drug administration, but they also may be used for intraoral injection (Fig. 5-11).

These syringes contain a Luer-Lok screw-on needle attachment with no aspirating tip. Aspiration can be accomplished by pulling back on the plunger of the syringe before or during injection. Because there is no thumb ring, aspiration with the plastic disposable syringe requires the use of both hands. In addition, these syringes do not accept dental cartridges. The needle, attached to the syringe, must be inserted into a vial or cartridge of local anesthetic drug and an appropriate volume of solution withdrawn. Care must be taken to avoid contaminating the multi-use vial during this procedure. Two- and 3-mL syringes with 25- or 27-gauge needles are recommended when the system is used for intraoral local anesthetic administration.

*Mizzy Inc., 616 Hollywood Ave., Cherry Hill, NJ 08002; 1-800-663-4700; www.keystoneind.com.

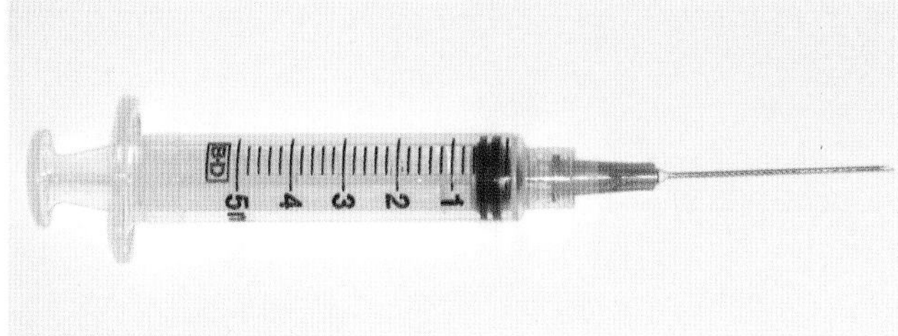

Figure 5-11. Plastic disposable syringe.

BOX 5-7 Advantages and Disadvantages of the Disposable Syringe

Advantages	Disadvantages
Disposable, single use	Does not accept prefilled dental cartridges
Sterile until opened	Aspiration difficult (requires two hands)
Lightweight (may feel awkward to the first-time user; tactile sensation better)	

The plastic, disposable, non–cartridge-containing syringe is not recommended for routine use. Its use should be considered only when a traditional syringe is not available or cannot be used. This system is also practical when diphenhydramine HCl is used as a local anesthetic in cases of presumed local anesthetic allergy (see Chapter 18). Box 5-7 lists the advantages and disadvantages of the disposable syringe.

Safety Syringes

Recent years have seen a move toward the development and introduction of *safety syringes* in both medicine and dentistry. Safety syringes minimize the risk of an accidental needle-stick injury occurring to a dental health provider with a contaminated needle after administration of a local anesthetic. These syringes possess a sheath that "locks" over the needle when it is removed from the patient's tissues, preventing accidental needle-stick.

Devices such as the UltraSafety Plus XL* and the 1 Shot Safety Syringe† were available as of January 2011. The UltraSafety Plus XL aspirating syringe system contains a syringe body assembly and a plunger assembly (Fig. 5-12, *A*). Once the syringe is properly assembled and the injection administered, the syringe may be made "safe" with one hand by gently moving the index and middle fingers against the front collar of the guard (Fig. 5-12, *B*). Once "guarded," the now contaminated needle is "safe," so that it is virtually impossible for dental health providers to be injured with the needle. Upon completion of the injection, the entire syringe is discarded into the proper receptacle (e.g., sharps container).

Dental safety syringes are designed as single-use items, although they permit reinjection. Reloading the syringe with a second anesthetic cartridge and reinjecting with the same syringe is discouraged because this obviates the important safety aspect of the device.

In 2000, Cuny and associates evaluated four dental safety syringe systems—Safe-Mate needle system (Septodont Inc.), Safety Plus syringe (Septodont Inc.), UltraSafe syringe (Septodont Inc.), and Hypo Safety syringe (Dentsply MPL Technologies, Franklin Park, Ill)—over a 1-year period at a U.S. dental school.[10] Their finding was that using these Food and Drug Administration (FDA)-approved devices resulted in an initial increase in needle-stick injuries. They stated that hands-on training, monitoring, and follow-up reminders appeared to be effective in reducing injuries associated with the change from traditional to safety needles.

Advantages and disadvantages of the safety syringe are listed in Box 5-8.

*UltraSafety Plus XL, Septodont Inc., 245C Quigley Blvd., New Castle, DE 19720; 1-800-872-8305; www.septodontinc.com.

†1 Shot Safety Syringe, Sultan Chemists, Englewood, NJ; 1-800-637-8582; www.sultanintl.com.

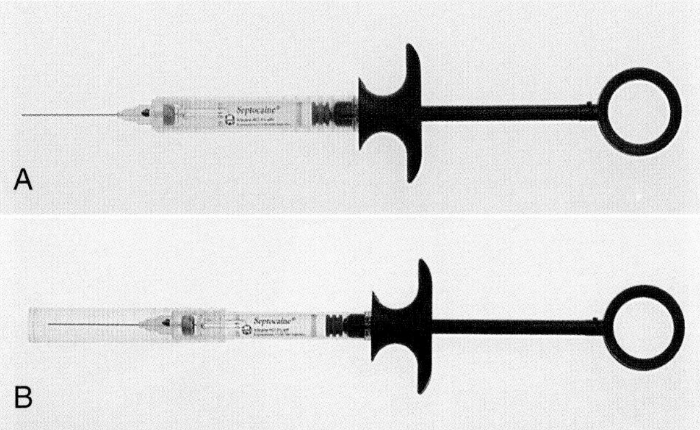

Figure 5-12. **A,** UltraSafety Plus XL aspirating syringe, ready for injection. **B,** UltraSafety Plus XL aspirating syringe; needle sheathed to prevent needle-stick injury.

BOX 5-8 Advantages and Disadvantages of the Safety Syringe

Advantages	Disadvantages
Disposable, single use	Cost: more expensive than reusable syringe
Sterile until opened	May feel awkward to a first-time user
Lightweight (better tactile sensation)	

Computer-Controlled Local Anesthetic Delivery (C-CLAD) Systems

The standard dental syringe described previously is a simple mechanical instrument that dates back to 1853, when Charles Pravaz patented the first syringe.[11] The dental syringe is a drug delivery device requiring that the operator simultaneously attempt to control the variables of drug infusion and

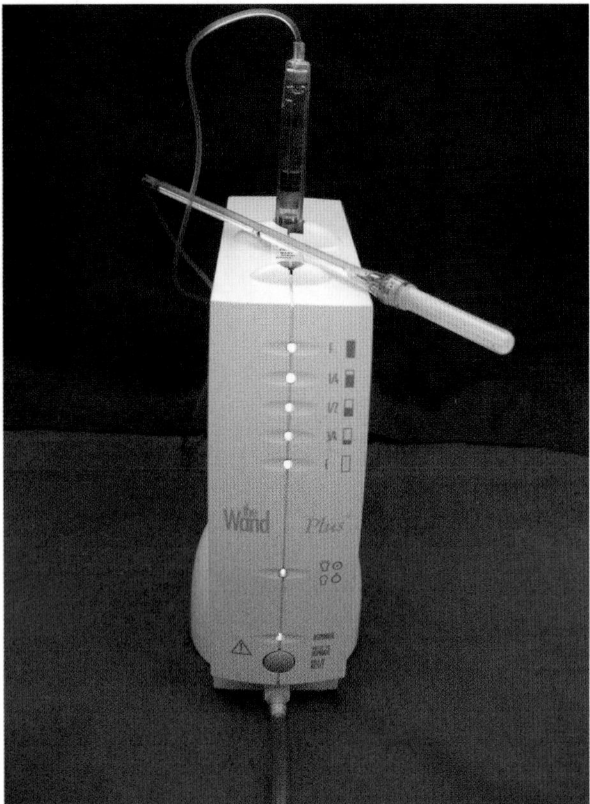

Figure 5-13. Computer-controlled local anesthetic delivery system—The Wand.

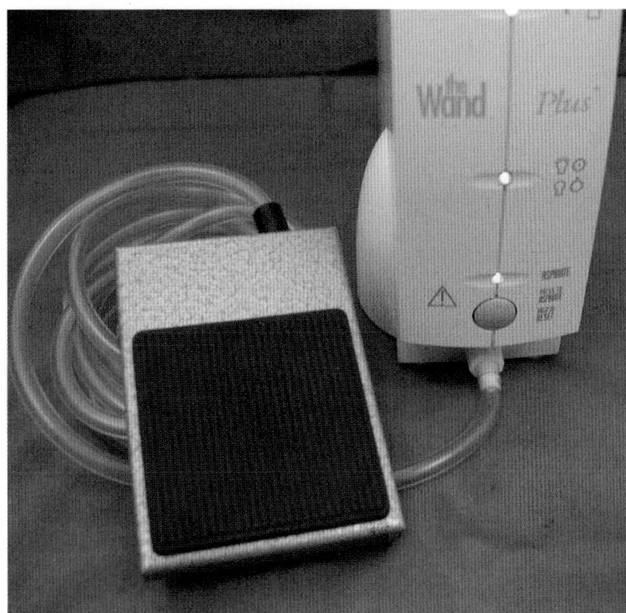

Figure 5-14. Foot-activated control of The Wand.

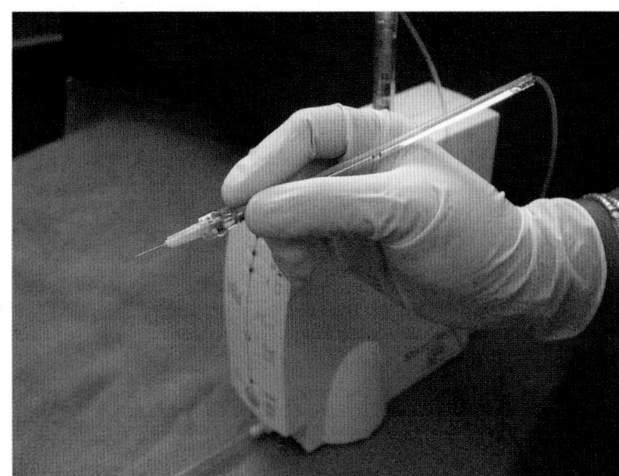

Figure 5-15. The Wand has a lightweight handpiece that provides improved tactile sensation and control.

the movement of a penetrating needle. The operator's inability to precisely control both of these activities during an injection can compromise an injection technique. In addition, a traditional syringe is handled with a palm-thumb grasp, which is not designed for ideal ergonomics or needle control during the injection. For certain practitioners—those with small hands—just holding a syringe with a full cartridge of anesthetic may be difficult.

In 1997 the first computer-controlled local anesthetic delivery (C-CLAD) system was introduced into dentistry. The Wand (Milestone Scientific Inc., Livingston, NJ) was designed to improve on the ergonomics and precision of the dental syringe (Fig. 5-13). This system enabled a dentist or hygienist to accurately manipulate needle placement with fingertip accuracy and deliver the local anesthetic with a foot-activated control (Fig. 5-14). A lightweight handpiece (Fig. 5-15), held in a penlike grasp, provides increased tactile sensation and control compared with the traditional syringe. Available flow rates of local anesthetic delivery are computer controlled and thus remain consistent from one injection to the next. C-CLAD systems represent a significant change in the manner in which a local anesthetic injection is administered. The operator is now able to focus attention on needle insertion and positioning, allowing the motor in the device to administer the drug at a preprogrammed rate of flow. It is likely that greater ergonomic control coupled with fixed flow rates is responsible for the improved injection experience demonstrated in many clinical studies conducted with these devices in dentistry.[12-16] Several clinical trials in medicine have demonstrated measurable benefits of this technology.[17,18]

Hochman and colleagues were the first to demonstrate a marked reduction in pain perception with injections using C-CLADs.[11] Fifty blindfolded dentists participated (they received the injection) in a controlled clinical study comparing the standard manual syringe with The Wand/CompuDent System for palatal injection. Forty-eight (96%) preferred injections with the C-CLADs. Overall pain perception was reduced two- to threefold when compared with the standard manual syringe.

Nicholson and associates conducted a randomized clinical study using two operators administering four different

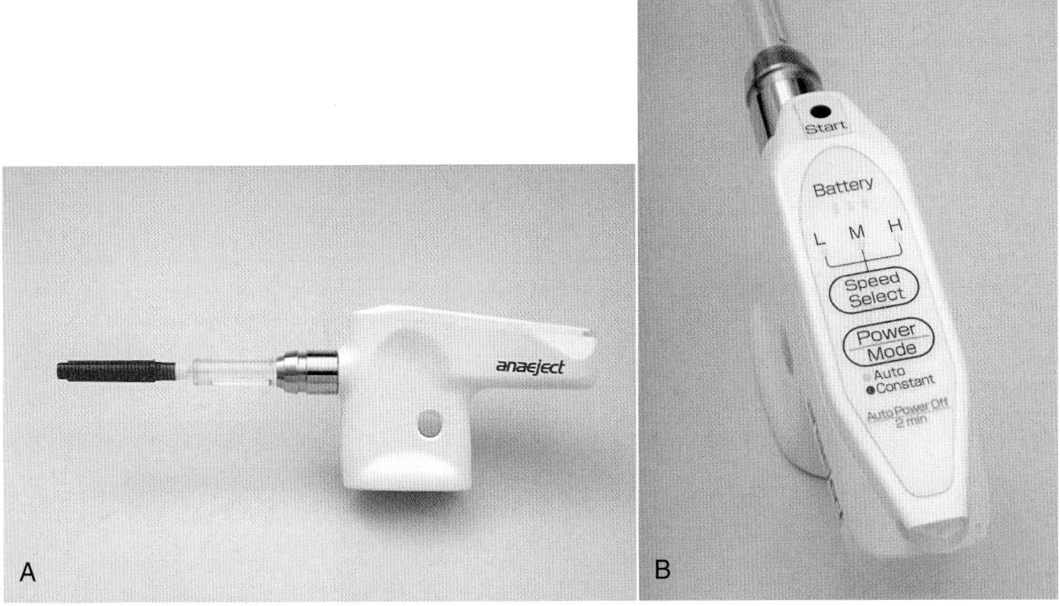

Figure 5-16. Anaeject computer-controlled local anesthetic delivery system.

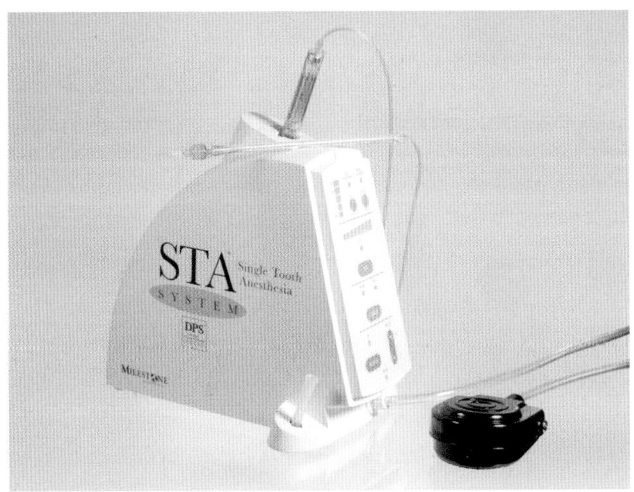

Figure 5-17. STA (Single Tooth Anesthesia) C-CLAD system.

types of dental injections to compare C-CLADs with the standard syringe.[13] Mean injection discomfort ratings were found to be consistently lower when C-CLADs were used compared with the manual syringe. Two thirds of patients preferred that future dental injections be performed with a C-CLAD system. Investigators in the study increasingly preferred to perform all injections with C-CLAD technology.

Perry and Loomer presented data from a single-blind crossover study comparing C-CLADs with traditional syringe delivery of local anesthetic for quadrant scaling and root planing. Twenty subjects received the anterior middle superior alveolar nerve block (AMSA) injection (described in Chapter 13). Scores for AMSA computer-controlled injection revealed highly significant differences in favor of the computer-controlled device ($P < .0001$).[14]

Fukayama and associates conducted a controlled clinical study to evaluate the pain perception of a C-CLAD device. Seventeen of 20 subjects reported a slight- or no-pain rating on a visual analog scale (VAS) for palatal injections administered with C-CLADs. Investigators concluded, "The new system provides comfortable anesthesia for patients and can be a good alternative for conventional manual syringe injection."[15]

At present, three C-CLADs are available in the North American market: The Wand/CompuDent System, The Wand/STA System, and the Comfort Control Syringe. Another system, the QuickSleeper, is marketed in Europe. Similar devices, such as the Anaeject, are marketed in Japan (Fig. 5-16).

The Wand/STA System. The STA-Single Tooth Anesthesia System (Milestone Scientific Inc., Livingston, NJ) represents a significant advance in C-CLAD technology (Fig. 5-17). The STA System was introduced in 2007. This third-generation C-CLAD instrument represents a new and meaningful innovation for subcutaneous injections performed both in dentistry and in medicine.[19] The technological advancement is related to the development of what is called *dynamic pressure-sensing technology* (DPS technology).[20] DPS technology enables the precise monitoring and control of fluid pressure at the needle tip when a subcutaneous injection is performed. Fluid exit-pressure at the needle tip is used to identify a given anatomic location and/or a specific tissue type based on this repeatable finding.[21] Exit-pressure information is provided to the clinician on a continuous basis in the form of spoken and/or audible sounds and visual indicators emitted from the STA instrument, thus providing continuous real-time feedback while a dental injection is performed (Fig. 5-18, *A* through *C*).[22]

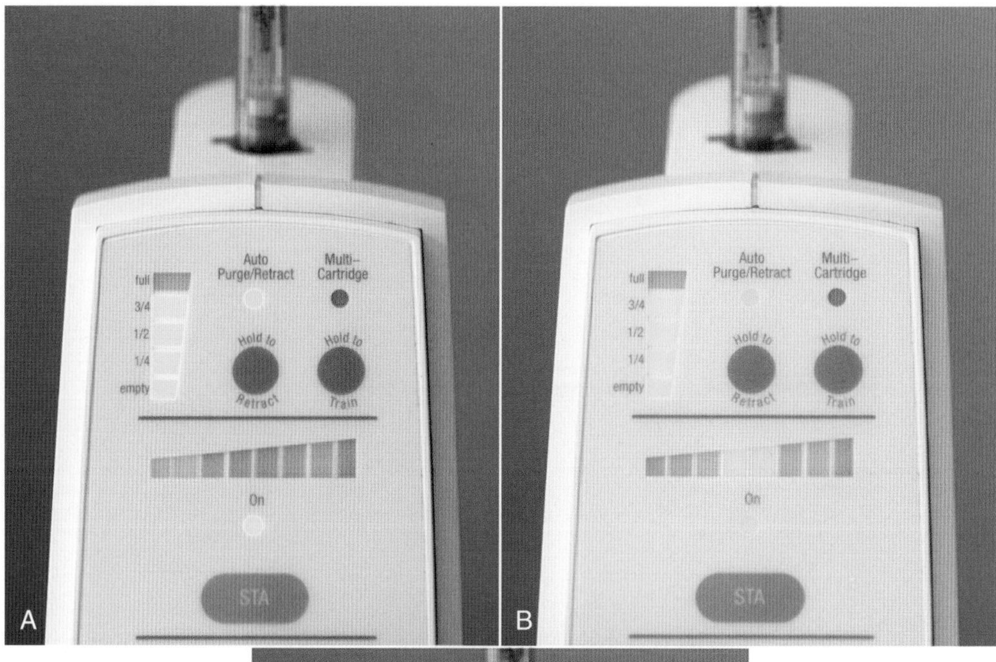

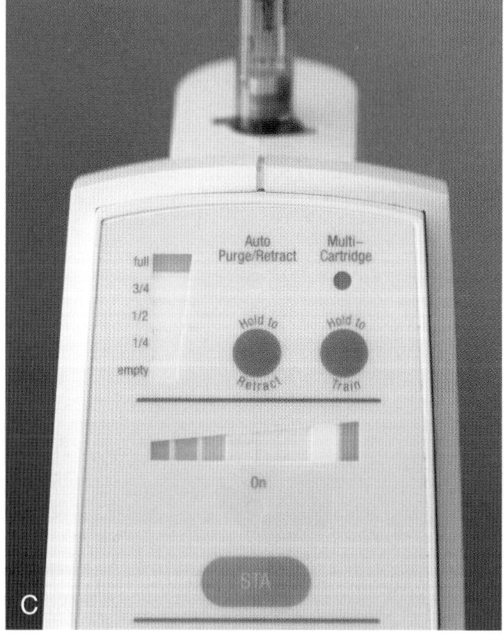

Figure 5-18. Dynamic Pressure Sensing (DPS) on the STA Single Tooth Anesthesia C-CLAD device provides both visual and audible feedback regarding placement of the needle tip during the periodontal ligament (PDL) injection. Horizontal color bars indicate pressure at the tip of the needle. **A,** Red—pressure is too low. **B,** Orange and dark yellow—increasing pressure but not yet adequate. **C,** Light yellow—correct pressure for PDL injection. At this point **(C)** the STA unit will also provide an audible clue "PDL, PDL, PDL" that the needle tip is properly situated.

The STA System instrument can perform all traditional injections, as well as several newer dental injection techniques as previously described with The Wand and CompuDent System instruments. In addition, the STA System offer a unique approach for performing PDL (intraligamentary) injection using DPS technology.[22] The instrument has been designed to accurately identify the precise anatomic location for the intraligamentary (PDL) injection.[23] The STA System audibly and visually "guides" placement of the needle tip into the anatomic entrance of the periodontal ligament space through DPS technology. Important to the success of the PDL injection is proper needle placement into its the PDL space. Use of a traditional syringe provides little or no information as to correct needle-tip location, so this can be considered a "blinded" approach to PDL injection. In contrast, using the DPS technology of the STA System informs the clinician of the status of needle position based on real-time information. This transforms the PDL injection technique into a "guided" technique that can be easily and accurately performed. Additionally, the STA instrument is capable of generating precise fluid pressures in ranges that are much lower in comparison with other injection devices. This ability to maintain lower pressures permits the absorption of greater volumes of anesthetic solution safely and effectively through the intraligamentary tissues—another benefit of this technology.[24] Allowing a greater volume of anesthetic to be safely administered results in a longer duration of anesthesia produced by the STA intraligamentary

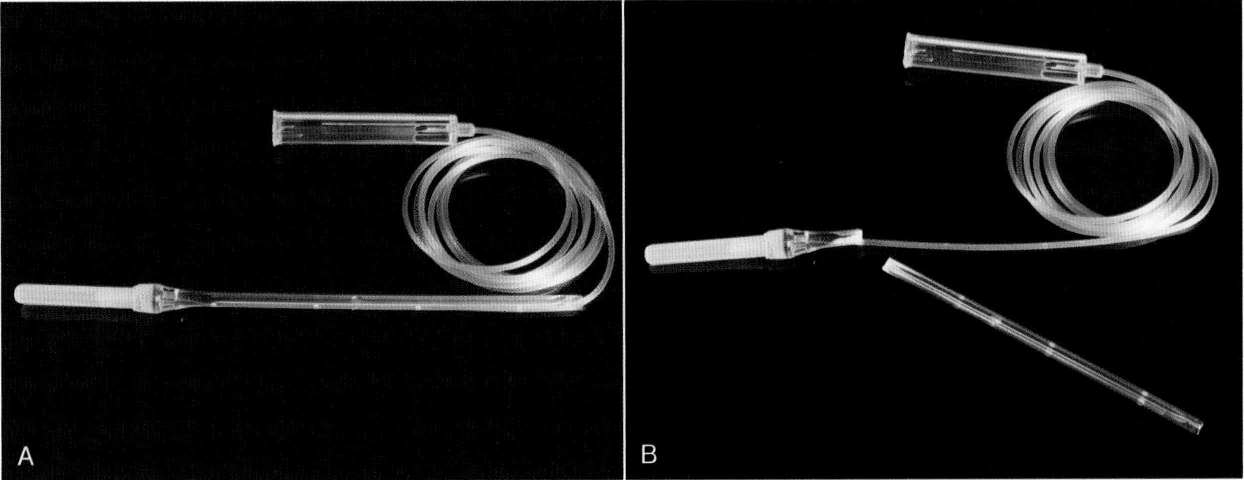

Figure 5-19. STA Wand handpiece is lightweight (less than 10 grams) **(A)** and can easily be shortened to aid in administration of some injections **(B)**, such as the AMSA or other palatal techniques.

injection compared with intraligamentary (PDL) injection performed using high-pressure syringes and/or other delivery instruments.[25]

Ferrari and coworkers published data on 60 patients receiving the intraligamentary (PDL) injection; they compared the STA System versus two other delivery instruments: a high-pressure mechanical syringe (Ligmaject, IMA Associates) and a conventional dental syringe.[25] Electrical pulp testing was performed on all teeth at regular intervals to determine success or failure when these different instruments are used. In addition, patient subjective pain responses were recorded post treatment. This study found the STA System to have a success rate of 100% in achieving effective pulpal anesthesia, as well as more rapid onset of anesthesia. The PDL injection in this study was performed as a primary injection for restorative dental care in mandibular teeth. The study also found subjective pain responses of "minimal or no pain" observed in all patients receiving PDL injections with the STA System. In contrast, PDL injections performed with the other two systems were found to have generally higher pain scores throughout testing. Investigators concluded that the STA instrument provided a more predictable, more reliable, and more comfortable PDL injection than a high-pressure mechanical syringe or a conventional dental syringe.

The STA System has two basic components: the STA Wand handpiece and the STA drive unit. The STA Wand handpiece is a single-use (per patient visit) lightweight handpiece (weighing less than 10 g) (Fig. 5-19, *A* and *B*). It provides excellent tactile control and use of a more desirable ergonomic grasp (Fig. 5-20). Clinicians have reported that a C-CLAD instrument, such as the STA System, is more comfortable to use and produces fewer musculoskeletal problems over the long term.[26]

STA Wand handpieces are available with many standard dental needle sizes: 30-gauge ½ inch, 27-gauge ½ inch, 30-gauge 1 inch, and 27-gauge 1¼ inch needle lengths. The STA Wand handpiece is a single-use sterilized handpiece

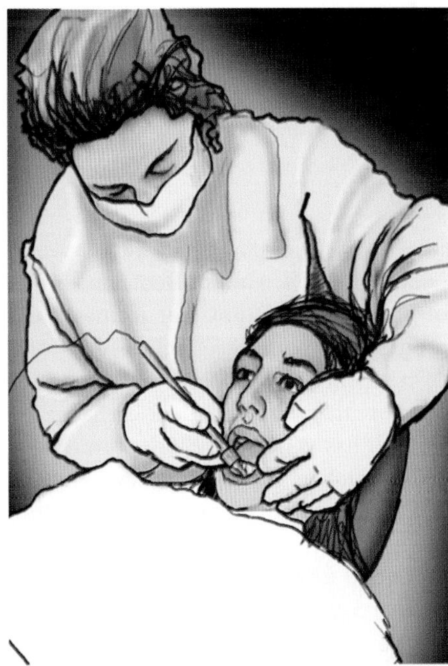

Figure 5-20. The STA Wand handpiece is held in an instrument grasp permitting the administrator greater tactile sensitivity during the injection.

(Fig. 5-21) that is available in two forms: one in which the handpiece has a preattached needle, and one in which a needle needs to be attached at the time of treatment. When the STA intraligamentary (PDL) injection is performed, it is suggested that a preattached needle handpiece be used. The STA Wand handpiece provides the general benefit of being easier and lighter to hold, allowing for greater access and ease of use as compared with the conventional syringe. Additionally, the STA Wand handpiece can be modified to different lengths for greater versatility of use (see Fig. 5-19, *B*).

The second component of the STA System is the drive unit itself. The drive unit integrates two cap holders into the base of the unit, thus allowing single-handed recapping of the needle from either side of the unit (see Fig. 5-17). New

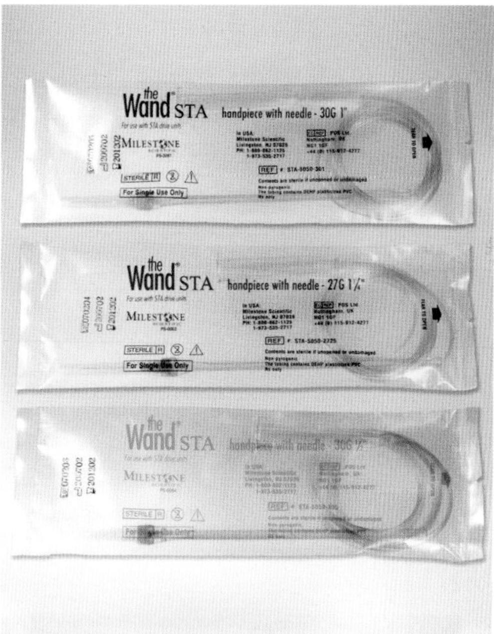

Figure 5-21. The STA Wand handpiece is presterilized, single-use and is available in a variety of needle gauge and lengths. Other Luer-Lok needles can also be sued on this handpiece.

BOX 5-9 Advantages and Disadvantages of The Wand/STA System

Advantages

Dynamic pressure-sensing (DPS) technology provides continuous real-time feedback when an injection is performed, resulting in a more predictable injection site location.
Allows the periodontal ligament (PDL) injection to be used as a predictable primary injection
Can be used for all traditional injection techniques
Recommended device for newer injection techniques such as anterior middle superior alveolar nerve block (AMSA), palatal anterior superior alveolar nerve block (P-ASA), and STA-intraligamentary injection
Reduces pain-disruptive behavior in children and adults
Reduces stress for patient
Reduces stress for operator

Disadvantages

Requires additional armamentarium
Cost

features not previously available with earlier versions of this C-CLAD device (Wand, CompuDent) include automatic purging of anesthetic solution that primes the handpiece before use, automatic plunger retraction after completion of use, and a multicartridge feature that reduces anesthetic waste when more than one anesthetic cartridge is used. The STA System also has a Training Mode feature that provides clinicians with spoken instructional guidance on its use, thereby minimizing the learning curve when the system is used for the first time.

Advantages and disadvantages of The Wand/STA System are listed in Box 5-9.

Comfort Control Syringe. Introduced several years after The Wand, the Comfort Control Syringe (CCS) System attempts to improve on the C-CLAD concept. The CCS System is an electronic, preprogrammed delivery device that provides the operator with the control needed to make the patient's local anesthetic injection experience as pleasant as possible (Fig. 5-22). As with other C-CLADs, this is achieved by depositing the local anesthetic more slowly and consistently than is possible manually. The CCS has a two-stage delivery system. Injection begins at an extremely slow rate to avoid the pain associated with rapid anesthetic delivery. After 10 seconds, the CCS automatically increases speed to a preprogrammed injection rate for the technique selected. Five preprogrammed injection rates are available for specific injections: Block, Infiltration, PDL, AMSA/palatal anterior superior alveolar nerve block (P-ASA), and Lingual Infiltration.

The handpiece controls are shown in Figure 5-23.

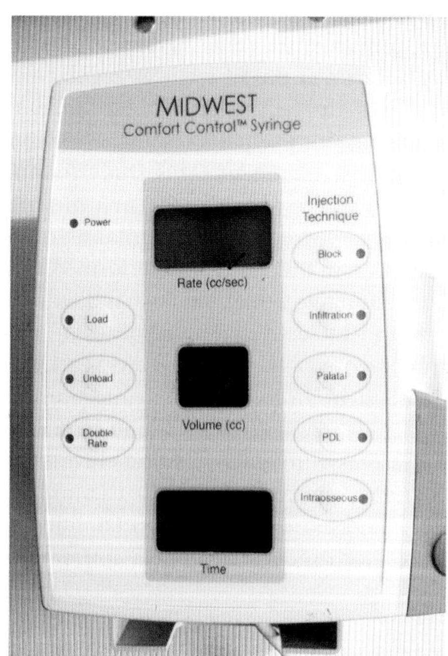

Figure 5-22. Comfort Control Syringe (CCS) body.

- The front button with the arrow and square controls the "Start/Stop" functions by initiating or terminating the selected program.
- The middle button activates the "Aspiration" function by slightly retracting the plunger.
- The rear button initiates "Double Rate" and operates in the same manner as the Double Rate button on the unit. It doubles the preprogrammed injection rate. Re-selecting it restores the preprogrammed speed.

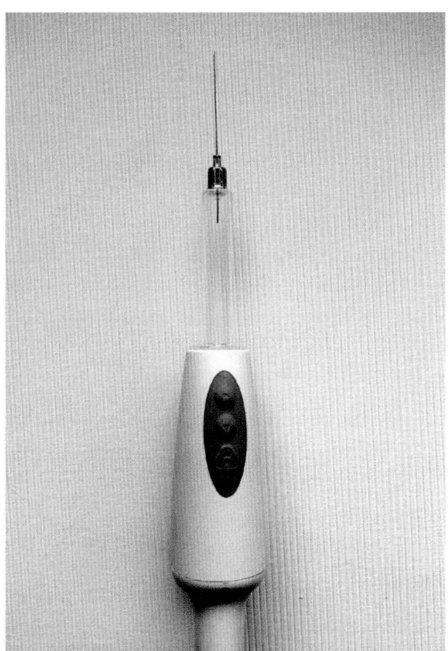

Figure 5-23. Comfort Control Syringe (CCS) handpiece.

BOX 5-10 Advantages and Disadvantages of the Comfort Control Syringe

Advantages	Disadvantages
Familiar "syringe" type of delivery system	Requires additional armamentarium
Easy to see exactly how much local anesthetic solution has been dispensed, just as on a manual syringe	More bulky than other computer-controlled local (C-CLAD) manual local anesthesia delivery devices
Inexpensive disposables (≈50¢/use)	Vibration may bother some users
All controls literally at the fingertips	Cost
Less costly than other C-CLADs	
Allows selection of various rates of delivery matched to the user injection technique utilized	

C-CLAD, Computer-controlled local anesthetic delivery.

Standard dental local anesthetic cartridges and dental needles may be used in the CCS. Box 5-10 lists advantages and disadvantages of the CCS.

C-CLADs allow local anesthetics to be administered comfortably to the patient in virtually all areas of the oral cavity. This is of greatest importance in the palate, where the level of patient discomfort can be significant. The nasopalatine nerve block, as well as other palatal injections (e.g., AMSA,[27] P-ASA[28]), can be administered atraumatically in most patients. It is reasonable to conclude that any injection technique that has even a remote possibility of being uncomfortable for the patient can be delivered more comfortably using a C-CLAD device.

CARE AND HANDLING OF SYRINGES

When properly maintained, metal and plastic reusable syringes are designed to provide long-term service. Following is a summary of manufacturers' recommendations concerning care of these syringes:

1. After each use, the syringe should be thoroughly washed and rinsed so as to be free of any local anesthetic solution, saliva, or other foreign matter. The syringe should be autoclaved in the same manner as other surgical instruments.
2. After every five autoclavings, the syringe should be dismantled and all threaded joints and the area where the piston contacts the thumb ring and the guide bearing should be lightly lubricated.
3. The harpoon should be cleaned with a brush after each use.
4. Although the harpoon is designed for long-term use, prolonged use will result in decreased sharpness and failure to remain embedded within the stopper of the cartridge. Replacement pistons and harpoons are readily available at low cost.

PROBLEMS

Leakage During Injection

When a syringe is reloaded with a second local anesthetic cartridge and a needle is already in place, care must be taken to ensure that the needle penetrates the center of the rubber diaphragm. An off-center perforation produces an ovoid puncture of the diaphragm, allowing leakage of the anesthetic solution around the outside of the metal needle and into the patient's mouth (Fig. 5-24). (For further information, see Chapter 7.)

Broken Cartridge

A badly worn syringe may damage the cartridge, leading to breakage. This also can result from a bent harpoon. A needle that is bent at its proximal end (Fig. 5-25) may not perforate the diaphragm on the cartridge. Positive pressure on the thumb ring increases pressure within the cartridge, which may cause the cartridge to break.

Bent Harpoon

The harpoon must be sharp and straight (Fig. 5-26). A bent harpoon produces an off-center puncture of the silicone rubber plunger, causing the plunger to rotate as it moves down the glass cartridge. This may result in cartridge breakage.

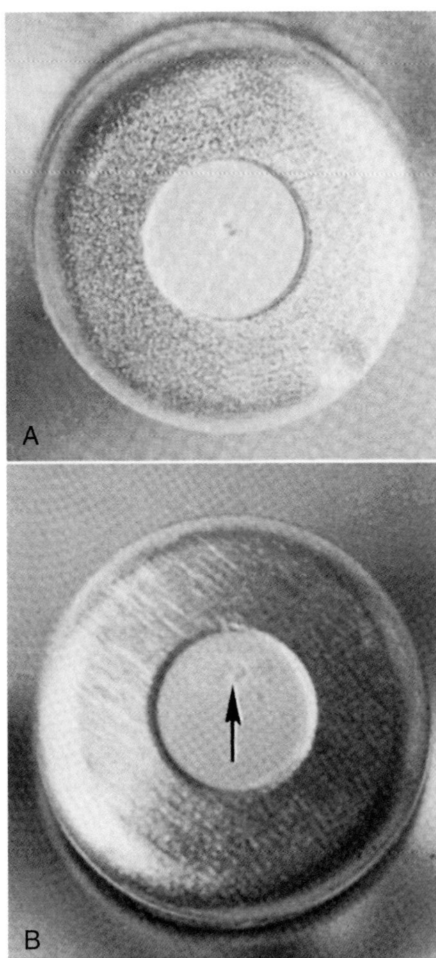

Figure 5-24. Eccentric perforation. **A,** Centric perforation of the diaphragm by a needle prevents leakage during injection. **B,** Off-center perforation *(arrow)* permits leakage of anesthetic solution into the patient's mouth.

Disengagement of the Harpoon from the Plunger During Aspiration

Disengagement occurs if the harpoon is dull or if the administrator applies too much pressure to the thumb ring during aspiration. If this happens, the harpoon should be cleansed and sharpened or replaced with a new sharp harpoon. Disengagement is most likely to occur when a 30-gauge dental needle is being used because significant resistance is produced within the needle lumen as aspiration is attempted. A very gentle backward motion of the plunger is all that is necessary for successful aspiration. Forceful action is not necessary. (See the discussion in Chapter 11.)

Surface Deposits

An accumulation of debris, saliva, and disinfectant solution interferes with syringe function and appearance. Deposits, which can resemble rust, may be removed with a thorough scrubbing. Ultrasonic cleaning will not harm syringes.

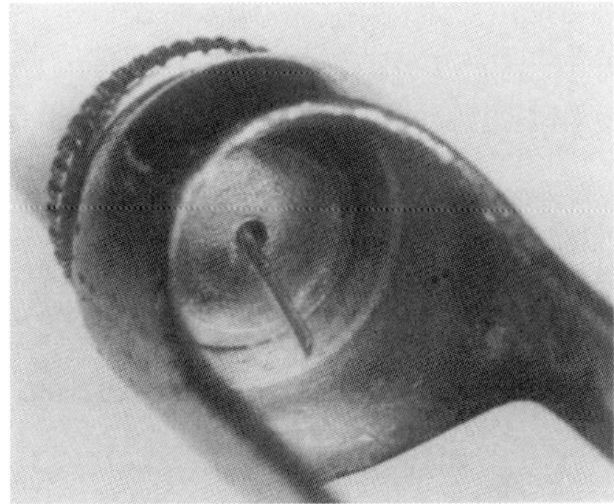

Figure 5-25. Bent needle. A needle bent at the proximal end may not perforate the cartridge diaphragm. Pressure on the thumb ring can lead to cartridge breakage.

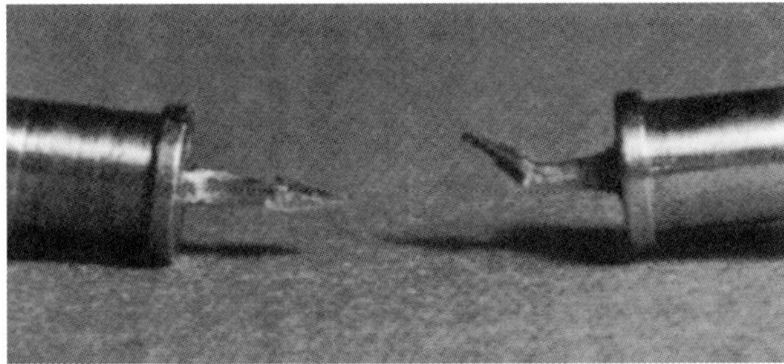

Figure 5-26. Note the bent harpoon of the syringe on the right.

RECOMMENDATIONS

No conclusive evidence indicates that any manufacturer's syringe is superior. Therefore the ultimate decision in selection of a syringe must be left to the discretion of the buyer. It is recommended, however, that before purchasing any syringe, the buyer place a full dental cartridge into it and pick up the syringe as if to use it. It should be noted whether the fingers (thumb to other fingers) are stretched maximally, because to aspirate with a harpoon-type syringe, one must be able to pull the thumb ring back several millimeters. If one is not able to do so, reliable aspiration is not possible. Although all syringes available today are of roughly the same dimensions, some variation is noted. Manufacturers market syringes with smaller thumb rings or shorter pistons. These modifications make aspiration easier to accomplish for persons with smaller hands.

Following are additional recommendations:

1. A safety syringe, minimizing the risk of accidental needle-stick injury, is recommended for use during all local anesthetic injections.
2. A self-aspirating syringe is recommended for practitioners with small hands.
3. Any syringe system used must be capable of aspiration. Nonaspirating syringes should never be used for local anesthetic injections.
4. All reusable syringes must be capable of being sterilized.
5. Nonreusable syringes must be disposed of properly.

References

1. Council on Dental Materials and Devices: New American National Standards Institute/American Dental Association specification no. 34 for dental aspirating syringes, J Am Dent Assoc 97:236–238, 1978.
2. Council on Dental Materials, Instruments, and Equipment: Addendum to American National Standards Institute/American Dental Association specification no. 34 for dental aspirating syringes, J Am Dent Assoc 104:69–70, 1982.
3. Bartlett SZ: Clinical observations on the effects of injections of local anesthetic preceded by aspiration, Oral Surg 33:520, 1972.
4. Malamed SF: Handbook of local anesthesia, St Louis, 1980, Mosby.
5. Meechan JG, Blair GS, McCabe JF: Local anaesthesia in dental practice. II. A laboratory investigation of a self-aspirating system, Br Dent J 159:109–113, 1985.
6. Meechan JG: A comparison of three different automatic aspirating dental cartridge syringes, J Dent 16:40–43, 1988.
7. Peterson JK: Efficacy of a self-aspirating syringe, Int J Oral Maxillofac Surg 16:241–244, 1987.
8. Figge FHJ, Scherer RP: Anatomical studies on jet penetration of human skin for subcutaneous medication without the use of needles, Anat Rec 97:335, 1947 (abstract).
9. Margetis PM, Quarantillo EP, Lindberg RB: Jet injection local anesthesia in dentistry: a report of 66 cases, US Armed Forces Med J 9:625–634, 1958.
10. Hoffmann-Axthelm W: History of dentistry, Chicago, 1981, Quintessence, p 339.
11. Hochman MN, Chiarello D, Hochman CB, et al: Computerized local anesthesia delivery vs. traditional syringe technique, NY State Dent J 63:24–29, 1997.
12. Gibson RS, Allen K, Hutfless S, et al: The Wand vs. traditional injection: a comparison of pain related behaviors, Pediatr Dent 22:458–462, 2000.
13. Nicholson JW, Berry TG, Summitt JB, et al: Pain perception and utility: a comparison of the syringe and computerized local injection techniques, Gen Dent 49:167–172, 2001.
14. Perry DA, Loomer PM: Maximizing pain control: the AMSA injection can provide anesthesia with few injections and less pain, Dimensions Dent Hyg 1:28–33, 2003.
15. Fukayama H, Yoshikawa F, Kohase H, et al: Efficacy of anterior and middle superior alveolar (AMSA) anesthesia using a new injection system: The Wand, Quint Int 34:737–741, 2003.
16. Tan PY, Vukasin P, Chin ID, et al: The Wand local anesthetic delivery system, Dis Colon Rectum 44:686–689, 2001.
17. Landsman A, DeFronzo D, Hedman J, McDonald J: A new system for decreasing the level of injection pain associated with local anesthesia of a toe, (abstract). Annual Meeting of the American Academy of Podiatric Medicine 2001.
18. Friedman MJ, Hochman MN: 21st century computerized injection for local pain control, Compend Contin Educ Dent 18:995–1003, 1997.
19. Kudo M, Ohke H, Katagiri K, et al: The shape of local anesthetic injection syringes with less discomfort and anxiety: evaluation of discomfort and anxiety caused by various types of local anesthetic injection syringes in high level trait-anxiety people, J Jpn Dent Soc Anesthesiol 29:173–178, 2001.
20. Hochman MN, Friedman MJ: In vitro study of needle deflection: a linear insertion technique versus a bi-directional rotation insertion technique, Quint Int 31:737–743, 2000.
21. Hochman MN, Friedman MJ: An in vitro study of needle force penetration comparing a standard linear insertion to the new bidirectional rotation insertion technique, Quint Int 32:789–796, 2001.
22. Pashley EL, Nelson R, Pashley DH: Pressures created by dental injections, J Dent Res 60:1742–1748, 1981.
23. Fuhs QM, Walker WA, Gouigh RW, et al: The periodontal ligament injection: histological effects on the periodontium in dogs, J Endodont 9:411–415, 1983.
24. Galili D, Kaufman E, Garfunkel AA, et al: Intraligamentary anesthesia: a histological study, Int J Oral Surg 12:511–516, 1984.
25. Albers DD, Ellinger RF: Histologic effects of high- pressure intraligamental injections on the periodontal ligament, Quint Int 19:361–363, 1988.
26. Froum SJ, Tarnow D, Caiazzo A, et al: Histologic response to intraligament injections using a computerized local anesthetic delivery system: a pilot study in Mini-Swine, J Periodont 71:1453–1459, 2000.
27. Friedman MJ, Hochman MN: The AMSA injection: a new concept for local anesthesia of maxillary teeth using a computer-controlled injection system, Quint Int 29:297–303, 1998.
28. Friedman MJ, Hochman MN: P-ASA block injection: a new palatal technique to anesthetize maxillary anterior teeth, J Esthet Dent 11:23–71, 1999.

CHAPTER 6

The Needle

TYPES

The needle is the vehicle that permits local anesthetic solution to travel from the dental cartridge into the tissues surrounding the needle tip. Most needles used in dentistry are stainless steel and disposable. Needles manufactured for dental intraoral injections are presterilized and disposable.

Reusable needles should not be used for injections.

Because the needle represents the most dangerous component of the armamentarium, the one most likely to produce injury to patient or doctor, *safety needles* are being developed.[1,2] Although these needles are not yet used to any appreciable degree in dentistry in the United States, it is likely that at some point in the not too distant future their use will become commonplace, if not mandatory.

ANATOMY OF A NEEDLE

The needle is composed of a single piece of tubular metal around which is placed a plastic or metal syringe adaptor and the needle hub (Fig. 6-1).

All needles have the following components in common: the bevel, the shaft, the hub, and the cartridge-penetrating end (Fig. 6-2).

The *bevel* defines the point or tip of the needle. Bevels are described by manufacturers as long, medium, and short. Several authors have confirmed that the greater the angle of the bevel with the long axis of the needle, the greater will be the degree of deflection as the needle passes through hydrocolloid (or the soft tissues of the mouth) (Fig. 6-3).[3-6] A needle whose point is centered on the long axis (e.g., the Huber point, the Truject needle; Fig. 6-4, *A*) will deflect to a lesser extent than a beveled-point needle, whose point is eccentric (Fig. 6-4, *B*) (Table 6-1).

Several manufacturers of dental needles have placed indicators on the plastic or metal hub to help orient the doctor to the position of the bevel during needle insertion and injection of the drug.

The *shaft* of the needle is one long piece of tubular metal running from the tip of the needle through the hub, and continuing to the piece that penetrates the cartridge (see Fig. 6-1). Two factors to be considered about this component of the needle are the diameter of its lumen (e.g., the needle gauge) and the length of the shaft from point to hub.

The *hub* is a plastic or metal piece through which the needle attaches to the syringe. The interior surface of metal-hubbed needles is prethreaded, as are most but not all plastic-hubbed needles.

The *cartridge-penetrating end* of the dental needle extends through the needle adaptor and perforates the diaphragm of the local anesthetic cartridge. Its blunt end rests within the cartridge.

When needles are selected for use in various injection techniques, two factors that must be considered are gauge and length.

GAUGE

Gauge refers to the diameter of the lumen of the needle: the smaller the number, the greater the diameter of the lumen. A 30-gauge needle has a smaller internal diameter than a 25-gauge needle. In the United States, needles are color-coded by gauge (Fig. 6-5).

There is a growing trend toward the use of smaller-diameter (higher-number gauge) needles, based on the assumption that they are less traumatic to the patient than needles with larger diameters (Table 6-2). This assumption is unwarranted.[7] Hamburg[8] demonstrated as far back as 1972 that patients cannot differentiate among 23-, 25-, 27-, and 30-gauge needles. Others have confirmed this finding.[9,10] A clinical experiment demonstrates this point:

1. Three needles—25-, 27-, and 30-gauge—are selected.
2. The buccal mucosa over the maxillary anterior teeth should be dried.
3. No topical anesthetic should be used.
4. The mucosa should be taut.
5. The mucosa should be gently penetrated (about 2 to 3 mm) with each of the three needles without revealing to the patient which needle is being used. A different site should be selected for each penetration.
6. Question the patient about his or her "feelings": Which one was felt the most? Which one the least?

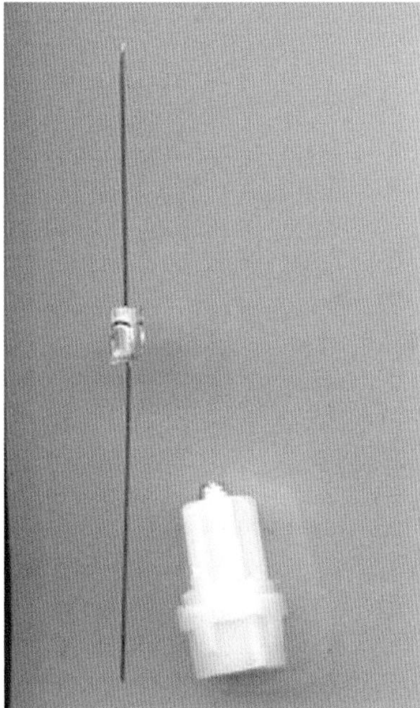

Figure 6-1. Metal disposable needle, dissembled.

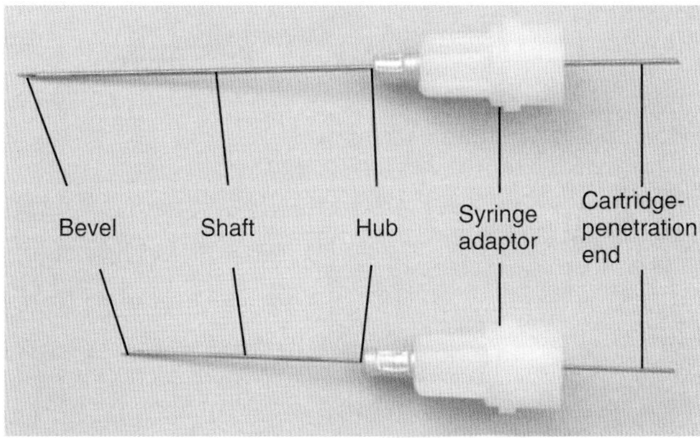

Figure 6-2. Components of dental local anesthetic needle. Long needle *(top)*; short needle *(bottom)*.

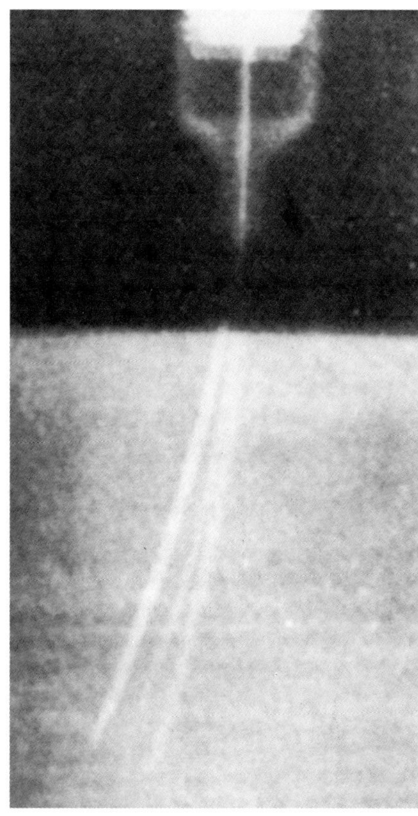

Figure 6-3. Radiograph demonstrating varying degrees of needle deflection with different gauges (*left to right,* 30-, 27-, and 25-). (From Robison SF, Mayhew RB, Cowan RD, et al: Comparative study of deflection characteristics and fragility of 25-, 27-, and 30-gauge short dental needles, *J Am Dent Assoc* 109:920-924, 1984.)

In literally hundreds of clinical demonstrations, no patient was able to correctly determine the gauge of each needle. The usual response has been that he or she could not discern any difference.

Larger-gauge needles (e.g., 25-gauge, 27-gauge) have distinct advantages over smaller ones (30-gauge) (Box 6-1): less deflection occurs as the needle passes through tissues (see Table 6-1 and Fig. 6-3). This leads to *greater accuracy* during needle insertion (it goes in a straighter line) and, it is hoped, to increased success rates, especially for techniques in which the depth of soft tissue penetrated is significant (e.g., inferior alveolar, Gow-Gates mandibular, Akinosi-Vazirani mandibular, anterior superior alveolar [ASA; infraorbital] nerve blocks). *Needle breakage,* although rare today with the use of disposable needles, is even less likely to occur with a larger needle. Numerous authors[11-14] have demonstrated that *aspiration of blood* is easier and more reliable through a larger lumen. Foldes and McNall[11] reported the following findings based on an unpublished study by Monheim:

1. One hundred percent positive aspirations were achieved from blood vessels with 25-gauge needles.
2. Eighty-seven percent positive aspirations were achieved from blood vessels with 27-gauge needles.
3. Two percent positive aspirations were achieved from blood vessels with 30-gauge needles.

Trapp and Davies[15] reported that in vivo human blood may be aspirated through 23-, 25-, 27-, and 30-gauge needles without a clinically significant difference in resistance to flow.

Despite this ambiguity concerning ability to aspirate blood through needles of various gauges, the use of larger needles (e.g., 25-gauge, 27-gauge) is recommended for any injection technique used in a highly vascular area, or when needle deflection through soft tissue would be a factor. Although blood may be aspirated through all 23- through 30-gauge needles, resistance to aspiration is greater when smaller-gauge needles are used, increasing the likelihood that the metal harpoon will become dislodged from the rubber plunger during aspiration, making the aspiration attempt futile.

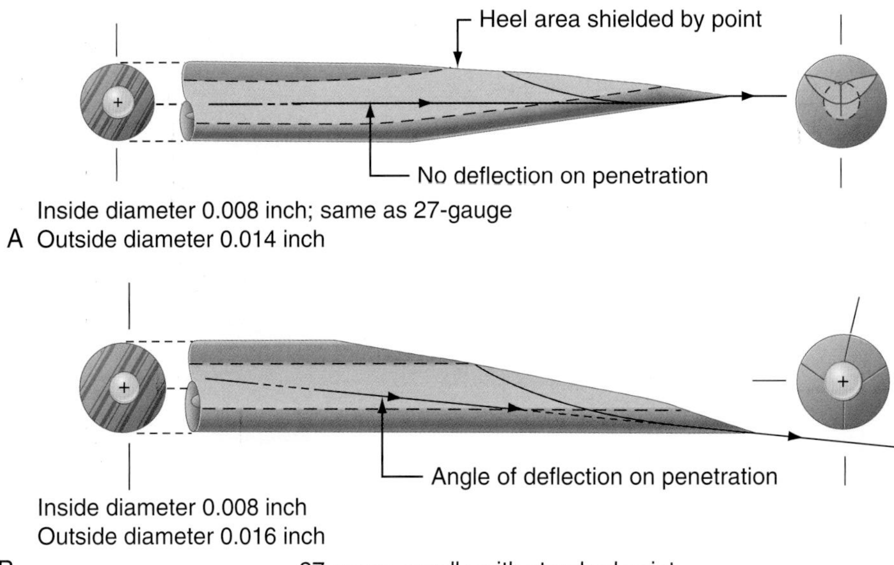

Figure 6-4. **A,** The tip of a nondeflecting needle is located in the center of the shaft, thereby minimizing deflection as the needle penetrates soft tissues. **B,** Conventional dental needle. The needle tip lies at the lower edge of the needle shaft, thereby producing deflection as the needle passes through soft tissue.

TABLE 6-1
Deflection of Needles Inserted in Hydrocolloid Tubes to Their Hubs

	Length (mm, Tip to Hub)	Maximum Tip Deflection (mm, ± SD)
25-Gauge long (conventional)	35	7.1 ± 0.81*
27-Gauge long (conventional)	36	8.4 ± 1.2*
27-Gauge short (conventional)	26	4.6 ± 0.97†
28-Gauge long (nondeflecting)	31	1.1 ± 0.82
28-Gauge short (nondeflecting)	22	0.8 ± 0.91

Data modified from Jeske AH, Boshart BF: Deflection of conventional versus non-deflecting dental needles in vitro, Anesth Prog 32:62-64, 1985.
*A statistically significant difference from the nondeflecting long needle ($P < .01$); n = 10 needles in each group.
†A statistically significant difference from the nondeflecting short needle ($P < .01$); n = 10 needles in each group.

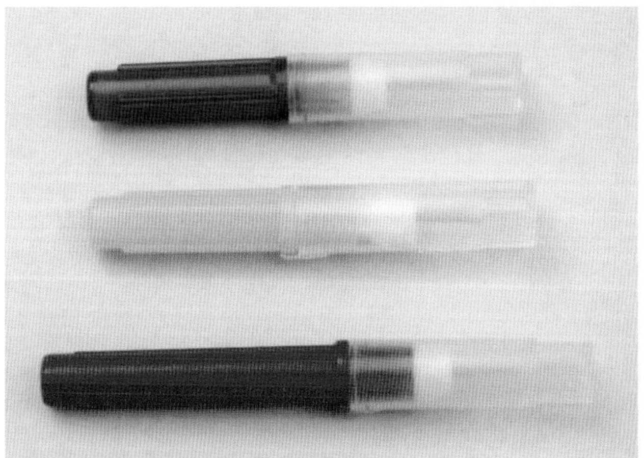

Figure 6-5. Color-coding by needle gauge: 25-gauge, red; 27-gauge, yellow; 30-gauge, blue.

BOX 6-1 Advantages of Larger-Gauge Needles Over Smaller-Gauge Needles

1. Less deflection, as needle advances through tissues
2. Greater accuracy of injection
3. Less chance of needle breakage
4. Easier aspiration
5. No perceptual difference in patient comfort

TABLE 6-2
Needle Purchases, U.S. Dentistry, 2006

		DATA PROVIDED BY			
Gauge	Length	Sullivan-Schein Inc. (2006)		Septodont Inc. (2006)	
25	Short	<1%	1%	0.6%	3%
	Long	1%		2.3%	
27	Short	10%	42%	13%	38%
	Long	32%		25%	
30	Short	50%	56%	51%	59%
	Extra short	6%		8%	

From Malamed SF, Reed KL, Poorsattar S: Needle breakage: incidence and prevention, Dent Clin North Am 54:745-756, 2010.

TABLE 6-3
Specifications for Needle Gauges*

Gauge	Outer Diameter, mm	Inner Diameter, mm
7	4.57	3.81
8	4.19	3.43
10	3.40	2.69
11	3.05	2.39
12	2.77	2.16
13	2.41	1.80
14	2.11	1.60
15	1.83	1.32
16	1.65	1.19
17	1.50	1.04
18	1.27	0.84
19	1.07	0.69
20	0.91	0.58
21	0.81	0.51
22	0.71	0.41
23	0.64	0.33
25	0.51	0.25
26	0.46	0.25
27	0.41	0.20
30	0.31	0.15

*Dental needle gauges highlighted.

Industry standards for needle gauge have been in place for years (Table 6-3); however, variations in internal diameter do exist between needle manufacturers. Larger-gauge needles (e.g., 25-gauge, 27-gauge) should be used when the risk of positive aspiration is increased, as during an inferior alveolar, posterior superior alveolar, or mental or incisive nerve block.

The most commonly used (e.g., most often purchased) needles in dentistry are the 30-gauge short and the 27-gauge long.[16] The 25-gauge (long or short) remains the preferred needle for all injections presenting a high risk of positive aspiration. The 27-gauge can be used for all other injection techniques, provided the aspiration percentage is low and tissue penetration depth is not great (increased deflection with this thinner needle). The 30-gauge needle is not specifically recommended for any injection, although it may be used in instances of localized infiltration, as when hemostasis is attained during periodontal therapy.

Deflection of the needle is a consideration when a needle must penetrate a greater thickness of soft tissue. On the standard dental needle (see Fig. 6-4, *B*), the tip of the point is located eccentrically. As the needle shaft penetrates soft tissue, the point of the needle is deflected by the tissue through which it passes. The greater the angle of the bevel, the greater is the degree of needle deflection. Every decade or so, a needle is introduced on which the tip of the point is located in the center of the lumen, thereby minimizing deflection as the needle passes through soft tissue (see Fig. 6-4, *A*). Jeske and Boshart[4] demonstrated the effectiveness of this "nondeflecting" needle (see Table 6-1). However, it needs to be demonstrated clinically that a lesser degree of needle deflection occurring as the needle passes through soft tissues actually results in an increased rate of successful anesthesia compared with that observed with standard needles. Over years of use, dentists become accustomed to the deflecting needles they use and gradually modify their injection techniques to accommodate this deflection (they "learn" to make the injections work even with deflection). Changing to a nondeflecting needle might initially lead to lower success rates.

Minimizing Needle Deflection: Bi-Rotational Insertion Technique (BRIT)

A new approach to reducing needle deflection has been described.[17] Rotational insertion (described as bi-rotational insertion technique [BRIT]), a technique in which the operator rotates the handpiece or needle in a back-and-forth rotational movement while advancing the needle through soft tissue, is similar to techniques used for acupuncture or endodontic instrumentation. Hochman and Friedman demonstrated that needle deflection could be virtually eliminated by using a rotational insertion technique during needle advancement.[17] An in-vitro study of 60 needle insertions into a tissue-like medium was performed with needles of three different gauges to compare rotational insertion versus the traditional linear nonrotating insertion technique. Investigators demonstrated that deflectional bending of a needle could be minimized or eliminated, regardless of the length or gauge of a needle, as long as the insertion was performed using the bi-rotational insertion technique.

Deflection of a needle is a consequence of resultant forces acting on the needle bevel during tissue penetration and advancement. An eccentric pointed beveled needle generates several different forces that act on it during insertion when a nonrotating linear insertion technique is used. A linear insertion technique is the conventional technique used with the traditional dental syringe, which is typically held with a palm-thumb grasp (Fig. 6-6). During this type of insertion, a force perpendicular to the forward directional movement (vector) acts on the surface of the beveled needle, causing the needle to bend (or deflect) in a direction opposite to

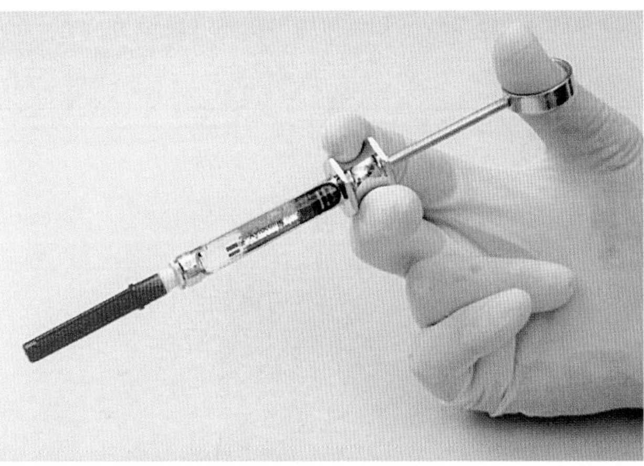

Figure 6-6. Traditional syringe held in palm-thumb grasp.

which the bevel faces (e.g., if the bevel faces "up," the advancing movement causes a beveled needle to deflect "downward"). The longer the needle length, the more exaggerated the bending or deflection becomes as a result of the greater distance traveled along the deflecting path. The smaller the diameter of the needle, the more exaggerated the bending or deflection, because a smaller-gauge needle is less capable of resisting the deflection or bending force on the surface of the beveled needle tip.

When the BRIT is used during needle insertion, the perpendicular force that causes deflection is eliminated or "neutralized" from the constant changing of bevel orientation as it is rotated (Fig. 6-7).[17] This allows eccentrically beveled needles to travel in a straight path. The traditional handheld syringe requires a palm-thumb grasp (see Fig. 6-6) that does not permit such a technique. A computer-controlled local anesthetic delivery (C-CLAD) device such as The Wand/CompuDent/STA (Milestone Scientific Inc., Livingston, NJ; discussed in Chapter 5) employs a lightweight handpiece that is held with a "penlike" or "dart" grasp that is easily rotated.

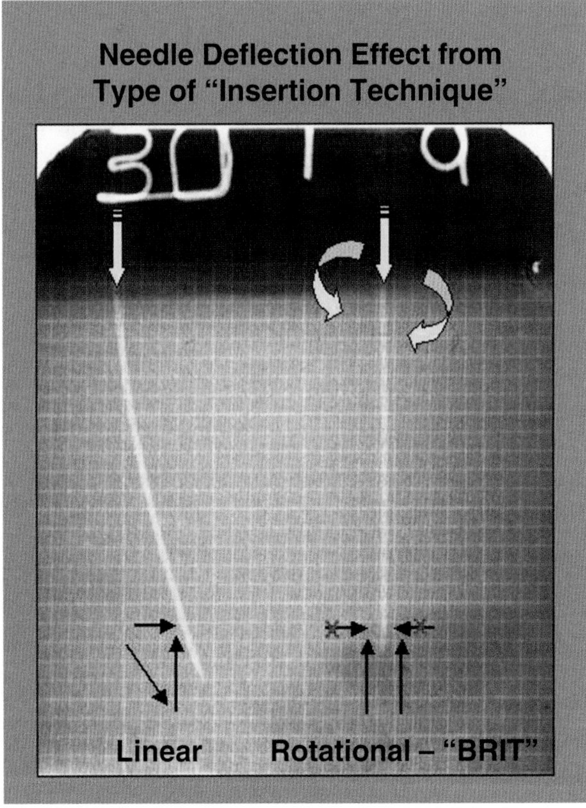

Figure 6-7. BRIT (bi-rotational insertion technique).

A subsequent study by the same authors demonstrated that the BRIT offers the added benefit of reducing the force necessary for needle penetration and advancement through tissues.[18] This is explained as follows. With rotational insertion, all resultant forces are directed toward the forward path of insertion because the deflecting or bending forces have been eliminated from the rotational insertion technique, as described earlier. This allows forward movement of the needle to occur more efficiently and with less effort (e.g., less force). In addition, rotation of the beveled needle allows the sharp cutting edge to contact the full circumference of the tissue surface, contributing to the reduction in force that is necessary during penetration and advancement. This is not unlike the rotational effect that a surgical drill bit has as it is boring through tissue or bone.

The BRIT, or bi-rotational insertion technique has been demonstrated to improve injection techniques because the deflection of a standard needle during insertion is minimized.[19]

LENGTH

Dental needles are available in three lengths: long, short and ultrashort. Ultrashort needles are available only as 30-gauge needles. Despite the claim for uniformity of length by manufacturers, significant differences are found (Table 6-4).

The length of a short needle is between 20 and 25 mm (measured hub to tip) with a standard of about 20 mm, and is 30 to 35 mm for the long dental needle, with a standard of about 32 mm (Fig. 6-8).

Needles should not be inserted into tissues all the way to their hubs unless this is absolutely necessary for the success of the injection. This statement has appeared in "standard" local anesthesia textbooks since the early to mid 1900s.[20-24] One reason for this precaution is needle breakage, which, although rare, does occur. The weakest portion of the needle

TABLE 6-4
Needle Lengths*

Manufacturer	25-Gauge Long	25-Gauge Short	27-Gauge Long	27-Gauge Short	30-Gauge Long	30-Gauge Short	30-Gauge Ultrashort
Industry standard	32	20	32	20			
Manufacturer A	30		30	21	25	21	
Manufacturer B	32 ± 1.5	22 ± 1.5	32 ± 1.5	22 ± 1.5		21 ± 1.5	12 ± 1.0
Manufacturer C			32	21	25	21	
Manufacturer D	35		35	25		25	10
Manufacturer E	32			21		19	

*All measurements obtained directly from needle manufacturers.

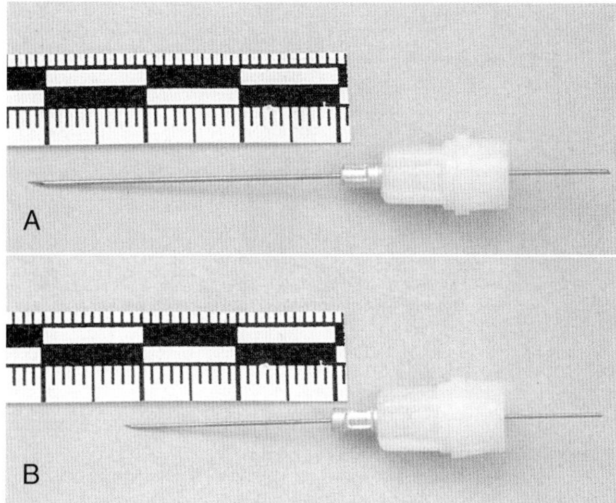

Figure 6-8. **A,** Long dental needle: length approximately 32 mm. **B,** Short dental needle: length approximately 20 mm.

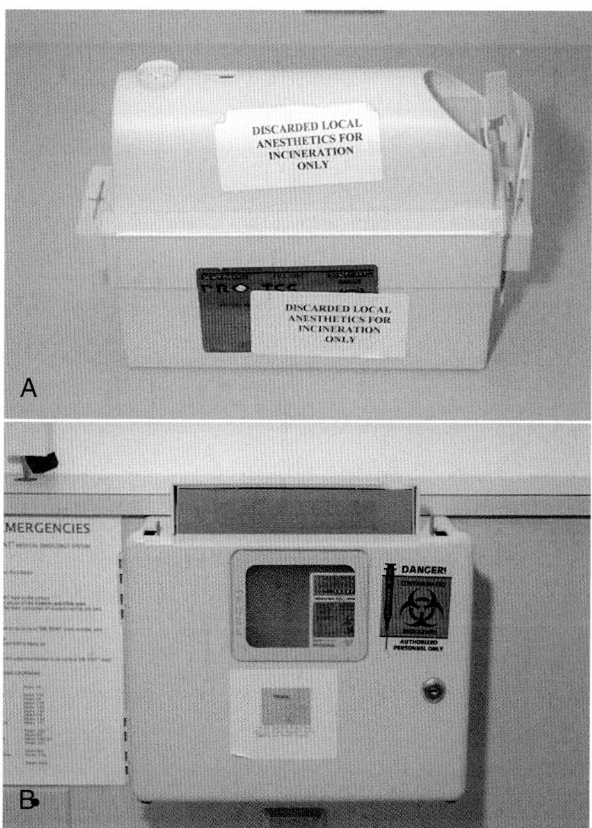

Figure 6-9. **A,** Container for disposal of discarded local anesthetic cartridges. **B,** "Sharps" container for disposal of contaminated needles.

(the most rigid, the part receiving the greatest stress during needle advancement through tissues) is at the hub, which is where needle breakage happens. When a needle that is inserted into the soft tissues to its hub breaks, the elastic properties of the tissues permit them to rebound and cover (bury) the needle remnant entirely. Retrieval is usually difficult (as discussed in Chapter 17). If even a small portion (5 mm or more) of the broken needle shaft remains visible within the oral cavity, it can usually be retrieved easily with a hemostat or pickup forceps.

A long needle is preferred for all injection techniques for which penetration of significant thicknesses of soft tissue (e.g., inferior alveolar, Gow-Gates mandibular, Akinosi mandibular, infraorbital, maxillary [V_2] nerve blocks) is required. Short needles may be used for any injection in any patient who does not require penetration of significant depths of soft tissue (e.g., close to or beyond 20 mm).

CARE AND HANDLING OF NEEDLES

Needles available to the dental profession today are presterilized and disposable. With proper care and handling, they should not be the cause of significant difficulties.

1. Needles must never be used on more than one patient.
2. Needles should be changed after several (three or four) tissue penetrations in the same patient.
   a. After three or four insertions, stainless steel disposable needles become dulled. Tissue penetration becomes increasingly traumatic with each insertion, producing pain on insertion and soreness when sensation returns after the procedure.
3. Needles should be covered with a protective sheath when not being used to prevent accidental needle-stick with a contaminated needle. (See the discussion in Chapter 9.)
4. Attention should always be paid to the position of the uncovered needle tip, whether inside or outside the patient's mouth. This minimizes the risk of potential injury to the patient and the administrator.
5. Needles must be properly disposed of after use to prevent possible injury or reuse by unauthorized individuals. Needles can be destroyed in any of the following ways:
   a. Contaminated needles (as well as all other items contaminated with blood or saliva, such as cartridges) should be disposed of in special "contaminated" or "sharps" containers (Fig. 6-9).
   b. Proper use of a self-sheathing ("safety" needle) needle or syringe unit (as discussed in Chapter 5) minimizes risk of accidental needle-stick.
   c. When needles are to be reused for subsequent injections (a practice unique to the dental profession vs. medicine or other health care professions, where second injections are rarely administered), recapping is accomplished using the "scoop" technique or a needle holder (Fig. 6-10).
   d. Contaminated needles should never be discarded into open trash containers.

In summary, in actual fact, only one local anesthetic needle is necessary in the dental office, the 25-gauge long, which can be used for all anesthetic techniques discussed in this text. It provides a rigidity that is not available with higher-gauge (smaller-diameter) needles and is necessary in

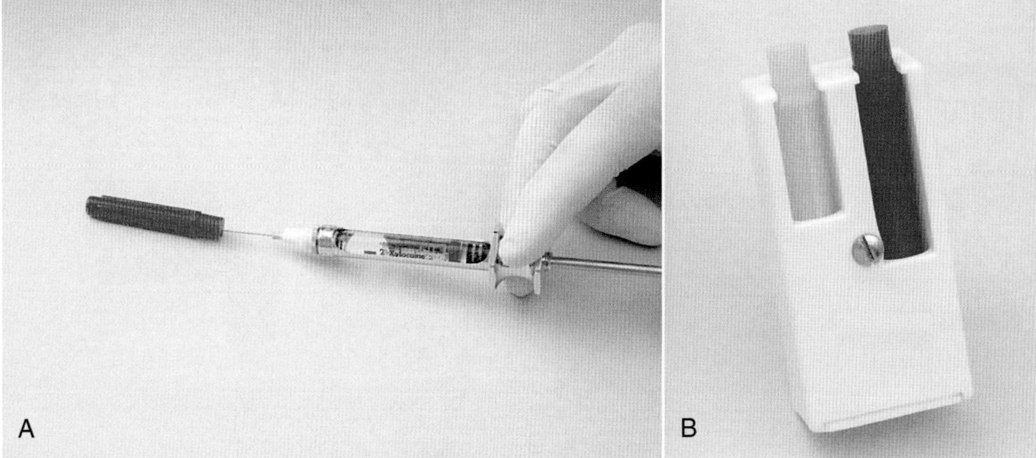

Figure 6-10. **A,** "Scoop" technique for recapping contaminated local anesthetic needle. **B,** Plastic needle cap holder.

the periodontal ligament (PDL) and for intraseptal injections; it deflects to a lesser degree than smaller needles and seemingly provides easier and more reliable aspiration. Because patient sensitivity is not increased with the 25-gauge long needle, its value is increased still further. In reality, however, it is practical to have a second needle available—the 25- or 27-gauge short needle—for use in injections in which the thickness of soft tissue to be penetrated is less than 20 mm, and where the risk of positive aspiration is minimal, as well as in areas of the oral cavity where stabilization of a long needle might prove difficult (e.g., maxillary anterior teeth, the palate).

PROBLEMS WITH NEEDLES

Pain on Insertion

Use of a dull needle can lead to pain on initial penetration of the mucosa. This pain may be prevented by using sharp, new, disposable needles and applying a topical anesthetic at the penetration site. The needle should be changed after three or four penetrations of mucosa if multiple insertions are necessary.

Breakage

Bending weakens needles, making them more likely to break on subsequent contact with hard tissues such as bone. Needles should not be bent if they are to be inserted into soft tissue to a depth greater than 5 mm. No injection technique used in dentistry (in which the needle enters into soft tissue) requires a needle to be bent for success of the injection. Most often, needles are bent by doctors administering an inferior alveolar nerve block (IANB), a posterior superior alveolar (PSA) nerve block, an intrapulpal injection, an injection into the PDL, or an intraosseous injection. The two nerve blocks mentioned (IANB, PSA) can be easily administered successfully with a straight (unbent) needle (see Chapters 13 and 14). The PDL and intrapulpal injections usually can be administered without bending the needle; however, occasions arise, such as at the distal root of a mandibular second molar (PDL), with root canals in posterior teeth (intrapulpal), or with injection into bone distal to a second molar (intraosseous), in which the injection site is not accessible with a straight needle. In these cases, bending of the needle is essential to success. Because the needle does not enter into soft tissue farther than 2 to 4 mm (PDL), or at all (intrapulpal), there is little danger of the needle being nonretrievable in the unlikely event that it breaks (Figs. 6-11 and 6-12).

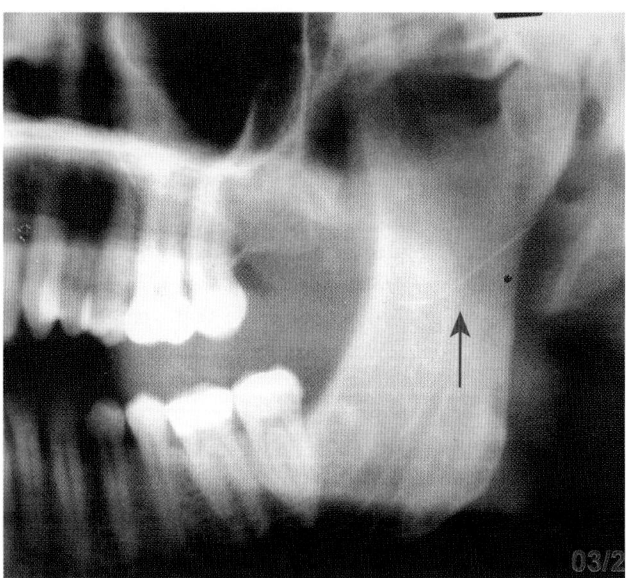

Figure 6-11. Retained broken needle after inferior alveolar nerve block *(arrow)*.

No attempt should be made to change the direction of a needle when it is embedded in tissue. If the direction of a needle must be changed, the needle should first be withdrawn *almost* completely from the tissue and then its direction altered.

No attempts should be made to force a needle against resistance (needles are not designed to penetrate bone). Smaller (30- and 27-gauge) needles are more likely to break than larger (25-gauge) needles. Of 105 broken needle cases this author has examined, 100 involved a 30-gauge short or ultrashort needle (95.23%). The remaining five needles were 27-gauge short.[99]

Needles recommended for specific injection techniques are presented in the following "Recommendations" section.

Pain on Withdrawal

Pain on withdrawal of the needle from tissue can be produced by "fishhook" barbs on the tip. Fishhook barbs may be produced during the manufacturing process, but it is much more likely that they will develop when the needle tip forcefully contacts a hard surface, such as bone. A needle should never be forced against resistance. If in doubt about the presence of barbs, change the needle between insertions.

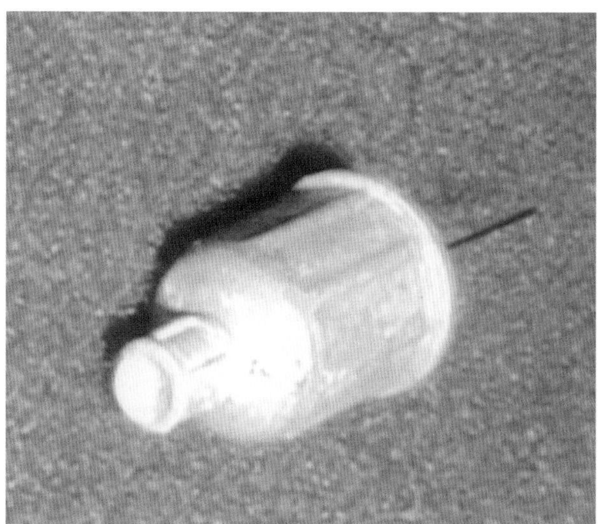

Figure 6-12. Remainder of retained local anesthetic needle shown in Figure 6-11.

Injury to the Patient or Administrator

Penetration of, with resultant injury to, areas of the body with the needle can occur unintentionally. A major cause is inattention by the administrator, although sudden unexpected movement by the patient is also a frequent cause. The needle should remain capped until it is to be used and should be made safe (sheathed or recapped) immediately after withdrawal from the mouth.

RECOMMENDATIONS

1. Sterile disposable needles should be used.
2. If multiple injections are to be administered, needles should be changed after three or four insertions in a single patient.
3. Needles must never be used on more than one patient.
4. Needles should not be inserted into tissue to their hub unless this is absolutely necessary for success of the injection.
5. The direction of a needle should not be changed while it is still in tissue.
6. A needle should never be forced against resistance.
7. Needles should remain capped until used and should be made safe immediately when withdrawn.
8. Needles should be discarded and destroyed after use to prevent injury or reuse by unauthorized persons.
9. The injection techniques presented in Table 6-5 are listed with their recommended needles (for the adult of average size).

TABLE 6-5
Recommended Needles for Injection Techniques

Technique	Needle Gauge	Needle Length
Supraperiosteal (infiltration)	27	Short
Posterior superior alveolar nerve block	27*	Short*
Middle superior alveolar nerve block	27	Short
Anterior middle superior alveolar (AMSA) nerve block	27	Short
Palatal approach anterior superior alveolar nerve block (P-ASA)	30†	Short
Buccal (long) nerve block	27‡	Short‡
Infiltration for hemostasis	27	Short
Periodontal ligament injection (PDL or intraligamentary [ILI])	27	Short
Intraseptal injection	27	Short
Intraosseous injection	27	Short
Intrapulpal injection	27	Short
Anterior superior alveolar nerve block ("infraorbital")	25 or 27	Long
Maxillary (V_2) nerve block	25 or 27	Long
Inferior alveolar ("mandibular") nerve block	25 or 27	Long
Gow-Gates mandibular nerve block	25 or 27	Long
Vazirani-Akinosi mandibular nerve block	25 or 27	Long

*In earlier editions of this book, the 25-gauge long needle was recommended. As a means of minimizing the risk of hematoma after the posterior superior alveolar injection, a short needle is now recommended. If available, a 25-gauge short needle should be used; where this is not available, the 27-gauge short needle is recommended. (See Chapter 13 for additional discussion.)

†The authors of the P-ASA paper recommend use of a 30-gauge ultrashort needle.[17,18]

‡In most clinical situations, the 25-gauge long needle, used for the inferior alveolar nerve block (IANB), is used for the buccal nerve block, which is administered immediately after the IANB.

References

1. Cuny EJ, Fredekind R, Budenz AW: Safety needles: new requirements of the Occupational Safety and Health Administration bloodborne pathogens rule, J Calif Dent Assoc 27:525–530, 1999.
2. Cuny E, Fredekind RE, Budenz AW: Dental sefety needles "effectiveness": results of a one-year evaluation, J Am Dent Assoc 131:1143–1148, 2000.
3. Aldous JA: Needle deflection: a factor in the administration of local anesthetics, J Am Dent Assoc 77:602–604, 1968.
4. Jeske AH, Boshart BF: Deflection of conventional versus non-deflecting dental needles in vitro, Anesth Prog 32:62–64, 1985.
5. Robison SF, Mayhew RB, Cowan RD, et al: Comparative study of deflection characteristics and fragility of 25-, 27-, and 30-gauge short dental needles, J Am Dent Assoc 109:920–924, 1984.
6. Delgado-Molina E, Tamarit-Borras M, Berini-Aytes L, et al: Comparative study of two needle models in terms of deflection during inferior alveolar nerve block, Med Oral Patol Oral Cir Bucal 14:440–444, 2009.
7. Jeske AH, Blanton PL: Misconceptions involving dental local anesthesia. Part 2. Pharmacology, Tex Dent J 119:310–314, 2002.
8. Hamburg HL: Preliminary study of patient reaction to needle gauge, NY State Dent J 38:425–426, 1972.
9. Farsakian LR, Weine FS: The significance of needle gauge in dental injections, Compendium 12:264–268, 1991.
10. Flanagan T, Wahl MI, Schmitt MM, et al: Size doesn't matter: needle gauge and injection pain, Gen Dent 55:216–217, 2007.
11. Foldes FF, McNall PG: Toxicity of local anesthetics in man, Dent Clin North Am 5:257–258, 1961.
12. Harris S: Aspirations before injection of dental local anesthetics, J Oral Surg 25:299–303, 1957.
13. Kramer H, Mitton V: Dental emergencies, Dent Clin North Am 17:443–460, 1973.
14. McClure DB: Local anesthesia for the preschool child, J Dent Child 35:441–448, 1968.
15. Trapp LD, Davies RO: Aspiration as a function of hypodermic needle internal diameter in the in-vivo human upper limb, Anesth Prog 27:49–51, 1980.
16. Malamed SF: Personal communications, Newark, Del, April 2006, Septodont Inc.
17. Hochman MN, Friedman MJ: In vitro study of needle deflection: a linear insertion technique versus a bi-directional rotation insertion technique, Quint Int 31:737–743, 2000.
18. Hochman MN, Friedman MJ: An in vitro study of needle force penetration comparing a standard linear insertion to the new bidirectional rotation insertion technique, Quint Int 32:789–796, 2001.
19. Aboushala A, Kugel G, Efthimiadis N, Krochak M: Efficacy of a computer-controlled injection system of local anesthesia in vivo, IADR Annual Meeting, 2000, Abstract 2775.
20. Cook-Waite Laboratories Inc.: Manual of local anesthesia in general dentistry, New York, 1936, Rensselaer & Springville, p 38.
21. Local anesthesia and pain control in dental practice, St Louis, 1957, CV Mosby, p 184.
22. Allen GD: Dental anesthesia and analgesia (local and general), ed 2, Baltimore, Md, 1979, Williams & Wilkins, p 133.
23. Yagiela JA, Jastack JT: Regional anesthesia of the oral cavity, St Louis, 1981, CV Mosby, p 105.
24. Malamed SF: Needles. In Handbook of local anesthesia, ed 5, St Louis, 2004, CV Mosby, p 103.
25. Malamed SF, Reed KL, Poorsattar S: Needle breakage: incidence and prevention, Dent Clin North Am 54:745–756, 2010.

CHAPTER 7

The Cartridge

The dental cartridge is a glass cylinder containing the local anesthetic drug, among other ingredients. In the United States and in many other countries, the glass cylinder itself can hold 2 mL of solution; however, as prepared today, the dental cartridge contains approximately 1.8 mL of local anesthetic solution. Local anesthetic products manufactured by Septodont (Lancaster, PA) list their volume as 1.7 mL (although in actuality they contain approximately 1.76 mL of local anesthetic solution). In other countries, notably the United Kingdom and Australia, the prefilled dental cartridge contains approximately 2.2 mL of local anesthetic solution; some countries including France and Japan have 1-mL dental cartridges (Fig. 7-1).

The dental cartridge is, by common usage, referred to by dental professionals as a *carpule*. The term *carpule* is actually a registered trade name for the dental cartridge prepared by Cook-Waite Laboratories, which introduced it into dentistry in 1920.

In recent years, local anesthetic manufacturers in some countries (but not as of yet in North America) have introduced a local anesthetic cartridge composed of plastic.[1] Plastic cartridges have several negative features, primarily leakage of solution during injection, the requirement for considerable force to be applied to the plunger of the syringe (e.g., periodontal ligament [PDL], nasopalatine),[1] and the fact that the plunger does not "glide" down the plastic cartridge as smoothly as it does down the glass cartridge, leading to sudden spurts of administration of local anesthetic, which can produce pain in the patient. Another problem with plastic cartridges is the fact that they are permeable to air. Exposure to oxygen leads to more rapid degradation of the vasoconstrictor in the cartridge and to a shorter shelf-life.[2]

COMPONENTS

The prefilled 1.8-mL dental cartridge consists of four parts (Fig. 7-2):

1. Cylindrical glass tube
2. Stopper (plunger, bung)
3. Aluminum cap
4. Diaphragm

The stopper (plunger, bung) is located at the end of the cartridge that receives the harpoon of the aspirating syringe. The harpoon is embedded into the silicone (non–latex-containing) rubber plunger with gentle finger pressure applied to the thumb ring of the syringe. The plunger occupies a little less than 0.2 mL of the volume of the entire cartridge. Until recently, the stopper was sealed with paraffin (wax) to produce an airtight seal against the glass walls of the cartridge. Glycerin was added in channels around the stopper as a lubricant, permitting it to traverse the glass cylinder more easily. Today, most local anesthetic manufacturers treat the stopper with silicone, eliminating both the paraffin and the glycerin. "Sticky stoppers" (stoppers that do not move smoothly down the glass cartridge) are infrequent today. Recent years have seen a move toward the use of a uniform black rubber stopper in all local anesthetic drug combinations. Virtually gone are the color-coded red, green, and blue stoppers that aided in identification of the drug. When black stoppers are used, a color-coding band, required by the American Dental Association (ADA) as of June 2003 for products to receive the ADA Seal of Approval, is found around the glass cartridge (Table 7-1).

In an intact dental cartridge (Fig. 7-3), the stopper is slightly indented from the lip of the glass cylinder. Cartridges whose plungers are flush with or extruded beyond the glass of the cylinder should not be used. This problem is discussed later in this chapter (see "Problems").

An aluminum cap is located at the opposite end of the cartridge from the rubber plunger. It fits snugly around the neck of the glass cartridge, holding the thin diaphragm in position. It is silver colored on most cartridges.

The diaphragm is a semipermeable membrane through which the needle penetrates into the cartridge. When properly prepared, the perforation of the needle is centrically located and round, forming a tight seal around the needle. Improper preparation of the needle and cartridge can produce an eccentric puncture with ovoid holes leading to leakage of the anesthetic solution during injection. The

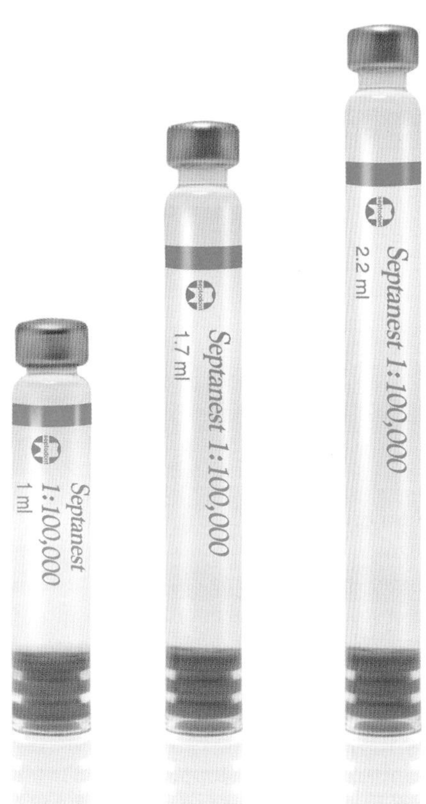

Figure 7-1. 1.0, 1.8-(1.7-), and 2.2-mL cartridges together.

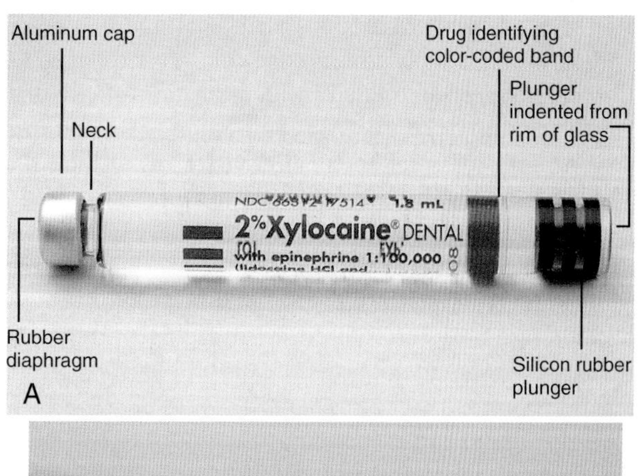

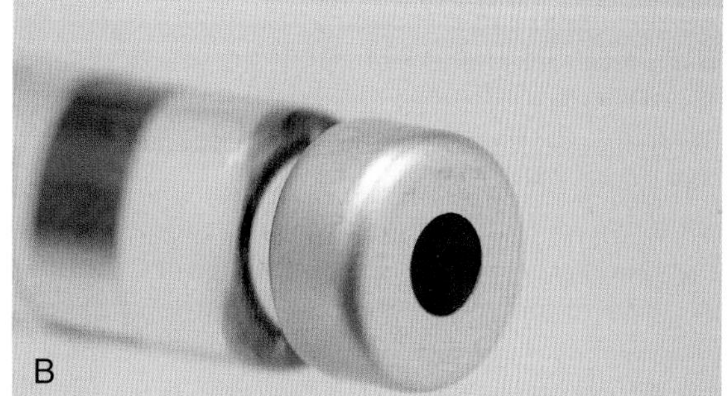

Figure 7-2. **A** and **B,** Components of the glass dental local anesthetic cartridge.

TABLE 7-1
Color-Coding of Local Anesthetic Cartridges, as per American Dental Association Council on Scientific Affairs

Local Anesthetic Solution	Color of Cartridge Band
Articaine HCl 4% with epinephrine 1:100,000	Gold
Bupivacaine 0.5% with epinephrine 1:200,000	Blue
Lidocaine HCl 2%	Light blue
Lidocaine HCl 2% with epinephrine 1:50,000	Green
Lidocaine HCl 2% with epinephrine 1:100,000	Red
Mepivacaine HCl 3%	Tan
Mepivacaine HCl 2% with levonordefrin 1:20,000	Brown
Prilocaine HCl 4%	Black
Prilocaine HCl 4% with epinephrine 1:200,000	Yellow

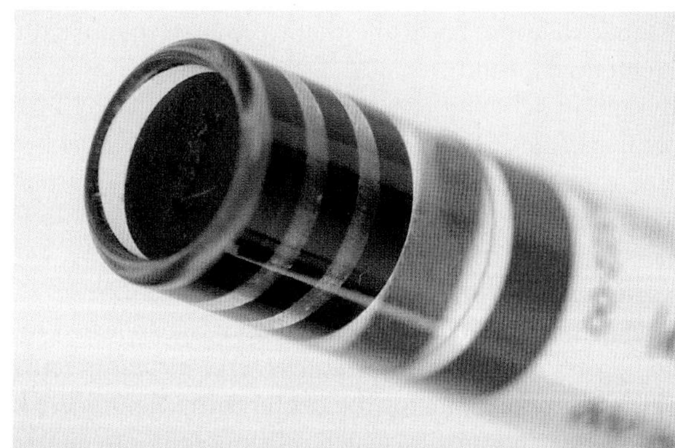

Figure 7-3. Silicone rubber plunger is slightly indented from the rim of the glass.

diaphragm is a semipermeable membrane that allows any solution in which the dental cartridge is immersed to diffuse into the cartridge, thereby contaminating the local anesthetic solution.

Persons with latex allergy may be at increased risk when administered a local anesthetic through a glass cartridge.[3] However, a recent literature review by Shojaei and Haas stated that although the possibility of an allergic reaction precipitated by latex in the dental local anesthetic cartridge does exist, "there are no reports of studies or cases in which a documented allergy was due to the latex component of cartridges for dental anesthesia."[4]

In recent years, latex-free dental cartridges have been introduced.

A thin Mylar plastic label applied to all cartridges (Fig. 7-4) serves to (1) protect the patient and the administrator in the event that the glass cracks, and (2) provide specifications about the enclosed drug. In addition, some manufacturers include a volume indicator on their labels, making it easier for the administrator to deposit precise volumes of anesthetic (see Fig. 7-4).

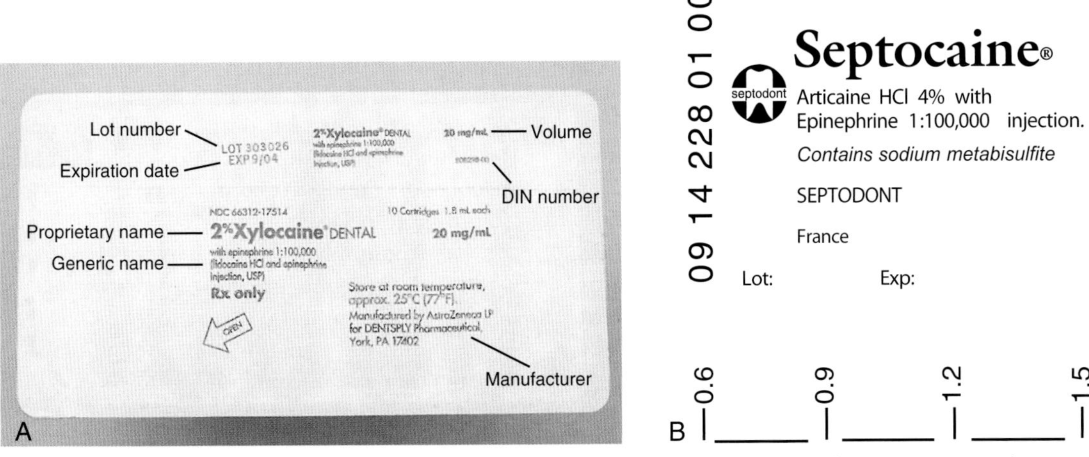

Figure 7-4. Mylar plastic label. Label with volume indicator. (Courtesy Septodont, Lancaster, PA.)

TABLE 7-2
Composition of Local Anesthetic Solution

Component	Function	"Plain" Local Anesthetic Solution	Vasopressor-Containing Local Anesthetic Solution
Local anesthetic drug (e.g., lidocaine HCl)	Blockade of nerve conduction	•	•
Sodium chloride	Isotonicity of the solution	•	•
Sterile water	Volume	•	•
Vasopressor (e.g., epinephrine, levonordefrin)	↑ Depth and ↑ duration of anesthesia; ↓ absorption of local anesthetic and vasopressor		•
Sodium (meta)bisulfite	Antioxidant		•
Methylparaben*	Bacteriostatic agent		

*Methylparaben is no longer included in single-use dental cartridges of local anesthetic; however, it is found in ALL multidose vials of injectable drugs.

TABLE 7-3
Calculation of Milligrams per Cartridge

Percent Solution	=	Milligrams (mg) per Milliliter (mL)	×	Volume of Cartridge	=	Milligrams per Cartridge
0.5	=	5	×	1.8	=	9
1.0	=	10	×	1.8	=	18
2.0	=	20	×	1.8	=	36
3.0	=	30	×	1.8	=	54
4.0	=	40	×	1.8	=	72

CARTRIDGE CONTENTS

The composition of the solution found in the dental cartridge varies depending on whether a vasopressor is included (Table 7-2).

The *local anesthetic drug* is the raison d'être for the entire dental cartridge. It interrupts the propagated nerve impulse, preventing it from reaching the brain. The drug contained within the cartridge is listed by its percent concentration. The number of milligrams of the local anesthetic drug can be calculated by multiplying the percent concentration (e.g., 2% = 20 mg/mL) by the volume: 1.8 (United States) or 2.2 (United Kingdom) (the number of milliliters in the cartridge). Thus a 1.8-mL cartridge of a 2% solution contains 36 mg (Table 7-3). The local anesthetic drug is stable and is capable of being autoclaved, heated, or boiled without breaking down. However, other components of the cartridge (e.g., vasopressor drug, cartridge seals) are more labile and are easily destroyed.

A *vasopressor drug* is included in most anesthetic cartridges to enhance safety and the duration and depth of action of the local anesthetic. The pH of dental cartridges containing vasopressors is lower (more acidic) than that of cartridges not containing vasopressors (pH of 3.5 [3.3 to 4.0] vs. 6.5). Because of this pH difference, plain local anesthetics have a somewhat more rapid onset of clinical action and are more comfortable (less "burning" on injection).[5-7]

Cartridges containing vasopressors also contain an *antioxidant*, most often sodium (meta)bisulfite. Sodium bisulfite prevents oxidation of the vasopressor by oxygen, which can be trapped in the cartridge during manufacture or can diffuse through the semipermeable diaphragm (or the walls of a plastic cartridge) after filling. Sodium bisulfite reacts with oxygen before the oxygen is able to destroy the vasopressor. When oxidized, sodium bisulfite becomes sodium bisulfate, having an even lower pH. The clinical relevance of this lies in the fact that increased burning (discomfort) is experienced by the patient on injection of an "older" cartridge of anesthetic with vasopressor compared with a fresher cartridge. Allergy to bisulfites must be considered in the medical evaluation of all patients before local anesthetic is administered[8,9] (see Chapter 10).

Sodium chloride is added to the cartridge to make the solution isotonic with the tissues of the body. In the past, isolated instances have been reported in which local anesthetic solutions containing too much sodium chloride (hypertonic solutions) produced tissue edema or paresthesia, sometimes lasting for several months, after drug administration.[10] This is no longer a problem.

Distilled water is used as a diluent to provide the volume of solution in the cartridge.

A significant change in cartridge composition in the United States and in many other countries was the removal of *methylparaben*, a bacteriostatic agent. A ruling by the Food and Drug Administration (FDA) mandated the removal of methylparaben from dental local anesthetic cartridges manufactured after January 1, 1984. Methylparaben possesses bacteriostatic, fungistatic, and antioxidant properties. It and related compounds (ethyl-, propyl-, and butylparaben) are commonly used as preservatives in ointments, creams, lotions, and dentifrices. In addition, paraben preservatives are found in all multiple-dose vials of drugs. Methylparaben is commonly used in a 0.1% concentration (1 mg/mL). Its removal from local anesthetic cartridges was predicated on two facts. First, dental local anesthetic cartridges are single-use items meant to be discarded and not reused. Therefore inclusion of a bacteriostatic agent is unwarranted. Second, repeated exposure to paraben has led to reports of increased allergic reactions in some persons.[11,12] Responses have been limited to localized edema, pruritus, and urticaria. Fortunately, to date there has not been a systemic allergic reaction to a paraben. Removal of methylparaben has further decreased an already minimal risk of allergy to local anesthetic drugs.

CARE AND HANDLING

Local anesthetics are marketed in vacuum-sealed tin containers of 50 cartridges and in blister packs of (usually) 10 cartridges. Although no manufacturer makes any claim of sterility about the exterior surface of the cartridge, bacterial cultures taken immediately on opening a container usually fail to produce any growth. Therefore it seems obvious that extraordinary measures related to cartridge sterilization are unwarranted. Indeed, the glass dental cartridge should not be autoclaved. The seals on the cartridge cannot withstand the extreme temperatures of autoclaving, and the heat-labile vasopressors are destroyed in the process. Plastic cartridges cannot be autoclaved.

Most commonly today, local anesthetics are marketed in cardboard boxes of approximately 50 cartridges. Within the box are 5 sealed units of 10 cartridges each (Fig. 7-5), called *blister packs*. Kept in this container until use, cartridges remain clean and uncontaminated.

Local anesthetic cartridges should be stored in their original container, preferably at room temperature (e.g., 21° C to 22° C), and in a dark place. There is no need to "prepare" a cartridge before use. The doctor or assistant should insert it into the syringe. However, many doctors feel compelled to somehow "sterilize" the cartridge. When this urge strikes, the doctor should apply an alcohol wipe moistened with undiluted 91% isopropyl alcohol or 70% ethyl alcohol to the rubber diaphragm (Fig. 7-6).

If a clear plastic cartridge dispenser is used, 1 day's supply of cartridges should be placed with the aluminum cap and diaphragm facing downward. Several (two or three) sterile dry 2 × 2-inch gauze wipes are placed in the center of the dispenser and are moistened with (not immersed in) 91% isopropyl alcohol or 70% ethyl alcohol. No liquid alcohol should be present around the cartridges. Before the syringe is loaded, the aluminum cap and the rubber diaphragm are rubbed against the moistened gauze.

Cartridges should not be permitted to soak in alcohol or other sterilizing solutions because the semipermeable diaphragm allows diffusion of these solutions into the dental cartridge, thereby contaminating it. Therefore, it is recommended that cartridges be kept in their original container until they are to be used.

Cartridge warmers are unnecessary. Indeed, occasionally they may produce problems. Overheating the local anesthetic solution can lead to (1) discomfort for the patient during injection, and (2) the more rapid degradation of a heat-labile vasopressor (producing a shorter duration of anesthesia with more burning on injection). It has been demonstrated that after the warmed glass cartridge is removed from the cartridge warmer and is placed in a metal syringe with the solution forced through a fine metal needle, its temperature has decreased almost to room temperature.[2,5,13,14]

Cartridge warmers, designed to maintain anesthetic solutions at "body temperature," are not needed and cannot be recommended. Local anesthetics in cartridges maintained at room temperature (20° C to 22° C) do not cause the patient any discomfort on injection into tissues, nor do patients complain of the solution being too cold.[14] On the other hand, warmed local anesthetic solutions at 27° C or above have a much greater incidence of being described as too hot or burning on injection.[13]

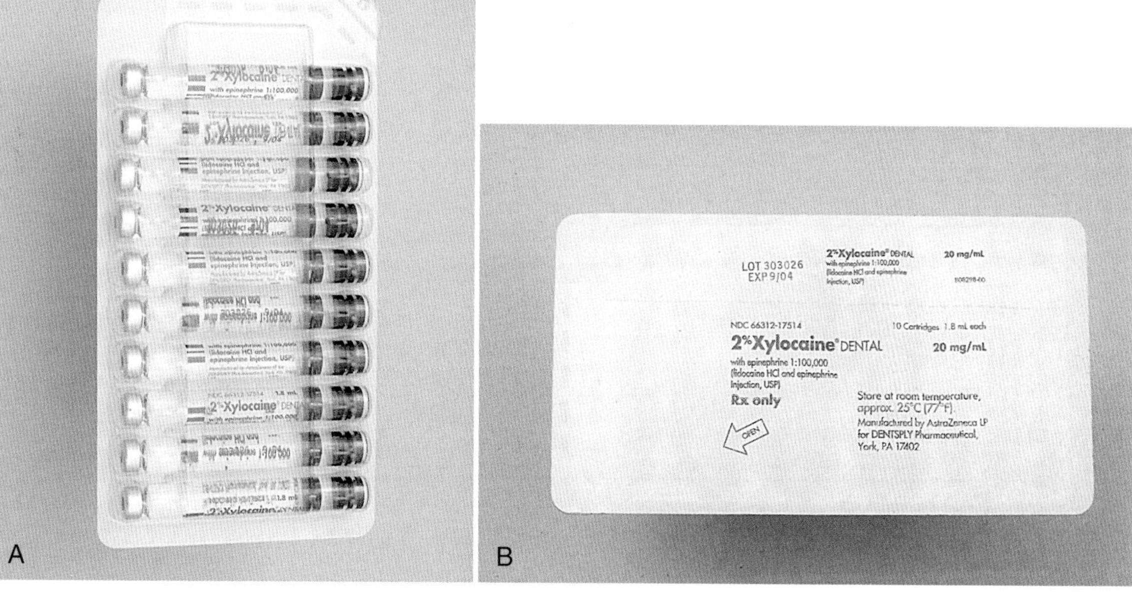

Figure 7-5. **A,** Ten local anesthetic cartridges are contained in a sealed "blister pack." **B,** Back of blister pack contains information about the drug.

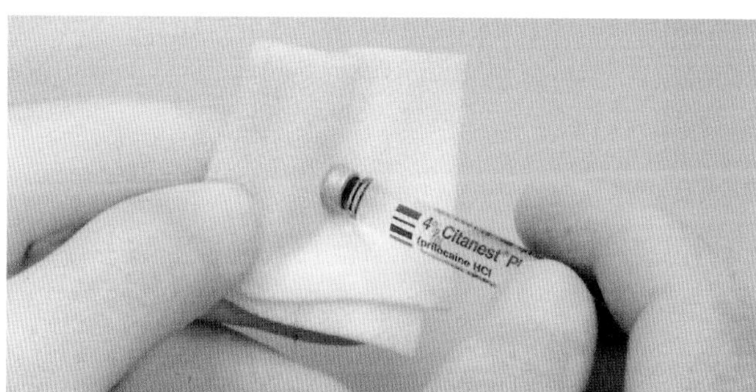

Figure 7-6. Preparing local anesthetic cartridge for use by wiping the rubber diaphragm with alcohol.

Local anesthetic cartridges should not be left exposed to direct sunlight because some contents may undergo accelerated deterioration. The primary clinical effect of this will be destruction of the vasopressor, with a corresponding decrease in the duration of clinical action of the anesthetic solution.

Included in every package of local anesthetic is an important document: the drug package insert. It contains valuable information about the product such as dosages, warnings, precautions, and care and handling instructions. All persons involved in the handling or administration of local anesthetics should review this document periodically (Fig. 7-7).

PROBLEMS

Occasionally problems develop with dental cartridges of local anesthetics. Although most are minor, producing slight inconvenience to the drug administrator, others are more significant and might prove harmful to the patient:

1. Bubble in the cartridge
2. Extruded stopper
3. Burning on injection
4. Sticky stopper
5. Corroded cap
6. "Rust" on the cap
7. Leakage during injection
8. Broken cartridge

Bubble in the Cartridge

A small bubble of approximately 1 to 2 mm diameter (described as "BB"-sized) frequently is found in the dental cartridge. It is composed of nitrogen gas, which was bubbled into the local anesthetic solution during its manufacture to prevent oxygen from being trapped inside the cartridge, potentially destroying the vasopressor. The nitrogen bubble may not always be visible in a normal cartridge (Fig. 7-8, *A*).

A larger bubble, which may be present with a plunger that is extruded beyond the rim of the cartridge, is the result of freezing of the anesthetic solution (Fig. 7-8, *B*). Such cartridges should not be used, because sterility of the solution cannot be assured. Instead, these cartridges should be returned to their manufacturer for replacement.

Extruded Stopper

The stopper can become extruded when a cartridge is frozen and the liquid inside expands. In this case, the solution no longer can be considered sterile and should not be used for injection. Frozen cartridges can be identified by the presence of a large (>2 mm) bubble, along with an extruded stopper.

An extruded stopper with no bubble is indicative of prolonged storage in a chemical disinfecting solution and

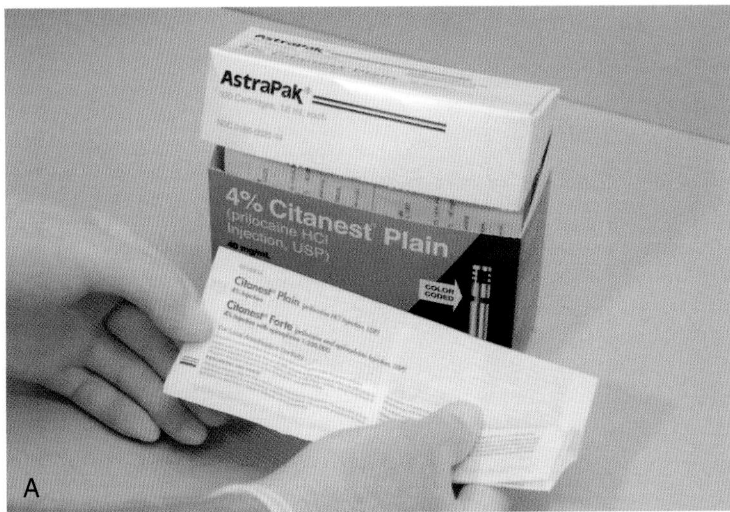

WARNINGS

DENTAL PRACTITIONERS WHO EMPLOY LOCAL ANESTHETICS IN THEIR OFFICES SHOULD BE WELL VERSED IN DIAGNOSIS AND MANAGEMENT OF EMERGENCIES WHICH MIGHT ARISE FROM THEIR USE. RESUSCITATIVE EQUIPMENT, OXYGEN, AND OTHER RESUSCITATIVE DRUGS SHOULD BE AVAILABLE FOR IMMEDIATE USE.

Reactions resulting in fatality have occurred on rare occasions with the use of local anesthetics, even in the absence of a history of hypersensitivity.

Figure 7-7. **A,** All local anesthetic containers have a product identification package insert, which should be read. **B,** Important information is contained in all package inserts.

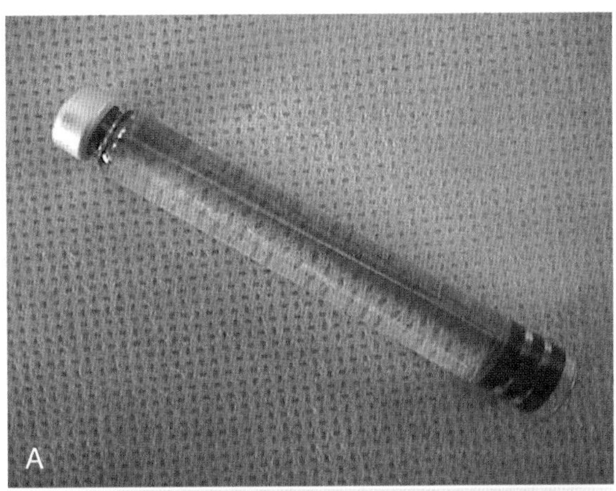

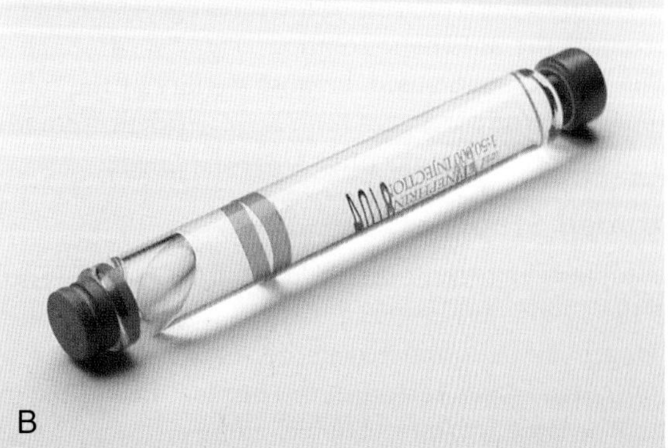

Figure 7-8. **A,** Normal cartridge with no bubble or a small BB-sized bubble. Note that the rubber stopper is indented from the glass rim. **B,** Local anesthetic cartridge with an extruded stopper and a large bubble caused by freezing.

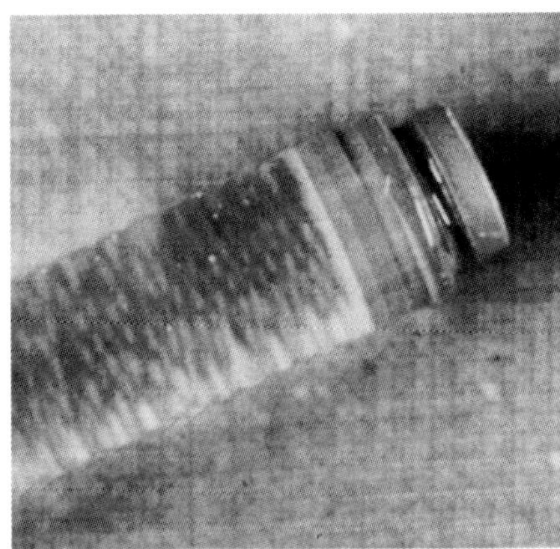

Figure 7-9. Extruded plunger on local anesthetic cartridge.

diffusion of the solution into the cartridge. Shannon and Wescott demonstrated that alcohol enters a cartridge through the diaphragm in measurable amounts within 1 day if the diaphragm is immersed in alcohol.[15] Local anesthetic solutions containing alcohol produce an uncomfortable burning on injection. Alcohol in sufficiently high concentration is a neurolytic agent capable of producing long-term paresthesia. The greatest concentration of alcohol reported to date in a dental cartridge has been 8% (Fig. 7-9), which is not likely to produce significant long-term injury.[16]

Antirust tablets should not be used in disinfectant solutions. The sodium nitrate (or similar agent) that they contain is capable of releasing metal ions, which have been related to an increased incidence of edema after local anesthetic administration.[17]

It should be remembered that small quantities of sterilizing solution can diffuse into a dental cartridge with no visible movement of the plunger. Care always must be taken in storage of local anesthetic cartridges.

Burning on Injection

A burning sensation on injection of anesthetic solution may be the result of one of the following:

1. Normal response to the pH of the drug
2. Cartridge containing sterilizing solution
3. Overheated cartridge
4. Cartridge containing a vasopressor

During the few seconds immediately after deposition of a local anesthetic solution, the patient may complain of a slight sensation of burning. This normal reaction is caused by the pH of the local anesthetic solution; it lasts a second or two, until the anesthetic takes effect, and is noted mainly by sensitive patients when receiving local anesthetics containing epinephrine or levonordefrin.

A more intense burning on injection is usually the result of diffusion of disinfecting solution into the dental cartridge and its subsequent injection into the oral mucous membranes. Although burning most often is a mere annoyance, the inclusion of disinfecting agents such as alcohol in dental cartridges can lead to more serious sequelae, such as postinjection paresthesia and tissue edema.[15,16]

Overheating of the solution in a cartridge warmer may produce burning on injection. The (Christmas tree) bulb-type cartridge warmer most often is at fault in this regard. Unless local anesthetic cartridges are unusually cold, there is little justification for use of a cartridge warmer. Local anesthetic solutions injected at room temperature are well tolerated by tissues and patients.

Use of a vasopressor-containing local anesthetic solution may be responsible for the sensation of burning on injection. The addition of a vasopressor and an antioxidant (sodium bisulfite) lowers the pH of the solution to approximately 3.5, making it significantly more acidic than solutions not containing a vasopressor (pH about 6.5).[5-7,17] Patients are more likely to feel the burning sensation with these solutions. A further decrease in the pH of the local anesthetic solution results as sodium bisulfite is oxidized to sodium bisulfate. This response can be minimized by careful checking of the expiration date on all cartridges before use. Conversely, increasing the pH of the anesthetic solution has the effect of making local anesthetic administration more comfortable for the patient.[17-19]

Sticky Stopper

The "sticky stopper" has become a rarity today, with the inclusion of silicone as a lubricant and the removal of paraffin as a sealant in the cartridge. In cases where paraffin is still used, difficulty in advancing the stopper may occur because the paraffin hardens on colder days. Using cartridges at room temperature minimizes this problem; using silicone-coated stoppers eliminates it. Plastic cartridges are associated with this problem to a greater degree than glass cartridges.

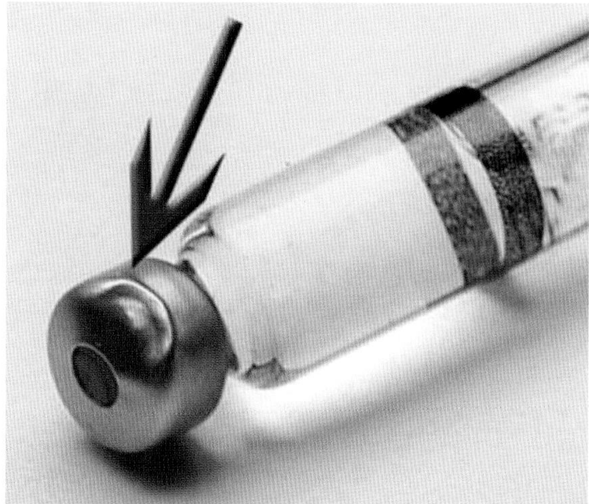

Figure 7-10. Local anesthetic cartridge with damaged cap. The glass around the neck of the cartridge should be examined carefully for cracks.

Corroded Cap

The aluminum cap on a local anesthetic cartridge can be corroded if immersed in disinfecting solutions that contain quaternary ammonium salts, such as benzalkonium chloride (e.g., "cold" sterilizing solution). These salts are electrolytically incompatible with aluminum. Aluminum-sealed cartridges should be disinfected in 91% isopropyl alcohol or 70% ethyl alcohol. Cartridges with corroded caps must not be used. Corrosion may be easily distinguished from rust, which appears as a red deposit on an intact aluminum cap.

Rust on the Cap

Rust found on a cartridge indicates that at least one cartridge in the tin container has broken or leaked. The "tin" container (actually steel dipped in molten tin) rusts, and the deposit comes off on the cartridges. Cartridges containing rust should not be used. If any cartridge contains rust a dented cap, or a visible crack (Fig. 7-10), all cartridges in the container must be carefully checked before use. With the introduction of nonmetal packaging, rust is rarely seen.

Leakage During Injection

Leakage of local anesthetic solution into the patient's mouth during injection occurs if the cartridge and the needle are prepared improperly and the needle puncture of the diaphragm is ovoid and eccentric. Properly placed on the syringe after the cartridge is inserted, the needle produces centric perforation of the diaphragm, which tightly seals itself around the needle. When pressure is applied to the plunger during injection, all of the solution is directed into the lumen of the needle. If the cartridge is placed in a

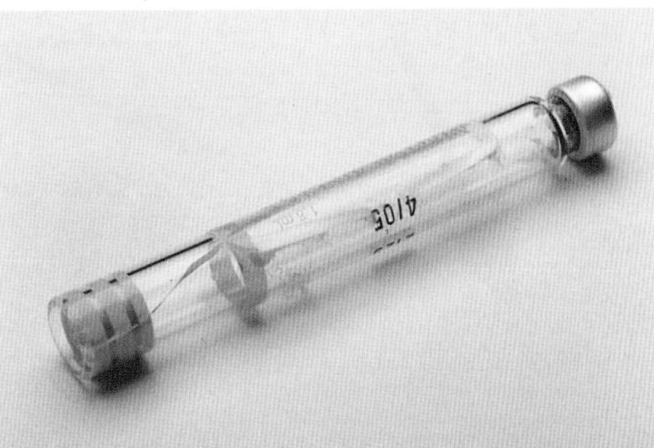

Figure 7-11. Cracked glass on dental cartridge.

breech-loading syringe after the needle, an eccentric ovoid perforation may occur; with pressure on the plunger, some solution is directed into the lumen of the needle, while some may leak out of the cartridge between the needle and the diaphragm and run into the patient's mouth (see Fig. 5-24). When the safety syringe is used, it is necessary to insert the cartridge after the needle has been attached; however, because the cartridge slides directly into the syringe, not from the side, leakage during injection is rarely a problem. Verbal and written communications from doctors using plastic cartridges indicate that the occurrence of leakage appears to be considerably greater when they are used.

The plastic dental cartridge does not withstand the application of injection pressure as well as the traditional glass cartridge. Meechan and associates applied pressures equal to those achieved during PDL injection with both glass and plastic local anesthetic cartridges.[1] Leakage of anesthetic occurred in 1.4% of glass cartridges, whereas leakage was noted in 75.1% of plastic cartridges.

Broken Cartridge

The most common cause of cartridge breakage is the use of a cartridge that has been cracked or chipped during shipping. Dented metal containers and damaged boxes should be returned to the supplier immediately for exchange. If a broken cartridge is found in a container, all remaining cartridges must be examined for hairline cracks or chips. Two areas that must be examined carefully are the thin neck of the cartridge where it joins the cap (see Fig. 7-10) and the glass surrounding the plunger (Fig. 7-11). Subjecting a cracked cartridge to the pressure of injection often causes the cartridge to shatter or "explode." If this occurs inside the patient's mouth, serious sequelae may result from ingestion of glass. It is essential to suction the patient's mouth thoroughly and consult with a physician or emergency department staff about follow-up therapy before discharging this patient. The addition of a thin Mylar plastic label to the glass cartridge minimizes such injury. Additionally, if the aluminum "cap" on the cartridge is damaged, the cartridge should not be used, because the underlying glass may have been damaged as well (see Fig. 7-10).

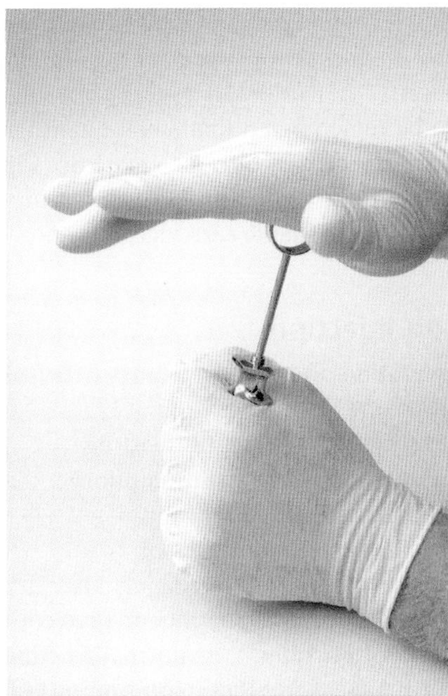

Figure 7-12. If force is necessary to embed the harpoon in the rubber plunger, the glass face of the syringe should be covered with the hand.

Plastic cartridges do not fracture when subjected to PDL injection pressures.[1]

Excessive force used to engage the aspirating harpoon in the stopper has resulted in numerous cases of shattered cartridges. Although they have not broken in the patient's mouth, injury to dental personnel has been reported. Hitting the thumb ring of the syringe in an attempt to engage the harpoon in the rubber stopper should be avoided. If this technique is essential to embed the harpoon in the rubber plunger (as it is with the plastic safety syringe), one hand should be used to cover the entire exposed glass face of the cartridge (Fig. 7-12). Proper preparation of the armamentarium (see Chapter 9) minimizes this problem.

Breakage also can occur as a result of attempting to use a cartridge with an extruded plunger. Extruded plungers can be forced back into the cartridge only with difficulty, if at all. Cartridges with extruded plungers should not be used.

Syringes with bent harpoons may cause cartridges to break (see Fig. 5-26). Bent needles that are no longer patent create a pressure buildup within the cartridge during attempted injection (see Fig. 5-25). No attempt should be made to force local anesthetic solution from a dental cartridge against significant resistance.

RECOMMENDATIONS

1. Dental cartridges must never be used on more than one patient.
2. Cartridges should be stored at room temperature.
3. It is not necessary to warm cartridges before use.

4. Cartridges should not be used beyond their expiration date.
5. Cartridges should be checked carefully for cracks, chips, and the integrity of the stopper and cap before use.

References

1. Meechan JG, McCabe JF, Carrick TE: Plastic dental anaesthetic cartridges: a laboratory investigation, Br Dent J 169:254–256, 1990.
2. Meechan JG, Donaldson D, Kotlicki A: The effect of storage temperature on the resistance to failure of dental local anesthetic cartridges, J Can Dent Assoc 61:143–144, 147–148, 1995.
3. Sussman GL, Beezhold DH: Allergy to latex rubber, Ann Intern Med 122:143–146, 1995.
4. Shojaei AR, Haas DA: Local anesthetic cartridges and latex allergy: a literature review, J Can Dent Assoc 68:10622–10626, 2002.
5. Jeske AH, Blanton PL: Misconceptions involving dental local anesthesia. Part 2, Pharmacology. Tex Dent J 119:4310–4314, 2002.
6. Wahl MJ, Schmitt MM, Overton DA, Gordon MK: Injection of bupivacaine with epinephrine vs. prilocaine plain, J Am Dent Assoc 133:111652–111656, 2002.
7. Wahl MJ, Overton DA, Howell J, et al: Pain on injection of prilocaine plain vs. lidocaine with epinephrine: a prospective double-blind study, J Am Dent Assoc 132:101396–101401, 2001.
8. Seng GF, Gay BJ: Dangers of sulfites in dental local anesthetic solutions: warning and recommendations, J Am Dent Assoc 113:769–770, 1986.
9. Perusse R, Goulet JP, Turcotte JY: Contraindications to vasoconstrictors in dentistry. Part II. Hyperthyroidism, diabetes, sulfite sensitivity, cortico-dependent asthma, and pheochromocytoma, Oral Surg 74:5687–5691, 1992.
10. Nickel AA: Paresthesia resulting from local anesthetics, J Oral Maxillofac Surg 42:52–79, 1984.
11. Wurbach G, Schubert H, Pillipp I: Contact allergy to benzyl alcohol and benzyl paraben, Contact Dermatitis 28:3187–3188, 1993.
12. Klein CE, Gall H: Type IV allergy to amide-type anesthetics, Contact Dermatitis 25:145–148, 1991.
13. Volk RJ, Gargiulo AV: Local anesthetic cartridge warmer-first in, first out, Ill Dent J 53:292–294, 1984.
14. Rogers KB, Fielding AF, Markiewicz SW: The effect of warming local anesthetic solutions prior to injection, Gen Dent 37:6496–6499, 1989.
15. Shannon IL, Wescott WB: Alcohol contamination of local anesthetic cartridges, J Acad Gen Dent 22:20–21, 1974.
16. Oakley J: Personal communications, 1985.
17. Moorthy AP, Moorthy SP, O'Neil R: A study of pH of dental local anesthetic solutions, Br Dent J 157:11394–11395, 1984.
18. Crose VW: Pain reduction in local anesthetic administration through pH buffering, J Ind Dent Assoc 70:224–225, 1991.
19. Hanna MN, Elhassan A, Veloso PM, et al: Efficacy of bicarbonate in decreasing pain on intradermal injection of local anesthetics: a meta-analysis, Reg Anesth Pain Med 34:122–125, 2009.

CHAPTER 8

Additional Armamentarium

In previous chapters, the three major components of the local anesthetic armamentarium—syringe, needle, and cartridge—have been discussed. Other important items are found in the local anesthetic armamentarium, however, including the following:

1. Topical antiseptic
2. Topical anesthetic
3. Applicator sticks
4. Cotton gauze (2 × 2 inches)
5. Hemostat

TOPICAL ANTISEPTIC

A topical antiseptic may be used to prepare the tissues at the injection site before the initial needle penetration. Its function is to produce a transient decrease in the bacterial population at the injection site, thereby minimizing any risk of postinjection infection.

The topical antiseptic, on an applicator stick, is placed at the site of injection for 15 to 30 seconds. There is no need to place a large quantity on the applicator stick; it should be sufficient just to moisten the cotton portion of the swab.

Available agents include Betadine (povidone-iodine) and Merthiolate (thimerosal). Topical antiseptics containing alcohol (e.g., tincture of iodine, tincture of Merthiolate) should not be used because the alcohol produces tissue irritation. In addition, allergy to iodine-containing compounds is common.[1,2] Before any iodine-containing topical antiseptic is applied to tissues, the patient should be questioned to determine whether adverse reactions to iodine have previously developed.

In a survey of local anesthetic techniques in dental practice,[3] 7.9% of dentists mentioned that they always used topical antiseptics before injection, 22.4% sometimes used them, and 69.7% never used them.

Postinjection infections can and do occur, and regular use of a topical antiseptic can virtually eliminate them. If a topical antiseptic is not available, a sterile gauze wipe should be used to prepare the tissues adequately before injection.

Application of a topical antiseptic is considered an optional step in tissue preparation before intraoral injection.

TOPICAL ANESTHETIC

Topical anesthetic preparations are discussed in depth in Chapter 4. Their use before initial needle penetration of the mucous membrane is strongly recommended. With proper application, initial penetration of mucous membrane anywhere in the oral cavity can usually be made without the patient's awareness.

For effectiveness, it is recommended that a minimal quantity of topical anesthetic be applied to the end of the applicator stick and placed directly at the site of penetration for approximately 1 minute. Gill and Orr have demonstrated that when topical anesthetics are applied according to the manufacturer's instructions (approximately 10 to 15 seconds), their effectiveness is no greater than that of a placebo, especially for palatal injections.[4] Stern and Giddon showed that application of a topical anesthetic to mucous membrane for 2 to 3 minutes leads to profound soft tissue analgesia.[5]

A variety of topical anesthetic agents are available for use today. Most contain the ester anesthetic benzocaine. The likelihood of occurrence of allergic reactions to esters, though minimal, is greater than that to amide topical anesthetics; however, because benzocaine is not absorbed systemically, allergic reactions are normally localized to the site of application. Of the amides, only lidocaine possesses topical anesthetic activity in clinically acceptable concentrations. The risk of overdose with amide topical anesthetics is greater than that with the esters and increases with the area of application of the topical anesthetic. Topical forms of lidocaine are available as ointments, gels, pastes, and sprays.

EMLA (eutectic mixture of local anesthetics) is a combination of lidocaine and prilocaine in a topical cream formulation, designed to provide surface anesthesia of intact skin. Its primary indications are for use before venipuncture and in pediatric surgical procedures, such as circumcision.[6,7]

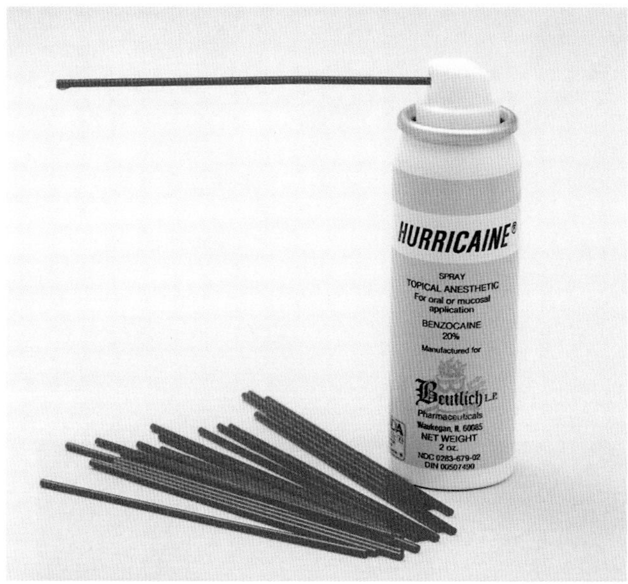

Figure 8-1. Disposable nozzle for topical anesthetic spray.

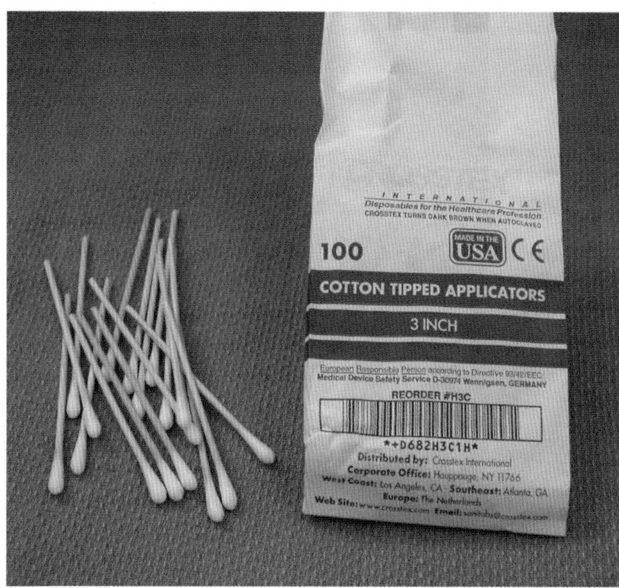

Figure 8-2. Cotton-tipped applicator sticks.

EMLA has been used effectively intraorally; however, it is not designed for intraoral administration, so it contains no flavoring agent and is bitter tasting.[8,9]

Unmetered sprays of topical anesthetics are potentially dangerous and are not recommended for routine use. Because topical anesthetics require greater concentration to penetrate mucous membranes, and because most topical anesthetics are absorbed rapidly into the cardiovascular system, only small measured doses should be administered. Topical anesthetic sprays that deliver a continuous stream of topical anesthetic until being deactivated are capable of delivering overly high doses of the topical anesthetic. If absorbed into the cardiovascular system, the resulting anesthetic blood level may approach overdose levels. Metered sprays that deliver a fixed dose with each administration, regardless of the length of time the nozzle is depressed, are preferred for topical formulations that are absorbed systemically. An example of this form of topical anesthetic spray is Xylocaine, which delivers 10 mg per administration.

Yet another potential problem with topical anesthetic sprays is difficulty keeping the spray nozzle sterile. This is a very important consideration when the form of topical anesthetic to be used is selected. Most topical anesthetic sprays today come with disposable applicator nozzles (Fig. 8-1).

It must be remembered that some topical anesthetic formulations contain preservatives, such as methylparaben, and other ingredients that may be significant in instances of allergy to local anesthetics.

APPLICATOR STICKS

Applicator sticks should be available as part of the local anesthetic armamentarium. They are wooden sticks with a cotton swab at one end. They can be used to apply topical antiseptic and anesthetic solutions to mucous membranes (Fig. 8-2) and compress tissue during palatal injections.

COTTON GAUZE

Cotton gauze is included in the local anesthetic armamentarium for (1) wiping the area of injection before needle penetration and (2) drying the mucous membrane to aid in soft tissue retraction for increased visibility.

Many dentists select gauze in lieu of topical antiseptic solution for cleansing the soft tissue at the site of needle penetration. Gauze effectively dries the injection site and removes any gross debris from the area (Fig. 8-3). It is not as effective as the topical antiseptic but is an acceptable substitute.

Retraction of lips and cheeks for improved access to, and visibility of, the injection site is important during all intraoral injections. Often this task becomes unnecessarily difficult if these tissues are moist, and it is made even more vexing by wearing gloves. Dry cotton gauze makes the tissues easier to grasp and to retract.

A variety of sizes of cotton gauze are available for tissue retraction, but the most practical and the most commonly used is the 2 × 2-inch size. Note that when gauze is placed intraorally to stop bleeding, it is recommended that 2 × 2-inch squares not be used. Larger, 4 × 4-inch gauze squares are much preferred. Additionally, whenever gauze is placed into and left in the mouth for a period of time, a length of dental floss should be tied around it, so that the gauze may be removed or retrieved from the mouth quickly, if necessary (Fig. 8-4).

HEMOSTAT

Although not considered an essential element of the local anesthetic armamentarium, a hemostat or pickup forceps should be readily available at all times in the dental office. Its primary function in local anesthesia is removal of a needle from the soft tissues of the mouth in the highly

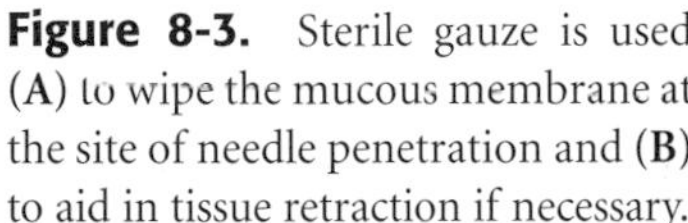

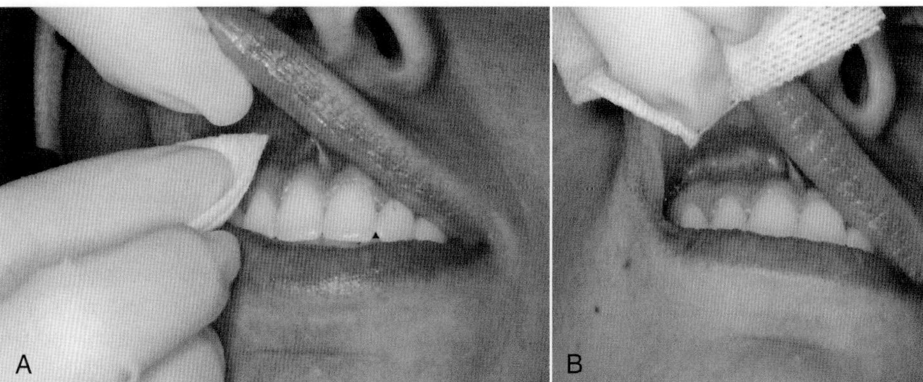

Figure 8-3. Sterile gauze is used (**A**) to wipe the mucous membrane at the site of needle penetration and (**B**) to aid in tissue retraction if necessary.

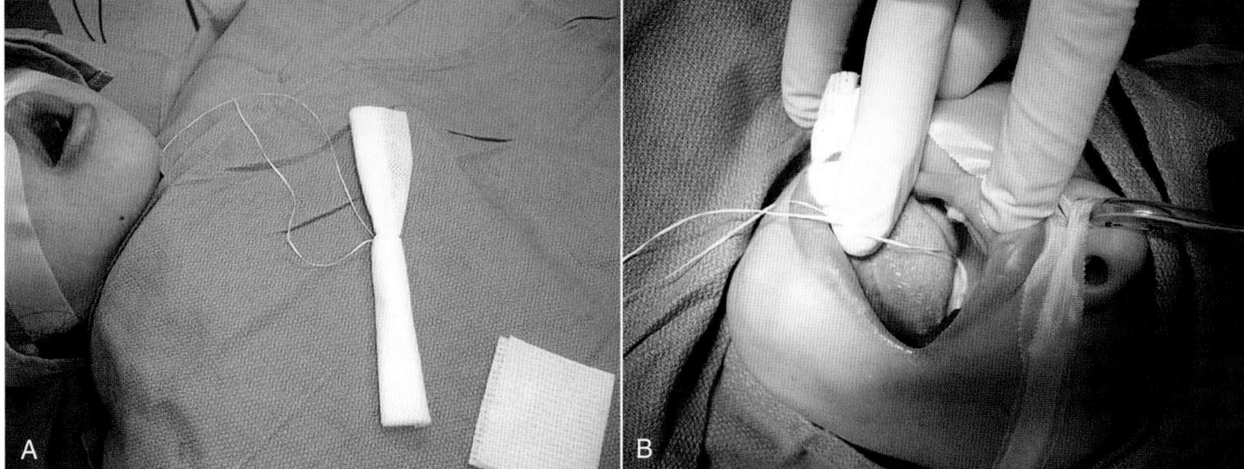

Figure 8-4. Floss tied around a gauze square aids easy retrieval.

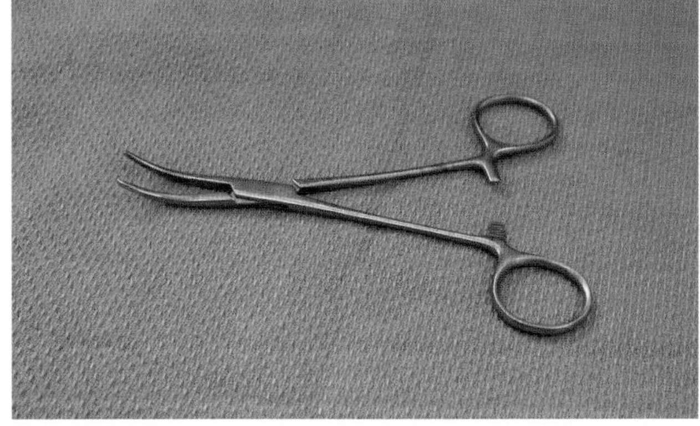

Figure 8-5. Hemostat.

unlikely event that the needle breaks off within tissues (Fig. 8-5).

References

1. Bennasr S, Magnier S, Hassan M, et al: Anaphylactic shock and low osmolarity contrast medium, Arch Pediatr 1:155–157, 1994.
2. Palobart C, Cros J, Orsel I, et al: Anaphylactic shock to iodinated povidone, Ann Fr Anesth Reanim 28(2):168–170, 2009.
3. Malamed SF: Handbook of local anesthesia, ed 1, St Louis, 1980, Mosby.
4. Gill CJ, Orr DL II: A double blind crossover comparison of topical anesthetics, J Am Dent Assoc 98:213–214, 1979.
5. Stern I, Giddon DB: Topical anesthesia for periodontal procedures, Anesth Prog 22:105–108, 1975.
6. Fetzer SJ: Reducing venipuncture and intravenous insertion pain with eutectic mixture of local anesthetic: a meta-analysis, Nurs Res 51:119–124, 2002.
7. Taddio A: Pain management for neonatal circumcision, Paediatr Drugs 3:101–111, 2001.
8. Bernardi M, Secco F, Benech A: Anesthetic efficacy of a eutectic mixture of lidocaine and prilocaine (EMLA) on the oral mucosa: prospective double-blind study with a placebo, Minerva Stomatol 48:39–43, 1999.
9. Munshi AK, Hegde AM, Latha R: Use of EMLA: is it an injection free alternative? J Clin Pediatr Dent 25:215–219, 2001.

CHAPTER 9

Preparation of the Armamentarium

Proper care and handling of the local anesthetic armamentarium can prevent or at least minimize the development of complications associated with the needle, syringe, and cartridge. Many of these have been discussed in the preceding chapters. Other complications and minor annoyances may be prevented through proper preparation of the armamentarium.

BREECH-LOADING, METALLIC OR PLASTIC, CARTRIDGE-TYPE SYRINGE

1. Remove the sterilized syringe from its container (Fig. 9-1).
2. Retract the piston fully before attempting to load the cartridge (Fig. 9-2).
3. Insert the cartridge, while the piston is fully retracted, into the syringe. Insert the rubber stopper end of the cartridge first (Fig. 9-3).
4. Engage the harpoon. While holding the syringe as if injecting, gently push the piston forward until the harpoon is firmly engaged in the plunger (Fig. 9-4). Excessive force is not necessary. Do NOT hit the piston in an effort to engage the harpoon because this frequently leads to cracked or shattered glass cartridges (Fig. 9-5).
5. Attach the needle to the syringe. Remove the white or clear protective plastic cap from the syringe end of the needle and screw the needle onto the syringe (Fig. 9-6). Most metal and plastic hubbed needles are prethreaded, making it easy for them to be screwed onto the syringe; however, some plastic hubbed syringes are not prethreaded, requiring the needle to be pushed toward the metal hub of the syringe while being turned.
6. Carefully remove the colored plastic protective cap from the opposite end of the needle, and expel a few drops of solution to test for proper flow.
7. The syringe is now ready for use.

Note: It is common practice in dentistry to attach the needle to the syringe before placing the cartridge. This sequence requires hitting the piston hard to engage the harpoon in the rubber stopper—a process that can lead to broken glass cartridges or leakage of anesthetic solution into the patient's mouth during the injection. The recommended sequence, as already described, virtually eliminates this possibility and should always be used.

Recapping the Needle

After removal of the syringe from the patient's mouth, the needle should be recapped immediately. Recapping is one of the two times when health professionals are most likely to be injured (stuck) with a needle*; it is probably the most dangerous time to be stuck because the needle is now contaminated with blood, saliva, and debris. Although a variety of techniques and devices for recapping have been suggested, the technique recommended by most state safety and health agencies is termed the *scoop technique* (Fig. 9-7), in which the uncapped needle is slid into the needle sheath lying on the instrument tray or table. Until a better method is designed, the scoop technique should be used for needle recapping.

Safety needles and syringes for use in dentistry are still in their developmental stage. Most systems currently available for dental use leave much to be desired.

Various needle cap holders are available—commercially made (Fig. 9-8) or self-made (from acrylic)—that hold the cap stationary while the needle is being inserted into it, making recapping somewhat easier to accomplish.

Unloading the Breech-Loading, Metallic or Plastic, Cartridge-Type Syringe

After administration of the local anesthetic, the following sequence is suggested for removing the used cartridge:

1. Retract the piston and pull the cartridge away from the needle with your thumb and forefinger as you retract the piston (Fig. 9-9), until the harpoon disengages from the plunger.

*The other common time for needle-stick injury is during injection, when a finger of the opposite hand is accidentally stuck as a result of sudden unexpected patient movement.

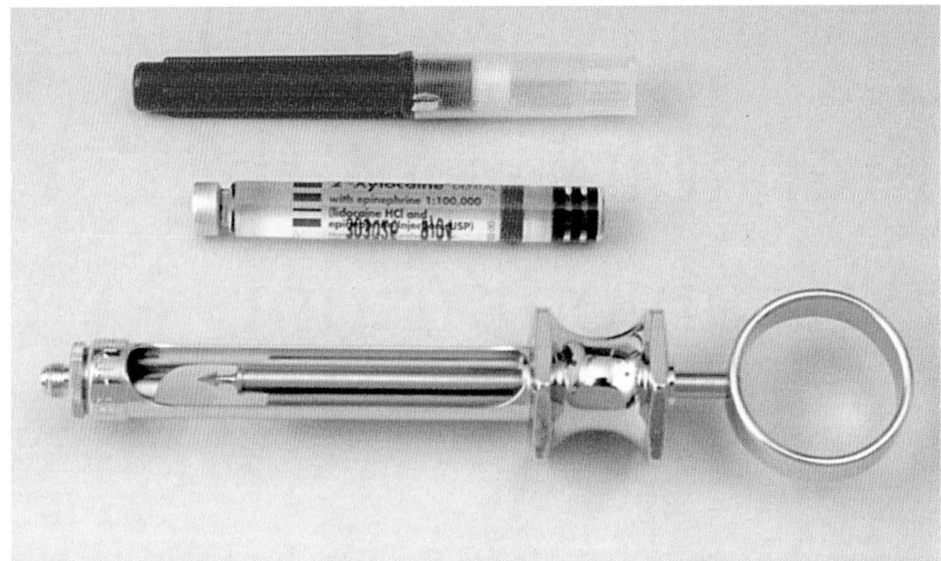

Figure 9-1. Local anesthetic armamentarium *(from top):* needle, cartridge, syringe.

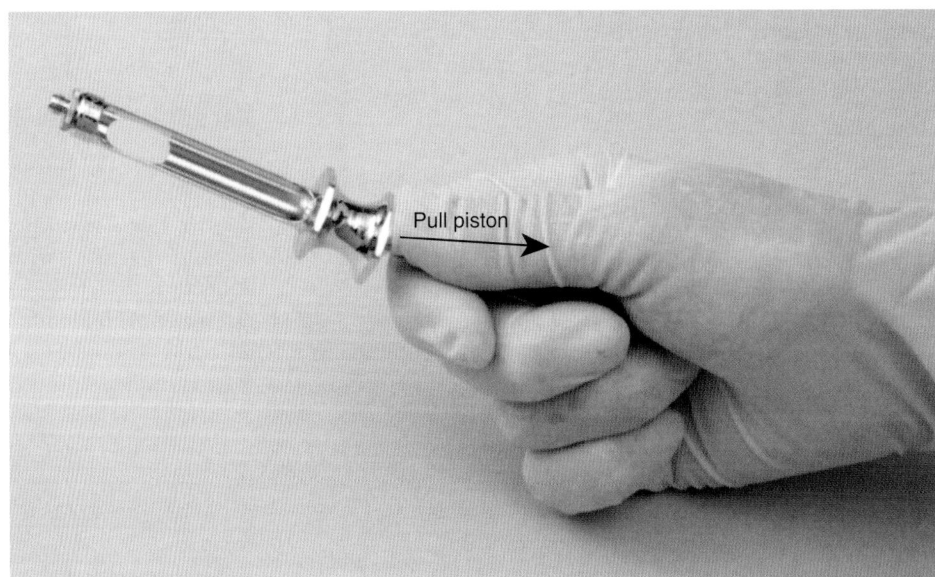

Figure 9-2. Retract the piston.

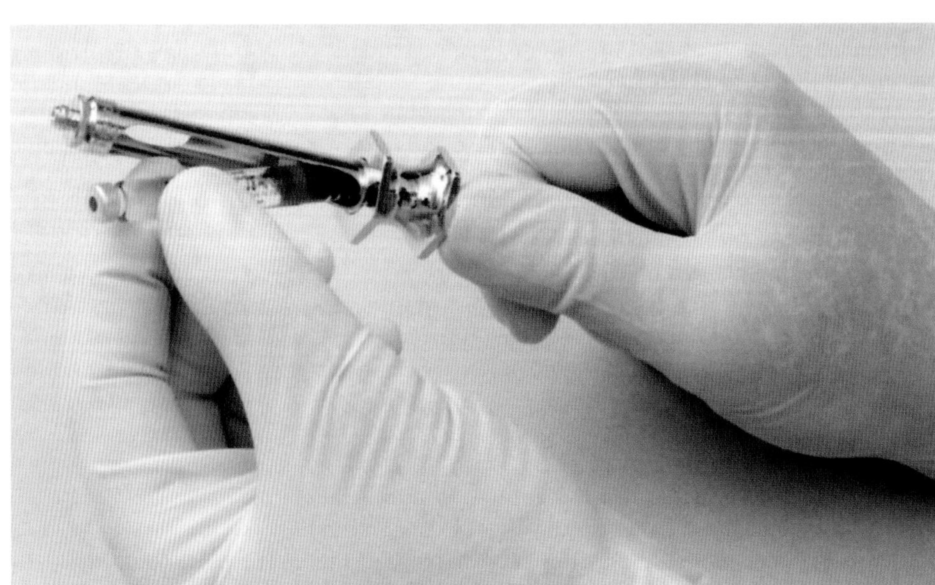

Figure 9-3. Insert the cartridge.

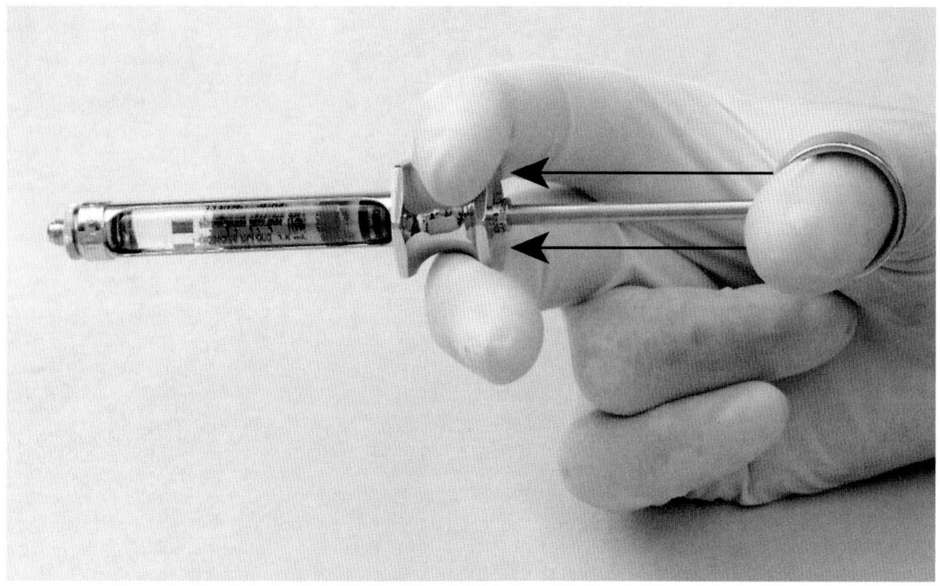

Figure 9-4. Engage the harpoon in the plunger with gentle finger pressure.

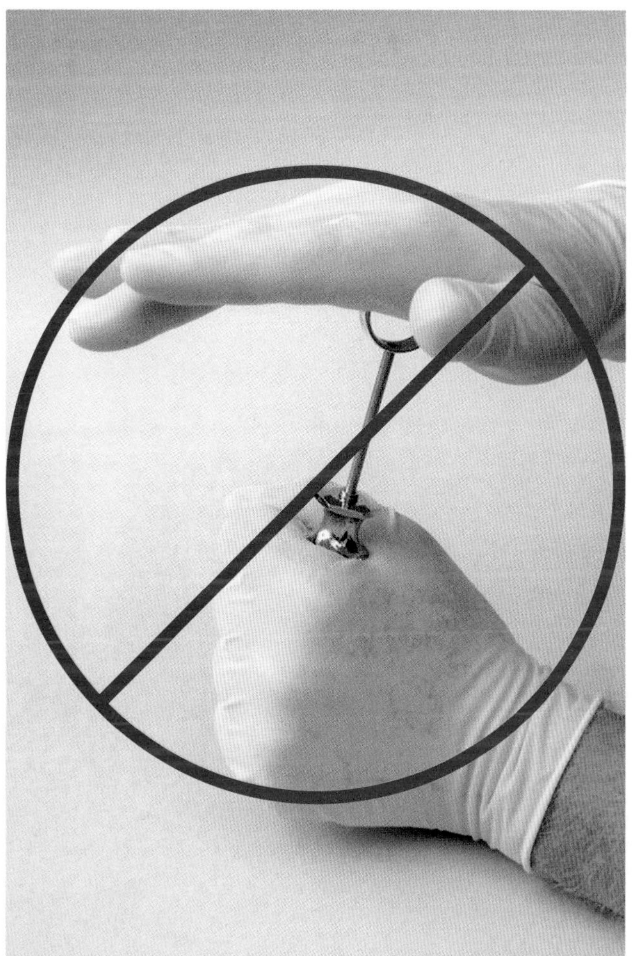

Figure 9-5. Do not exert force on the plunger; the glass may crack.

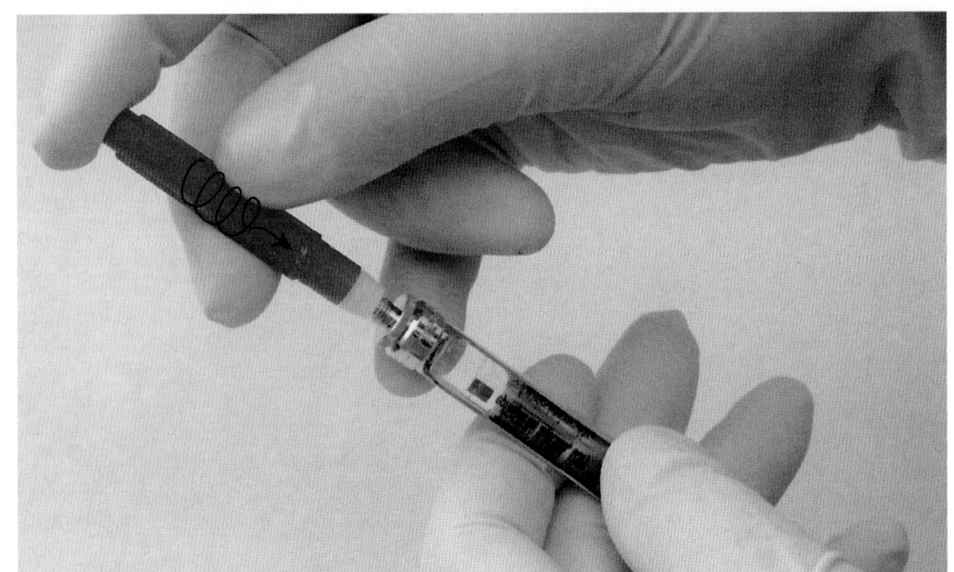

Figure 9-6. If the plastic hubbed needle is not prethreaded, it must be screwed onto the syringe while simultaneously being pushed into the metal needle adaptor of the syringe.

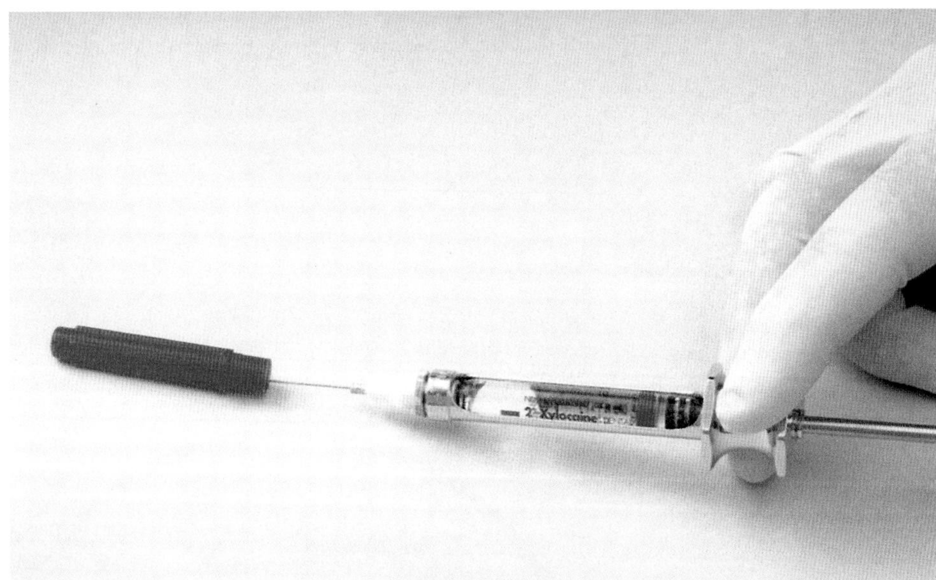

Figure 9-7. "Scoop" technique for recapping a needle after use.

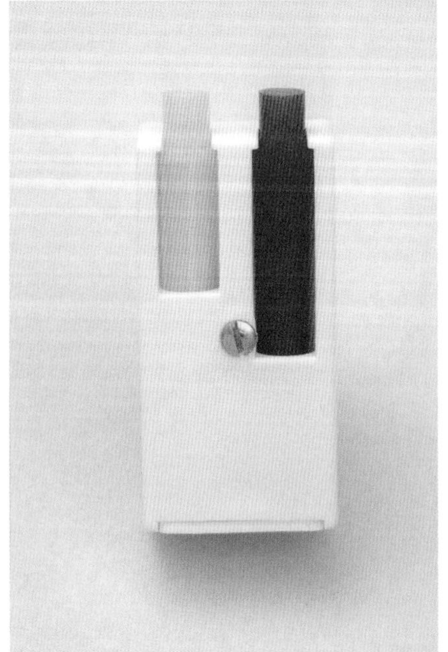

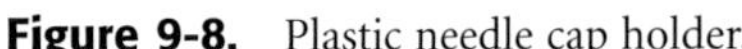

Figure 9-8. Plastic needle cap holder.

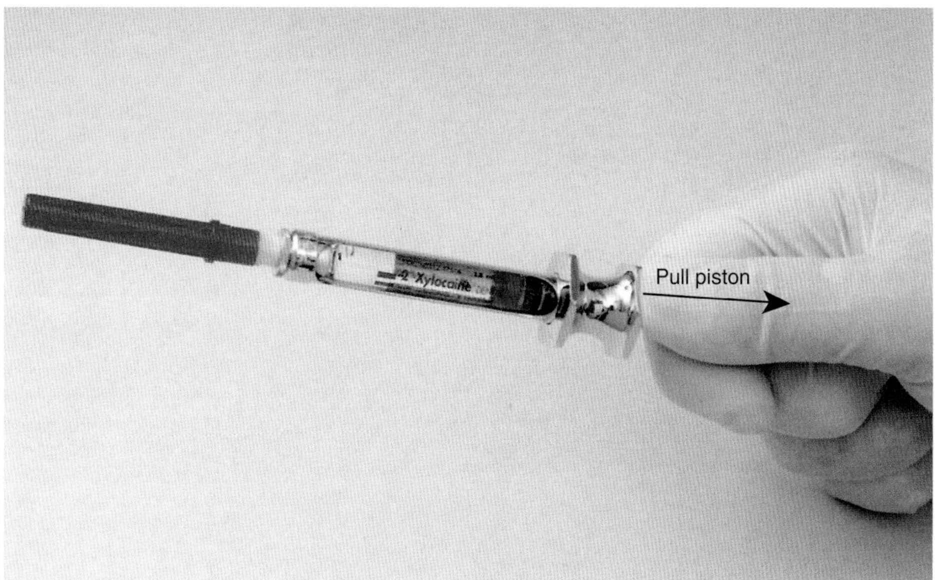

Figure 9-9. Retract the piston.

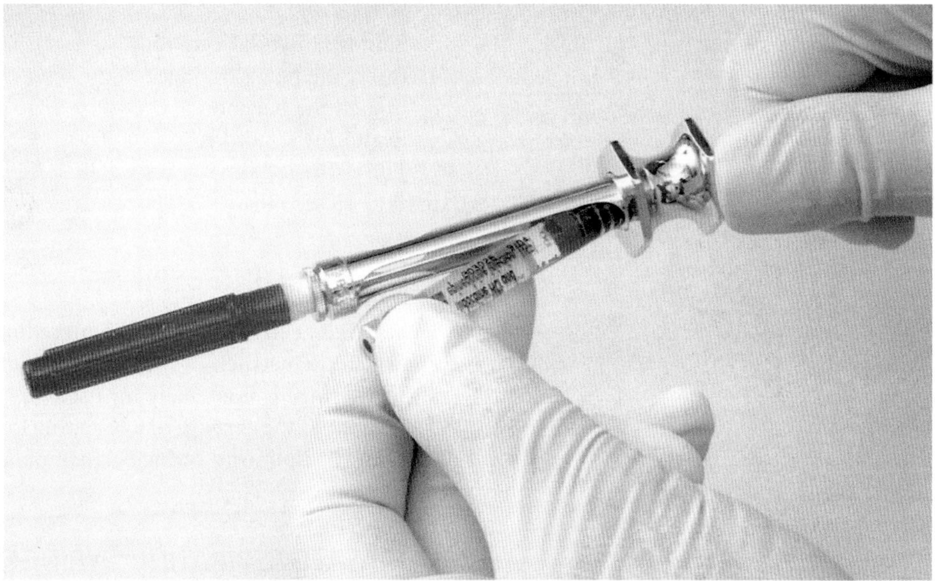

Figure 9-10. Remove the used cartridge.

2. Remove the cartridge from the syringe by inverting the syringe, permitting the cartridge to fall free (Fig. 9-10).
3. Properly dispose of the used needle. All needles must be discarded after use to prevent injury or intentional misuse by unauthorized persons. Carefully unscrew the now recapped needle, being careful not to accidentally discard the metal needle adaptor (Fig. 9-11). The use of a sharps container is recommended (Fig. 9-12) for needle disposal.

PLACING AN ADDITIONAL CARTRIDGE IN A (TRADITIONAL) SYRINGE

On occasion it is necessary to deposit an additional cartridge of local anesthetic solution. To do this, the following sequence is suggested with the metallic or plastic breech-loading syringe:

1. Recap the needle using the scoop (or other appropriate) technique, and remove it from the syringe.
2. Retract the piston (disengaging the harpoon from the rubber stopper).

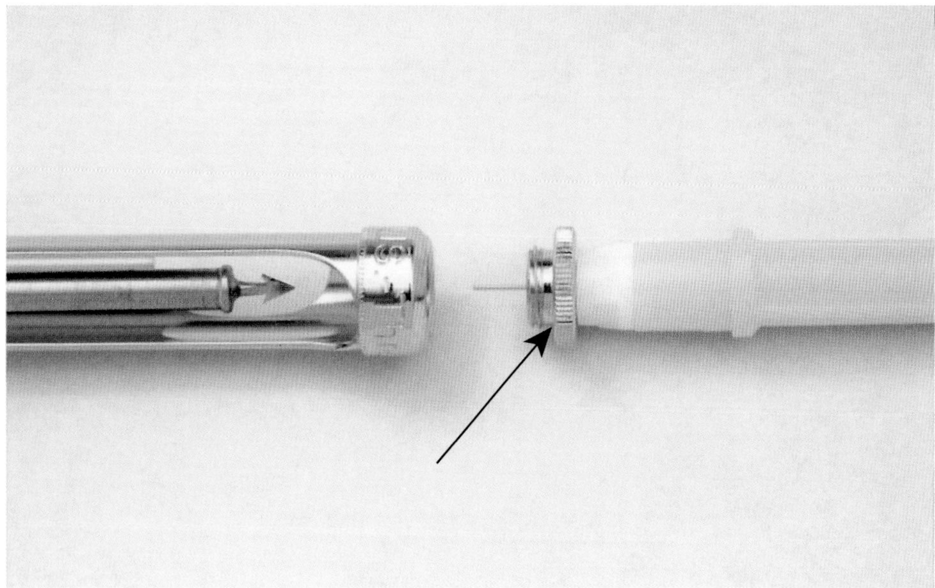

Figure 9-11. When discarding the needle, check to be sure that the metal needle adaptor from the syringe is not inadvertently discarded also *(arrow).*

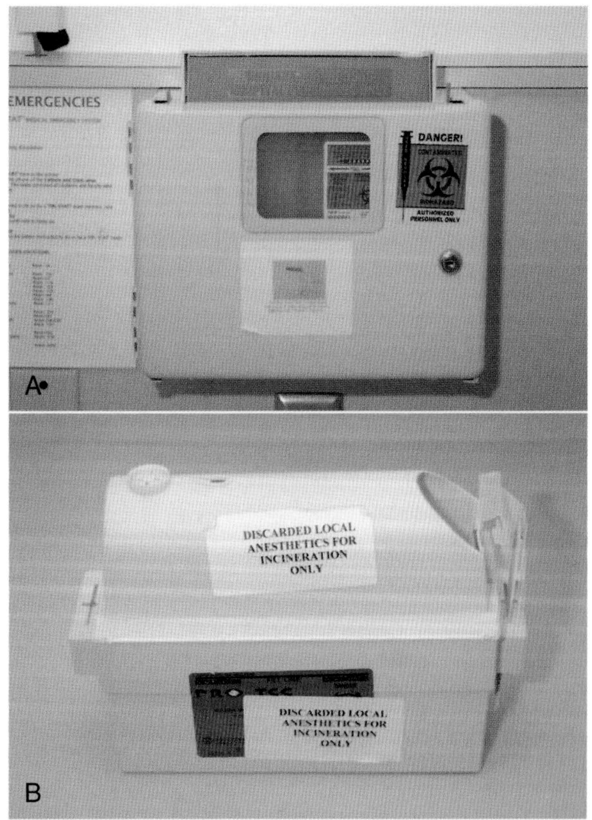

Figure 9-12. **A,** A sharps container is required for storage of discarded contaminated needles. **B,** A separate sealed container is recommended for discarded local anesthetic cartridges.

3. Remove the used cartridge.
4. Insert the new cartridge.
5. Embed the harpoon.
6. Reattach the needle.

The estimated time necessary to complete this procedure is 10 to 15 seconds.

SELF-ASPIRATING SYRINGE*

1. Insert the cartridge (as in the preceding instructions).
2. Attach the needle.
3. The syringe is now ready for use.

Because of the absence of a harpoon, loading and unloading the self-aspirating syringe are simple procedures.

ULTRASAFE ASPIRATING SYRINGE†

Loading the Safety Syringe

1. While gripping the barrel firmly, fully insert the anesthetic cartridge into the open end of the injectable system (Fig. 9-13).
2. Grip the plunger handle, putting the thumb behind the finger holder. Introduce the handle tip into the barrel of the injectable system, behind the cartridge (Fig. 9-14).
3. Next, slide the sheath protecting the needle backward, toward the handle, until it CLICKS (the click is made as

*From Dentsply, www.dentsply.com. This is a portion of the instructions that Dentsply encloses with its syringes.
†From Safety Syringes, Arcadia, Calif (www.safetysyringes.com). This is a portion of the instructions that Safety Syringes encloses with its syringes.

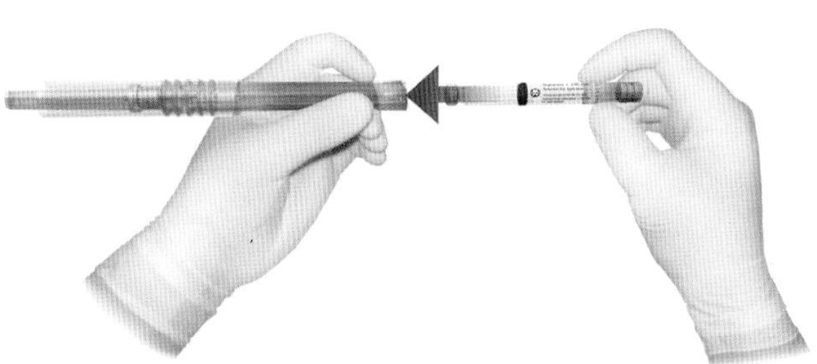

Figure 9-13. Insert the local anesthetic cartridge into the safety syringe. (Courtesy Septodont, Inc., Lancaster, PA.)

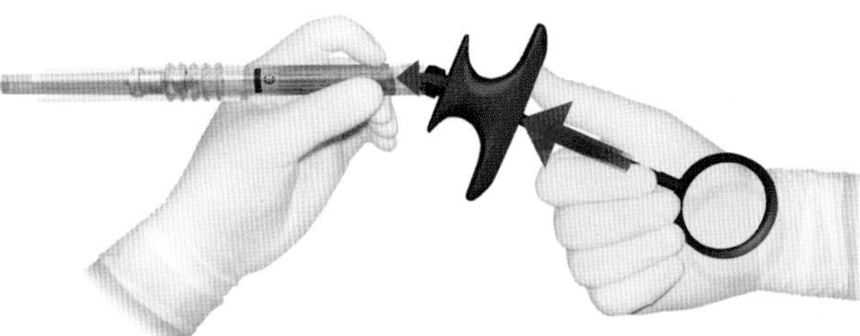

Figure 9-14. Introduce the handle tip into the barrel of the injectable system, behind the cartridge. (Courtesy Septodont, Inc., Lancaster, PA.)

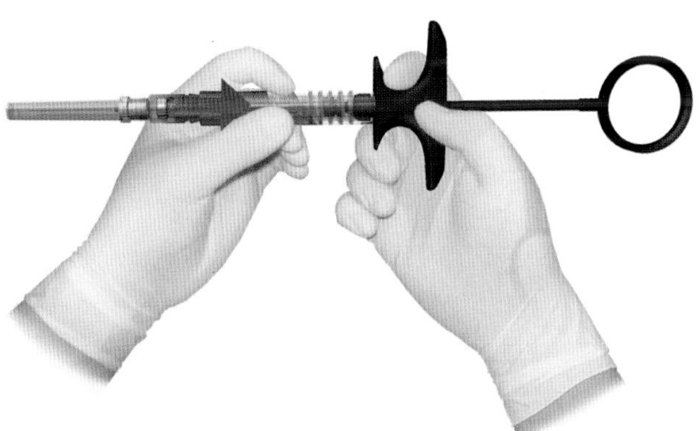

Figure 9-15. While protecting the needle, slide the sheath backward toward the handle until it CLICKS. (Courtesy Septodont, Inc., Lancaster, PA.)

the sheath hits the handle and locks the unit together) (Fig. 9-15).

4. All movements now are away from the needle. Remove the needle cap and discard. The system is now ready to use (Fig. 9-16).

Aspiration

Passive Aspiration (Self-Aspiration). At the base of the cartridge barrel of the injectable system, you will see there is a small protuberance. It appears as a blob of glue holding the centered needle, the needle-end that penetrates the diaphragm of the cartridge when inserted. At the start of the injection, the diaphragm is pressed against the protuberance; a depression occurs, and when released (injection stopped), the diaphragm moves back away from the protuberance and aspiration occurs (Fig. 9-17, *A*).

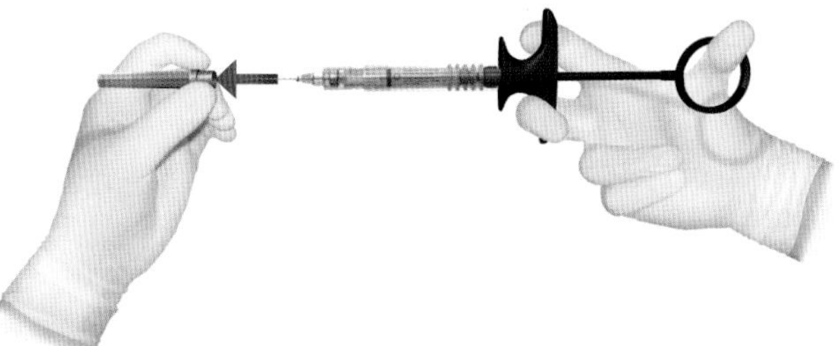

Figure 9-16. Remove the needle cap and discard. (Courtesy Septodont, Inc., Lancaster, PA.)

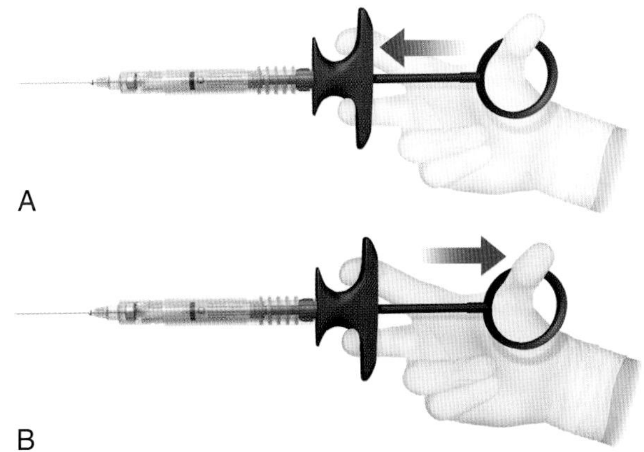

Figure 9-17. **A,** Passive aspiration. **B,** Active aspiration. (Courtesy Septodont, Inc., Lancaster, PA.)

Active Aspiration. Active aspiration is obtained by the silicone top of the plunger handle creating a vacuum when, thumb in ring, the practitioner pulls back (Fig. 9-17, *B*). The bung follows the plunger tip, providing active aspiration, which is best observed when a minimum of 0.25 to 0.35 mL of solution (providing space) has been expelled or used from the cartridge.

5. When using only one cartridge:

   Note: During multiple injection procedures using one cartridge, the practitioner may safely retain the syringe for further use by moving the sheath toward the needle until it reaches the holding position (Fig. 9-18). Should you need to insert a second cartridge, follow from step 7 onward.

To complete the procedure, slide the protective sheath toward the locking position, which is the second notch at the end of the barrel (Fig. 9-19, *A* and *B*). This has now locked the needle safely in the protective sheath.

6. Remove the plunger handle after use. After you have locked the injectable system in the *(B)* position, hold the barrel of the injectable system with one hand, and,

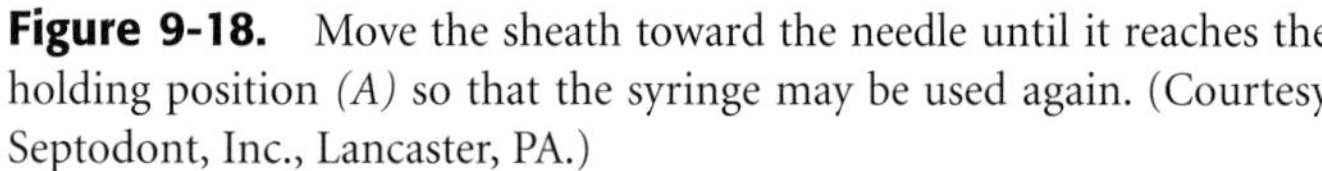

Figure 9-18. Move the sheath toward the needle until it reaches the holding position *(A)* so that the syringe may be used again. (Courtesy Septodont, Inc., Lancaster, PA.)

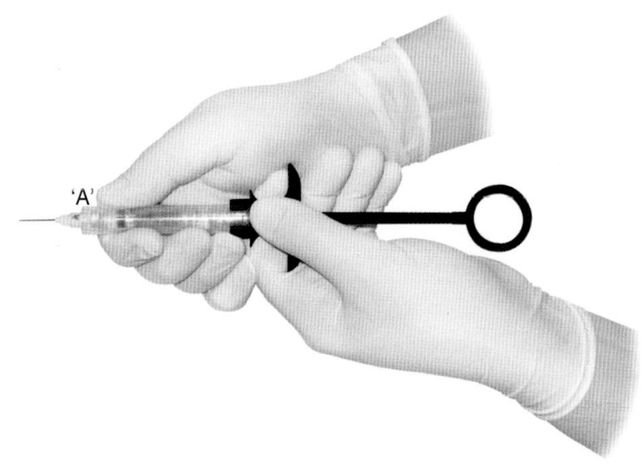

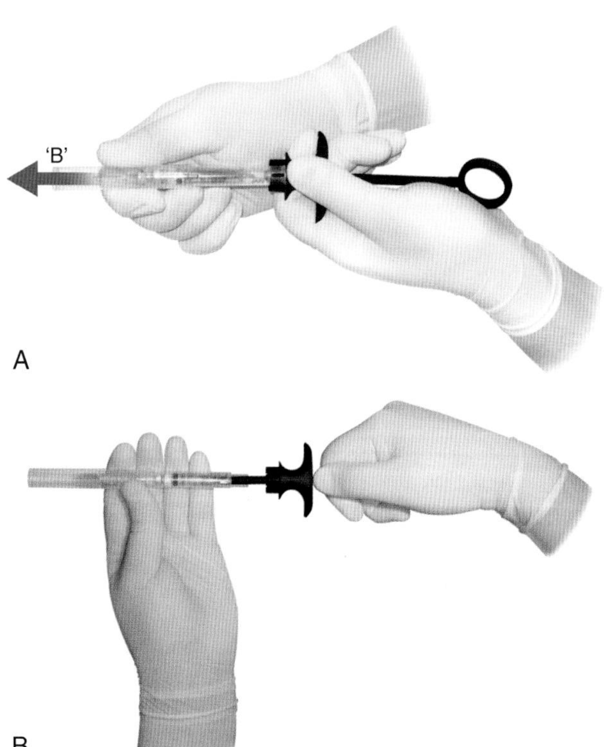

Figure 9-19. **A,** To lock the syringe, slide the protective sheath toward the locking position *(B)*, which is the second notch at the end of the barrel. **B,** Locked safety syringe. (Courtesy Septodont, Inc., Lancaster, PA.)

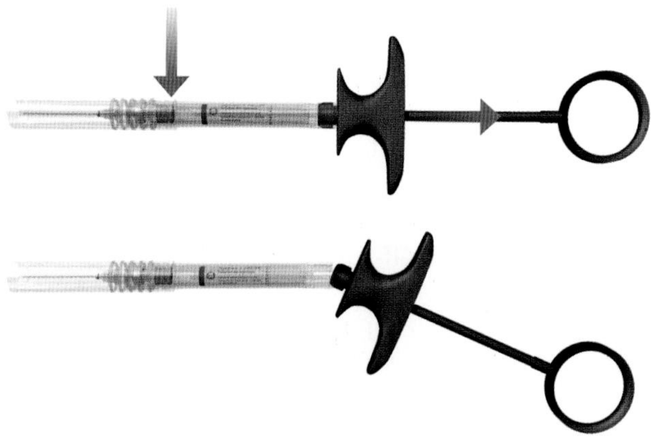

Figure 9-20. Remove the plunger handle after use. After locking the injectable system in the *(B)* position (see Fig. 9-19, *A*), hold the barrel of the injectable system with one hand, and while using the other hand, place a finger in the ring of the plunger handle and pull backward until the plunger is fully retracted. After you have fully retracted the plunger, peel off the handle in one movement. (Courtesy Septodont, Inc., Lancaster, PA.)

while using the other hand, place a finger in the ring of the plunger handle and pull backward until the plunger is fully retracted. After you have fully retracted the plunger, peel off the handle in one movement (Fig. 9-20). Now the injectable system can be disposed of safely and the handle autoclaved.

7. When inserting a second cartridge:

Note: During procedures that require more than one cartridge, retract the sheath to the holding position *(A)* as a needle-stick prevention device. *Should the system be inadvertently fully locked into position* (B), *no attempt whatsoever should be made to unlock it.* Use a new injection system.

Hold the barrel of the injectable system with one hand, and, while using the other hand, place a finger in the ring of the plunger handle and pull backward until the plunger is fully retracted. Now that you have fully retracted the plunger, peel off the handle in one movement.

8. Take hold of the plunger handle of the injection system, and pull the grip handle back toward the ring. Now insert the tip of the plunger into the empty cartridge, which is inside the injectable system. Pull out the cartridge attached to the plunger by the silicone tip, remove the cartridge from the plunger, and dispose of safely. You are now ready to insert a fresh cartridge and proceed as from step 1.

IN THIS PART

PART III

Techniques of Regional Anesthesia in Dentistry

The anatomy of the head, neck, and oral cavity is presented as a prelude to detailed descriptions of the techniques of regional anesthesia. Techniques that are commonly used in dentistry are presented. Although many of the techniques described in these chapters also may be carried out successfully with an extraoral approach, the author has limited descriptions to intraoral techniques, primarily because of the extremely limited use of extraoral nerve blocks in contemporary dental practice. The interested reader is referred to textbooks that describe extraoral techniques at some length.[1,2]

Each injection technique usually has several variations. Subtle differences are noted when techniques are taught to students by different persons. The reader must always keep in mind that there is never only one "correct" technique. Goals in the administration of local anesthesia are to provide clinically adequate pain control without unnecessarily increasing risk or provoking any immediate or delayed complications in the patient. Any technique that meets these two criteria is acceptable. The techniques presented in this section are those that this author finds most acceptable. In several situations, alternative approaches to the technique are also described.

A subject that is all too often neglected—the requirements for pain control and local anesthesia within the dental specialties—is discussed after these basic injection techniques are described. These requirements vary somewhat from endodontics to pediatric dentistry to periodontics to prosthodontics to oral and maxillofacial surgery and require special attention (Chapter 16). Administration of local anesthetics to the geriatric patient, a significant and growing segment of the population, is also reviewed.

The beginning of this section, Chapters 10 and 11, addresses two important subjects related to all injections: the physical and psychological evaluation of the patient before injection and basic injection technique (e.g., preparation of the patient and tissues for administration of any local anesthetic, the procedure for an atraumatic [painless] injection).

References

1. Hadzic A, Vloka JD: Peripheral nerve blocks: principles and practice, New York, 2004, McGraw-Hill.
2. Chelly J: Peripheral nerve blocks: a color atlas, ed 3, Philadelphia, 2009, Lippincott Williams & Wilkins.

CHAPTER 10

Physical and Psychological Evaluation

Before starting any dental procedure, the doctor or hygienist must determine whether the patient can tolerate the planned dental procedure in relative safety. If this is not the case, the specific treatment modifications necessary to decrease the risk presented by the patient must be determined. This is especially important whenever drugs are to be administered during treatment, such as analgesics, sedatives, inhalation sedation (N_2O-O_2) agents, and local anesthetics. Before administering local anesthetics, the administrator must determine the relative risk presented by the patient. This is important because local anesthetics, like all drugs, exert actions on many parts of the body (see Chapter 2). Actions of local anesthetics include depressant effects on excitable membranes (e.g., central nervous system [CNS], cardiovascular system [CVS]). Because local anesthetics undergo biotransformation primarily in the liver (amides) or blood (esters) the functional status of these systems must be determined before drug administration. Because a small percentage of all injected local anesthetic is excreted in an active (unmetabolized) form in the kidneys, kidney function must be evaluated. Other questions should be asked: Has the patient ever received a local anesthetic for medical or dental care? If so, were any adverse reactions observed?

Most undesirable reactions to local anesthetics are produced not by the drugs themselves but as a response to the act of drug administration.[1] These reactions are commonly psychogenic and have the potential to be life threatening if not recognized and managed promptly. The two most commonly occurring psychogenic reactions are vasodepressor syncope and hyperventilation. Other psychogenically induced reactions noted as a response to local anesthetic administration may include tonic–clonic convulsions, bronchospasm, and angina pectoris.

However, local anesthetics are not absolutely innocuous drugs, nor is the act of local anesthetic administration entirely benign. The doctor must seek to uncover as much information as possible concerning the patient's physical and mental status before administration of a local anesthetic. Fortunately the means to do so exist in the form of the medical history questionnaire, the dialogue history, and the physical examination of the patient. Adequate use of these tools can lead to an accurate determination of a patient's physical status and can prevent up to 90% of all life-threatening medical emergencies in dental practice.[2]

GOALS OF PHYSICAL AND PSYCHOLOGICAL EVALUATION

In the following discussion, a comprehensive but easy-to-use program of physical evaluation is described.[3,4] Used as recommended, it allows the dental team to accurately determine any potential risk presented by the patient before the start of treatment. This system can be used to meet the following goals:

1. To determine the patient's ability to tolerate *physically* the stresses involved in the planned dental treatment
2. To determine the patient's ability to tolerate *psychologically* the stresses involved in the planned dental treatment
3. To determine whether treatment modification is indicated to enable the patient to better tolerate the stresses of dental treatment
4. To determine whether the use of psychosedation is indicated
5. To determine which technique of sedation is most appropriate for the patient
6. To determine whether contraindications exist to (a) the planned dental treatment or (b) any of the drugs to be used.

The first two goals involve the patient's ability to tolerate the stress involved in the planned dental care. Stress may be of a physiologic or psychological nature. Patients with underlying medical problems may be less able to tolerate the usual levels of stress associated with various types of dental care. These patients are more likely to experience an acute exacerbation of their underlying medical problem(s) during periods of increased stress. Such disease processes include angina pectoris, seizure disorders, asthma, and sickle cell disease. Although most of these patients will be able to tolerate the planned dental care in relative safety, it is the obligation of the dental team to determine whether a problem does exist and the severity of the problem and to decide how it might impact the proposed dental treatment plan.

Excessive stress can prove detrimental to the non–medically compromised (i.e., "healthy") patient. Fear, anxiety, and acute pain produce abrupt changes in the homeostasis of the body that may prove detrimental. Many "healthy" patients suffer from fear-related emergencies, including hyperventilation and vasodepressor syncope (also known as vasovagal syncope and "fainting").

The third goal is to determine whether the usual treatment regimen for a patient should be modified to enable the patient to better tolerate the stress of treatment. In some cases, a healthy patient will be psychologically unable to tolerate the planned treatment. Treatment may be modified to minimize the stress faced by this patient. The medically compromised patient will also benefit from treatment modification aimed at minimizing stress. The stress reduction protocols (SRPs) outlined in this chapter are designed to aid the dentist and the hygienist in minimizing treatment-related stress for both healthy and medically compromised patients.

When it is believed that the patient will require some assistance in coping with his or her dental treatment, the use of psychosedation should be considered. The last three goals involve determination of the need for use of psychosedation, selection of the most appropriate technique, and selection of the most appropriate drug(s) for patient management.

PHYSICAL EVALUATION

The term *physical evaluation* is used to describe the steps involved in fulfilling the aforementioned goals. Physical evaluation in dentistry consists of the following three components:

1. Medical history questionnaire
2. Physical examination
3. Dialogue history

With the information (database) collected from these three steps, the dentist and the hygienist will be better able to (1) determine the physical and psychological status of the patient (establish a risk factor classification for the patient); (2) seek medical consultation, if indicated; and (3) appropriately modify the planned dental treatment, if indicated. Each of the three steps in the evaluation process is discussed in general terms, with specific emphasis placed on its importance in the evaluation of the patient for whom local anesthesia is to be administered.

Medical History Questionnaire

The use of a written, patient-completed medical history questionnaire is a moral and legal necessity in the practice of both medicine and dentistry. Such questionnaires provide the dentist and the hygienist with valuable information about the physical and in some cases the psychological condition of the prospective patient.

Many types of medical history questionnaires are available; however, most are simply modifications of two basic types: the "short" form and the "long" form. The *short form* medical history questionnaire provides basic medical history information and is best suited for use by a dentist or hygienist with considerable clinical experience in physical evaluation. When using the short-form history, the dentist or hygienist must have a firm grasp of the appropriate dialogue history required to aid in determination of the relative risk presented by the patient. The dentist or the hygienist should be experienced in the use of techniques of physical evaluation and interpretation of findings. Unfortunately, most dentist offices use the short form or a modification of it primarily as a convenience for their patient and themselves. The *long form,* on the other hand, results in a more detailed database concerning the physical condition of the prospective patient. It is used most often in teaching situations and represents a more ideal instrument for teaching physical evaluation.

In recent years, computer-generated medical history questionnaires have been developed.[5] These questionnaires permit patients to enter their responses to questions electronically on a computer. Whenever a positive response is given, the computer asks additional questions related to the positive response. In effect, the computer asks the questions called for in the dialogue history.

Any medical history questionnaire can prove to be extremely valuable or entirely worthless. The ultimate value of the questionnaire resides in the ability of the dentist or hygienist to interpret the significance of the answers and to elicit additional information through physical examination and dialogue history.

In this sixth edition of *Local Anesthesia,* the prototypical adult health history questionnaire that has been developed by the University of the Pacific (UOP) School of Dentistry in conjunction with MetLife has been included (Fig. 10-1).[6] Figure 10-2 is an example of a pediatric medical history questionnaire.

This health history has been translated into 36 different languages, constituting the languages spoken by 95% of the persons on this planet. The cost of the translation was supported by several organizations including the California Dental Association, but most extensively by MetLife Dental. The health history (see Fig. 10-1), translations of the health history (Fig. 10-3), the interview sheet (Fig. 10-4), the medical consultation form (Fig. 10-5), and protocols for the dental management of medically complex patients may be found on the University of the Pacific Website at www.dental.pacific.edu under "Dental Professionals" and then under "Health History Forms." Protocols for the management of medically complex patients can be found at the same Website under "Pacific Dental Management Protocols." Translations of the medical history form can be found at www.metdental.com under "Multilanguage Medical Health History Forms Available."

Text continued on p. 131

MetLife **HEALTH HISTORY** English **University of the Pacific**

Patient Name:____________________ Patient Identification Number:__________
Birth Date:__________

I. CIRCLE APPROPRIATE ANSWER (leave blank if you do not understand question):

1.	Yes	No	Is your general health good?
2.	Yes	No	Has there been a change in your health within the last year?
3.	Yes	No	Have you been hospitalized or had a serious illness in the last three years? If YES, why?__________
4.	Yes	No	Are you being treated by a physician now? For what? __________ Date of last medical exam?__________ Date of last dental exam __________
5.	Yes	No	Have you had problems with prior dental treatment?
6.	Yes	No	Are you in pain now?

II. HAVE YOU EXPERIENCED:

7.	Yes	No	Chest pain (angina)?	18.	Yes	No	Dizziness?
8.	Yes	No	Swollen ankles?	19.	Yes	No	Ringing in ears?
9.	Yes	No	Shortness of breath?	20.	Yes	No	Headaches?
10.	Yes	No	Recent weight loss, fever, night sweats?	21.	Yes	No	Fainting spells?
11.	Yes	No	Persistent cough, coughing up blood?	22.	Yes	No	Blurred vision?
12.	Yes	No	Bleeding problems, bruising easily?	23.	Yes	No	Seizures?
13.	Yes	No	Sinus problems?	24.	Yes	No	Excessive thirst?
14.	Yes	No	Difficulty swallowing?	25.	Yes	No	Frequent urination?
15.	Yes	No	Diarrhea, constipation, blood in stools?	26.	Yes	No	Dry mouth?
16.	Yes	No	Frequent vomiting, nausea?	27.	Yes	No	Jaundice?
17.	Yes	No	Difficulty urinating, blood in urine?	28.	Yes	No	Joint pain, stiffness?

III. DO YOU HAVE OR HAVE YOU HAD:

29.	Yes	No	Heart disease?	40.	Yes	No	AIDS
30.	Yes	No	Heart attack, heart defects?	41.	Yes	No	Tumors, cancer?
31.	Yes	No	Heart murmurs?	42.	Yes	No	Arthritis, rheumatism?
32.	Yes	No	Rheumatic fever?	43.	Yes	No	Eye diseases?
33.	Yes	No	Stroke, hardening of arteries?	44.	Yes	No	Skin diseases?
34.	Yes	No	High blood pressure?	45.	Yes	No	Anemia?
35.	Yes	No	Asthma, TB, emphysema, other lung diseases?	46.	Yes	No	VD (syphilis or gonorrhea)?
36.	Yes	No	Hepatitis, other liver disease?	47.	Yes	No	Herpes?
37.	Yes	No	Stomach problems, ulcers?	48.	Yes	No	Kidney, bladder disease?
38.	Yes	No	Allergies to: drugs, foods, medications, latex?	49.	Yes	No	Thyroid, adrenal disease?
39.	Yes	No	Family history of diabetes, heart problems, tumors?	50.	Yes	No	Diabetes?

IV. DO YOU HAVE OR HAVE YOU HAD:

51.	Yes	No	Psychiatric care?	56.	Yes	No	Hospitalization?
52.	Yes	No	Radiation treatments?	57.	Yes	No	Blood transfusions?
53.	Yes	No	Chemotherapy?	58.	Yes	No	Surgeries?
54.	Yes	No	Prosthetic heart valve?	59.	Yes	No	Pacemaker?
55.	Yes	No	Artificial joint?	60.	Yes	No	Contact lenses?

V. ARE YOU TAKING:

61.	Yes	No	Recreational drugs?	63.	Yes	No	Tobacco in any form?
62.	Yes	No	Drugs, medications, over-the-counter medicines (including aspirin), natural remedies?	64.	Yes	No	Alcohol?

Please list:__________

VI. WOMEN ONLY:

65.	Yes	No	Are you or could you be pregnant or nursing?	66.	Yes	No	Taking birth control pills?

VII. ALL PATIENTS:

67. Yes No Do you have or have you had any other diseases or medical problems NOT listed on this form?
If so, please explain:__________

To the best of my knowledge, I have answered every question completely and accurately. I will inform my dentist of any change in my health and/or medication.

Patient's signature:__________ Date:__________

RECALL REVIEW:

1. Patient's signature__________ Date:__________
2. Patient's signature__________ Date:__________
3. Patient's signature__________ Date:__________

The Health History is created and maintained by the University of the Pacific School of Dentistry, San Francisco, California.
Support for the translation and dissemination of the Health Histories comes from MetLife Dental Care.

Figure 10-1. Adult health history questionnaire. (Reprinted with permission from University of the Pacific Arthur A. Dugoni School of Dentistry, San Francisco.)

Child's Name: ____________ Date of Birth: ________ Age ______ Date: ______
Address: ____________ Telephone: ( )______
Physician's name (Medical Doctor): ____________ Telephone: ( )______

Please circle the appropriate answer.

1. Does your child have a health problem? .... YES NO
2. Was your child a patient in a hospital? .... YES NO
3. Date of last physical exam: ____________
4. Is your child now under medical care? .... YES NO
5. Is your child taking medication now? .... YES NO
   If so, for what? ____________.
6. Has your child ever had a serious illness or operation? YES NO
7. If so, explain: ____________
8. Does your child have (or ever had) any of the following diseases?
   a. Rheumatic fever or rheumatic heart disease ... YES NO
   b. Congenital heart disease .... YES NO
   c. Cardiovascular disease (heart trouble, heart attack, coronary insufficiency, coronary occlusion, high blood pressure, arteriosclerosis, stroke) .... YES NO
   d. Allergy? Food ☐ Medicine ☐ Other ☐ .. YES NO
   e. Asthma ☐ Hay Fever ☐ .... YES NO
   f. Hives or a skin rash .... YES NO
   g. Fainting spells or seizures .... YES NO
   h. Hepatitis, jaundice or liver disease .... YES NO
   i. Diabetes .... YES NO
   j. Inflammatory rheumatism (painful or swollen joints) .... YES NO
   k. Arthritis .... YES NO
   l. Stomach ulcers .... YES NO
   m. Kidney trouble .... YES NO
   n. Tuberculosis (TB) .... YES NO
   o. Persistent cough or cough up blood .... YES NO
   p. Veneral disease .... YES NO
   q. Epilepsy .... YES NO
   r. Sickle cell disease .... YES NO
   s. Thyroid disease .... YES NO
   t. AIDS .... YES NO
   u. Emphysema .... YES NO
   v. Psychiatric treatment .... YES NO
   w. Cleft lip/palate .... YES NO
   x. Cerebral palsy .... YES NO
   y. Mental retardation .... YES NO
   z. Hearing disability .... YES NO
   aa. Developmental disability .... YES NO
   If yes, explain: ____________
   bb. Was your child premature? .... YES NO
   If yes, how many weeks ____________
   cc. Other: ____________
9. Does your child have to urinate (pass water) more than six times a day? .... YES NO
10. Is your child thirsty much of the time? .... YES NO
11. Has your child had abnormal bleeding associated with previous surgery, extractions or accidents? .... YES NO
12. Does he/she bruise easily? .... YES NO
13. Has he/she ever required a blood transfusion? ..... YES NO
14. Does he/she have any blood disorders such as anemia, etc.? .... YES NO
15. Has he/she ever had surgery, x-ray or chemotherapy for a tumor, growth, or other condition? .... YES NO
16. Does your child have a disability that prevents treatment in a dental office? .... YES NO
17. Is he/she taking any of the following?
    a. Antibiotics or sulfa drugs .... YES NO
    b. Anticoagulants (blood thinners) .... YES NO
    c. Medicine for high blood pressure .... YES NO
    d. Cortisone or steroids .... YES NO
    e. Tranquilizers .... YES NO
    f. Aspirin .... YES NO
    g. Dilantin or other anticonvulsant .... YES NO
    h. Insulin, tolbutamide, Orinase, or similar drug ... YES NO
    i. Any other? ____________
18. Is he/she allergic to, or has he/she ever reacted adversely to, any of the following?
    a. Local anesthetics .... YES NO
    b. Penicillin or other antibiotics .... YES NO
    c. Sulfa drugs .... YES NO
    d. Barbituates, sedatives, or sleeping pills .... YES NO
    e. Aspirin .... YES NO
    f. Any other? ____________
19. Has he/she any serious trouble associated with any previous dental treatment? .... YES NO
    If so, please explain: ____________
20. Has your child been in any situation which could expose him/her to x-rays or other ionizing radiators? ...... YES NO
21. Last date of dental examination: ____________
22. Has he/she ever had orthodontic treatment (worn braces)? .... YES NO
23. Has he/she ever been treated for any gum diseases (gingivitis, periodontitis, trenchmouth, pyorrhea)? .... YES NO
24. Does his/her gums bleed when brushing teeth? .... YES NO
25. Does he/she grind or clench teeth? .... YES NO
26. Has he/she often had toothaches? .... YES NO
27. Has he/she had frequent sores in his/her mouth? .. YES NO
28. Has he/she had any injuries to his/her mouth or jaws? YES NO
    If yes, explain: ____________
29. Does he/she have any sores or swellings of his/her mouth or jaws? .... YES NO
30. Have you been satisfied with your child's previous dental care? .... YES NO

ADOLESCENT WOMEN:

31. Are you pregnant now, or think you may be? .... YES NO
32. Do you anticipate becoming pregnant? .... YES NO
33. Are you taking the pill? .... YES NO

To the best of my knowledge, all of the preceding answers are true and correct. If my child ever has a change in his/her health or his/her medicines change, I will inform the doctor at the next appointment without fail.

Parent's Signature: ____________ Date ______

MEDICAL HISTORY/ PHYSICAL EXAMINATION REVIEW

Date	Addition	Student/Faculty Signatures	

Figure 10-2. Pediatric medical history questionnaire. (From Malamed SF: Medical emergencies in the dental office, ed 6, St Louis, 2007, Mosby.)

MetLife | **Historia Médica** Spanish | University of the Pacific

Nombre del paciente:__________ No. de Ident. del Paciente: __________
Fecha de nacimiento: __________

I. MARQUE CON UN CÍRCULO LA RESPUESTA CORRECTA (Deje en BLANCO si no entiende la pregunta):

1. Sí No ¿Está en buena salud general?
2. Sí No ¿Han habido cambios en su salud durante el último año?
3. Sí No ¿Ha estado hospitalizado/a o ha tenido de una enfermedad grave en los últimos tres años?
   ¿Si Sí, por qué? __________
4. Sí No ¿Se encuentra actualmente bajo tratamiento médico? ¿Para qué? __________
   Fecha de su último examen médico: __________ Fecha de su última cita dental: __________
5. Sí No ¿Ha tenido problemas con algún tratamiento dental en el pasado?
6. Sí No ¿Tiene algún dolor ahora?

II. HA NOTADO:

7. Sí No ¿Dolor de pecho (angina)?
8. Sí No ¿Los tobillos hinchados?
9. Sí No ¿Falta de aliento?
10. Sí No ¿Reciente pérdida de peso, fiebre, sudor en la noche?
11. Sí No ¿Tos persistente o tos con sangre?
12. Sí No ¿Problemas de sangramiento, moretes?
13. Sí No ¿Problemas nasales (sinusitis)?
14. Sí No ¿Dificultad al tragar?
15. Sí No ¿Diarrea, estreñimiento, sangre en las heces?
16. Sí No ¿Vómitos con frecuencia, náuseas?
17. Sí No ¿Dificultad al orinar, sangre en la orina?
18. Sí No ¿Mareos?
19. Sí No ¿Ruidos o zumbidos en los oídos?
20. Sí No ¿Dolores de cabeza?
21. Sí No ¿Desmayos?
22. Sí No ¿Vista borrosa?
23. Sí No ¿Convulsiones?
24. Sí No ¿Sed excesiva?
25. Sí No ¿Orina con frecuencia?
26. Sí No ¿Boca seca?
27. Sí No ¿Ictericia?
28. Sí No ¿Dolor o rigidez en las articulaciones?

III. TIENE O HA TENIDO:

29. Sí No ¿Enfermedades del corazón?
30. Sí No ¿Infarto de corazón, defectos en el corazón?
31. Sí No ¿Soplos en el corazón?
32. Sí No ¿Fiebre reumática?
33. Sí No ¿Apoplejía, endurecimiento de las arterias?
34. Sí No ¿Presión sanguínea alta?
35. Sí No ¿Asma, tuberculosis, enfisema, otras enfermedades pulmonares?
36. Sí No ¿Hepatitis, otras enfermedades del hígado?
37. Sí No ¿Problemas del estómago, úlceras?
38. Sí No ¿Alergias a remedios, comidas, medicamentos látex?
39. Sí No ¿Familiares con diabetes, problemas de corazón, tumores?
40. Sí No ¿SIDA?
41. Sí No ¿Tumores, cáncer?
42. Sí No ¿Artritis, reuma?
43. Sí No ¿Enfermedades de los ojos?
44. Sí No ¿Enfermedades de la piel?
45. Sí No ¿Anemia?
46. Sí No ¿Enfermedades venéreas (sífilis o gonorrea)?
47. Sí No ¿Herpes?
48. Sí No ¿Enfermedades renales (riñón), vejiga?
49. Sí No ¿Enfermedades de tiroides o glándulas suprarrenales?
50. Sí No ¿Diabetes?

VI. TIENE O HA TENIDO:

51. Sí No ¿Tratamiento psiquiátrico?
52. Sí No ¿Tratamientos de radiación?
53. Sí No ¿Quimioterapia?
54. Sí No ¿Válvula artificial del corazón?
55. Sí No ¿Articulación artificial?
56. Sí No ¿Hospitalizaciones?
57. Sí No ¿Transfusiones de sangre?
58. Sí No ¿Cirugías?
59. Sí No ¿Marcapasos?
60. Sí No ¿Lentes de contacto?

V. ESTÁ TOMANDO:

61. Sí No ¿Drogas de uso recreativo?
62. Sí No ¿Remedios, medicamentos, medicamentos sin receta (incluyendo aspirina)?
63. Sí No ¿Tabaco de cualquier tipo?
64. Sí No ¿Alcohol (bebidas alcohólicas)?

Liste por favor:__________

VI. SÓLO PARA MUJERES:

65. Sí No ¿Está o podría estar embarazada o dando pecho?
66. Sí No ¿Está tomando pastillas anticonceptivas?

VII. PARA TODOS LOS PACIENTES:

67. Sí No ¿Tiene o ha tenido alguna otra enfermedad o problema médico que NO está en este cuestionario?

Si la respuesta es afirmativa, explique: __________

Que yo sepa, he respondido completamente y correctamente todas las preguntas. Informaré a mi dentista si hay algún cambio en mi salud y/o en los medicamentos que tomo.

Firma del Paciente __________ Fecha __________

REVISIÓN SUPLEMENTARIA:

1. Firma del Paciente __________ Fecha __________
2. Firma del Paciente __________ Fecha __________
3. Firma del Paciente __________ Fecha __________

The Health History is created and maintained by the University of the Pacific School of Dentistry, San Francisco, California.
Support for the translation and dissemination of the Health Histories comes from MetLife Dental Care.

Figure 10-3. Spanish health history questionnaire. (Reprinted with permission from University of the Pacific Arthur A. Dugoni School of Dentistry, San Francisco.)

MetLife

HEALTH HISTORY INTERVIEW

University of the Pacific

Patient Name:______________________________________

SIGNIFICANT MEDICAL FINDINGS	DENTAL MANAGEMENT CONSIDERATIONS	DATE

Record below the number and details of any YES response noted on the Health History, plus details of any YES response to questions A through F.

A.	yes/no	Cardiovascular
B.	yes/no	Infectious diseases
C.	yes/no	Allergy to medicines
D.	yes/no	Hematologic, bleeding
E.	yes/no	Medications
F.	yes/no	Other medical problems not asked?

__________ ______________________________

Date Doctor's Signature

This Health History Interview form is created and maintained by the University of the Pacific School of Dentistry, San Francisco, California. Support for the translation and dissemination of the Health Histories comes from MetLife Dental Care.

Figure 10-4. Health history interview sheet. (Reprinted with permission from University of the Pacific Arthur A. Dugoni School of Dentistry, San Francisco.)

MetLife **MEDICAL CONSULTATION REQUEST** **University of the Pacific**

To: Dr.____________________ Please complete the form below and return it to

____________________ Dr.____________________

____________________ ____________________

RE: ____________________ ____________________

____

Date of Birth

Phone # ____________________

Fax # ____________________

Our patient has presented with the following medical problem(s):____________________

____

____

The following treatment is scheduled in our clinic:____________________

____

Most patients experience the following with the above planned procedures:

bleeding: • minimal (<50ml) • significant (>50ml)
stress and anxiety: • low • medium • high

____________________ ____________________
Dentist signature Date

PHYSICIAN'S RESPONSE

Please provide any information regarding the above patient's need for antibiotic prophylaxis, current cardiovascular condition, coagulation ability, and the history and status of infectious diseases. Ordinarily, local anesthesia is obtained with 2% lidocaine, 1:100,000 epinephrine. For some surgical procedures, the epinephrine concentration may be increased to 1:50,000 for hemostasis. The epinephrine dose NEVER exceeds 0.2 mg total.

*CHECK **ALL** THAT APPLY*

- **OK** to **PROCEED** with dental treatment; **NO** special precautions and **NO** prophylactic antibiotics are needed.
- Antibiotic prophylaxis **IS** required for dental treatment according to the current American Heart Association and/or American Academy of Orthopedic Surgeons guidelines.
- Other precautions are required (please list):____________________

  ____
- **DO NOT** proceed with treatment. (Please give reason.)____________________

  ____

  Treatment may proceed on (Date)____________
- Patient has an infectious disease:
  - AIDS (please provide current lab results)
  - TB (PPD+/active)
  - Hepatitis, type ______(acute/carrier)
  - Other (explain)____________
- Requested relevant medical and/or laboratory information is attached.

____________________ ____________________
Physician signature Date

PATIENT CONSENT

I agree to the release of my medical information to the University of the Pacific School of Dentistry.

____________________ ____________________
Patient signature Date

This Medical Consultation form is created and maintained by the University of the Pacific School of Dentistry, San Francisco, California. Support for the translation and dissemination of the health histories comes from MetLife Dental Care.

Figure 10-5. Medical consultation form. (Reprinted with permission from University of the Pacific Arthur A. Dugoni School of Dentistry, San Francisco.)

The health history has been translated while keeping the same question numbering sequence. Thus a dentist who speaks English and is caring for a patient who does not can ask the patient to complete the health history in his or her own language. The dentist then compares the English health history with the patient's translated health history, scanning the translated version for YES responses. When a YES is found, the dentist is able to look at the question number and match it to the question number on the English version. For example, the dentist would know that a YES response to question No. 34 on the non-English version is the same as this response to question No. 34 on the English version, which relates to high blood pressure (HBP). For that matter, a Mandarin Chinese–speaking dentist could use the multilanguage health history with an English-speaking patient and have the same cross-referenced information. A dentist who speaks Spanish could use the multilanguage health history with a patient who speaks French. With the uniform health history question sequence, these health history translations can serve patients and dentists all around the world.

The health history is divided into sections related to signs and symptoms ("Have you experienced?"), diagnosed diseases ("Do you have or have you had?"), medical treatments (including drugs and other physiologically active compounds), and several other questions.

Although both long- and short-form medical history questionnaires are valuable in determining a patient's physical condition, one criticism of most available health history questionnaires is the absence of questions related to the patient's attitudes toward dentistry. It is recommended therefore that one or more questions be included that relate to this all-important subject:

1. Do you feel very nervous about having dental treatment?
2. Have you ever had a bad experience in the dental office?

Question Nos. 5 and 6 on the UOP medical history questionnaire address these points.

Following is the UOP medical history questionnaire with a discussion of the significance of each point.

I. CIRCLE APPROPRIATE ANSWER: *(Leave blank if you do not understand the question.)*

1. Is Your General Health Good?

Comment: General survey questions seek patients' general impression of their health. Studies have demonstrated that a YES response to this question does not necessarily correlate with the patient's actual state of health.[7]

2. Has There Been a Change in Your Health Within the Last Year?

3. Have You Been Hospitalized or Had a Serious Illness in the Last 3 Years? If YES, Why?

4. Are You Being Treated by a Physician Now? For What?

Date of last medical exam?

Date of last dental exam?

Comment: Question Nos. 2, 3, and 4 seek information regarding recent changes in the patient's physical condition. In all instances of a positive response, an in-depth dialogue history must ensue to determine the precise nature of the change in health status, the type of surgical procedure or illness, and the names of any medications the patient may now be taking to help manage the problem.

5. Have You Had Problems With Prior Dental Treatment?

Comment: Many adults are reluctant to verbally admit to the dentist, hygienist, or assistant their fears about treatment, for fear of being labeled a "baby." This is especially true of young men in their late teens or early twenties; they attempt to "take it like a man" or "grin and bear it" rather than admit their fears. Because the most common fear mentioned by dental patients is fear of injection (the "shot," in their words), all too often, such macho behavior results in an episode of vasodepressor syncope. Whereas many such patients will not offer verbal admissions of fear, many of these same patients will volunteer this information in writing.

6. Are You in Pain Now?

Comment: The primary aim of this question is related to the need for immediate dental care. Its purpose is to determine what prompted the patient to seek dental care. If pain is present, the dentist may need to treat the patient immediately on an emergency basis, whereas in the more normal situation, treatment can be delayed until future visits. This may affect the use of local anesthesia, in that effective pain control can be more difficult to achieve in the presence of infection and chronic, albeit, now acute, pain in the fearful patient.

II. HAVE YOU EXPERIENCED:

7. Chest Pain (Angina)?

Comment: A history of angina (defined, in part, as chest pain brought on by exertion and alleviated by rest) usually indicates the presence of coronary artery disease with attendant ischemia of the myocardium. The risk factor for the typical patient with stable angina is ASA 3 (American Society of Anesthesiologists' [ASA] physical status classification system).* In the presence of dental fears, sedation is absolutely indicated in the anginal patient. Inhalation sedation with N_2O-O_2 is preferred. Effective pain control—local anesthesia with vasoconstrictor included—is absolutely indicated. Patients with unstable or recent-onset angina represent ASA 4 risks.

*The ASA physical status classification system is discussed in detail later in this chapter.

8. Swollen Ankles?

Comment: Swollen ankles (pitting edema or dependent edema) indicate possible heart failure (HF). However, varicose veins, pregnancy, and renal dysfunction are other causes of ankle edema. Healthy persons who stand on their feet for long periods (e.g., mail carriers, dental staff members) may develop ankle edema that is not life threatening, merely esthetically unpleasing.

9. Shortness of Breath?

Comment: Although the patient may respond negatively to specific questions (questions No. 29 to No. 35 in Section III) regarding the presence of various heart and lung disorders (e.g., angina, HF, pulmonary emphysema), clinical signs and symptoms of heart or lung disease may be evident. A positive response to this question does not always indicate that the patient suffers such a disease. To more accurately determine the patient's status before the start of dental care, further evaluation is suggested.

10. Recent Weight Loss, Fever, Night Sweats?

Comment: The question refers primarily to an unexpected gain or loss of weight, not to intentional weight loss (e.g., dieting). Unexpected weight change may indicate HF, hypothyroidism (increased weight), hyperthyroidism, widespread carcinoma, uncontrolled diabetes mellitus (weight loss), or a number of other disorders. The presence of fever and/or night sweats should be pursued to determine whether they are innocent or perhaps clues to the presence of a more significant problem, such as tuberculosis.

11. Persistent Cough, Coughing Up Blood?

Comment: A positive response mandates an in-depth dialogue history to determine the cause of the persistent cough or hemoptysis (blood-tinged sputum). The most common causes of hemoptysis are bronchitis and bronchiectasis, neoplasms, and tuberculosis.

A chronic cough can indicate active tuberculosis or other chronic respiratory disorders, such as chronic bronchitis. Cough associated with an upper respiratory infection confers an ASA 2 classification on the patient, whereas chronic bronchitis in a patient who has smoked more than one pack of cigarettes daily for many years may indicate chronic lung disease and confer on the patient an ASA 3 risk.

12. Bleeding Problems, Bruising Easily?

Comment: Bleeding disorders, such as hemophilia, are associated with prolonged bleeding or frequent bruising and can lead to modification of certain forms of dental therapy (e.g., surgery, technique of local anesthetic administration, venipuncture) and therefore must be made known to the dentist before treatment is begun.

Before a needle is inserted into the vascular soft tissues of the oral cavity, it should be determined whether the patient is at risk of excessive bleeding. In the presence of coagulopathies or other bleeding disorders, injection techniques with a greater incidence of positive aspiration should be avoided, if possible, in favor of supraperiosteal, periodontal ligament (PDL), intraosseous (IO), or other techniques less likely to produce bleeding. Techniques that might be avoided when bleeding disorders are present include the maxillary (V_2) nerve block (high tuberosity approach), the posterior superior alveolar nerve block (PSA), the inferior alveolar nerve block (IANB), and probably both the Gow-Gates and the Akinosi-Vazirani mandibular nerve blocks. Although the latter two techniques have relatively low positive aspiration rates, bleeding following their administration is likely to occur deep in the tissues and therefore may be more difficult to manage. Modifications should be listed in the patient's chart.

13. Sinus Problems?

Comment: Sinus problems can indicate the presence of an allergy (ASA 2), which should be pursued in the dialogue history, or an upper respiratory tract infection (URI) (ASA 2), such as a common cold. The patient may experience some respiratory distress when placed in a supine position; distress may also be present if a rubber dam is used. Specific treatment modifications—postponing treatment until the patient is able to breathe more comfortably, limiting the degree of recline in the dental chair, and foregoing use of a rubber dam—are advisable.

14. Difficulty Swallowing?

Comment: Dysphagia, or the inability to swallow, can have many causes. Before the start of any dental treatment, the dentist should seek to determine the cause and severity of the patient's complaint.

15. Diarrhea, Constipation, Blood in Stools?

Comment: This is an evaluation to determine whether gastrointestinal (GI) problems are present, many of which require patients to be medicated. Causes of blood in feces can range from benign, self-limiting events to serious life-threatening disease. Common causes include anal fissures, aspirin-containing drugs, bleeding disorders, esophageal varices, foreign body trauma, hemorrhoids, neoplasms, use of orally administered steroids, the presence of intestinal polyps, and thrombocytopenia.

16. Frequent Vomiting, Nausea?

Comment: A multitude of causes can lead to nausea and vomiting. Medications, however, are among the most common causes of nausea and vomiting.[8-10] Opiates, digitalis, levodopa, and many cancer drugs act on the chemoreceptor trigger zone in the area postrema to induce vomiting. Drugs that frequently induce nausea include nonsteroidal anti-inflammatory drugs (NSAIDs), erythromycin, cardiac antidysrhythmics, antihypertensive drugs, diuretics, oral antidiabetic agents, oral contraceptives, and many GI drugs, such as sulfasalazine.[8-10]

GI and systemic infections, viral and bacterial, are the second most common cause of nausea and vomiting.

17. Difficulty Urinating, Blood in Urine?

Comment: Hematuria, the presence of blood in the urine, requires evaluation to determine the cause; it is potentially indicative of urinary tract infection or obstruction.

18. Dizziness?

Comment: A positive response may indicate chronic postural (orthostatic) hypotension, symptomatic hypotension or anemia, or transient ischemic attack (TIA), a form of pre-stroke. In addition, patients with certain types of seizure disorders, such as the "drop attack," may report fainting or dizzy spells. The dentist may be advised to perform further evaluation, including a consultation with the patient's primary care physician. A transient ischemic attack represents an ASA 3 risk, whereas chronic postural hypotension normally represents an ASA 2 or 3 risk.

19. Ringing in Ears?

Comment: Tinnitus (an auditory sensation in the absence of sound heard in one or both ears, such as ringing, buzzing, hissing, or clicking) is a common side effect of certain drugs including salicylates, indomethacin, propranolol, levodopa, aminophylline, and caffeine. It may be seen with multiple sclerosis, tumor, and ischemic infarction.

20. Headaches?

Comment: The presence of headache should be evaluated to determine the cause. Common causes include chronic daily headaches, cluster headaches, migraine headaches, and tension-type headaches. If necessary, consultation with the patient's primary care physician is warranted. Determine the drug(s) used by the patient to manage his or her symptoms, because many of these agents can have an effect on the clotting of blood that could influence choice of local anesthetic technique (e.g., avoidance of those with a higher positive aspiration rate).

21. Fainting Spells?

Comment: Fainting (vasodepressor syncope) is the most common medical emergency in dentistry. It is most likely to occur during administration of a local anesthetic as a result of needle phobia (trypanophobia[11]). Prior recognition of needle phobia can usually result in prevention of the syncopal episode.

22. Blurred Vision?

Comment: Blurred vision is an increasingly common finding as patients age. Leading causes of blurred vision and blindness include glaucoma, diabetic retinopathy, and macular degeneration. Double vision, or diplopia, usually results from extraocular muscle imbalance, the cause of which must be sought. Common causes include damage to third, fourth, or sixth cranial nerves secondary to myasthenia gravis, vascular disturbance, and intracranial tumor.

23. Seizures?

Comment: Seizures are common emergencies in the dental environment. The most likely candidate to have a seizure is the epileptic patient. Even epileptics who are well controlled with antiepileptic drugs may suffer seizures in stressful situations, such as might occur in the dental office. The dentist must determine the type of seizure, the frequency of occurrence, and the drug(s) used to prevent the seizure before starting dental treatment. Treatment modification using SRPs (discussed later in this chapter) is desirable for patients with known seizure disorders. Sedation is highly recommended in the fearful epileptic dental patient as a means of preventing a seizure from developing during treatment. Epileptics whose seizures are under control (occur infrequently) are ASA 2 risks; those with more frequent seizures represent ASA 3 or 4 risk. A classic overdose of local anesthetic manifests as tonic–clonic seizure activity.

24. Excessive Thirst?

Comment: Polydipsia, or excessive thirst, is oftentimes seen in diabetes mellitus, diabetes insipidus, and hyperparathyroidism.

25. Frequent Urination?

Comment: Polyuria, or frequent urination, may be benign (too much fluid intake) or may be a symptom of diabetes mellitus, diabetes insipidus, Cushing syndrome, or hyperparathyroidism.

26. Dry Mouth?

Comment: Fear is a common cause of a dry mouth, especially in the dental environment. Many other causes of xerostomia are known, including Sjögren syndrome.

27. Jaundice?

Comment: Jaundice, or yellowness of skin, the whites of the eyes, and mucous membranes, is due to deposition of bile pigment resulting from an excess of bilirubin in the blood (hyperbilirubinemia). It is frequently caused by obstruction of bile ducts, excessive destruction of red blood cells (hemolysis), or disturbances in the functioning of liver cells. Jaundice is a sign that might be indicative of a benign problem, such as a gallstone obstructing the common bile duct, or it may be due to pancreatic carcinoma involving the opening of the common bile duct into the duodenum. Because amide local anesthetics undergo primary biotransformation in the liver, the presence of significant hepatic dysfunction (e.g., ASA 4) may represent a relative or absolute contraindication to administration of these drugs. Articaine HCl, which undergoes biotransformation both in the liver and in the blood (plasma cholinesterase), is preferred in these patients because it has an elimination half-life of 27 minutes (vs. 90 minutes for most other amide local anesthetics).

28. Joint Pain, Stiffness?

Comment: A history of joint pain and stiffness (arthritis) may be associated with long-term use of salicylates (aspirin) or other NSAIDs, some of which may alter blood clotting. Arthritic patients who are receiving long-term corticosteroid therapy may suffer increased risk of acute adrenal insufficiency, especially the patient who has recently stopped taking the steroid. Such patients may require a short course of steroid therapy or a modification (increase) in corticosteroid dose during dental treatment, so that their body is better able to respond to any additional stress that might be associated with the treatment.

Because of possible difficulties in positioning the patient comfortably, modifications may be necessary to accommodate the patient's physical disability. Most patients receiving corticosteroids are categorized as ASA 2 or 3 risk depending on the reason for the medication and the degree of disability present. Patients with significantly disabling arthritis are ASA 3 risks. Problems secondary to arthritis may require modification in positioning during local anesthetic injection.

III. DO YOU HAVE OR HAVE YOU HAD:

29. Heart Disease?

Comment: This represents a survey question seeking to detect the presence of any and all types of heart disease. In the presence of a YES answer, the dentist must seek more specific detailed information as to the nature and severity of the problem and a list of any medications taken by the patient to manage the condition. Because many forms of heart disease are exacerbated in the presence of stress, consideration of the SRP becomes increasingly important.

30. Heart Attack, Heart Defects?

Comment: Heart attack is the lay term for myocardial infarction (MI). The dentist must determine the time that has elapsed since the patient suffered the MI, the severity of the MI, and the degree of residual myocardial damage to decide whether treatment modifications are indicated. Elective dental care traditionally has been withheld for the first 6 months after an MI,[12] although recent evidence demonstrates that many patients are able to tolerate stress in as few as 3 to 4 weeks after experiencing an MI.[13,14] Most post-MI patients are considered to be ASA 3 risks 6 months or more after the event; however, a patient who has experienced an MI within 6 months before the planned dental treatment should be considered an ASA 4 risk until medical consultation with his or her cardiologist is obtained. When little or no residual damage to the myocardium is present, the patient may be considered an ASA 2 risk after 6 months.

Heart failure: The degree of heart failure (weakness of the "pump") present must be assessed through the dialogue history. When a patient has a more serious condition, such as congestive heart failure (CHF) or dyspnea (labored breathing) at rest, specific treatment modifications are warranted. In this situation, the dentist must consider whether the patient requires supplemental O_2 during treatment. Whereas most HF patients are classified according to the ASA physical status classification system as ASA 2 (mild HF without disability) or ASA 3 (disability developing with exertion or stress) risks, the presence of dyspnea at rest represents an ASA 4 risk. Effective pain control is essential in the ASA 2 and 3 HF patient, but care must be taken in selecting the appropriate drugs and technique to prevent significant increases in the cardiac workload. Local anesthetics containing vasopressors are definitely indicated in these patients because they are more likely to provide successful pain control for dental procedures compared with "plain" local anesthetics.

Congenital heart lesions: An in-depth dialogue history is required to determine the nature of the lesion and the degree of disability present. Patients can represent ASA 2, 3, or 4 risk. The dentist may recommend medical consultation, especially for the pediatric patient, to judge the severity of the lesion. Some dental treatments require prophylactic antibiotics.

31. Heart Murmurs?

Comment: Heart murmurs are common, but not all murmurs are clinically significant. The dentist should determine whether a murmur is functional (nonpathologic, or ASA 2), whether clinical signs and symptoms of valvular stenosis or regurgitation are present (ASA 3 or 4), and whether antibiotic prophylaxis is warranted. A major clinical symptom of a significant (organic) murmur is undue fatigue. Table 10-1 provides guidelines for antibiotic prophylaxis (most recently revised in 2007).[15] Box 10-1 categorizes cardiac problems as to their requirements for antibiotic prophylaxis, and Box 10-2 addresses prophylaxis and dental procedures specifically. As noted in the Guidelines, antibiotic prophylaxis is NOT indicated for the administration of routine dental injection techniques through noninfected tissues. Guidelines for antibiotic prophylaxis in orthopedic patients with total joint replacements were published initially in 2003[16] and were last revised in 2010.[17]

32. Rheumatic Fever?

Comment: A history of rheumatic fever should prompt the dentist to perform an in-depth dialogue history for the presence of rheumatic heart disease (RHD). In the presence of RHD, antibiotic prophylaxis may be indicated as a means of minimizing the risk of developing subacute bacterial endocarditis (SBE). Depending on the severity of the disease and the presence of a disability, RHD patients can be an ASA 2, 3, or 4 risk. Additional treatment modifications may be advisable.

33. Stroke, Hardening of Arteries?

Comment: The dentist must pay close attention to stroke, cerebrovascular accident (CVA), or "brain attack" (the term increasingly used to confer on the lay public and health care professionals the urgency needed in prompt management of

TABLE 10-1
Antibiotic Prophylaxis 2007*

Situation	Agent	Adults	Children
Oral	Amoxicillin	2 g	50 mg/kg
Unable to take oral medication	Ampicillin *or*	2 g IM or IV†	50 mg/kg IM or IV
	Cefazolin or ceftriaxone	1 g IM or IV	50 mg/kg IM or IV
Allergic to penicillins or ampicillin Oral	Cephalexin‡§	2 g	50 mg/kg
	or		
	Clindamycin	600 mg	20 mg/kg
	or		
	Azithromycin or clarithromycin	500 mg	15 mg/kg
Allergic to penicillins or ampicillin and unable to take oral medication	Cefazolin or ceftriaxone§	1 g IM or IV	50 mg/kg IM or IV
	or		
	Clindamycin	600 mg IM or IV	20 mg/kg IM or IV

From Wilson W, Taubert KA, Gewitz M, et al: Prevention of infective endocarditis: guidelines from the American Heart Association: a guideline from the American Heart Association Rheumatic Fever, Endocarditis, and Kawasaki Disease Committee, Council on Cardiovascular Disease in the Young, and the Council on Clinical Cardiology, Council on Cardiovascular Surgery and Anesthesia, and the Quality of Care and Outcomes Research Interdisciplinary Working Group, Circulation 116:1736–1754, 2007.

*Regimen: single dose 30 to 60 minutes before procedure.

†*IM*, Intramuscular; *IV*, intravenous.

‡Or other first- or second-generation oral cephalosporin in equivalent adult or pediatric dosage.

§Cephalosporins should not be used in an individual with a history of anaphylaxis, angioedema, or urticaria with penicillins or ampicillin.

BOX 10-1 Cardiac Conditions Associated With the Highest Risk of Adverse Outcome from Endocarditis for Which Prophylaxis With Dental Procedures Is Recommended

- Prosthetic cardiac valve
- Previous infective endocarditis
- Congenital heart disease (CHD)*
- Unrepaired cyanotic CHD, including palliative shunts and conduits
- Completely repaired congenital heart defect with prosthetic material or device, whether placed by surgery or by catheter intervention, during the first 6 mo after the procedure†
- Repaired CHD with residual defects at the site or adjacent to the site of a prosthetic patch or prosthetic device (which inhibits endothelialization)
- Cardiac transplantation recipients who develop cardiac valvulopathy

†Prophylaxis is recommended because endothelialization of prosthetic material occurs within 6 mo after the procedure.

*Except for the conditions listed previously, antibiotic prophylaxis is no longer recommended for any form of CHD.

BOX 10-2 Dental Procedures for Which Endocarditis Prophylaxis Is Recommended for Patients

All dental procedures that involve manipulation of gingival tissue or the periapical region of teeth or perforation of the oral mucosa.*

*The following procedures and events do not need prophylaxis: routine anesthetic injections through noninfected tissue, taking of dental radiographs, placement of removable prosthodontic or orthodontic appliances, adjustment of orthodontic appliances, placement of orthodontic brackets, shedding of deciduous teeth, and bleeding from trauma to the lips or oral mucosa.

the victim of a CVA). A patient who has suffered a CVA is at greater risk of suffering another CVA or a seizure should he or she become hypoxic. The importance of effective pain control, through administration of local anesthetic solutions with vasopressors, cannot be overstated. Epinephrine concentrations should be minimized (e.g., 1:200,000) but this agent should be included as it increases anesthetic effectiveness. The dentist should be especially sensitive to the presence of transient cerebral ischemia (TCI), a precursor to CVA; TCI represents an ASA 3 risk. The post-CVA patient is an ASA 4 risk within 6 months of the CVA, becoming an ASA 3 risk 6 or more months after the incident (if the recovery is uneventful). In rare cases, the post-CVA patient can be an ASA 2 risk.

34. High Blood Pressure?

Comment: Elevated blood pressure (BP) measurements are frequently encountered in the dental environment secondary to the added stress that many patients associate with a visit to the dental office. With a history of HBP, the dentist must determine the drugs the patient is taking, the potential side effects of those medications, and any possible interactions with other drugs that might be used during dental treatment. Guidelines for clinical evaluation of risk (ASA categories) based on adult BP values are presented later in this chapter. The SRP is a significant factor in minimizing further elevation in BP during treatment.

35. Asthma, Tuberculosis (TB), Emphysema, Other Lung Disease?

Comment: Determining the nature and severity of respiratory problems is an essential part of patient evaluation. Many acute problems developing in the dental environment are stress related, increasing the workload of the cardiovascular system and the O_2 requirements of many tissues and organs in the body. The presence of severe respiratory disease can greatly influence the planned dental treatment and the choice of drugs and technique if sedation is required.

Asthma (bronchospasm) is marked by a partial obstruction of the lower airway. The dentist must determine the nature of the asthma (intrinsic [allergic] vs. extrinsic [nonallergic]), the frequency of acute episodes, causal factors, the method of management of acute episodes, and drugs the patient may be taking to minimize the occurrence of acute episodes. Stress is a common precipitating factor in acute asthmatic episodes. The well-controlled asthmatic patient represents an ASA 2 risk, whereas the well-controlled but stress-induced asthmatic patient is an ASA 3 risk. Patients whose acute episodes are frequent and/or difficult to terminate (requiring hospitalization [status asthmaticus]) are ASA 3 or 4 risk.

With a history of *tuberculosis,* the dentist must first determine whether the disease is active or arrested. (Arrested tuberculosis represents an ASA 2 risk.) Medical consultation and dental treatment modification are recommended when such information is not easily determined.

Emphysema is a form of chronic obstructive pulmonary disease (COPD), also called *chronic obstructive lung disease* (COLD). The emphysematous patient has a decreased respiratory reserve from which to draw if cells of the body require additional O_2, which they do during stress. Supplemental O_2 therapy during dental treatment is recommended in severe cases of emphysema; however, the severely emphysematous (ASA 3 and 4) patient should not receive more than 3 L of O_2 per minute.[18] This flow restriction helps to ensure that the dentist does not eliminate the hypoxic drive, which is the emphysematous patient's primary stimulus for breathing. The emphysematous patient is an ASA 2, 3, or 4 risk, depending on the degree of disability.

36. Hepatitis, Other Liver Disease?

Comment: Liver diseases may be transmissible (hepatitis A and B) or may indicate the presence of hepatic dysfunction. A history of blood transfusion or of past or present drug addiction should alert the dentist to a probable increase in the risk of hepatic dysfunction. (Hepatic dysfunction is a common finding in the parenteral drug abuse patient.) Hepatitis C is responsible for more than 90% of cases of posttransfusion hepatitis, but only 4% of cases are attributable to blood transfusion; up to 50% of cases are related to IV drug use. Incubation of hepatitis C averages 6 to 7 weeks. The clinical illness is mild, usually asymptomatic, and characterized by a high rate (>50%) of chronic hepatitis.[19] Because most drugs undergo biotransformation in the liver, care must be taken when specific drugs and techniques of administration are selected for the patient with significant hepatic dysfunction. In general, local anesthetics and vasopressors are indicated for use, with consideration of minimizing the dose in patients with severe hepatic dysfunction (e.g., ASA 4).

37. Stomach Problems, Ulcers?

Comment: The presence of stomach or intestinal ulcers may be indicative of acute or chronic anxiety and the possible use of medications such as tranquilizers, H_1-inhibitors, and antacids. Knowledge of which drugs are taken is important before additional drugs are administered in the dental office. A number of H_1-inhibitors are now over-the-counter (OTC) drugs. Because many patients do not consider OTC drugs "real" medications, the dentist must specifically question the patient about them. The presence of ulcers does not itself represent increased risk during treatment. In the absence of additional medical problems, the patient may represent an ASA 1 or 2 risk.

38. Allergies to: Drugs, Foods, Medications, Latex?

Comment: The dentist must evaluate a patient's allergies thoroughly before administering dental treatment or drugs. The importance of this question and its full evaluation cannot be overstated. A complete and vigorous dialogue history must be undertaken before any dental treatment is begun, especially when a presumed or documented history of drug allergy is present. Adverse drug reactions (ADRs) are not uncommon. Many, if not most, ADRs are labeled as "allergy" by the patient and also on occasion by his or her health care professional. However, despite the great frequency with which allergy is reported, true documented and reproducible allergic drug reactions are relatively rare. A recent review of food allergy revealed 30% self-reporting of "food allergy" by the studied population, when the reality is that true food allergy is seen in 8% of children and 5% of adults.[20]

All ADRs must be evaluated thoroughly, especially when the dentist plans to administer or prescribe closely related medications for the patient during dental treatment. Alleged "allergy to Novocaine" is frequently reported.

The incidence of true, documented, reproducible allergy to the amide local anesthetics is virtually nil.[21,22] However, reports of alleged allergy to local anesthetics is common.[23,24] Thorough investigation of the alleged allergy is essential if the patient is not to be assigned the label of "allergic to all -caine drugs," thereby precluding dental (and surgical) care in a normal manner. Avoidance of dental care or receipt of care under general anesthesia is the alternative in these cases.

Reports of allergy to "epinephrine" or "adrenaline" also must be carefully evaluated. Most often, such reports prove to be simply an exaggerated physiologic response by the patient to the injected epinephrine or, more commonly, to endogenous catecholamine release in response to the act of receiving the injection (the "adrenal squeeze," as a colleague called it recently).

Two essential questions that must be asked in all instances of alleged allergy are these: (1) Describe your reaction, and (2) How was it managed?

The presence of allergy alone represents an ASA 2 risk. No emergency situation is as frightening to health care professionals as the acute, systemic allergic reaction known as *anaphylaxis*. Prevention of this life-threatening situation is more gratifying than treatment of anaphylaxis once it develops.

Investigation into a patient's report of "allergy to local anesthesia" is so important that it is discussed in depth in Chapter 18.

39. Family History of Diabetes, Heart Problems, Tumors?

Comment: Knowledge of family history can assist in determining the presence of a number of disorders that have some hereditary component.

40. Acquired Immunodeficiency Syndrome (AIDS)?

Comment: Patients who have a positive test result for human immunodeficiency virus (HIV) are representative of every area of the population. The usual barrier techniques should be employed to minimize risk of cross-infection for both patient and staff members. Patients who are HIV positive are considered ASA 2, 3, 4, or 5 risk depending on the current status of their infection.

Proper care and handling of the local anesthetic syringe/needle must be observed, as in all situations, to avoid accidental needle-stick injury.

41. Tumors, Cancer?

Comment: The presence or prior existence of cancer of the head or neck may require specific modification of dental therapy. Irradiated tissues have decreased resistance to infection, diminished vascularity, and reduced healing capacity. No specific contraindication exists to administration of drugs for the management of pain or anxiety in these patients; however, techniques of local anesthetic drug administration may, on rare occasion, be contraindicated if the tissues in the area of deposition have been irradiated. Many persons with cancer may be receiving long-term therapy with CNS depressants, such as antianxiety drugs, hypnotics, and opioids. Consultation with the patient's oncologist is recommended before dental treatment is begun. A past or current history of cancer does not necessarily increase ASA risk status. However, patients who are cachectic or hospitalized or are in poor physical condition may represent ASA 4 or 5 risk.

42. Arthritis, Rheumatism?

Comment: See *Comment* for question No. 28.

43. Eye Disease?

Comment: For patients with *glaucoma*, the need to administer a drug that diminishes salivary gland secretions will have to be addressed. Anticholinergics, such as atropine, scopolamine, and glycopyrrolate, are contraindicated in patients with acute narrow angle glaucoma because these drugs produce an increase in intraocular pressure. Patients with glaucoma are usually ASA 2 risks. There is no contraindication to local anesthetic administration with or without vasopressors.

44. Skin Diseases?

Comment: Skin represents an elastic, rugged, self-regenerating, protective covering for the body. The skin also represents our primary physical presentation to the world and as such displays a myriad of clinical signs of disease processes, including allergy and cardiac, respiratory, hepatic, and endocrine disorders.[25]

45. Anemia?

Comment: Anemia is a relatively common adult ailment, especially among young adult women (iron deficiency anemia). The dentist must determine the type of anemia present. The ability of the blood to carry O_2 or to give up O_2 to other cells is decreased in anemic patients. This decrease can become significant during procedures in which hypoxia is likely to develop. There is no contraindication to local anesthetic administration with or without vasopressors.

Sickle cell anemia is seen exclusively in black patients. Periods of unusual stress or of O_2 deficiency (hypoxia) may precipitate sickle cell crisis. Administration of supplemental O_2 during treatment is strongly recommended for patients with sickle cell disease. Persons with sickle cell trait represent ASA 2 risk, whereas those with sickle cell disease are 2 or 3 risks.

In addition, congenital or idiopathic methemoglobinemia, although rare, represents a relative contraindication to administration of the amide local anesthetic prilocaine.[26]

46. VD (Syphilis or Gonorrhea)?

47. Herpes?

Comment: When treating patients with sexually transmitted diseases (STDs), dentists and staff members are at risk of infection. In the presence of oral lesions, elective dental care might be postponed. Standard barrier techniques, such as protective gloves, eyeglasses, and masks, provide operators with a degree of (but not total) protection. Such patients usually represent ASA 2 and 3 risks but may be 4 or 5 risks in extreme situations.

48. Kidney, Bladder Disease?

Comment: The dentist should evaluate the nature of the renal disorder. Treatment modifications including antibiotic prophylaxis may be appropriate for several chronic forms of renal disease. Functionally anephric patients are ASA 3 or 4 risks, whereas patients with most other forms of renal dysfunction may be ASA 2 or 3 risks. Box 10-3 shows a sample dental referral letter for a patient on long-term hemodialysis treatment as the result of chronic kidney disease.

BOX 10-3 Hemodialysis Letter

Dear Doctor:

The patient who bears this note is undergoing long-term chronic hemodialysis treatment because of chronic kidney disease. In providing dental care to this patient, please observe the following precautions:

1. Dental treatment is most safely done 1 day after the last dialysis treatment or at least 8 hours thereafter. Residual heparin may make hemostasis difficult. (Some patients are on long-term anticoagulant therapy.)
2. We are concerned about bacteremic seeding of the arteriovenous shunt devices and heart valves. We recommend prophylactic antibiotics before and after dental treatment. Antibiotic selection and dosage can be tricky in renal failure.

We recommend 3 g of amoxicillin 1 hour before the procedure and 1.5 g 6 hours later. For patients with penicillin allergies, 1 g of erythromycin 1 hour before the procedure and 500 mg 6 hours later is recommended.

Sincerely,

49. Thyroid, Adrenal Disease?

Comment: The clinical presence of thyroid or adrenal gland dysfunction—hyperfunction or hypofunction—should prompt the dentist to use caution in administering certain drug groups (e.g., epinephrine to hyperthyroid patients, CNS depressants to hypothyroid patients). In most instances, however, the patient has previously seen a physician and has undergone treatment for thyroid disorder by the time he or she seeks dental treatment. In this case, the patient is likely to be in a euthyroid state (normal blood levels of thyroid hormone) because of surgical intervention, irradiation, or drug therapy. The euthyroid state represents an ASA 2 risk, whereas clinical signs and symptoms of hyperthyroidism or hypothyroidism represent ASA 3 or, in rare instances, ASA 4 risk. Patients who are clinically hyperthyroid are more likely to hyper-respond to "usual" doses of epinephrine (e.g., develop tachycardia, have elevated blood pressure). Vital signs should be monitored preoperatively, perioperatively, and postoperatively in these situations.

Patients with hypofunctioning adrenal cortices have Addison disease and receive daily replacement doses of glucocorticosteroids. In stressful situations, their body may be unable to respond appropriately, leading to loss of consciousness. Hypersecretion of cortisone, Cushing syndrome, rarely results in an acute life-threatening situation. Consideration of sedation, in the presence of dental anxiety, is recommended.

50. Diabetes?

Comment: A patient who responds positively to this question requires further inquiry to determine the type, severity, and degree of control of his or her diabetic condition. A patient with type 1 (insulin-dependent diabetes mellitus, or IDDM) or type 2 (non–insulin-dependent diabetes mellitus, or NIDDM) diabetes mellitus is rarely at great risk from dental care or commonly administered dental drugs (e.g., local anesthetics, epinephrine, antibiotics, CNS depressants). The NIDDM patient is usually an ASA 2 risk; the well-controlled IDDM patient, an ASA 3 risk; and the poorly controlled IDDM patient, an ASA 3 or 4 risk.

The greatest concerns during dental treatment relate to the possible effects of the dental care on subsequent eating and development of hypoglycemia (low blood sugar). Patients leaving a dental office with residual soft tissue anesthesia, especially in the mandible (e.g., tongue, lips), usually defer eating until sensation returns, a period potentially of 5 (lidocaine, mepivacaine, articaine, prilocaine with vasoconstrictor) or more (up to 12) hours (bupivacaine with vasoconstrictor). Diabetic patients have to modify their insulin doses if they do not maintain normal eating habits. Administration of the local anesthetic reversal agent, phentolamine mesylate, at the conclusion of dental treatment can significantly minimize the duration of residual soft tissue anesthesia.[27,28]

IV. DO YOU HAVE OR HAVE YOU HAD:

51. Psychiatric Care?

Comment: The dentist should be aware of any nervousness (in general or specifically related to dentistry) or history of psychiatric care before treating the patient. Such patients may be receiving a number of drugs to manage their disorders that might interact with drugs the dentist uses to control pain and anxiety (Table 10-2). Medical consultation should be considered in such cases. Extremely fearful patients are ASA 2 risks, whereas patients receiving psychiatric care and drug therapy represent ASA 2 or 3 risk.

52. Radiation Treatments?

53. Chemotherapy?

Comment: Therapies for cancer. See *Comment* for question No. 41.

54. Prosthetic Heart Valve?

Comment: Patients with prosthetic (artificial) heart valves are no longer uncommon. The dentist's primary concern is to determine whether antibiotic prophylaxis is required. Antibiotic prophylactic protocols were presented earlier in this chapter.[15] The dentist should be advised to consult with the patient's physician (e.g., the cardiologist, the cardiothoracic surgeon) before providing treatment. Patients with prosthetic heart valves usually represent ASA 2 or 3 risk. Administration of local anesthetic drugs and vasopressors is indicated for these patients. Antibiotic prophylaxis is not indicated for the administration of routine dental injection techniques through noninfected tissues.[15]

TABLE 10-2
Dental Drug Interactions With Local Anesthetics and Vasopressors*

Dental Drug	Interacting Drug	Consideration	Action
Local anesthetics (LAs)	Cimetidine, β-adrenergic blocker (propranolol)	Hepatic metabolism of amide LA may be depressed	Use LAs cautiously, especially repeat dosages
	Antidysrhythmics (mexiletine, tocainide)	Additive CNS, CVS depression	Use LAs cautiously—keep dose as low as possible to achieve anesthesia
	CNS depressants: alcohol, antidepressants, antihistamines, benzodiazepines, antipsychotics, centrally acting antihypertensives, muscle relaxants, other LAs, opioids	Possible additive or supra-additive CNS, respiratory depression	Consider limiting maximum dose of LAs, especially with opioids
	Cholinesterase inhibitors: antimyasthenics, antiglaucoma drugs	Antimyasthenic drug dosage may require adjustment because LA inhibits neuromuscular transmission	Physician consultation
Vasoconstrictors; epinephrine	α-Adrenergic blockers (phenoxybenzamine, prazosin); antipsychotics (haloperidol, entacapone)	Possible hypotensive response following large dose of epinephrine	Use vasoconstrictor cautiously—as low a dose as possible
	Catecholamine-*O*-methyltransferase inhibitors (tolcapone, entacapone)	May enhance systemic actions of vasoconstrictors	Use vasoconstrictor cautiously—as low a dose as possible
	CNS stimulants (amphetamine, methylphenidate); ergot derivatives (dihydroergotamine, methysergide)	Effects of stimulant or vasoconstrictor may occur	Use vasoconstrictor cautiously—as low a dose as possible
	Cocaine	Effects of vasoconstrictors; can result in cardiac arrest	Avoid use of vasoconstrictor in patient under influence of cocaine
	Digitalis glycosides (digoxin, digitoxin)	Risk of cardiac dysrhythmias	Physician consultation
	Levodopa, thyroid hormones (levothyroxine, liothyronine)	Large doses of either (beyond replacement doses) may risk cardiac toxicity	Use vasoconstrictor cautiously—as low a dose as possible
	Tricyclic antidepressants (amitriptyline, doxepin, imipramine)	May enhance systemic effects of vasoconstrictor	Avoid use of levonordefrin or norepinephrine; use epinephrine cautiously as low a dose as possible
	Nonselective β-blockers (propranolol, nadolol)	May lead to hypertensive responses, especially to epinephrine	Monitor BP after initial LA injection

From Ciancio SG: ADA/PDR guide to dental therapeutics, ed 5, Chicago, 2010, American Dental Association.
BP, Blood pressure; *CNS,* central nervous system; *CVS,* cardiovascular system.
*Drug–drug interactions of greater clinical significance are emboldened for emphasis.

55. Artificial Joint?

Comment: More than 1,000,000 total joint arthroplasties are performed annually in the United States.[17] An expert panel of dentists, orthopedic surgeons, and infectious disease specialists convened by the American Dental Association (ADA) and the American Academy of Orthopaedic Surgeons performed a thorough review of available data to determine the need for antibiotic prophylaxis to prevent hematogenous prosthetic joint infection in dental patients who have undergone total joint arthroplasty. The panel concluded that antibiotic prophylaxis is not recommended for dental patients with pins, plates, and screws, or for those who have undergone total joint replacement. However, dentists should consider antibiotic premedication in a small number of patients who may be at increased risk for the development of hematogenous total joint infection (Table 10-3).[16]

56. Hospitalization?

57. Blood Transfusions?

58. Surgeries?

Comment: Determine the reason for hospitalization, the duration of the hospital stay, and any medications prescribed that the patient may currently be taking.

Determine the reason for the blood transfusion (e.g., prolonged bleeding, accident, type of surgery).

TABLE 10-3
Orthopedic Prophylaxis

Patient Type	Condition Placing Patient at Risk
All patients during first 2 years following joint replacement	NA
Immunocompromised/ immunosuppressed patients	Inflammatory arthropathies such as rheumatoid arthritis, systemic lupus erythematosus
Patients with comorbidities*	Previous prosthetic joint infection Malnourishment Hemophilia HIV infection Insulin-dependent (type 1) diabetes Malignancy

Data from American Dental Association, American Academy of Orthopedic Surgeons: Antibiotic prophylaxis for dental patients with total joint replacements, J Am Dent Assoc 134:895-898, 2003.
HIV, Human immunodeficiency virus; *NA,* not applicable.
*Patients potentially at increased risk of experiencing hematogenous total joint infection.

Determine the nature (elective, emergency) and type of surgery (cosmetic, GI, cardiac, etc.) and the patient's physical status at the present time.

59. Pacemaker?

Comment: Cardiac pacemakers are implanted beneath the skin of the upper chest or the abdomen with pacing wires extending into the myocardium. The most frequent indication for the use of a pacemaker is the presence of a clinically significant dysrhythmia. Fixed-rate pacemakers provide a regular, continuous heart rate regardless of the heart's inherent rhythm, whereas the more commonly used demand pacemaker is activated only when the rhythm of the heart falls into an abnormal range. Although there is little indication for antibiotic administration in these patients, medical consultation is suggested before the start of treatment to obtain the specific recommendations of the patient's physician. The patient with a pacemaker is commonly an ASA 2 or 3 risk during dental treatment.

In recent years, persons who represent a significant risk of sudden unexpected death (e.g., cardiac arrest) as a result of electrical instability of the myocardium (e.g., ventricular fibrillation) have had implantable cardioverter-defibrillators (ICDs) placed below the skin of their chest. Medical consultation is strongly recommended for these patients.

60. Contact Lenses?

Comment: Contact lenses are commonly worn by persons with visual disturbances. Dental considerations for patients with contact lenses include removal of the lenses during administration of any sedation technique. Sedated patients may not close their eyes as frequently as unsedated patients, thereby increasing the likelihood of irritating the sclera and cornea of the eye. This is particularly recommended when inhalation sedation (N_2O-O_2) is employed because any leakage of gases from the nasal hood is likely to irritate the eyes.

V. ARE YOU TAKING:

61. Recreational Drugs?

Comment: Although most patients will not admit to the use of recreational drugs, it is important to ask the question. This becomes particularly important when the dentist is considering the use of CNS-depressant drugs for sedation or local anesthetics with or without a vasoconstrictor, such as epinephrine.

62. Drugs, Medications, Over-the-Counter Medicines (Including Aspirin), Natural Remedies?

Comment: Because many patients make a distinction between the terms *drug* and *medication,* questionnaires should use both terms to determine what drugs (pharmaceutically active substances) a patient has taken. Unfortunately, in today's world, the term *drug* often connotes the illicit use of medications (e.g., opioids). In the minds of many patients, people "do" drugs but "take" medications for the management of medical conditions. Additionally, natural remedies contain active substances, some of which may interact with drugs commonly used in dentistry.[29,30]

The dentist must be aware of all medications and drugs that their patients take to control and treat medical disorders. Frequently, patients take medications without knowing the condition the medications are designed to treat; many patients do not even know the names of drugs that they are taking. It becomes important therefore for dentists to have available one or more means of identifying these medications and of determining their indications, side effects, and potential drug interactions. Many excellent sources are available, including online services, such as MD Consult,* Lexi-Comp,† and Epocrates.‡ The *Physicians' Desk Reference* (PDR),[31] both in hard copy and online, offers a picture section that aids in identification of commonly prescribed drugs. The PDR also offers the *Physicians' Desk Reference for Herbal Medicines.*[31] The *ADA Guide to Dental Therapeutics* is another valuable reference to those drugs commonly employed in dentistry and to the medications most often prescribed by physicians. Potential complications and drug interactions are stressed.[31a]

Knowledge of the drugs and medications patients are taking permits dentists to identify medical disorders, possible side effects—some of which may be of significance in dental treatment (e.g., postural hypotension)—and possible interactions between those medications and the drugs administered during dental treatment (see Table 10-2).

63. Tobacco in Any Form?

*MD Consult: www.mdconsult.com.
†Lexi-Comp: www.lexi.com.
‡Epocrates: www.epocrates.com.

64. Alcohol?

Comment: Chronic use of tobacco and/or alcohol over extended periods can lead to the development of potentially life-threatening problems including neoplasms, hepatic dysfunction, and, in women, complications during pregnancy.

VI. WOMEN ONLY:

65. Are You or Could You Be Pregnant or Nursing?

66. Taking Birth Control Pills?

Comment: Pregnancy represents a relative contraindication to extensive elective dental care, particularly during the first trimester. Consultation with the patient's obstetrician-gynecologist (OBGYN) is recommended before the start of any dental treatment. Administration of local anesthetics with or without epinephrine is acceptable during pregnancy. Food and Drug Administration (FDA) pregnancy categories are presented in Box 10-4, and known fetal effects of local anesthetics and vasopressors are presented in Table 10-4.

VII. ALL PATIENTS:

67. Do You Have or Have You Had Any Other Diseases or Medical Problems *Not* Listed on This Form?

Comment: The patient is encouraged to comment on specific matters not previously mentioned. Examples of several possibly significant disorders include acute intermittent porphyria, methemoglobinemia, atypical plasma cholinesterase, and malignant hyperthermia.

To the best of my knowledge, I have answered every question completely and accurately. I will inform my dentist of any change in my health and/or medication.

Comment: This final statement is important from a medicolegal perspective because although instances of purposeful lying on health histories are rare, they do occur. This statement should be accompanied by the date on which the history was completed and the signatures of both the patient (or the parent or guardian if the patient is a minor or is not legally competent) and the dentist who reviews the history. This in effect becomes a contract obliging the patient, parent, or guardian to report any changes in the patient's health or medications. Brady and Martinoff[7] demonstrated that a patient's analysis of personal health frequently is overly optimistic, and that pertinent health matters sometimes are not immediately reported.

The medical history questionnaire should be updated on a regular basis, approximately every 3 to 6 months or after any prolonged lapse in treatment. In most instances, the entire medical history questionnaire need not be redone. The dentist or dental hygienist need only ask the following questions:

1. Have you experienced any change in your general health since your last dental visit?
2. Are you now under the care of a physician? If so, what is the condition being treated?
3. Are you currently taking any drugs, medications, or over-the-counter products?

If any of these questions elicits a positive response, a detailed dialogue history should follow. For example, a patient may answer that no change has occurred in general health but may want to notify the dentist of a minor change in condition, such as the end of a pregnancy (It's a girl!) or a recent diagnosis of NIDDM or asthma.

In either situation, a written record of having updated the history should be appended to the patient's progress notes or on the health history form. When the patient's health status has changed significantly since the last history was completed, the entire history should be redone (e.g., if a patient was recently diagnosed with cardiovascular disease and is managing it with a variety of drugs that he or she was not previously taking).

In reality, most persons do not undergo significant changes in their health with any regularity. Thus one health history questionnaire can remain current for many years. Therefore the ability to demonstrate that a patient's medical history has been updated on a regular basis becomes all the more important.

The medical history questionnaire should be completed in ink. Corrections and deletions are made by drawing a single line through the original entry without obliterating it.

BOX 10-4 FDA Pregnancy Categories

- **A** Studies have failed to demonstrate a risk to the fetus in any trimester.
- **B** Animal reproduction studies fail to demonstrate a risk to the fetus; no human studies available
- **C** Only given after risks to the fetus are considered; animal reproduction studies have shown adverse effects on fetus; no human studies available
- **D** Definite human fetal risks; may be given in spite of risks if needed in life-threatening conditions
- **X** Absolute fetal abnormalities; not to be used at any time during pregnancy because risks outweigh benefits

From FDA pregnancy risk categories for local anesthetics: B—lidocaine, prilocaine; C—articaine, bupivacaine, mepivacaine. Available at: www.epocrates.com. Accessed October 28, 2010.

TABLE 10-4
Known Fetal Effects of Drugs

Drug	Effect
Anesthetics, local	No adverse effects in dentistry
Articaine	No adverse effects reported in dentistry
Bupivacaine	Does not cross placenta readily; no adverse effects in dentistry
Epinephrine	No adverse effects reported for dental use
Lidocaine	No adverse effects reported in dentistry
Mepivacaine	No adverse effects reported in dentistry
Prilocaine	No adverse effects reported in dentistry

The change is then added along with the date of the change. The dentist initials the change.

A written notation should be placed in the chart whenever a patient reveals significant information during the dialogue history. As an example, when a patient answers affirmatively to the question about a "heart attack", the dentist's notation may read "2008" (the year the MI occurred).

PHYSICAL EXAMINATION

The medical history questionnaire is quite important to the overall assessment of a patient's physical and psychological status. However, the questionnaire has limitations. For the questionnaire to be valuable, the patient must (1) be aware of the presence of any medical condition and (2) be willing to share this information with the dentist.

Most patients do not knowingly deceive their dentist by omitting important information from the medical history questionnaire, although cases in which such deception has occurred are on record. A patient seeking treatment for an acutely inflamed tooth decides to withhold from the dentist that he had an MI 2 months earlier because he knows that to tell the dentist would mean that he would likely not receive the desired treatment (e.g., extraction).

The other factor, a patient's knowledge of his or her physical condition, is a much more likely cause of misinformation on the questionnaire. Most "healthy" persons do not visit their physician regularly for routine checkups. Recent information has suggested that annual physical examination should be discontinued in the younger healthy patient because it has not proved as valuable an aid in preventive medicine, as was once thought.[32a] In addition, most patients simply do not visit their physician on a regular basis, doing so instead whenever they become ill. From this premise, it stands to reason that the true state of the patient's physical condition may be unknown to the patient. Feeling well, although usually a good indicator of health, is not a guarantor of good health.[7] Many disease entities may be present for a considerable length of time without exhibiting overt signs or symptoms that alert the patient of their presence (e.g., HBP, diabetes mellitus, cancer). When signs and symptoms are present, they are frequently mistaken for other, more benign problems. Although they may answer questions on the medical history questionnaire to the best of their knowledge, patients cannot give a positive response to a question unless they are aware that they have the condition. The first few questions on most histories refer to the length of time since the patient's last physical examination. The value of the remaining answers, dealing with specific disease processes, can be gauged from the patient's responses to these initial questions.

Because of these problems, which are inherent in the use of a patient-completed medical history questionnaire, the dentist must look for additional sources of information about the physical status of the patient. Physical examination of the patient provides much of this information. This consists of the following:

1. Monitoring of vital signs
2. Visual inspection of the patient
3. Function tests, as indicated
4. Auscultation of heart and lungs and laboratory tests, as indicated

Minimal physical evaluation for all potential patients should consist of (1) measurement of vital signs and (2) visual inspection of the patient.

The primary value of the physical examination is that it provides the dentist with important (up-to-the-minute) information concerning the physical condition of the patient immediately before the start of treatment, as contrasted with the questionnaire, which provides historical (dated) information. The patient should undergo a minimal physical evaluation at the initial visit to the office before the start of any dental treatment. Readings obtained at this time, called *baseline vital signs,* are recorded on the patient's chart.

Vital Signs

The six vital signs are as follows:
1. Blood pressure (BP)
2. Heart rate (pulse) and rhythm
3. Respiratory rate
4. Temperature
5. Height
6. Weight

Vital signs and guidelines for their interpretation follow.

Blood Pressure

Technique. The following technique is recommended for the accurate manual determination of BP.[33] A stethoscope and a sphygmomanometer (blood pressure cuff) are the required equipment. The most accurate and reliable of these devices is the mercury-gravity manometer. The aneroid manometer, probably the most frequently used, is calibrated to be read in millimeters of mercury (mm Hg) and is quite accurate if well maintained. Rough handling of the aneroid manometer may lead to erroneous readings. It is recommended that the aneroid manometer be recalibrated at least annually. Use of automatic BP monitors has become common because their accuracy has increased while their cost has decreased, ranging from well under $100 to several thousand dollars. Likewise, their accuracy varies. The use of automatic monitors simplifies the monitoring of vital signs, but dentists should be advised to check the accuracy of these devices periodically (comparing values with those of the more accurate mercury or aneroid manometer).

Although they are most accurate, the use of mercury manometers has become increasingly rare because they are too bulky for easy carrying and mercury spills are potentially dangerous.[34] Aneroid manometers are easy to use, are somewhat less accurate than mercury manometers, and are more delicate, requiring recalibration at least annually or when dropped or bumped.[34]

Automatic devices containing all equipment in one unit negate the need for a separate stethoscope and manometer.

TABLE 10-5
Guidelines for Blood Pressure (Adult)

Blood Pressure, mm Hg, or torr	ASA Classification	Dental Therapy Consideration
<140 and <90	1	1. Routine dental management 2. Recheck in 6 mo, unless specific treatment dictates more frequent monitoring.
140-159 and/or 90-94	2	1. Recheck BP before dental treatment for three consecutive appointments; if all exceed these guidelines, medical consultation is indicated. 2. Routine dental management 3. SRP as indicated
160-199 and/or 95-114	3	1. Recheck BP in 5 min. 2. If BP is still elevated, medical consultation before dental therapy is warranted. 3. Routine dental therapy 4. SRP
200+ and/or 115+	4	1. Recheck BP in 5 min. 2. Immediate medical consultation if still elevated 3. No dental therapy, routine or emergency,* until elevated BP is corrected 4. Refer to hospital if immediate dental therapy is indicated.

ASA, American Society of Anesthesiologists; *BP,* blood pressure; *SRP,* stress reduction protocol.
*When the BP of the patient is slightly above the cutoff for category 4 and anxiety is present, inhalation sedation may be employed in an effort to diminish the BP (via the elimination of stress).

Most are easy to use, whereas more expensive devices have automatic inflation and deflation systems and readable printouts of both BP and heart rate. As with the aneroid manometer, automatic BP systems are somewhat fragile, requiring recalibration on a regular schedule or when bumped or dropped. Body movements may influence accuracy, and even the most accurate devices do not work on certain people.[34]

Automatic BP monitors that fit on the patient's wrist are available and easy to use. However, BP measurements at the wrist may not be as accurate as those taken at the upper arm, and systematic error can occur as a result of differences in the position of the wrist relative to the heart (see later discussion).[35,36] The technique of blood pressure monitoring is discussed in extensive detail in other textbooks.[37]

For the adult patient with a baseline BP in the ASA 1 range (<140/<90 mm Hg), it is suggested that BP be recorded every 6 months unless specific dental procedures demand more frequent monitoring. The parenteral administration of any drug (*local anesthesia*; IM, IV, or inhalation sedation; or general anesthesia) mandates more frequent recording of vital signs.

Patients with BPs in the ASA 2, 3, or 4 category should be monitored more frequently (e.g., at every appointment), as outlined in Table 10-5. Patients with known HBP should have their BP monitored at each visit to determine whether BP is adequately controlled. It is impossible to gauge BP by "looking" at a person, or by asking, "How do you feel?" Routine monitoring of BP in all patients according to treatment guidelines will effectively minimize the occurrence of acute complications of HBP (e.g., hemorrhagic CVA).

The normal range of BP in younger patients is somewhat lower than that in adults. Table 10-6 presents a normal range of BP in infants and children.

TABLE 10-6
Normal Vital Signs According to Age

Age	Heart Rate (beats/min)	Blood Pressure (mm Hg)	Respiratory Rate (breaths/min)
3-6 mo	90-120	70-90/50-65	30-45
6-12 mo	80-120	80-100/55-65	25-40
1-3 yr	70-110	90-105/55-70	20-30
3-6 yr	65-110	95-110/60-75	20-25
6-12 yr	60-95	100-120/60-75	14-22
12+ yr	55-85	110-135/65-85	12-18

Modified from Hartman ME, Cheifitz IM: Pediatric emergencies and resuscitation. In Kliegman RM, Stanton BF, St. Geme JW III, Schor NF, et al, eds: Nelson textbook of pediatrics, ed 19, Philadelphia, 2011, Saunders.

Heart Rate and Rhythm

Technique. Heart rate (pulse) and rhythm may be measured at any readily accessible artery. Most commonly used for routine measurement are the brachial artery, which is located on the medial aspect of the antecubital fossa, and the radial artery, which is located on the radial and ventral aspects of the wrist.

Guidelines for Clinical Evaluation. Three factors should be evaluated while the pulse is monitored:
1. The heart rate (recorded as beats per minute)
2. The rhythm of the heart (regular or irregular)
3. The quality of the pulse (thready, weak, bounding, full)

The heart rate should be evaluated for a minimum of 30 seconds, ideally for 1 minute. The normal resting heart rate for an adult ranges from 60 to 110 beats per minute. It is often lower in a well-conditioned athlete (physiologic [sinus] bradycardia) and elevated in the fearful individual (sinus tachycardia). However, clinically significant disease may also produce slow (bradycardia [<60 per minute]) or rapid (tachycardia [>110 per minute]) heart rates. It is suggested that any heart rate below 60 or above 110 beats per minute (adult) should be evaluated (initially via dialogue history). Where no obvious cause is present (e.g., endurance sports, anxiety), medical consultation should be considered.

The healthy heart maintains a relatively regular rhythm. Irregularities in rhythm should be confirmed and evaluated via dialogue history and/or medical consultation before the start of treatment. The occasional *premature ventricular contraction (PVC)* is so common that it is not necessarily considered abnormal. Clinically, PVCs detected by palpation appear as a break in a generally regular rhythm in which a longer-than-normal pause (a "skipped beat") is noted, followed by resumption of regular rhythm. PVCs may be produced by smoking, fatigue, stress, various drugs (e.g., epinephrine, caffeine), and alcohol. Frequent PVCs are usually associated with a damaged or an ischemic myocardium.

Disturbances in the regularity of heart rhythm should be evaluated before the start of dental treatment, particularly when drugs (e.g., local anesthetics, sedatives) are to be administered. Table 10-6 presents the range of normal heart rates in children of various ages.

Administration of epinephrine-containing local anesthetics is relatively contraindicated in patients with ventricular dysrhythmias unresponsive to medical therapy. Dysrhythmias frequently are induced by an ischemic or irritable myocardium. Epinephrine and other catecholamines may provoke further irritability, leading to potentially more serious, possibly fatal dysrhythmias.

Respiratory Rate

Guidelines for Clinical Evaluation. Normal respiratory rate for an adult is 14 to 18 breaths per minute. Bradypnea (abnormally slow rate) may be produced by, among other causes, opioid administration, whereas tachypnea (abnormally rapid rate) is seen with fever, fear (hyperventilation), and alkalosis. The most common change in ventilation noted in the dental environment is hyperventilation, an abnormal increase in the rate and depth of respiration. It is also seen, but much less frequently, in diabetic acidosis. The most common cause of hyperventilation in dental and surgical settings is extreme psychological stress, which is not infrequent during local anesthetic administration (e.g., "the shot").

Any significant variation in respiratory rate should be evaluated before treatment. Table 10-6 presents the normal range of respiratory rates at different ages.

BP, heart rate and rhythm, and respiratory rate provide information about the functioning of the cardiorespiratory system. It is recommended that they be recorded as part of the routine physical evaluation for all potential dental patients. Recording of the remaining vital signs—temperature, height, and weight—although desirable, may be considered optional. However, when parenteral drugs are to be administered, including local anesthetics, especially in lighter-weight, younger, or older patients, actual recording of a patient's weight becomes considerably more important.

TABLE 10-7
Acceptable Weight (in Pounds) for Men and Women*

	AGE	
Height	**19-34 Years**	**35 Years and Older**
5 ft 0 in	97-128	108-138
5 ft 1 in	101-132	111-143
5 ft 2 in	104-137	115-148
5 ft 3 in	107-141	119-152
5 ft 4 in	111-146	122-157
5 ft 5 in	114-150	126-162
5 ft 6 in	118-156	130-167
5 ft 7 in	121-160	134-172
5 ft 8 in	125-164	138-178
5 ft 9 in	129-169	142-183
5 ft 10 in	132-174	146-188
5 ft 11 in	136-179	151-194
6 ft 0 in	140-184	155-199
6 ft 1 in	144-189	159-205
6 ft 2 in	148-195	164-210

Department of Health & Human Services (HHS) and Department of Agriculture (USDA): Dietary guidelines for Americans, Washington, DC, 2005, HHS/USDA.
*Weights based on weighing in without shoes or clothes.

Height and Weight

Technique. Patients should be asked to state their height and weight. The range of normal height and weight is quite variable and is available on charts developed by various insurance companies. New guidelines for range of normal height and weight have been published (Table 10-7).

In pediatric patients, especially those weighing less than 30 kg (66 lb), it is strongly suggested that the patient be weighed before receiving local anesthetic or CNS-depressant drugs (e.g., sedatives).

For the dentist who treats younger, lighter-weight (less than 30 kg [66 lb]) patients, it is strongly suggested that a scale be available in the office. If the child will not willingly step onto the scale for measurement, the doctor can, after weighing himself or herself, hold the patient, obtain their combined weight, then subtract his or her own weight to accurately calculate the patient's weight. Parents are not usually accurate informers about their child's weight.

Visual Inspection of the Patient

Visual observation of the patient provides the dentist with valuable information concerning the patient's medical status and level of apprehension toward the planned treatment. Observation of the patient's posture, body movements, speech, and skin can assist in the diagnosis of possibly significant disorders that may have gone undetected previously. The reader is referred to other textbooks for a more detailed discussion of visual inspection of the dental patient.[37-39]

Additional Evaluation Procedures

Following completion of these three steps (medical history questionnaire, vital signs, and physical examination), it occasionally will be necessary to follow up with additional evaluation for specific medical disorders. This examination may include auscultation of the heart and lungs, testing for blood glucose levels, retinal examination, function tests for cardiorespiratory status (e.g., breath-holding test, match test), electrocardiographic examination, and blood chemistries. Many of these tests are used in dental offices but do not represent a standard of care in dentistry.

Dialogue History

After patient information has been collected, the dentist reviews with the patient any positive responses on the questionnaire, seeking to determine the severity of these disorders and any potential risk that they might represent during the planned treatment. This process, the *dialogue history,* is an integral part of patient evaluation. The dentist must put to use all available knowledge of the disease to assess the degree of risk to the patient.

One example of dialogue history is presented below. For a more in-depth description of dialogue history for specific disease states, the reader is referred to *Medical Emergencies in the Dental Office,* 6th edition.[37]

The following is a dialogue history to be initiated with a positive reply to angina pectoris:

1. What precipitates your angina?
2. How frequently do you experience anginal episodes?
3. How long do your anginal episodes last?
4. Describe a typical anginal episode.
5. How does nitroglycerin affect the anginal episode?
6. How many tablets or sprays do you normally need to terminate the episode?
7. Are your anginal episodes stable (similar in nature), or has there been a recent change in their frequency, intensity, radiation pattern of pain, or response to nitroglycerin (seeking unstable or preinfarction angina)?

Dialogue history should be completed for every positive response noted on the medical history. A written note should be included on the questionnaire that summarizes the patient's response to the questions. For example, "heart attack" is circled. Written by the dentist next to this on the questionnaire is the statement "June 2008," implying that the patient stated that the heart attack occurred in June 2008.

Dialogue history related to the administration of local anesthetic in patients with alleged allergy is presented in Chapter 18.

Determination of Medical Risk

Having completed all components of the physical evaluation and a thorough dental examination, the dentist next takes all of this information and answers the following questions:

1. Is the patient capable, physically and psychologically, of tolerating in relative safety the stresses involved in the proposed treatment?
2. Does the patient represent a greater risk (of morbidity or mortality) than normal during this treatment?
3. If the patient does represent an increased risk, what modifications will be necessary in the planned treatment to minimize this risk?
4. Is the risk too great for the patient to be managed safely as an outpatient in the medical or dental office?

In an effort to answer these questions, the Herman Ostrow School of Dentistry of USC developed a physical evaluation system that attempts to assist the dentist in categorizing patients from the standpoint of risk factor orientation.[40] Its function is to assign the patient an appropriate risk category so that dental care can be provided to the patient in comfort and with increased safety. The system is based on the ASA physical status classification system, which is described next.

PHYSICAL STATUS CLASSIFICATION SYSTEM

In 1962 the American Society of Anesthesiologists (ASA) adopted what is now referred to as the ASA physical status (ASA PS) classification system.[41] This system represents a means of estimating medical risk presented by a patient undergoing a surgical procedure. The system has been in continual use since 1962, virtually without change, and has proved to be a valuable method of determining surgical and anesthetic risk before the actual procedure.[42,43] The classification system follows:

Class 1. A healthy patient (no physiologic, physical, or psychological abnormalities)

Class 2. A patient with mild systemic disease without limitation of daily activities

Class 3. A patient with severe systemic disease that limits activity but is not incapacitating

Class 4. A patient with incapacitating systemic disease that is a constant threat to life

Class 5. A moribund patient not expected to survive 24 hours with or without the operation

Class 6. A brain-dead patient whose organs are being removed for donor purposes

When this system was adapted for use in a typical outpatient dental or medical setting, ASA 5 and 6 were eliminated and an attempt made to correlate the remaining four classifications with possible treatment modifications for dental treatment. Figure 10-6 illustrates the USC physical evaluation form on which a summary of the patient's physical and psychological status is presented along with planned treatment modifications.

In the discussion of the ASA categories to follow, the term *normal* or *usual* activity is used along with the term *distress.* Definitions of these terms follow: *Normal* or *usual* activity is defined as the ability to climb one flight of stairs or to walk two level city blocks; *distress* is defined as undue fatigue, shortness of breath, or chest pain. Figure 10-7 illustrates the ASA classification system based on the ability to climb one flight of stairs.

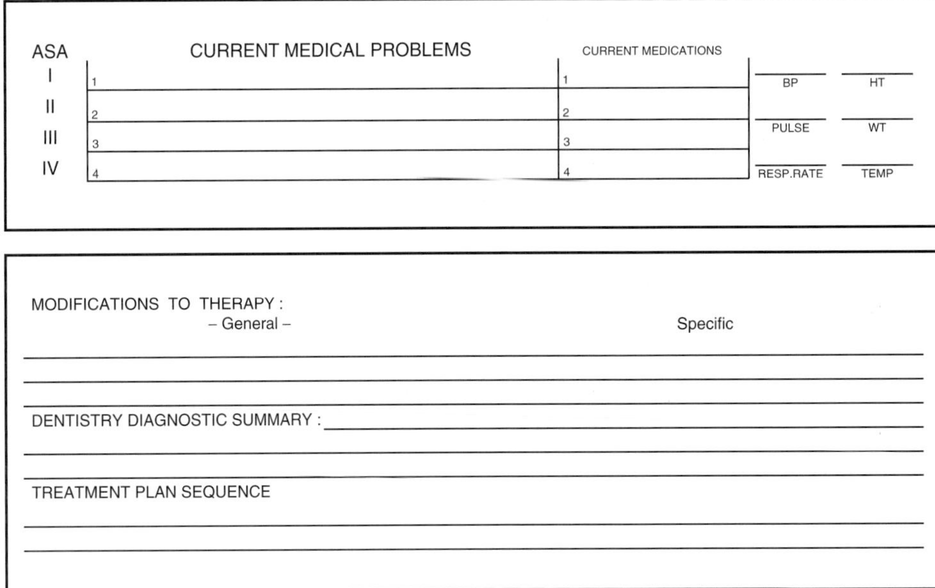

ASA | CURRENT MEDICAL PROBLEMS | CURRENT MEDICATIONS
I 1 | 1 | BP | HT
II 2 | 2 | PULSE | WT
III 3 | 3 | RESP.RATE | TEMP
IV 4 | 4

MODIFICATIONS TO THERAPY:
– General – Specific

DENTISTRY DIAGNOSTIC SUMMARY:

TREATMENT PLAN SEQUENCE

Figure 10-6. The Herman Ostrow School of Dentistry of University of Southern California (USC) physical evaluation (PE) summary form.

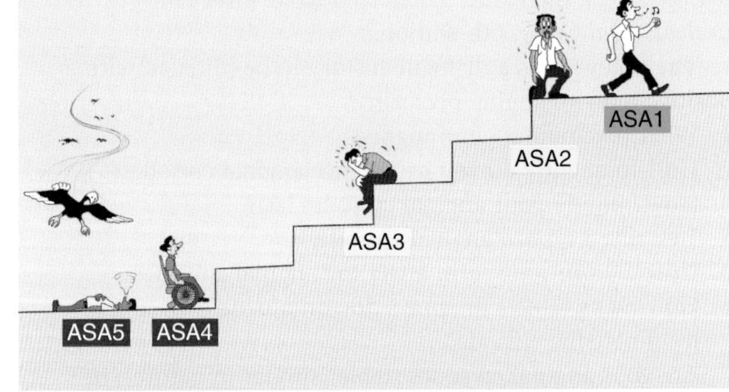

Figure 10-7. ASA classification. (Courtesy Dr. Lawrence Day.)

ASA 1

A patient in the ASA 1 category is defined as normal and healthy. After reviewing the available information, the dentist determines that the patient's heart, lungs, liver, kidneys, and central nervous system are healthy and that his or her blood pressure is below 140/90 millimeters of mercury. The patient is not unduly phobic and is younger than 60 years. A patient in the ASA 1 category is an excellent candidate for elective surgical or dental care, with minimal risk of experiencing an adverse medical event during treatment.

ASA 2

Patients in the ASA 2 category have a mild systemic disease or are healthy patients (ASA 1) who demonstrate extreme anxiety and fear toward dentistry or are older than 60 years. Patients classified as ASA 2 generally are somewhat less able to tolerate stress than are patients classified as ASA 1; however, they still are at minimal risk during dental treatment. An ASA 2 classification represents a yellow light for the dentist (proceed with caution). Elective dental care is warranted, with minimal increased risk to the patient during treatment. However, the dentist should consider possible treatment modifications.

ASA 3

A patient in the ASA 3 category has severe systemic disease that limits activity but is not incapacitating. At rest, a patient in the ASA 3 category does not exhibit signs and symptoms of distress (such as undue fatigue, shortness of breath, and chest pain); however, when stressed, physiologically or psychologically, the patient does exhibit such signs and symptoms. An example is a patient with angina who is pain free while in the waiting room but develops chest pain when seated in the dental chair. Similar to ASA 2, the ASA 3 classification indicates that the dentist should proceed with caution. Elective dental care is not contraindicated, although the patient is at increased risk during treatment. The dentist should give serious consideration to implementing treatment modifications.

ASA 4

A patient in the ASA 4 category has an incapacitating systemic disease that is a constant threat to life. Patients with this classification have a medical problem or problems of greater significance than the planned dental treatment. The dentist postpones elective dental care until the patient's physical condition has improved to at least an ASA 3 classification. A patient in the ASA 4 category exhibits clinical signs and symptoms of disease at rest. This classification represents a red light, a warning that the risk involved in treating the patient is too great to permit elective care. In dental emergencies, such as cases of infection or pain, clinicians should treat patients conservatively in the dental office until their medical condition improves. When possible, emergency treatment should be noninvasive, consisting of drugs such as analgesics for pain and antibiotics for infection. When the dentist believes that immediate intervention is required (e.g., incision and drainage, extraction, pulpal extirpation), it is suggested that the patient receive care in an acute care facility (i.e., a hospital) whenever possible.

ASA 5

An ASA 5 classification indicates a moribund patient not expected to survive 24 hours without surgery. Patients in this category almost always are hospitalized and terminally ill. In many institutions, these patients are not to be resuscitated if they experience respiratory or cardiac arrest (they are termed "DNR" ["Do Not Resuscitate"]. Elective dental treatment is contraindicated; however, emergency care in the realm of palliative treatment (i.e., relief of pain and/or infection) may be necessary. An ASA 5 classification is a red light with regard to dental care.

The ASA PS classification system is not meant to be inflexible; rather, it is meant to function as a relative value system based on a dentist's clinical judgment and assessment of available relevant clinical data.[40] When the dentist is unable to determine the clinical significance of one or more diseases, consultation with the patient's physician or other medical or dental colleagues is recommended. In all cases, however, the treating dentist makes the final decision regarding whether to treat or postpone treatment. The ultimate responsibility for the health and safety of a patient lies solely with the dentist, who decides to treat or not treat the patient.

Table 10-8 summarizes the ASA physical status classification system as modified for use in dentistry.

DRUG–DRUG INTERACTIONS AND CONTRAINDICATIONS

Potential drug–drug interactions involving local anesthetics or vasopressors, and three relative contraindications to the administration of local anesthetics—malignant hyperthermia (malignant hyperpyrexia), atypical plasma cholinesterase, and idiopathic or congenital methemoglobinemia—are detailed in the following discussion. A fourth—allergy (an absolute contraindication)—is discussed in Chapter 18.

The importance of each potential interaction is listed in its significance rating as designed by Moore and associates.[44] The rating system is defined in Box 10-5.

Drug–Drug Interactions

Amide Local Anesthetics With Inhibitors of Metabolism (e.g., Cimetidine, Lidocaine) (Significance Rating = 5). The H_2-receptor blocker cimetidine (Tagamet) modifies the

TABLE 10-8
American Society of Anesthesiologists Physical Status (ASA PS) Classification System

ASA PS	Definition	Example	Treatment Recommendations
1	Healthy patient	—	No special precautions
2	Patient with mild systemic disease	Pregnancy, well-controlled type 2 diabetes, epilepsy, asthma, thyroid dysfunction, BP 140-159/90-94 mm Hg	Elective care okay; consider treatment modification
3	Patient with severe systemic disease that limits activity but is not incapacitating	Stable angina pectoris, post myocardial infarction >6 months, post CVA >6 months, exercise-induced asthma, type 1 diabetes (controlled), epilepsy (less well controlled), symptomatic thyroid dysfunction, BP 160-199/95-114 mm Hg	Elective care okay; serious consideration of treatment modification
4	Patient with an incapacitating systemic disease that is a constant threat to life	Unstable angina pectoris, post myocardial infarction <6 months, uncontrolled seizures, BP >200/>115 mm Hg	Elective care contraindicated; emergency care: noninvasive (e.g., drugs) or in a controlled environment
5	Moribund patient not expected to survive 24 hours without operation	End-stage cancer, end-stage infectious disease, end-stage cardiovascular disease, end-stage hepatic dysfunction	Palliative care

Modified from Malamed SF: Knowing your patient, J Am Dent Assoc 141:3S–7S, 2010.
BP, Blood pressure; *CVA,* cerebrovascular accident; *mm Hg,* millimeters of mercury.

BOX 10-5 Significance Ratings for Dental Drug Interactions

Rating	Definition
1	Major reactions that are established, probable, or suspected
2	Moderate reactions that are established, probable, or suspected
3	Minor reactions that are established, probable, or suspected
4	Major or minor reactions that are possible
5	Minor reactions that are possible; all reactions that are unlikely

Severity Rating

Major: Potentially life threatening or capable of causing permanent damage

Moderate: Could cause deterioration of patient's clinical status; additional treatment or hospitalization might be necessary

Minor: Mild effects that are bothersome or unnoticed; should not significantly affect therapeutic outcome

Documentation Rating

Established: Proved to occur in well-controlled studies

Probable: Very likely, but not proved clinically

Suspected: Could occur; some good data exist, but more study is needed

Possible: Could occur; data are very limited

Unlikely: Doubtful; there is no consistent and reliable evidence of an altered clinical effect

biotransformation of lidocaine by competing with it for binding to hepatic oxidative enzymes. Other H_2-receptor blockers, such as ranitidine and famotidine, do not inhibit lidocaine biotransformation.[45,46] The net result of this interaction with cimetidine is an increase in the half-life of the circulating local anesthetic. With typical dental practice usage of local anesthetics, this interaction is of little clinical significance. The interaction between amide local anesthetics and cimetidine might be of greater clinical significance in the presence of a history of HF (ASA 3 or greater), where the percentage of cardiac output delivered to the liver falls while the percentage of cardiac output delivered to the brain increases.[47] With greater blood levels of lidocaine secondary to cimetidine, and an increased percentage in blood being delivered to the brain, the risk of local anesthetic overdose is increased. Inhibition of local anesthetic metabolism has little effect on peak plasma levels of the local anesthetic when given as a single injection.[48] This combination of factors—cimetidine and ASA 3 + HF—represents a relative contraindication to the use of amide local anesthetics. Minimal doses of amide local anesthetics should be administered.

Summation Interactions With Local Anesthetics (Significance Rating = 1). Combinations of local anesthetics may be administered together without unnecessary increase in risk of development of a toxic reaction (overdose). Toxicity of local anesthetics is additive when they are administered in combination. To minimize this risk, the total dose of all local anesthetics administered should not exceed the lowest of the maximum recommended therapeutic doses (MRTD) of each of the administered local anesthetics.

Sulfonamides and Esters (Significance Rating = 5). Ester local anesthetics, such as procaine and tetracaine, may inhibit the bacteriostatic action of the sulfonamides. With the uncommon use of sulfonamides today, along with the extremely rare administration of ester local anesthetics in dentistry, this potential drug interaction is unlikely to be noted. As a rule, ester local anesthetics should not be administered to patients receiving sulfonamides.

Local Anesthetics With Opioid Sedation (Significance Rating = 1). Sedation with opioid analgesics may increase the risk of local anesthetic overdose. This is of primary concern in younger, lighter-weight children. Therefore the dosage of local anesthetic should, as always, be minimized.

Local Anesthetic–Induced Methemoglobinemia (Significance Rating = 4). Methemoglobin may result when prilocaine is administered in excessive dosages.[49] Local anesthetic–induced methemoglobinemia is discussed later in this chapter.

Vasoconstrictor and Tricyclic Antidepressant (e.g., Levonordefrin and Amitriptyline) (Significance Rating = 1). Tricyclic antidepressants (TCAs) are commonly prescribed in the management of major depression. TCAs may enhance the cardiovascular actions of exogenously administered vasopressors. This enhancement of activity is approximately fivefold to tenfold with levonordefrin and norepinephrine, but is only twofold with epinephrine and phenylephrine.[50] This interaction has been reported to have resulted in a series of hypertensive crises, one of which led to the death of a patient (after a small dose of norepinephrine [norepinephrine is not available in dental local anesthetics in North America]).[51] Administration of norepinephrine and levonordefrin should be avoided in patients receiving TCAs. Patients receiving epinephrine-containing local anesthetics should be administered the smallest effective dose. Yagiela and associates recommend limiting the epinephrine dose to patients receiving TCAs in a dental appointment to 0.05 mg or 5.4 mL of a 1 : 100,000 epinephrine concentration.[52] Commonly prescribed TCAs are listed in Box 10-6.

Vasoconstrictors and Nonselective β-Adrenoceptor Antagonist (β-Blocker) (e.g., Propranolol and Epinephrine) (Significance Rating = 1). Administration of vasopressors in patients being treated with nonselective β-blockers increases the likelihood of a serious elevation in blood

BOX 10-6 Antidepressant Medications

Tricyclic Antidepressants	Monoamine Oxidase Inhibitors
Amitriptyline (Elavil)	Isocarboxazid (Marplan)
Nortriptyline (Aventyl, Pamelor)	Phenelzine (Nardil)
Imipramine (Tofranil)	Tranylcypromine (Parnate)
Doxepin (Sinequan)	Trimipramine (Surmontil)
Amoxapine (Asendin)	
Desipramine (Norpramin)	
Protriptyline (Vivactil)	
Clomipramine (Anafranil)	

BOX 10-7 β-Adrenoceptor Antagonists (β-Blockers)

Nonselective (β_1- and Cardioselective β_2-Adrenoreceptors)
Penbutolol (Levatol)
Carteolol (Cartrol)
Pindolol (Visken)
Timolol (Blocadren)
Sotalol (Betapace)
Nadolol (Corgard)
Propranolol (Inderal, Betachron)

β_1-Adrenoreceptors
Atenolol (Tenormin)
Betaxolol (Kerlone)
Metoprolol (Lopressor)
Acebutolol (Sectral)
Esmolol (Brevibloc)
Bisoprolol (Zebeta)

pressure accompanied by a reflex bradycardia. Several cases have been reported in the medical literature and appear to be dose related.[53,54] Reactions have occurred with epinephrine doses ranging from 0.04 to 0.32 mg, the equivalent of the administration of 4 to 32 mL of local anesthetic with a 1:100,000 epinephrine concentration.[55] Box 10-7 lists both nonselective and cardioselective β-blockers.

Monitoring of preoperative vital signs—specifically, blood pressure, heart rate, and rhythm—is strongly recommended for all patients, but is especially recommended in patients receiving β-blockers. Re-recording these vital signs at 5 to 10 minutes after administration of a vasopressor-containing local anesthetic is strongly suggested.

Vasoconstrictor With Hydrocarbon Inhalation Anesthetic (e.g., Halothane or Enflurane and Epinephrine) (Significance Rating = 1). There is an increased possibility of cardiac dysrhythmias when patients receiving certain halogenated general anesthetic gases are administered epinephrine.[56,57] Discussion with the anesthesiologist before local anesthetic administration during general anesthesia is suggested.

Vasoconstrictor With Cocaine (Significance Rating = 1). Cocaine is a local anesthetic drug that possesses significant stimulatory properties on the CNS and CVS. Cocaine stimulates norepinephrine release and inhibits its reuptake in adrenergic nerve terminals, thus producing a state of catecholamine hypersensitivity.[58,59] Tachycardia and hypertension frequently are observed with cocaine administration, both of which increase cardiac output and myocardial oxygen requirements.[60] When this results in myocardial ischemia, potentially lethal dysrhythmias, anginal pain, myocardial infarction, or cardiac arrest may ensue.[61-63] The risk of such problems is elevated in dentistry when a local anesthetic containing a vasopressor is accidentally administered intravascularly in a patient with already high cocaine blood levels. After intranasal application of cocaine, peak blood levels develop within 30 minutes and usually disappear after 4 to 6 hours.[64] Whenever possible, local anesthetics containing vasopressors should not be administered to patients who have used cocaine on the day of their dental appointment.[65] Unfortunately, it is the rare abuser of cocaine who will volunteer this vital information to the dentist. The use of epinephrine-impregnated gingival retraction cord, although not recommended for use in any dental patient, is absolutely contraindicated in the cocaine abuser.

Administration of local anesthetics to cocaine abusers also can increase the risk of local anesthetic overdose. If there is any suspicion about a patient having used cocaine recently, the patient should be questioned directly. If cocaine has been used within 24 hours of the dental appointment, or if it is suspected that cocaine has been used within 24 hours, the planned dental treatment should be postponed.[66,67]

Vasoconstrictor With Antipsychotic or Another α-Adrenoceptor Blocker (Significance Rating = 4). α-Adrenoceptor blockers such as phenoxybenzamine and prazosin (Minipress), and antipsychotic drugs such as haloperidol (Haldol) and thioridazine (Mellaril), may produce significant hypotension as a result of overdose. This hypotensive effect may be intensified with large doses of vasoconstrictors. Vasoconstrictors should be used with caution.[68]

Vasoconstrictor With Adrenergic Neuronal Blocker (Significance Rating = 4). Sympathomimetic effects may be enhanced. The vasoconstrictor should be used cautiously.[69] Phenothiazines are psychotropic drugs usually prescribed for the management of serious psychotic disorders. The most commonly observed side effect of phenothiazines involving the cardiovascular system is postural hypotension. Phenothiazines suppress the vasoconstricting actions of epinephrine, permitting its milder vasodilating actions to work unopposed. This response is not likely to develop when local anesthetics are administered extravascularly; however, accidental intravascular administration of a vasopressor-containing local anesthetic could lead to hypotension in patients receiving phenothiazines.[67]

Local anesthetics containing vasopressors are not contraindicated in patients receiving phenothiazines; however, it is recommended that the smallest volume of vasopressor-containing local anesthetic that is compatible with clinically adequate pain control be administered.

Commonly prescribed phenothiazines include chlorpromazine (Thorazine) and promethazine (Phenergan).

Vasoconstrictor With Thyroid Hormone (e.g., Epinephrine and Thyroxine) (Significance Rating = 4). Summation of effects is possible when thyroid hormones are taken in excess. Vasoconstrictors should be used with caution when clinical signs and symptoms indicating hyperthyroidism are present.[70,71]

Vasoconstrictor and Monoamine Oxidase Inhibitors (Significance Rating = 5). Monoamine oxidase inhibitors (MAOIs) are prescribed in the management of major depression, certain phobic-anxiety states, and obsessive-compulsive disorders (Box 10-8).[67] They are capable of potentiating the actions of vasopressors used in dental local anesthetics by inhibiting their biodegradation by the enzyme monoamine oxidase (MAO) at the presynaptic neuron level.[58]

Historically, the administration of local anesthetics containing vasopressors has been absolutely contraindicated for patients receiving MAOIs because of the increased risk of hypertensive crisis. However, Yagiela and others demonstrated that such an interaction among epinephrine, levonordefrin, norepinephrine, and MAO did not occur.[52,67] Such a response, hypertensive crisis, did develop with phenylephrine, a vasopressor not used at present in dental local anesthetic solutions.

Therefore, it seems appropriate to state, "there seems to be no restriction, from a theoretical basis, to use local anesthetic with vasoconstrictor other than phenylephrine in patients currently treated with MAOIs."[67]

BOX 10-8 Monoamine Oxidase Inhibitors

Generic	Proprietary
Clorygyline	—
Isocarboxazid	Marplan
Moclobemide	Aurorix
Pargyline	Eutonyl
Phenelzine	Nardil
Selegiline	Deprenyl, Eldepryl
Tranylcypromine	Parnate
Brofaromine	Consonar
Iproniazid	Marsilid
Isoniazid	—
MDMA	—
Fluoxetine	Prozac

For a thorough review of potentially significant drug interactions occurring in dentistry, the reader is referred to the excellent series of papers that appeared in 1999 in the *Journal of the American Dental Association.*[44,48,72-74]

• • •

Most known drug–drug interactions involving local anesthetics or vasopressors occur with CNS and CVS depressants. Whenever a potential drug–drug interaction is known, doses of local anesthetics should be decreased. There is no formula for the correct degree of reduction. Prudence dictates, however, that the smallest dose of local anesthetic or vasopressor that is clinically effective should be used.

Knowledge of all drugs and medications, including prescription and nonprescription drugs, as well as herbal remedies, being taken by a patient better enables the doctor to evaluate the patient's overall physical and psychological well-being. Drug references such as *Mosby's Drug Consult, Compendium of Pharmaceuticals and Specialties* (CPS) (Canada), Lexi-Comp,* and Epocrates.com† are valuable resources in determining drug information, including the potential for drug–drug interactions. Current medications should be listed in the dental record.

MALIGNANT HYPERTHERMIA

Malignant hyperthermia (MH; malignant hyperpyrexia) is one of the most intense and life-threatening complications associated with the administration of general anesthesia. It is rare: 1:15,000 incidence among children receiving general anesthesia and 1:50,000 incidence in adults.[75] The syndrome is transmitted genetically by an autosomally dominant gene. Reduced penetrance and variable expressivity in siblings of families inheriting the syndrome are also characteristic of its genetic transmission. MH is seen more frequently in males than females—a finding that increases with increasing age. To date, the youngest reported case of MH occurred in a boy aged 2 months and the oldest in a 78-year-old man.

Reports of MH in North America appear to be clustered in three regions: Toronto (in Canada) and Wisconsin and Nebraska (in the United States). Most persons with MH are functionally normal, the presence of MH becoming known only when the individual is exposed to triggering agents or through specific testing.

For many years, it was thought that MH could be triggered when susceptible patients were exposed to amide local anesthetics.[76] Indeed, in both the first and second editions of this textbook, MH was considered an absolute contraindication to amide local anesthetics. However, recent findings[77-79] and publications by the Malignant Hyperthermia Association of the United States (MHAUS)[80] have demonstrated that amide local anesthetics are not likely to trigger such episodes; thus MH has been re-categorized as a relative contraindication in the third and subsequent editions.

*Lexi-Comp (www.lexi.com).
†Epocrates.com.

Causes

All reported cases of MH (associated with drug administration) have developed during the administration of general anesthesia.[81] No association with the type of surgical procedure being performed has been noted. Several cases of MH have been reported among patients receiving general anesthesia for dental care, including one case in a dental office.[82,83]

Anesthetic agents that have been associated with cases of MH are as follows (several of these drugs, such as lidocaine and mepivacaine, have been associated with MH only anecdotally): succinylcholine, halothane, enflurane, isoflurane, desflurane, and sevoflurane.

Two drugs have been associated with a preponderance of MH cases: succinylcholine, a skeletal muscle relaxant (77% of all cases), and the inhalation anesthetic halothane (60%).[84] Of significance to dentistry is the fact that the two most commonly used (amide) local anesthetics, lidocaine and mepivacaine, had been administered along with other potential trigger agents in cases in which MH developed. At one time, a history of documented MH or a high risk of MH was considered to be an absolute contraindication to the administration of all amide local anesthetics. However, recent evidence demonstrates that MH is not a likely occurrence with amide local anesthetics as used in dentistry, and therefore should be considered a relative contraindication. The Malignant Hyperthermia Association of the United States (MHAUS; www.mhaus.org) has a policy statement on the use of local anesthetics[85]: "Based on limited clinical and laboratory evidence, all local anesthetic drugs appear to be safe for MH susceptible individuals." This statement followed several reports in the literature, including one by Adragna,[86] which stated, "After an extensive search of the literature, I have been unable to find any reports of any malignant hyperthermic crisis caused solely by the use of amide local anesthetics without epinephrine...In fact, lidocaine has been used successfully to treat the arrhythmias of a severe MH reaction and, in fact, lidocaine has been used routinely as a local anesthetic without problems on [MH syndrome] MHS patients in at least one institution...The question I am posing is clear. Is there any evidence that amide local anesthetics are contraindicated in MHS patients, or is our habit of avoiding them just a habit?" Because the MH syndrome has yet to be reported in a situation in which local anesthetic was the sole drug administered, it is reasonable for the dentist to manage the dental needs of such patients using amide or ester local anesthetics. Prior consultation with the patient's physician is strongly suggested.

Adriani and Sundin reported that in susceptible patients, MH may be precipitated by factors other than the drugs just listed.[87] These include emotional factors (excitement and stress) and physical factors (mild infection, muscle injury, vigorous exercise, and elevated environmental temperatures). It appears then that the dental office could be a site where the susceptible patient, exposed to excessive stresses such as pain and fear, might exhibit symptoms of MH.

Recognition of the High-Risk Malignant Hyperthermia Patient

No questions on medical history questionnaires currently used in dentistry specifically address MH. The only ones on the health history questionnaire that might elicit this information are as follows: ***Question No. 56:*** Do you have, or have you had hospitalization? ***Question No. 58:*** Do you have, or have you had surgeries? And ***question No. 67:*** Do you have, or have you had any other diseases or medical problems NOT listed on this form? The patient with MH or a family member at risk usually will volunteer this information to his or her doctor at an early visit.

Family members are usually evaluated for their risk after the occurrence of MH. Initial evaluation involves determination of the blood levels of creatinine phosphokinase (CPK).[88] Elevated CPK levels are seen when muscle damage has occurred. With an elevated CPK, a second phase of evaluation is required, involving the histologic examination of a biopsy specimen taken from the quadriceps muscle (with the patient under a type of anesthesia known to be safe) and testing of the specimen for an increased contracture response when exposed to halothane and caffeine.

Dental Management of the Malignant Hyperthermia Patient

On disclosure of the presence of MH, or when the risk of its occurrence is high, it is recommended that the dentist contact the patient's primary care physician to discuss treatment options.

Dental management on an outpatient basis with local anesthetics as the only drugs administered is indicated in most cases, but with higher-risk patients, it might be prudent to conduct such treatment within the confines of a hospital, where immediate emergency care is available should the MH syndrome be triggered. "Normal" doses of amide local anesthetics may be used with little increase in risk.[85] Vasoconstrictors may be included to provide longer periods of pain control or hemostasis.

Box 10-9 lists the MHAUS list of safe anesthetic agents for MH patients.

ATYPICAL PLASMA CHOLINESTERASE

Choline–ester substrates, such as the depolarizing muscle relaxant succinylcholine and the ester local anesthetics, are hydrolyzed in the blood by the enzyme plasma cholinesterase, which is produced in the liver. Hydrolysis of these chemicals is usually quite rapid, their blood levels decreasing rapidly, thereby terminating the drug's action (succinylcholine) or minimizing the risk of overdose (ester local anesthetics).

Approximately 1 out of every 2820 persons possesses an atypical form of plasma cholinesterase, transmitted as an inherited autosomal recessive trait.[89] Although many genetic variations of atypical plasma cholinesterase are identifiable, not all produce clinically significant signs and symptoms.

BOX 10-9 Safe Anesthetics for MH-Susceptible Patients

Barbiturates/Intravenous Anesthetics
Diazepam
Etomidate (Amidate)
Hexobarbital
Katamine (Ketalar)
Methohexital (Bervital)
Midazolam
Narcobarbital
Propofol (Diprivan)
Thiopental (Pentothal)

Inhaled Non-Volatile General Anesthetic
Nitrous Oxide

Local Anesthetics
Amethocaine
Articaine
Bupivicaine
Dibucaine
Etidocaine
Eucaine
Lidocaine (Xylocaine)
Levobupivacaine
Mepivicaine (Carbocaine)
Procaine (Novocain)
Prilocaine (Citanest)
Ropivacaine
Stovaine

Narcotics (Opioids)
Alfentanil (Alfenta)
Anileridine
Codeine (Methyl Morphine)
Diamorphine
Fentanyl (Sublimaze)
Hydromorphone (Dilaudid)
Meperidine (Demerol)
Methadone
Morphine
Naloxone
Oxycodone
Phenoperidine
Remifentanil
Sufentanil (Sufenta)

Safe Muscle Relaxants
Arduan (Pipecuronium)
Curare (The active ingredient is Tubocurraine.)
Gallamine
Metocurine
Mivacron (Mivacurium)
Neuromax (Doxacurium)
Nimbex (Cisatracurium)
Norcuron (Vecuronium)
Pavulon (Pancuronium)
Tracrium (Atracurium)
Zemuron (Rocuronium)

Anxiety Relieving Medications
Ativan (Lorazepam)
Centrax
Dalmane (Flurazepam)
Halcion (Triazolam)
Klonopin
Librax
Librium (Chlordiazepoxide)
Midazolam (Versed)
Paxipam (Halazepam)
Restoril (Temazepam)
Serax (Oxazepam)
Tranxene (Clorazepate)
Valium (Diazepam)

Data from Malignant Hyperthermia Association of the United States: Anesthetic list for MH-susceptible patients. Available at: www.medical.mhaus.org. Accessed June 2008.
MH, Malignant hyperthermia.

Determination

In most cases, the presence of atypical plasma cholinesterase is determined through the patient's response to succinylcholine, a depolarizing skeletal muscle relaxant. Succinylcholine is commonly administered during the induction of general anesthesia to facilitate intubation of the trachea. Apnea is produced for a brief time with spontaneous ventilation returning as the succinylcholine is hydrolyzed by plasma cholinesterase. When atypical plasma cholinesterase is present, the apneic period is prolonged from minutes to many hours. Patient management simply involves the maintenance of controlled ventilation until effective spontaneous respiratory efforts return. After recovery, the patient and family members are tested for a serum cholinesterase survey. The dibucaine number is determined from a sample of blood. Normal patients have dibucaine numbers between 66 and 86. Atypical plasma cholinesterase patients exhibiting prolonged response to succinylcholine have dibucaine numbers as low as 20, with other genetic variants exhibiting intermediate values. Patients with low dibucaine numbers are more likely to exhibit prolonged succinylcholine-induced apnea.[90]

Significance in Dentistry

The presence of atypical plasma cholinesterase should alert the doctor to the increased risk of prolonged apnea in patients receiving succinylcholine during general anesthesia. Also, and of greater significance in the typical ambulatory dental patient not receiving general anesthesia or succinylcholine, is the increased risk of developing elevated blood levels of the ester local anesthetics. Signs and symptoms of local anesthetic overdose are more apt to be noted in these patients, even with "normal" dosages. Because injectable ester local anesthetics are rarely used in dentistry anymore, the presence of atypical plasma cholinesterase represents a relative contraindication to their administration. Because they undergo biotransformation in the liver, amide local anesthetics do not present an increased risk of overly high blood levels in these patients. Ester anesthetics may be administered, if deemed necessary by the doctor, but their doses should be minimized.

METHEMOGLOBINEMIA

Methemoglobinemia is a condition in which a cyanosis-like state develops in the absence of cardiac or respiratory abnormalities. When the condition is severe, blood appears chocolate brown, and clinical signs and symptoms, including respiratory depression and syncope, may be noted. Death, although unlikely, can result. Methemoglobinemia may occur through inborn errors of metabolism or may be acquired through administration of drugs or chemicals that increase the formation of methemoglobin. The local anesthetic prilocaine has been shown to produce clinically significant methemoglobinemia when administered in large doses to patients with subclinical methemoglobinemia.[91,92]

Administration of prilocaine to patients with congenital methemoglobinemia or other clinical syndromes in which the oxygen-carrying capacity of blood is reduced should be avoided because of the increased risk of producing clinically significant methemoglobinemia. The topical anesthetic benzocaine also can induce methemoglobinemia, but only when administered in very large doses.[93,94]

Causes

Iron is normally present in the reduced or ferrous state (Fe^{++}) in the hemoglobin molecule. Each hemoglobin molecule contains four ferrous atoms, each loosely bound to a molecule of oxygen. In the ferrous state, hemoglobin can carry oxygen that is available to the tissues. Because hemoglobin in the erythrocyte is inherently unstable, it is continuously being oxidized to the ferric form (Fe^{+++}), in which state the oxygen molecule is more firmly attached and cannot be released to the tissues. This form of hemoglobin is called *methemoglobin.* To permit an adequate oxygen-carrying capacity in the blood, an enzyme system is present that continually reduces the ferric form to the ferrous form. In usual clinical situations, approximately 97% to 99% of hemoglobin is found in the more functional ferrous state, and 1% to 3% is found in the ferric state. This enzyme system is known commonly as *methemoglobin reductase* (erythrocyte nucleotide diaphorase), and it acts to reconvert iron from the ferric to the ferrous state at a rate of 0.5 g/dl/hr, thus maintaining a level of less than 1% methemoglobin (0.15 g/dl) in the blood at any given time. As blood levels of methemoglobin increase, clinical signs and symptoms of cyanosis and respiratory distress may become noticeable. In most instances, they are not observed until a methemoglobin blood level of 1.5 to 3.0 g/dl (10% to 20% methemoglobin) is reached.[95]

Acquired Methemoglobinemia

Although prilocaine can produce elevated methemoglobin levels, other chemicals and substances can also do this, including acetanilid, aniline derivatives (e.g., crayons, ink, shoe polish, dermatologicals), benzene derivatives, cyanides, methylene blue in large doses, nitrates (antianginals), para-aminosalicylic acid, and sulfonamides.[26] Sarangi and Kumar reported the case of a fatality that occurred because of a chemically induced methemoglobinemia from writing ink.[96] Daly and associates reported the case of a child born with 16% (2.3 g/dl) methemoglobin that supposedly resulted because the mother, while still pregnant, had stood with wet bare feet on a bath mat colored with aniline dye.[97] In these situations, nitrates in the pen and dye were absorbed and converted to nitrites, which oxidized the ferrous atoms to ferric atoms and thus produced methemoglobinemia.

Acquired Methemoglobinemia—Prilocaine

The production of methemoglobin by prilocaine is dose related. Toluene is present in the prilocaine molecule, which as the drug is biotransformed becomes *o*-toluidine, a compound capable of oxidizing ferrous iron to ferric iron and of blocking the methemoglobin reductase pathways. Peak blood levels of methemoglobin develop approximately 3 to 4 hours after drug administration and persist for 12 to 14 hours.

Clinical Signs and Symptoms and Management

Signs and symptoms of methemoglobinemia usually appear 3 to 4 hours after administration of large doses of prilocaine to healthy patients, or of smaller doses in patients with the congenital disorder. Most dental patients will have left the office by this time, thus provoking a worried telephone call to the doctor. Although signs and symptoms vary with blood levels of methemoglobin, typically the patient appears lethargic and in respiratory distress; mucous membranes and nail beds will be cyanotic and the skin pale gray (ashen). Diagnosis of methemoglobinemia is made on the presentation of cyanosis unresponsive to oxygen administration and a distinctive brown color of arterial blood.[86] Administration of 100% oxygen does not lead to significant improvement (ferric atoms cannot surrender oxygen to tissues). Venous blood (gingival puncture) may appear chocolate brown and will not turn red when exposed to oxygen. Definitive treatment of this situation requires the slow IV administration of 1% methylene blue (1.5 mg/kg or 0.7 mg/lb). This dose may be repeated every 4 hours if cyanosis persists or returns. Methylene blue acts as an electron acceptor in the transfer of electrons to methemoglobin, thus hastening conversion of ferric to ferrous atoms. However, methylene blue, if administered in excess, can itself cause methemoglobinemia.

Another treatment, although not as rapid-acting as methylene blue and therefore not as popular, is the IV or IM administration of ascorbic acid (100 to 200 mg/day). Ascorbic acid accelerates the metabolic pathways that produce ferrous atoms.

Methemoglobinemia should not develop in a healthy ambulatory dental patient, provided doses of prilocaine HCl remain within recommended limits. The presence of congenital methemoglobinemia remains a relative contraindication to the administration of prilocaine. Although prilocaine may be administered, if absolutely necessary, its dose must be minimized. Whenever possible, alternate local anesthetics should be used.

The maximum recommended dose of prilocaine is listed by the manufacturer as 8.0 mg/kg (3.6 mg/lb). Methemoglobinemia is unlikely to develop at doses below this level.

References

1. Daublander M, Muller R, Lipp MD: The incidence of complications associated with local anesthesia in dentistry, Anesth Prog 44:132–141, 1997.
2. McCarthy FM: Essentials of safe dentistry for the medically compromised patient, Philadelphia, 1989, WB Saunders.
3. McCarthy FM: Stress reduction and therapy modifications, J Calif Dent Assoc 9:41–47, 1981.
4. McCarthy FM, Malamed SF: Physical evaluation system to determine medical risk and indicated dental therapy modifications, J Am Dent Assoc 99:181–184, 1979.
5. Berthelsen CL, Stilley KR: Automated personal health inventory for dentistry: a pilot study, J Am Dent Assoc 131:59–66, 2000.
6. Jacobsen PL, Fredekind R, Budenz AW, et al: The medical health history in dental practice: MetLife quality resource guide, Bridgewater, NJ, July 2003, MetLife.
7. Brady WF, Martinoff JT: Validity of health history data collected from dental patients and patient perception of health status, J Am Dent Assoc 101:642–645, 1980.
8. Jeske AH, editor: Mosby's dental drug reference, ed 9, St Louis, 2009, Mosby.
9. Fukuda K: Intravenous anesthetics. In Miller RD, editor: Miller's anesthesia, ed 6, Philadelphia, 2005, Elsevier.
10. Skidmore-Roth L: Mosby's 2010 nursing drug reference, St Louis, 2010, Mosby.
11. Hamilton JG: Needle phobia—a neglected diagnosis, J Fam Pract 41:169–175, 1995.
12. Gottlieb SO, Flaherty JT: Medical therapy of unstable angina pectoris, Cardiol Clin 9:19–98, 1991.
13. Little JW: Ischemic heart disease. In Little JW, Falace DA, Miller CS, et al, editors: Dental management of the medically compromised patient, ed 7, St Louis, 2007, Mosby.
14. Shah KB, Kleinman BS, Sami H, et al: Reevaluation of perioperative myocardial infarction in patients with prior myocardial infarction undergoing noncardiac operations, Anesth Analg 71:231–235, 1990.
15. Wilson W, Taubert KA, Gewitz M, et al: Prevention of infective endocarditis: guidelines from the American Heart Association: a guideline from the American Heart Association Rheumatic Fever, Endocarditis, and Kawasaki Disease Committee, Council on Cardiovascular Disease in the Young, and the Council on Clinical Cardiology, Council on Cardiovascular Surgery and Anesthesia, and the Quality of Care and Outcomes Research Interdisciplinary Working Group, Circulation 116:1736–1754, 2007.
16. American Dental Association, American Academy of Orthopedic Surgeons: Antibiotic prophylaxis for dental patients with total joint replacements, J Am Dent Assoc 134:895–898, 2003.
17. Public Relations Department, American Academy of Orthopedic Surgeons: Information statement 1033: antibiotic prophylaxis for bacteremia in patients with joint replacements, Rosemont, Ill, February 2009, Revised June 2010, American Academy of Orthopedic Surgeons.
18. National Collaborating Centre for Chronic Conditions, Chronic Obstructive Pulmonary Disease: National clinical guideline on management of chronic obstructive pulmonary disease in adults in primary and secondary care, Thorax 59(Suppl 1):1–232, 2004.
19. Yakahane Y, Kojima M, Sugai Y, et al: Hepatitis C virus infection in spouses of patients with type C chronic liver disease, Ann Intern Med 120:748–752, 1994.
20. Chafen JJ, Newberry SJ, Riedl MA, et al: Diagnosing and managing common food allergies: a systematic review, JAMA 303:1848–1856, 2010.
21. Haas DA: An update on local anesthetics in dentistry, J Can Dent Assoc 68:546–551, 2002.
22. Yagiela JA: Injectable and topical local anesthetics. In ADA/PDR guide to dental therapeutics, ed 5, Chicago, 2010, American Dental Association.
23. Jackson D, Chen AH, Bennett CR: Identifying true lidocaine allergy, J Am Dent Assoc 125:1362–1366, 1994.
24. Shojaei AR, Haas DA: Local anesthetic cartridges and latex allergy: a literature review, J Can Dent Assoc 68:622–626, 2002.
25. Seidel HM, Ball JW, Dains J, editors: Mosby's guide to physical examination, St Louis, 2012, CV Mosby.
26. Wilburn-Goo D, Lloyd LM: When patients become cyanotic: acquired methemoglobinemia, J Am Dent Assoc 130:826–831, 1999.
27. Hersh EV, Moore PA, Papas AS, et al, and the Soft Tissue Anesthesia Recovery Group: Reversal of soft tissue local anesthesia with phentolamine mesylate, J Am Dent Assoc 139:1080–1093, 2008.
28. Malamed SF: Reversing local anesthesia, Inside Dent 4:2–3, 2008.
29. DerMarderosian A, Beutler JA, editors: The review of natural products, St Louis, 2005, Facts and Comparisons.
30. Fetrow CH, Avila JR: Professional's handbook of complementary and alternative medicine, Philadelphia, 2003, Lippincott Williams & Wilkins.
31. 2011 Physicians' desk reference, ed 65, Oradell, NJ, 2011, Medical Economics.

31a. Gruenwald J, Brendler T, Jaenicke C, editors: 2011 Physicians' desk reference for herbal medicines, Oradell, NJ, 2011, Medical Economics.

32. American Dental Association: ADA/PDR guide to dental therapeutics, ed 5, Chicago, 2010, The Association.

32a. Smith DM, Lombardo JA, Robinson JB: The preparticipation evaluation, primary care, Clin Off Pract 18:777–807, 1991.

33. American Heart Association: Recommendations for human blood pressure determination by sphygmomanometry, Dallas, 1967, The Association.
34. Pickering TG, Hall JE, Appel LJ, et al: Recommendations for blood pressure measurement in humans and experimental animals. Part 1. Blood pressure measurement in humans: a statement for professionals from the Subcommittee of Professional and Public Education of the American Heart Association Council on High Blood Pressure Research, Hypertension 45:142–161, 2005.
35. Mitchell PT, Parlin RW, Blackburn H: Effect of vertical displacement of the arm on indirect blood pressure measurement, N Engl J Med 271:72–74, 1964.

36. Wonka F, Thummler M, Schoppe A: Clinical test of a blood pressure measurement device with a wrist cuff, Blood Press Monit 1:361–366, 1996.
37. Malamed SF. Prevention. In Malamed SF, editor: Medical emergencies in the dental office, ed 6, St Louis, 2007, Mosby Elsevier.
38. Little JW, Falace DA, Miller CS, et al: Dental management of the medically compromised patient, ed 7, St Louis, 2007, Mosby.
39. Seidel HM, Ball JW, Dains J, editors: Mosby's guide to physical examination, St Louis, 2006, CV Mosby.
40. McCarthy FM, Malamed SF: Physical evaluation system to determine medical risk and indicated dental therapy modifications, J Am Dent Assoc 99:181–184, 1979.
41. American Society of Anesthesiologists: New classification of physical status, Anesthesiology 24:111, 1963.
42. Lagasse RS: Anesthesia safety: model or myth? A review of the published literature and analysis of current original data, Anesthesiology 97:1609–1617, 2002.
43. Fleisher LA: Risk of anesthesia. In Miller RD, Fleisher LA, Johns RA, editors: Miller's anesthesia, ed 6, New York, 2005, Churchill Livingstone.
44. Moore PA, Gage TW, Hersh EV, et al: Adverse drug interactions in dental practice: professional and educational implications, J Am Dent Assoc 130:17–54, 1999.
45. Kishikawa K, Namiki A, Miyashita K, et al: Effects of famotidine and cimetidine on plasma levels of epidurally administered lignocaine, Anaesthesia 45:719–721, 1990.
46. Wood M: Pharmacokinetic drug interactions in anaesthetic practice, Clin Pharmacokinet 21:85–307, 1991.
47. Wu FL, Razzaghi A, Souney PE: Seizure after lidocaine for bronchoscopy: case report and review of the use of lidocaine in airway anesthesia, Pharmacotherapy 13:12–78, 1993.
48. Moore PA: Adverse drug interactions in dental practice: interactions associated with local anesthetics, sedatives and anxiolytics. Part IV of a series, J Am Dent Assoc 130:441–554, 1999.
49. Wilburn-Goo D, Lloyd LM: When patients become cyanotic: acquired methemoglobinemia, J Am Dent Assoc 130:26–31, 1999.
50. Jastak JT, Yagiela JA: Vasoconstrictors and local anesthesia: a review and rational use, J Am Dent Assoc 107:623–630, 1983.
51. Boakes AJ, Laurence DR, Lovel KW, et al: Adverse reactions to local anesthetic vasoconstrictor preparations: a study of the cardiovascular responses to xylestesin and hostcain with noradrenalin, Br Dent J 133:137–140, 1972.
52. Yagiela JA, Duffin SR, Hunt LM: Drug interactions and vasoconstrictors used in local anesthetic solutions, Oral Surg 59:565–571, 1985.
53. Hansbrough JF, Near A: Propranolol-epinephrine antagonism with hypertension and stroke, Ann Intern Med 92:717, 1980 (letter).
54. Kram J, Bourne HR, Melmon KL, et al: Propranolol, Ann Intern Med 80:282, 1974 (letter).
55. Foster CA, Aston SJ: Propranolol-epinephrine interaction: a potential disaster, Reconstr Surg 72:74–78, 1983.
56. Ghoneim MM: Drug interactions in anaesthesia: a review, Can Anaesthet Soc J 18:353–375, 1971.
57. Reichle FM, Conzen PF: Halogenated inhalational anaesthetics: best practice and research, Clin Anaesthesiol 17:19–46, 2003.
58. Hardman JG, Limbird LE, editors: Goodman and Gilman's the pharmacological basis of therapeutics, ed 10, New York, 2001, McGraw-Hill.
59. Hoffman BB, Lefkowitz RJ, Taylor P: Neurotransmission: the autonomic and somatic motor nervous systems. In Goodman and Gilman's the pharmacological basis of therapeutics, ed 9, New York, 1996, McGraw-Hill.
60. Benzaquen BS, Cohen V, Eisenberg MJ: Effects of cocaine on the coronary arteries, Am Heart J 142:302–410, 2001.
61. Gradman AH: Cardiac effects of cocaine: a review, Biol Med 61:137–141, 1988.
62. Vasica G, Tennant CC: Cocaine use and cardiovascular complications, Med J Austral 177:260–262, 2002.
63. Hahn IH, Hoffman RS: Cocaine use and acute myocardial infarction, Emerg Med Clin North Am 19:493–510, 2001.
64. Myerburg RJ: Sudden cardiac death in persons with normal (or near normal) hearts, Am J Cardiol 79:3–9, 1997.
65. Van Dyke D, Barash PG, Jatlow P, et al: Cocaine: plasma concentrations after intranasal application in man, Science 191:859–861, 1976.
66. Friedlander AH, Gorelick DA: Dental management of the cocaine addict, Oral Surg 65:45–48, 1988.
67. Perusse R, Goulet J-P, Turcotte J-Y: Contraindications to vasoconstrictors in dentistry. Part III. Pharmacologic interactions, Oral Surg Oral Med Oral Pathol 74:592–697, 1992.
68. Debruyne FM: Alpha blockers: are all created equal? Urology 56(5 Suppl 1):20–22, 2000.
69. Emmelin N, Engstrom J: Supersensitivity of salivary glands following treatment with bretylium or guanethidine, Br J Pharmacol Chemother 16:15–319, 1961.
70. McDevitt DG, Riddel JG, Hadden DR, et al: Catecholamine sensitivity in hyperthyroidism and hypothyroidism, Br J Clin Pharmacol 6:97–301, 1978.
71. Johnson AB, Webber J, Mansell P, et al: Cardiovascular and metabolic responses to adrenaline infusion in patients with short-term hypothyroidism, Clin Endocrinol 43:647–751, 1995.
72. Yagiela JA: Adverse drug interactions in dental practice: interactions associated with vasoconstrictors. Part V of a series, J Am Dent Assoc 130:501–709, 1999.
73. Hersh EV: Adverse drug interactions in dental practice: interactions involving antibiotics. Part II of a series, J Am Dent Assoc 130:236–251, 1999.
74. Haas DA: Adverse drug interactions in dental practice: interactions associated with analgesics. Part III of a series. J Am Dent Assoc 130:397–407, 1999.
75. Rosenberg H, Fletcher JE: An update on the malignant hyperthermia syndrome, Ann Acad Med Singapore 23(Suppl 6):84–97, 1994.
76. Carson JM, Van Sickels JE: Preoperative determination of susceptibility to malignant hyperthermia, J Oral Maxillofac Surg 40:432–435, 1982.
77. Gielen M, Viering W: 3-in-1 lumbar plexus block for muscle biopsy in malignant hyperthermia patients: amide local anaesthetics may be used safely, Acta Anaesthesiol Scand 30:581–583, 1986.
78. Paasuke RT, Brownell AKW: Amine local anaesthetics and malignant hyperthermia, Can Anaesth Soc J 33:126–129, 1986 (editorial).
79. Ording H: Incidence of malignant hyperthermia in Denmark, Anesth Analg 64:700–704, 1985.

80. Malignant Hyperthermia Association of the United States: Anesthetic list for MH-susceptible patients. www.mhaus.org. Accessed September 9, 2011.
81. Jurkat-Rott K, McCarthy T, Lehmann-Horn F: Genetics and pathogenesis of malignant hyperthermia, Muscle Nerve 23:1–17, 2000.
82. Steelman R, Holmes D: Outpatient dental treatment of pediatric patients with malignant hyperthermia: report of three cases, ASDC J Dent Child 59:12–65, 1992.
83. Amato R, Giordano A, Patrignani F, et al: Malignant hyperthermia in the course of general anesthesia in oral surgery: a case report, J Int Assoc Dent Child 12:15–28, 1981.
84. The European Malignant Hyperpyrexia Group: A protocol for the investigation of malignant hyperpyrexia (MH) susceptibility, Br J Anaesth 56:1267–1269, 1984.
85. Malignant Hyperthermia Association of the United States: MHAUS Professional Advisory Council adopts new policy statement on local anesthetics, Communicator 3:4, 1985.
86. Adragna MG: Medical protocol by habit: avoidance of amide local anesthetics in malignant hyperthermia susceptible patients, Anesthesiology 62:99–100, 1985 (letter).
87. Adriani J, Sundin R: Malignant hyperthermia in dental patients, J Am Dent Assoc 108:180–184, 1984.
88. Kaus SJ, Rockoff MA: Malignant hyperthermia, Pediatr Clin North Am 41:121–237, 1994.
89. Williams FM: Clinical significance of esterases in man, Clin Pharmacokinet 10:392–403, 1985.
90. Abernethy MH, George PM, Herron JL, et al: Plasma cholinesterase phenotyping with use of visible-region spectrophotometry, Clin Chem 32(1 Pt 1):194–197, 1986.
91. Prilocaine-induced methemoglobinemia-Wisconsin, 1993, MMWR Morb Mortal Wkly Rep 43:555–657, 1994.
92. Bellamy MC, Hopkins PM, Hallsall PJ, et al: A study into the incidence of methaemoglobinaemia after "three-in-one" block with prilocaine, Anaesthesia 47:1084–1085, 1992.
93. Guertler AT, Pearce WA: A prospective evaluation of benzocaine-associated methemoglobinemia in human beings, Ann Emerg Med 24:426–630, 1994.
94. Rodriguez LF, Smolik LM, Zbehlik AJ: Benzocaine-induced methemoglobinemia: a report of a severe reaction and review of the literature, Ann Pharmacother 28:543–649, 1994.
95. Eilers MA, Garrison TE: General management principles. In Marx J, Hockberger R, Walls R, editors: Rosen's emergency medicine: concepts and clinical practice, ed 5, St Louis, 2002, Mosby.
96. Sarangi MP, Kumar B: Poisoning with writing ink, Indian Pediatr 31:756–857, 1994.
97. Daly DJ, Davenport J, Newland MC: Methemoglobinemia following the use of prilocaine, Br J Anaesth 36:737–739, 1964.

CHAPTER 11

Basic Injection Technique

Absolutely nothing that is done for patients by their dentist is of greater importance than the administration of a drug that prevents pain during dental treatment.[1] Yet the very act of administering a local anesthetic commonly induces great anxiety or is associated with pain in the recipient. Patients frequently mention that they would prefer anything to the injection or "shot" (to use patients' term for the local anesthetic injection). Not only can the injection of local anesthetics produce fear and pain, it is also a factor in the occurrence of emergency medical situations. In a review of medical emergencies developing in Japanese dental offices, Matsuura determined that 54.9% of emergency situations arose either during administration of the local anesthetic or in the 5 minutes immediately after its administration.[2] Most of these emergency situations were directly related to increased stress associated with receipt of the anesthetic (the injection) and not to the drug being used. Moreover, in a survey on the occurrence of medical emergencies in dental practices in North America, 4309 dentists responded that a total of more than 30,000 emergency situations had developed in their offices over the previous 10 years.[3] Ninety-five percent of respondents stated that they had experienced a medical emergency in their office in this time period. More than half of these emergencies (15,407) were vasodepressor syncope (common faint), most of which occurred during or immediately after administration of the local anesthetic.

Local anesthetics can and should be administered in a nonpainful, or atraumatic, manner. Most dental students' first injections were given to classmate "patients," who then gave the same injection to the student who had just injected them. Most likely, these students went out of their way to make their injection as painless as possible. At the Herman Ostrow School of Dentistry of U.S.C., these first injections usually are absolutely atraumatic. Students are routinely surprised by this, some having experienced the more usual (e.g., painful) injection at some time in the past when they were "real" dental patients. Why should there be a difference in dental injections and in the degree of pain between injections administered by an inexperienced beginning student and those given by a more experienced practitioner? All too often, local anesthetic administration becomes increasingly traumatic for the patient the longer a dentist has been out of school. Can this discouraging situation be corrected?

Local anesthetic administration need not, and should not, be painful. Every one of the local anesthetic techniques presented in the following chapters can be done atraumatically, including the administration of local anesthetics on the palate (the most sensitive area in the oral cavity). Several skills and attitudes are required of the drug administrator, the most important of which is probably empathy. If the administrator truly believes that local anesthetic injections do not have to be painful, then through a conscious or subconscious effort, it is possible to make minor changes in technique that will cause formerly traumatic procedures to be less painful for the patient.

Additionally, the ability to buffer the pH of the local anesthetic solution to a more physiologic 7.35 to 7.5 from the pH of 3.5 in the cartridge has greatly aided in the process of atraumatic injection.[4,5]

An atraumatic injection has two components: a technical aspect and a communicative aspect.

◆ **Step 1:** Use a sterilized sharp needle. Stainless steel disposable needles currently used in dentistry are sharp and rarely produce any pain on insertion or withdrawal. However, because these needles are machine manufactured, occasionally (rarely) a fishhook-type barb may appear on the tip. This results in atraumatic insertion of the needle followed by painful withdrawal as the barb tears the unanesthetized tissue. This may be avoided by the use of sterile 2 × 2-inch gauze. Place the needle tip against the gauze and draw the needle backward. If the gauze is snagged, a barb is present and the needle should not be used. (This procedure is optional and may be omitted if fear of needle contamination is great.)

Disposable needles are sharp on first insertion. However, with each succeeding penetration, their sharpness diminishes. By the third or fourth penetration, the operator can feel an increase in tissue resistance to needle penetration.

Clinically, this is evidenced by increased pain on penetration and increased postanesthetic tissue discomfort. Therefore it is recommended that stainless steel disposable needles be changed after every three or four tissue penetrations.

The gauge of the needle should be determined solely by the injection to be administered. Pain caused by needle penetration in the absence of adequate topical anesthesia can be eliminated in dentistry through the use of needles not larger than 25 gauge. Multiple studies have demonstrated that patients cannot differentiate among 25-, 27-, and 30-gauge needles inserted into mucous membranes, even without the benefit of topical anesthesia.[6-8] Needles of 23 gauge and larger are associated with increased pain on initial insertion.

◆ **Step 2:** Check the flow of local anesthetic solution. After the cartridge is properly loaded into the syringe, and with the aspirator tip (harpoon) embedded into the silicone rubber stopper (if appropriate), a few drops of local anesthetic should be expelled from the cartridge. This ensures a free flow of solution when it is deposited at the target area. The stoppers on the anesthetic cartridge are made of a silicone rubber to ensure ease of administration. Only a few drops of the solution should be expelled from the needle to determine whether a free flow of solution occurs.

◆ **Step 3:** Determine whether to warm the anesthetic cartridge or syringe. If the cartridge is stored at room temperature (approximately 22° C, 72° F), there is no reason for a local anesthetic cartridge to be warmed before its injection into soft tissues. The patient will not perceive local anesthetic solution stored at room temperature as too cold or too hot when it is injected.

Most complaints concerning overly warm local anesthetic cartridges pertain to those stored in cartridge warmers heated by a (Christmas tree–type) light bulb. Temperatures within these cartridges frequently become excessive, leading to patient discomfort and adverse effects on the contents of the cartridge[9] (see Chapter 7).

Cartridges stored in refrigerators or other cool areas should be brought to room temperature before use.

Some persons advocate slight warming of the metal syringe before its use. The rationale is that a cold metal object is psychologically more disturbing to the patient than is the same object at room temperature. It is recommended that both the local anesthetic cartridge and the metal syringe be as close to room temperature as possible, preferably without the use of any mechanical devices to achieve these temperatures. Holding the loaded metal syringe in the palm of one's hand for half a minute before injection warms the metal. Plastic syringes do not pose this problem.

◆ **Step 4:** Position the patient. Any patient receiving local anesthetic injections should be in a physiologically sound position before and during the injection.

Vasodepressor syncope (common faint), the most commonly seen medical emergency in dentistry, most often occurs before, during, and, on occasion, immediately after local anesthetic administration. The primary pathophysiologic component of this situation is cerebral ischemia secondary to an inability of the heart to supply the brain with an adequate volume of oxygenated blood. When a patient is seated in an upright position, the effect of gravity is such that the blood pressure in cerebral arteries is decreased by 2 mm Hg for each inch above the level of the heart.

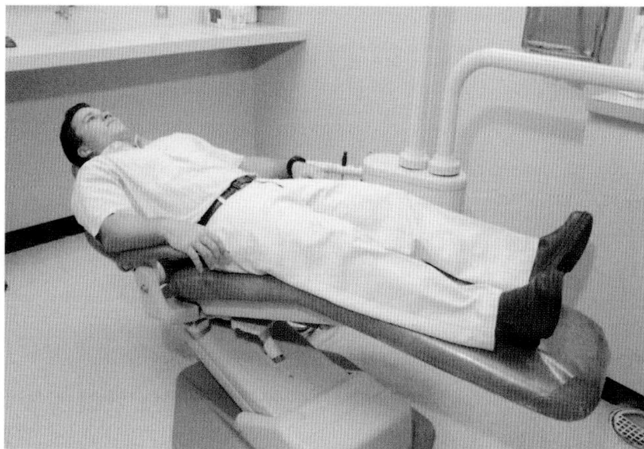

Figure 11-1. Physiologic position of patient for receipt of local anesthetic injection.

In the presence of anxiety, blood flow is increasingly directed toward the skeletal muscles at the expense of other organ systems such as the gastrointestinal tract (the "fight-or-flight" response). In the absence of muscular movement ("I can take it like a man!"), the increased volume of blood in skeletal muscles remains there, decreasing venous return to the heart and decreasing the volume of blood available to be pumped by the heart (uphill) to the brain. Decreased cerebral blood flow is evidenced by the appearance of signs and symptoms of vasodepressor syncope (e.g., lightheadedness, dizziness, tachycardia, palpitations). If this situation continues, cerebral blood flow declines still further, and consciousness is lost.

To prevent this, it is recommended that during local anesthetic administration, the patient should be placed in a supine position (head and heart parallel to the floor) with the feet elevated slightly (Fig. 11-1). Although this position may vary according to the dentist's and the patient's preference, the patient's medical status, and the specific injection technique, all techniques of regional block anesthesia can be carried out successfully with the patient in this position.

◆ **Step 5:** Dry the tissue. A 2 × 2-inch gauze should be used to dry the tissue in and around the site of needle penetration and to remove any gross debris (Fig. 11-2). In addition, if the lip must be retracted to attain adequate visibility during the injection, it too should be dried to ease retraction (Fig. 11-3).

◆ **Step 6:** Apply topical antiseptic (optional). After the tissues are dried, a suitable topical antiseptic should be

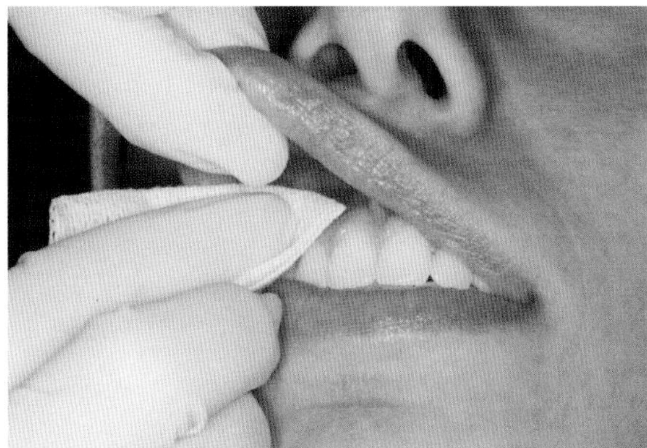

Figure 11-2. Sterilized gauze is used to gently wipe tissue at site of needle penetration.

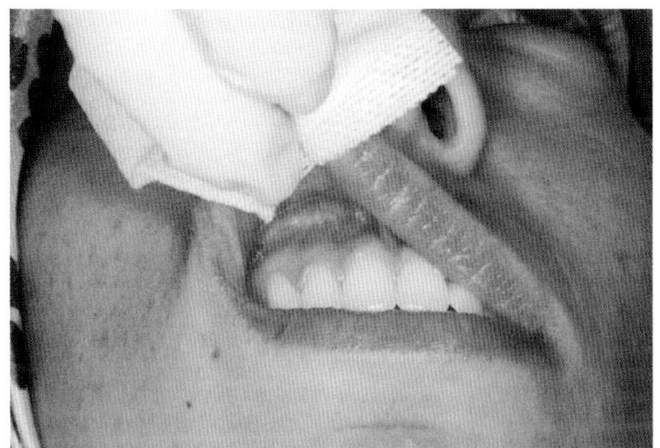

Figure 11-3. Sterilized gauze also may be used as an aid in tissue retraction.

applied at the site of injection. This further decreases the risk of introducing septic materials into the soft tissues, producing inflammation or infection. Antiseptics include Betadine (povidone-iodine) and Merthiolate (thimerosal). Alcohol-containing antiseptics can cause burning of the soft tissue and should be avoided. (This step is optional; however, the preceding step [No. 5] of drying the tissue must not be eliminated.)

◆ **Step 7A:** Apply topical anesthetic. A topical anesthetic is applied after the topical antiseptic. As with the topical antiseptic, it should be applied only at the site of needle penetration. All too often, excessive amounts of topical anesthetic are used on large areas of soft tissue, producing undesirably wide areas of anesthesia (e.g., the soft palate, the pharynx), an unpleasant taste, and, perhaps even more important with some topical anesthetics (such as lidocaine), rapid absorption into the cardiovascular system (CVS), leading to higher local anesthetic blood levels, which increase the risk of overdose. Only a small quantity of topical anesthetic should be placed on the cotton applicator stick and applied directly at the injection site (Fig. 11-4).

Topical anesthetics produce anesthesia of the outermost 2 or 3 mm of mucous membrane; this tissue is quite

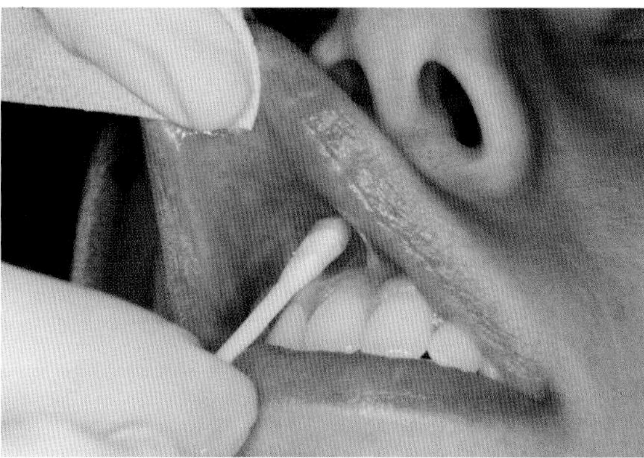

Figure 11-4. A small quantity of topical anesthetic is placed at the site of needle penetration and is kept in place for at least 1 minute.

sensitive. Ideally the topical anesthetic should remain in contact with the tissue for 2 minutes to ensure effectiveness.[10,11] A minimum application time of 1 minute is recommended.

◆ **Step 7B:** Communicate with the patient. During the application of topical anesthetic, it is desirable for the operator to speak to the patient about the reasons for its use. Tell the patient, "I'm applying a topical anesthetic to the tissue so that the remainder of the procedure will be much more comfortable." This statement places a positive idea in the patient's mind concerning the upcoming injection.

Note that the words *injection, shot, pain,* and *hurt* are not used. These words have a negative connotation; they tend to increase a patient's fears. Their use should be avoided if at all possible. More positive (e.g., less threatening) words can be substituted in their place. "Administer the local anesthetic" is used in place of "Give an injection" or "Give a shot." The latter is a particularly poor choice of words and must be avoided. Commonly used by Canadian dentists is the word *freeze,* as in "I'm going to freeze you now." A statement such as, "This will not hurt" also should be avoided. Patients hear only the word *hurt,* ignoring the rest of the statement. The same is true for the word *pain.* An alternative to this is the word *discomfort.* Although their meanings are similar, discomfort is much less threatening and produces less fear.

◆ **Step 8:** Establish a firm hand rest. After the topical anesthetic swab is removed from the tissue, the prepared local anesthetic syringe should be picked up (see Chapter 9). It is essential to maintain complete control over it at all times. To do so requires a steady hand so that tissue penetration may be accomplished readily, accurately, and without inadvertent nicking of tissues. A firm hand rest is necessary. The types of hand rest vary according to the practitioner's likes, dislikes, and physical abilities. Persons with long fingers can use finger rests on the patient's face for many injections; those with shorter fingers may need elbow rests. Figures 11-5 to 11-7 illustrate a variety of hand and finger rests that can be used to stabilize the local anesthetic syringe.

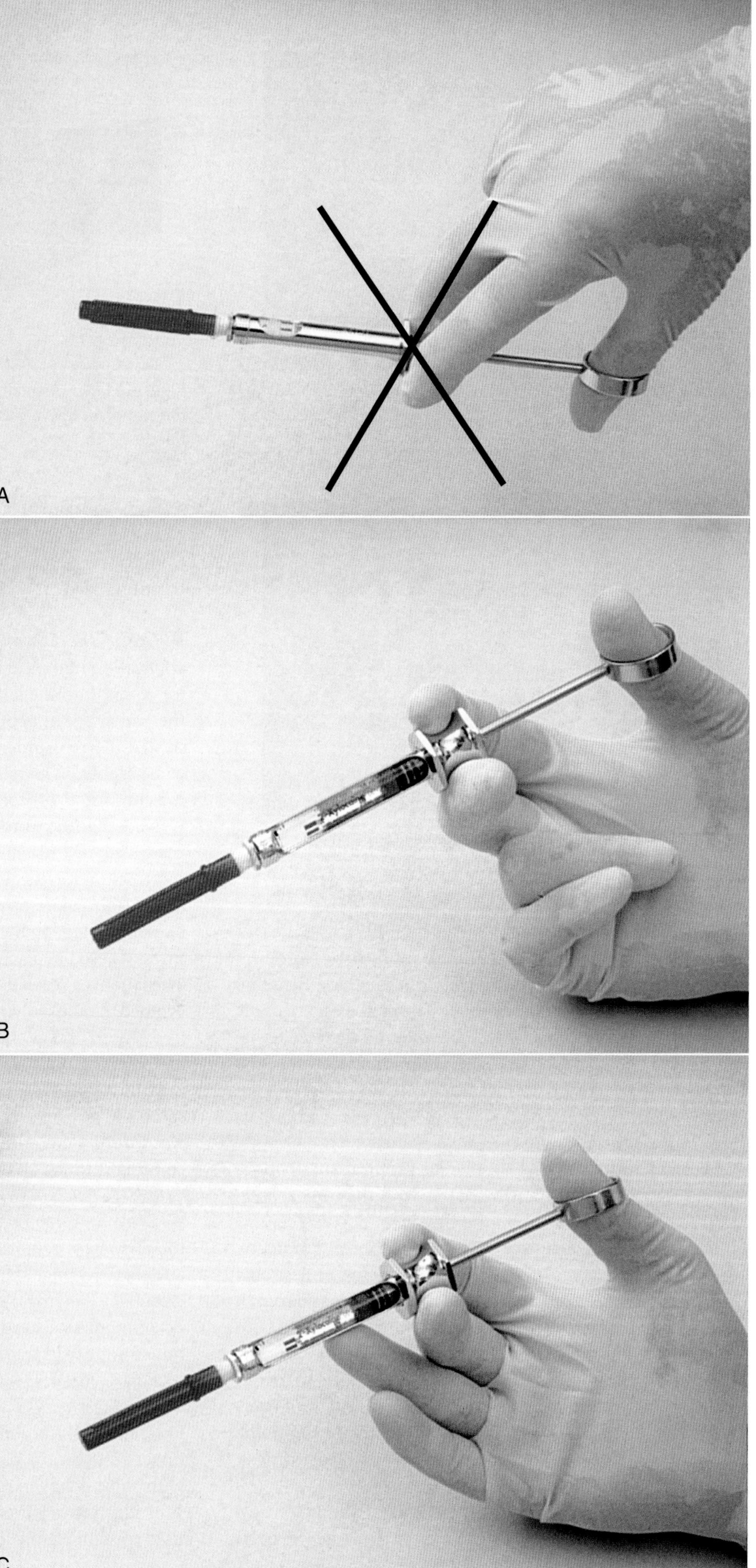

Figure 11-5. Hand positions for injections. **A,** Palm down: poor control over the syringe; not recommended. **B,** Palm up: better control over the syringe because it is supported by the wrist; recommended. **C,** Palm up and finger support: greatest stabilization; highly recommended.

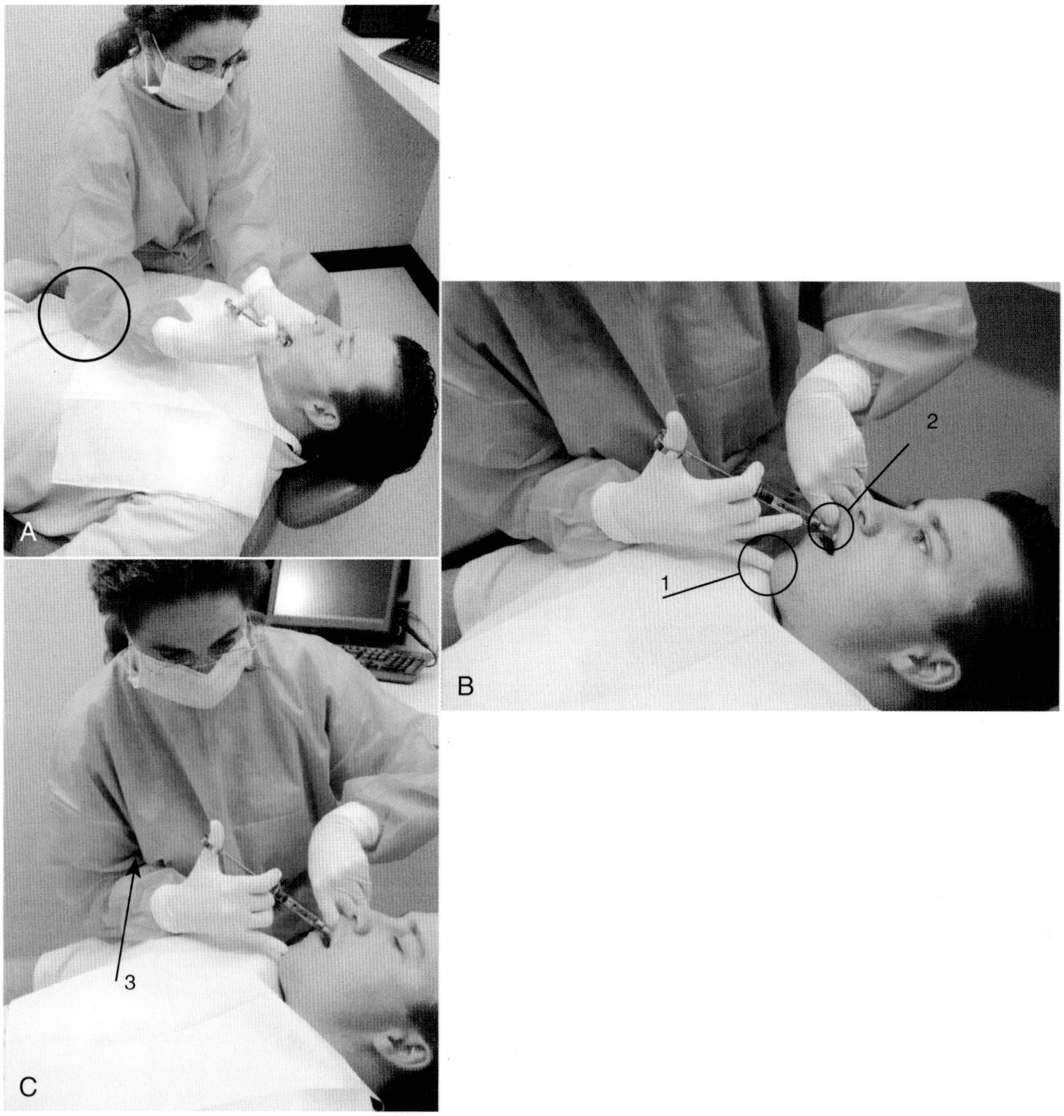

Figure 11-6. **A,** Use of the patient's chest for stabilization of syringe during right inferior alveolar nerve block *(circle)*. Never use the patient's arm to stabilize a syringe. **B,** Use of the chin (1) as a finger rest, with the syringe barrel stabilized by the patient's lip (2). **C,** When necessary, stabilization may be increased by drawing the administrator's arm in against his or her chest (3).

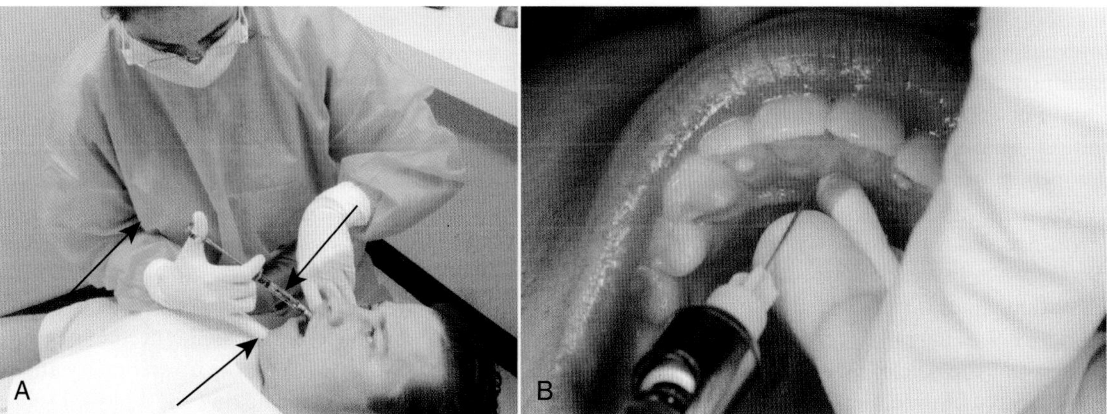

Figure 11-7. **A,** Syringe stabilization for a right posterior superior alveolar nerve block: syringe barrel on the patient's lip, one finger resting on the chin and one on the syringe barrel *(arrows)*, upper arm kept close to the administrator's chest to maximize stability. **B,** Syringe stabilization for a nasopalatine nerve block: index finger used to stabilize the needle, syringe barrel resting in the corner of the patient's mouth.

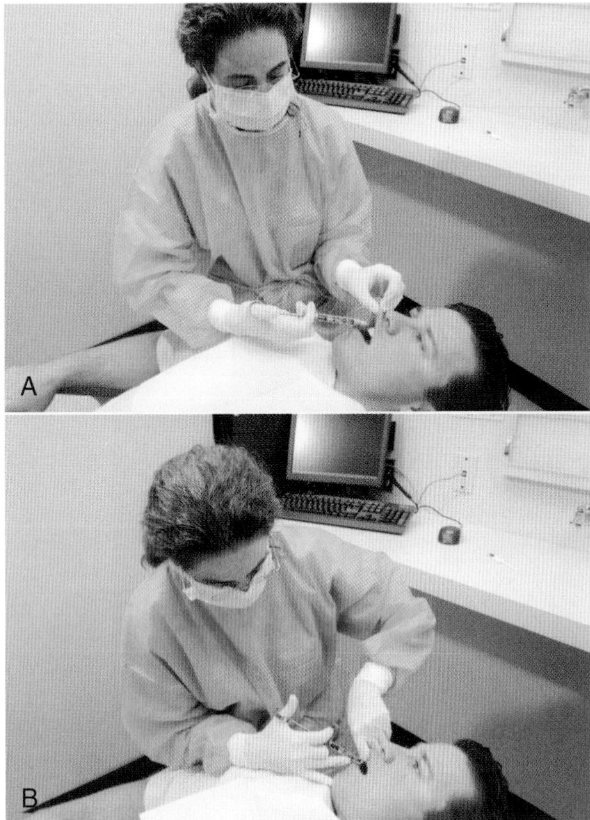

Figure 11-8. **A,** Incorrect position: no hand or finger rest for stabilization of syringe. **B,** Incorrect position: administrator resting elbow on patient's arm.

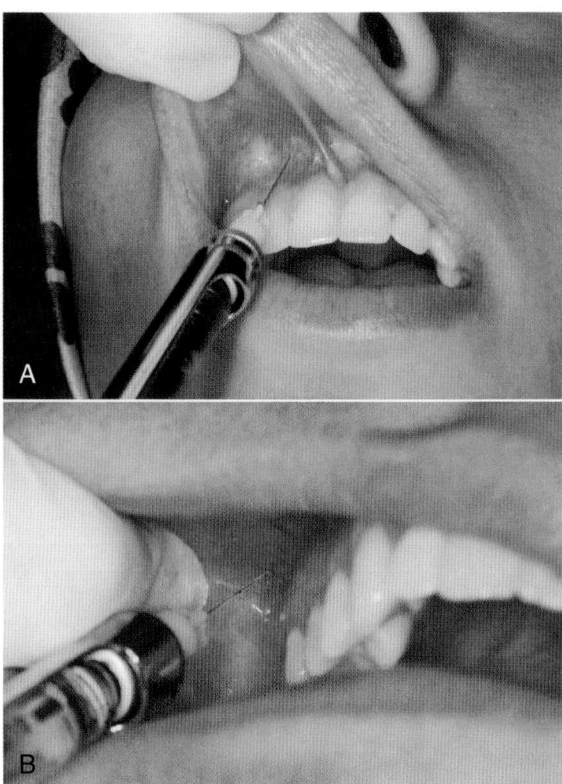

Figure 11-9. **A,** Tissue at needle penetration site is pulled taut, aiding both visibility and atraumatic needle insertion. **B,** Taut tissue provides excellent visibility of the penetration site for a posterior superior alveolar nerve block.

Any finger or hand rest that permits the syringe to be stabilized without increasing risk to a patient is acceptable. Two techniques to be avoided are (1) using no syringe stabilization of any kind, and (2) placing the arm holding the syringe directly onto the patient's arm or shoulder (Fig. 11-8). In the first situation, it is highly unlikely that a needle can be adequately stabilized without the use of some form of rest. The operator has less control over the syringe, thereby increasing the possibility of inadvertent needle movement and injury. Resting on a patient's arm or shoulder is also dangerous and can lead to patient or administrator needle-stick injury. If the patient inadvertently moves during the injection, damage can occur as the needle tip moves around within the mouth. Apprehensive patients, especially children, frequently move their arms during local anesthetic administration.

◆ **Step 9:** Make the tissue taut. The tissues at the site of needle penetration should be stretched before insertion of the needle (Fig. 11-9). This can be accomplished in all areas of the mouth except the palate (where the tissues are naturally quite taut). Stretching of the tissues permits the sharp stainless steel needle to cut through the mucous membrane with minimal resistance. Loose tissues, on the other hand, are pushed and torn by the needle as it is inserted, producing greater discomfort on injection and increased postoperative soreness.

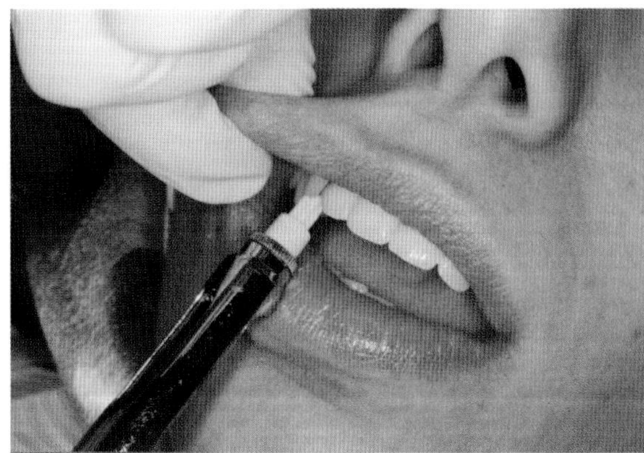

Figure 11-10. When soft tissues are pulled over the needle, visualization of the injection site is impaired.

Techniques of distraction also are effective in this regard. Some dentists jiggle the lip as the needle is inserted; others recommend leaving the needle tip stationary and pulling the soft tissues over the needle tip (Fig. 11-10). Devices that are attached to the syringe that produce vibration as the injection is given are available. Two examples are DentalVibe (BING Innovations LLC, Boca Raton, Fla; Fig. 11-11) and

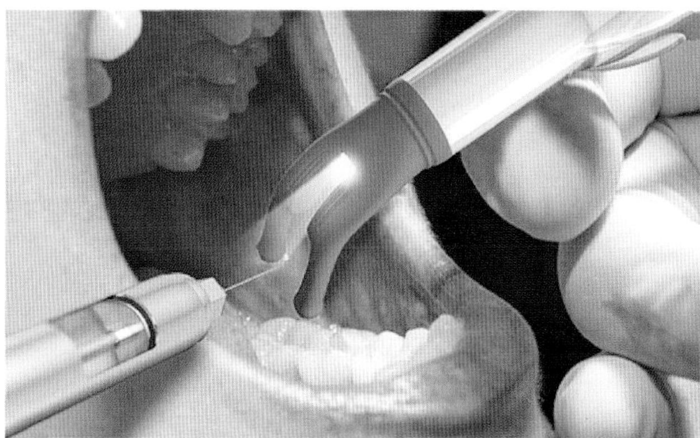

Figure 11-11. DentalVibe.

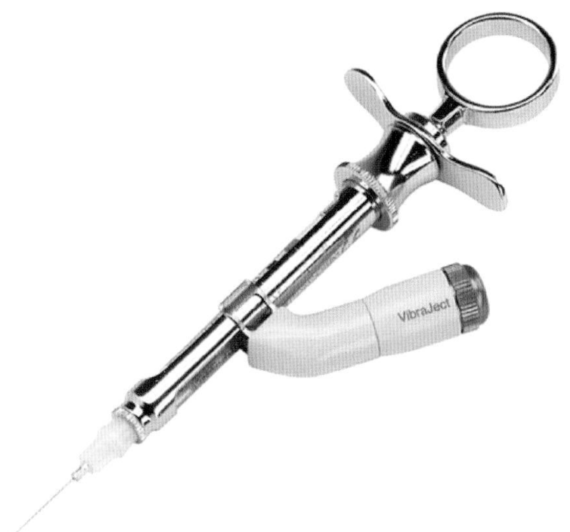

Figure 11-12. VibraJect.

VibraJect (Newport Coast, Calif; Fig. 11-12). Although nothing is inherently wrong with distraction techniques, there generally is no need for them. Because the operator should maintain sight of the needle tip at all times, needles should not be inserted blindly into tissues, as is necessitated by many of the distraction techniques (e.g., pulling lip over needle tip).

Proper application of topical anesthetic, taut tissues, and a firm hand rest can produce an unnoticed initial penetration of tissues virtually 100% of the time.

◆ **Step 10:** Keep the syringe out of the patient's line of sight. With the tissue prepared and the patient positioned, the assistant should pass the syringe to the administrator out of the patient's line of sight either behind the patient's head or across and in front of the patient. A right-handed practitioner administrating a right-side injection can sit facing the patient (Fig. 11-13) or, if administering a left-side injection, facing in the same direction as the patient (Fig. 11-14). In all cases, it is better if the syringe is not visible to the patient.

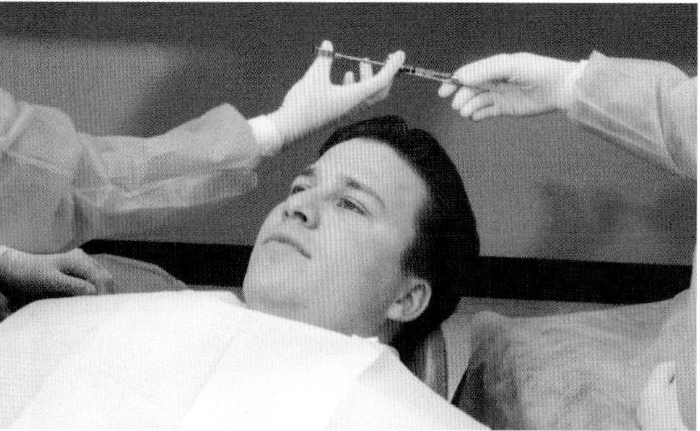

Figure 11-13. Passing syringe from assistant to administrator behind the patient, out of his or her line of sight.

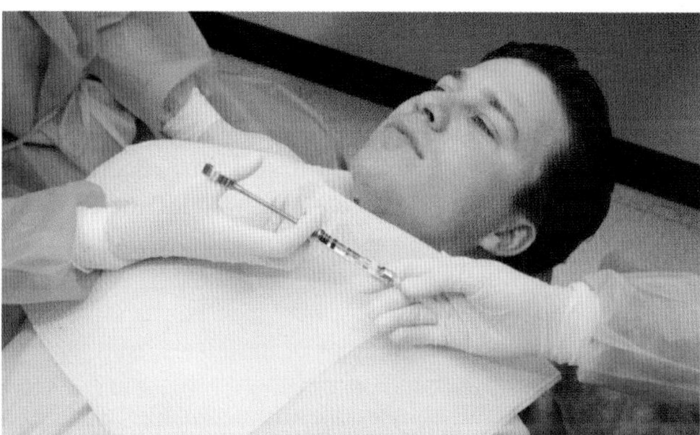

Figure 11-14. Passing syringe from assistant to administrator below the patient's line of sight.

Proper positioning for left-handed operators is a mirror image of that for right-handed ones. (Specific recommendations for administrator positioning during local anesthetic injections are discussed in Chapters 13 and 14.)

◆ **Step 11A:** Insert the needle into the mucosa. With the needle bevel properly oriented (see specific injection technique for bevel orientation; however, as a general rule, the bevel of the needle should be oriented toward bone), insert the needle gently into the tissue at the injection site (where the topical anesthetic was placed) to the depth of its bevel. With a firm hand rest and adequate tissue preparation, this potentially traumatic procedure is accomplished without the patient ever being aware of it.

◆ **Step 11B:** Watch and communicate with the patient. During Step 11A, the patient should be watched and communicated with; the patient's face should be observed for evidence of discomfort during needle penetration. Signs such as furrowing of the brow or forehead and blinking of the eyes may indicate discomfort (Fig. 11-15). More frequently, no change will be noticed in the patient's facial expression at this time (indicating a painless, or atraumatic, needle insertion).

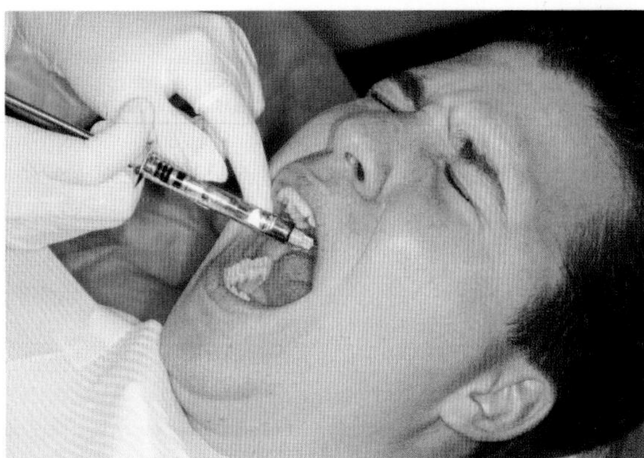

Figure 11-15. The patient's face should be observed during administration of local anesthetic; any squinting of the eyes or furrowing of the brows, indicating discomfort, should be noted.

The practitioner should communicate with the patient as Step 11A is carried out. The patient should be told in a positive manner, "I don't expect you to feel this," as the needle penetrates the tissues. The words, "This will not hurt," should be avoided; this is a negative statement, and the patient hears only the word (hurt).

◆ **Step 12:** Inject several drops of local anesthetic solution (optional).

◆ **Step 13:** Slowly advance the needle toward the target. Steps 12 and 13 are carried out together. The soft tissue in front of the needle may be anesthetized with a few drops of local anesthetic solution. After 2 or 3 seconds are allowed for anesthesia to develop, the needle should be advanced into this area and a little more anesthesia deposited. The needle should then be advanced again. These procedures may be repeated until the needle reaches the desired target area. Use of a buffered local anesthetic will increase patient comfort during injection as a result of (1) the increased pH of the anesthetic solution (7.35 to 7.5) and (2) the presence of CO_2 in the buffered solution. CO_2 possesses anesthetic properties.[12]

In most patients, however, injection of local anesthetic during insertion of the needle toward the target area is entirely unnecessary. Pain is rarely encountered between the surface mucosa and the mucoperiosteum. If patients are asked post injection what they felt as the needle was being advanced through soft tissue (as in an inferior alveolar or posterior superior alveolar nerve block), the usual reply is that they were aware that something was there, but that it did not hurt.

On the other hand, patients who are apprehensive about injections of local anesthetics are likely to react to any sensation as though it were painful. These patients are said to have a lowered pain reaction threshold (PRT). Apprehensive patients should be told, "To make you more comfortable, I will deposit a little anesthetic as I advance (the needle) toward the target." Minimal amounts of the local anesthetic should be injected as the process continues. In an injection such as the inferior alveolar nerve block, for which the average depth of needle insertion is 20 to 25 mm, not more than $\frac{1}{8}$ of a cartridge of local anesthetic should be deposited as the soft tissues are penetrated. Aspiration does not need to be performed at this stage because of the small amount of anesthetic solution that is being continually deposited over a changing injection site. If a vessel were to be penetrated during this procedure, only a drop or two (<1 mg) of anesthetic would be deposited intravascularly. As the needle is advanced further, it leaves the vessel. However, aspiration should always be carried out before any significant volume of solution is deposited (Steps 15 and 16).

When treating patients who are more sensitive, or when injecting into more sensitive tissues, the use of buffered local anesthetic solutions can be of great benefit in making penetration of soft tissues more comfortable for the patient.

◆ **Step 14:** Deposit several drops of local anesthetic before touching the periosteum. In techniques of regional block anesthesia in which the needle touches or comes close to the periosteum, several drops of solution should be deposited just before contact. The periosteum is richly innervated, and contact with the needle tip produces pain. Anesthetizing the periosteum permits atraumatic contact. Regional block injection techniques that require this are the inferior alveolar, Gow-Gates mandibular, and anterior superior alveolar (infraorbital) nerve blocks.

Knowledge of when to deposit the local anesthetic comes with experience. The depth of penetration of soft tissue at any injection site varies from patient to patient; therefore the periosteum may be contacted inadvertently. However, a keen tactile sense is developed with repetition, enabling the needle to be used gently as a probe. This enables the administrator to detect subtle changes in tissue density as the needle nears bone. With experience and development of this tactile sense, a small volume of local anesthetic solution may be deposited just before gentle contact with the periosteum.

◆ **Step 15:** Aspirate. Aspiration must always be carried out before a volume of local anesthetic is deposited at any site. Aspiration dramatically minimizes the possibility of an intravascular injection. The goal of aspiration is to determine where the tip of the needle tip is situated (within a blood vessel or without). To aspirate, one must create negative pressure within the dental cartridge. The self-aspirating syringe does this whenever the operator stops applying positive pressure to the thumb ring (plunger). With the traditional harpoon-aspirating syringe, the administrator must make a conscious effort to create this negative pressure within the cartridge.

Adequate aspiration requires that the tip of the needle remain unmoved, neither pushed farther into nor pulled out of the tissues, during the aspiration test. Adequate stabilization is mandatory. Beginners have a tendency to pull the syringe out of the tissues while attempting to aspirate.

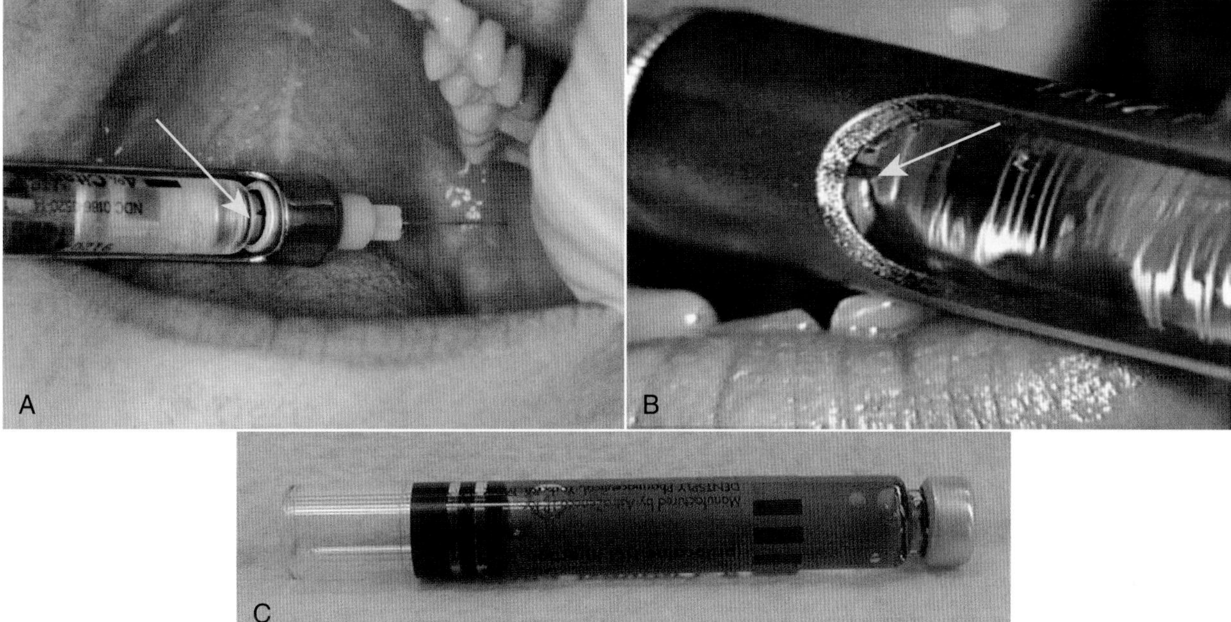

Figure 11-16. **A,** Negative aspiration. With the needle in position at the injection site, the administrator pulls the thumb ring of the harpoon-aspirating syringe 1 or 2 mm. The needle tip should not move. Check the cartridge at the site where the needle penetrates the diaphragm *(arrow)* for a bubble or blood. **B,** Positive aspiration. A slight reddish discoloration at the diaphragm end of the cartridge *(arrow)* on aspiration usually indicates venous penetration. Reposition the needle, reaspirate, and, if negative, deposit the solution. **C,** Positive aspiration. Bright red blood rapidly filling the cartridge usually indicates arterial penetration. Remove the syringe from the mouth, change the cartridge, and repeat the procedure.

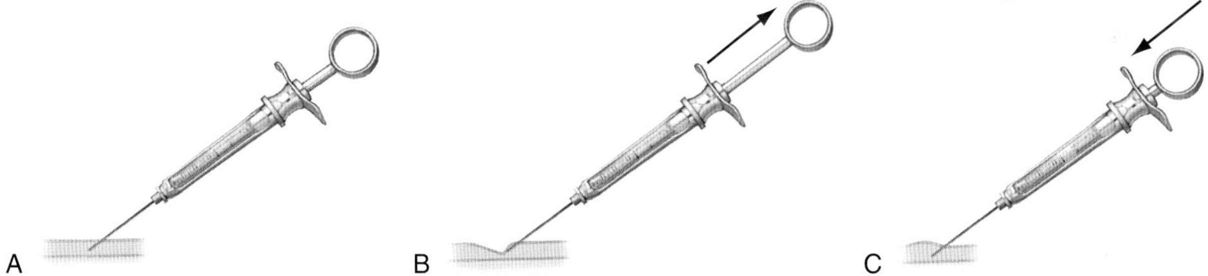

Figure 11-17. **A,** Needle tip within blood vessel but bevel abuts the wall of the vein. **B,** On aspiration vein wall is sucked into needle tip producing a false negative aspiration test. **C,** Rotating syringe 45 degrees and reaspirating will provide a true "positive" aspiration in this scenario.

When the harpoon-aspirating syringe is used, the thumb ring should be pulled back gently. Movement of only 1 or 2 mm is needed. This produces negative pressure within the cartridge that then translates to the tip of the needle. Whatever is lying in the soft tissues around the needle tip (e.g., blood, tissue [or air, if tested out of the mouth]) will be drawn back into the anesthetic cartridge. By observing the needle end visible within the cartridge for signs of blood return, the administrator can determine whether positive aspiration has occurred. Any sign of blood is a positive aspiration, and local anesthetic solution should not be deposited at that site (Fig. 11-16). No return at all, or a small air bubble, indicates a negative aspiration. Aspiration should be performed at least twice before the larger volume of local anesthetic is administered (as required by the injection technique being employed), with the orientation of the bevel changed (rotate barrel of syringe about 45 degrees for second aspiration test) to ensure that the bevel of the needle is not located inside a blood vessel but is abutting against the wall of the vessel, providing a false-negative aspiration (Fig. 11-17). Several additional aspiration tests are suggested during administration of the anesthetic drug. This serves two functions: (1) to slow down the rate of anesthetic administration, and (2) to preclude the deposition of large volumes of anesthetic into the cardiovascular system.

A major factor determining whether aspiration can be performed reliably is the gauge of the needle. Larger-gauge needles (e.g., 25) are recommended more often than smaller-gauge needles (e.g., 27, 30) whenever a greater risk of positive aspiration exists.

◆ **Step 16A:** Slowly deposit the local anesthetic solution. With the needle in position at the target area and aspirations completed and negative, the administrator should begin pressing gently on the plunger to start administering the predetermined (for the injection technique) volume of anesthetic. Slow injection is vital for two reasons: (1) of utmost significance is the safety factor (discussed in greater detail in Chapter 18); and (2) slow injection prevents the solution from tearing the tissue into which it is deposited. Rapid injection results in immediate discomfort (for a few seconds) followed by prolonged soreness (days) when the numbness provided by the local anesthetic dissipates later.

Slow injection is defined ideally as the deposition of 1 mL of local anesthetic solution in not less than 60 seconds. Therefore a full 1.8 mL cartridge requires approximately 2 minutes to be deposited. Through slow deposition, the solution is able to diffuse along normal tissue planes without producing discomfort during or following injection.

Most local anesthetic administrators tend to administer these drugs too rapidly. In a survey of 209 dentists, 84% stated that the average time spent to deposit 1.8 mL of local anesthetic solution was less than 20 seconds.[13]

In actual clinical practice, it therefore seems highly improbable to expect doctors to change their rate of injection from less than 20 seconds to a safe and comfortable 2 minutes per cartridge. A more realistic time span in a clinical situation is 60 seconds for a full 1.8 mL cartridge. This rate of deposition of solution does not produce tissue damage during or after anesthesia and, in the event of accidental intravascular injection, does not produce an extremely serious reaction. Few injection techniques require the administration of 1.8 mL for success.

For many years, the author has used one particular method to slow the rate of injection. After two negative aspirations, he deposits a volume of solution (approximately one fourth of the total to be deposited) and then aspirates again. If the aspiration is negative, he deposits another fourth of the solution, reaspirates, and continues this process until the total volume of solution for the given injection is deposited. This enables him to do two positive things during injection: (1) to reaffirm through multiple negative aspirations that the solution is in fact being deposited extravascularly, and (2) to stop the injection for aspiration; this automatically slows the rate of deposit and thereby minimizes patient discomfort. In the first situation, if positive aspiration occurs after deposition of one-fourth of a cartridge, only 9 mg of a 2% solution, or 13.5 mg of a 3% solution, or 18 mg of a 4% solution will have been deposited intravascularly—doses unlikely to provoke a drug-related adverse reaction. The needle tip should be repositioned, negative aspiration (×2) achieved, and the injection continued. The risk of an adverse reaction secondary to intravascular injection is greatly minimized in this manner.

◆ **Step 16B:** Communicate with the patient. The patient should be communicated with during deposition of the local anesthetic. Most patients are accustomed to receiving their local anesthetic injections rapidly. Statements such as, "I'm depositing the solution (or "I'm doing this") slowly so it will be more comfortable for you, but you're not receiving any more than is usual" go far to allay a patient's apprehension at this time. The second part of the statement is important, because some patients might not realize that there is a fixed volume of anesthetic solution in the syringe. A reminder that they are not receiving any more than is usual is a comfort to the patient.

◆ **Step 17:** Slowly withdraw the syringe. After completion of the injection, the syringe should be slowly withdrawn from the soft tissues and the needle made safe by capping it immediately with its plastic sheath via the scoop technique.

Concerns about the possibility of needle-stick injury and the spread of infection caused by inadvertent sticking with contaminated needles have led to the formulation of guidelines for the recapping of needles for health care providers.[14] It has been demonstrated that the time health professionals are most apt to be injured with needles is when recapping after administration of an injection.[15,16] At this time, the needle is contaminated with blood, tissue, and (after intraoral injection) saliva. A number of devices have been marketed to aid the health professional in recapping the needle safely.[17] Needle guards, placed over the needle cap before injection, prevent fingers from being stuck during recapping. Although guidelines are not yet in effect, the following are most often mentioned for preventing accidental needlestick: Needles should not be reused. After their use, needles should immediately be discarded into a sharps container. This policy, although applicable in almost all nondental hospital situations in which only one injection is administered is, in many clinical situations, impractical in dentistry, where multiple injections are commonplace. The "scoop" technique (Fig. 11-18)—in which the needle cap has been placed on the instrument tray, and after injection the administrator simply slides the needle tip into the cap (without physically touching the cap), scooping up the needle cap—can be used for multiple injections without increased risk. The capped needle is then discarded in a sharps container (Fig. 11-19). An acrylic needle holder that holds the cap upright during injection can be purchased or fabricated. The needle then can be reinserted into the cap without difficulty after injection (Fig. 11-20).

◆ **Step 18:** Observe the patient. After completion of the injection, the doctor, hygienist, or assistant should remain with the patient while the anesthetic begins to take effect (and its blood level increases). Most true adverse drug reactions, especially those related to intraorally administered local anesthetics, develop either during the injection or within 5 to 10 minutes of its completion. All too often, reports are heard of situations in which a local anesthetic was administered and the doctor left the patient alone for a few minutes only to return to find the patient seizing or unconscious. Matsuura reported that 54.9% of all medical

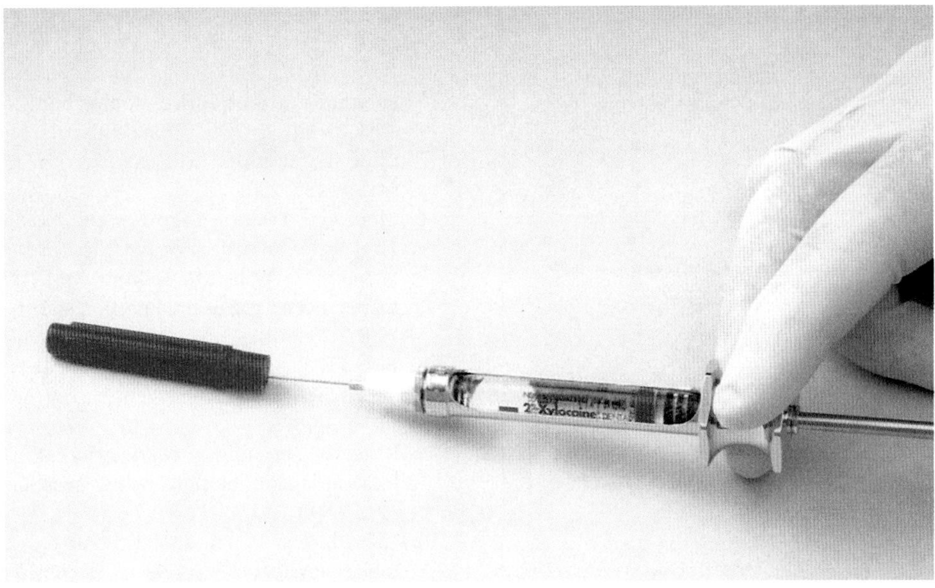

Figure 11-18. "Scoop" technique for recapping needle after use.

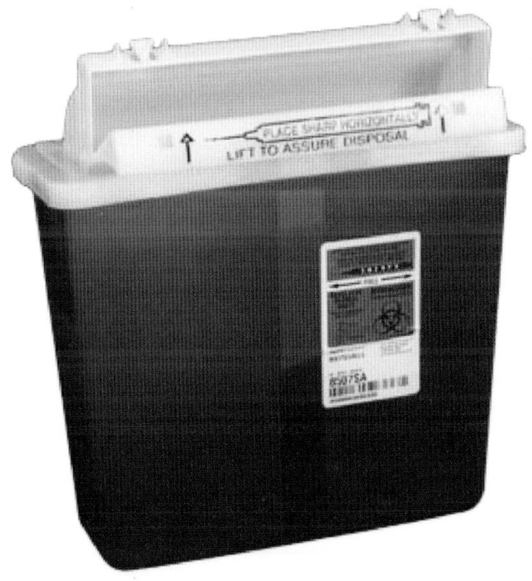

Figure 11-19. Sharps container for needle.

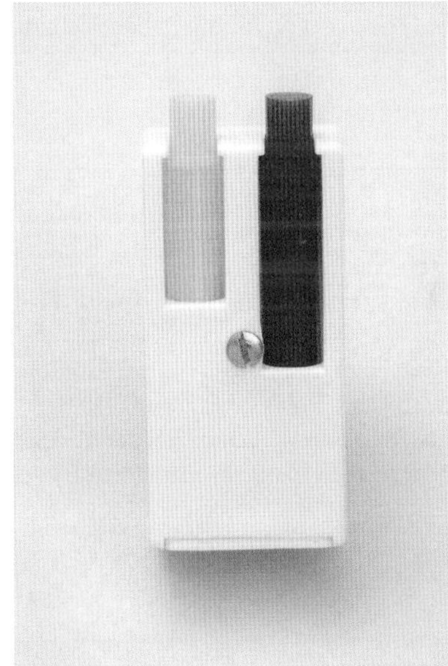

Figure 11-20. Plastic needle cap holder.

emergencies arising in Japanese dental offices developed either during the injection of local anesthetics or in the 5 minutes immediately after their administration.[2] Patients should not be left unattended after administration of a local anesthetic.

◆ **Step 19:** Record the injection on the patient's chart. An entry must be made of the local anesthetic drug used, the vasoconstrictor used (if any), the dose (in milligrams) of the solution(s) used, the needle(s) used, the injection(s) given, and the patient's reaction. For example, in the patient's dental progress notes, the following might be inscribed: R-IANB, 25-long, 2% lido + 1 : 100,000 epi, 36 mg. Tolerated procedure well.

The administrator of local anesthetics who adheres to these steps develops a reputation among patients as a "painless dentist." It is not possible to guarantee that every injection will be absolutely atraumatic because the reactions of both patients and doctors are far too variable. However, even when they feel some discomfort, patients invariably state that the injection was better than any other they had previously experienced. This should be the goal sought with every local anesthetic injection.

The atraumatic injection technique was developed over many years by Dr. Nathan Friedman and the Department of Human Behavior at the University of Southern California School of Dentistry. These principles are incorporated into this section.

ATRAUMATIC INJECTION TECHNIQUE

1. Use a sterilized sharp needle.
2. Check the flow of local anesthetic solution.
3. Determine whether to warm the anesthetic cartridge or syringe.
4. Position the patient.
5. Dry the tissue.
6. Apply topical antiseptic (optional).
7a. Apply topical anesthetic.
7b. Communicate with the patient.
8. Establish a firm hand rest.
9. Make the tissue taut.
10. Keep the syringe out of the patient's line of sight.
11a. Insert the needle into the mucosa.
11b. Watch and communicate with the patient.
12. Inject several drops of local anesthetic solution (optional).
13. Slowly advance the needle toward the target.
14. Deposit several drops of local anesthetic before touching the periosteum.
15. Aspirate ×2.
16a. Slowly deposit the local anesthetic solution.
16b. Communicate with the patient.
17. Slowly withdraw the syringe. Cap the needle and discard.
18. Observe the patient after the injection.
19. Record the injection on the patient's chart.

References

1. de St Georges J: How dentists are judged by patients, Dent Today 23:96, 98–99, 2004.
2. Matsuura H: Analysis of systemic complications and deaths during dental treatment in Japan, Anesth Prog 36:219–228, 1989.
3. Malamed SF: Emergency medicine: preparation and basics of management, Dent Today 20:64, 66–67, 2001.
4. Hanna MN, Elhassan A, Veloso PM, et al: Efficacy of bicarbonate in decreasing pain on intradermal injection of local anesthetics: a meta-analysis, Reg Anesth Pain Med 34:122–125, 2009.
5. Burns CA, Ferris G, Feng C, et al: Decreasing the pain of local anesthesia: a prospective, double-blind comparison of buffered, premixed 1% lidocaine with epinephrine versus 1% lidocaine freshly mixed with epinephrine, J Am Acad Dermatol 54:128–131, 2006.
6. Mollen AJ, Ficara AJ, Provant DR: Needles—25 gauge versus 27 gauge—can patients really tell? Gen Dent 29:417–418, 1981.
7. Flanagan T, Wahl MJ, Schmitt MM, Wahl JA: Size doesn't matter: needle gauge and injection pain, Gen Dent 55:216–217, 2007.
8. Benko K, Fiechtl J, Gray-Eurom K, et al: Fixing faces painlessly: facial anesthesia in emergency medicine, Emerg Med Pract 11:1–19, 2009.
9. Rogers KB, Fielding AF, Markiewicz SW: The effect of warming local anesthetic solutions before injection, Gen Dent 37:496–499, 1989.
10. Gill CJ, Orr DL: A double blind crossover comparison of topical anesthetics, J Am Dent Assoc 98:213, 1979.
11. Jeske AH, Blanton PL: Misconceptions involving dental local anesthesia. Part 2. Pharmacology, Tex Dent J 119:310–314, 2002.
12. Catchlove RF: The influence of CO_2 and pH on local anesthetic action, J Pharm Exp Ther 181:298–309, 1972.
13. Malamed SF: Results of a survey of 209 dentists. In Handbook of local anesthesia, ed 4, St Louis, 1997, Mosby.
14. Goldwater PN, Law R, Nixon AD, et al: Impact of a recapping device on venipuncture-related needlestick injury, Infect Control Hosp Epidemiol 10:11–25, 1989.
15. McCormick RD, Maki DG: Epidemiology of needle-stick injuries in hospital personnel, Am J Med 70:928–932, 1981.
16. Berry AJ, Greene ES: The risk of needlestick injuries and needlestick-transmitted diseases in the practice of anesthesiology, Anesthesiology 77:1007–1021, 1992.
17. Cuny E, Fredekind RE, Budenz AW: Dental safety needles' effectiveness: results of a one-year evaluation, J Am Dent Assoc 131:1443–1448, 2000.

CHAPTER 12

Anatomic Considerations

TRIGEMINAL NERVE

An understanding of the management of pain in dentistry requires thorough knowledge of the fifth (V) cranial nerve (Fig. 12-1). The right and left trigeminal nerves provide, among other functions, an overwhelming majority of sensory innervation from teeth, bone, and soft tissues of the oral cavity. The trigeminal nerve is the largest of the twelve cranial nerves. It is composed of a small motor root and a considerably larger (tripartite) sensory root. The motor root supplies the muscles of mastication and other muscles in the region. The three branches of the sensory root supply the skin of the entire face and the mucous membrane of the cranial viscera and oral cavity, except for the pharynx and base of the tongue. Table 12-1 summarizes the functions of the trigeminal nerve and the 11 other cranial nerves.

Motor Root

The motor root of the trigeminal nerve arises separately from the sensory root, originating in the motor nucleus within the pons and medulla oblongata (Fig. 12-2). Its fibers, forming a small nerve root, travel anteriorly along with, but entirely separate from, the larger sensory root to the region of the semilunar (or gasserian) ganglion. At the semilunar ganglion, the motor root passes in a lateral and inferior direction under the ganglion toward the foramen ovale, through which it leaves the middle cranial fossa along with the third division of the sensory root, the mandibular nerve (Figs. 12-3 and 12-4). Just after leaving the skull, the motor root unites with the sensory root of the mandibular division to form a single nerve trunk.

Motor fibers of the trigeminal nerve supply the following muscles:

1. Masticatory
   a. Masseter
   b. Temporalis
   c. Pterygoideus medialis
   d. Pterygoideus lateralis
2. Mylohyoid
3. Anterior belly of the digastric
4. Tensor tympani
5. Tensor veli palatini

Sensory Root

Sensory root fibers of the trigeminal nerve constitute the central processes of ganglion cells located in the trigeminal (semilunar or gasserian) ganglion. Two ganglia are present, one innervating each side of the face. They are located in Meckel's cavity, on the anterior surface of the petrous portion of the temporal bone (see Fig. 12-3). The ganglia are flat and crescent shaped and measure approximately 1.0 × 2.0 cm; their convexities face anteriorly and downward. Sensory root fibers enter the concave portion of each crescent, and the three sensory divisions of the trigeminal nerve exit from the convexity:

1. The ophthalmic division (V_1) travels anteriorly in the lateral wall of the cavernous sinus to the medial part of the superior orbital fissure, through which it exits the skull into the orbit.
2. The maxillary division (V_2) travels anteriorly and downward to exit the cranium through the foramen rotundum into the upper portion of the pterygopalatine fossa.
3. The mandibular division (V_3) travels almost directly downward to exit the skull, along with the motor root, through the foramen ovale. These two roots then intermingle, forming one nerve trunk that enters the infratemporal fossa.

On exiting the cranium through their respective foramina, the three divisions of the trigeminal nerve divide into a multitude of sensory branches.

Each of the three divisions of the trigeminal nerve is described, but more attention is devoted to the maxillary and mandibular divisions because of their greater importance in pain control in dentistry. Figure 12-5 illustrates the sensory distribution of the trigeminal nerve.

Ophthalmic Division (V_1). The ophthalmic division is the first branch of the trigeminal nerve. It is purely sensory and is the smallest of the three divisions. It leaves the cranium

Text continued on p. 175

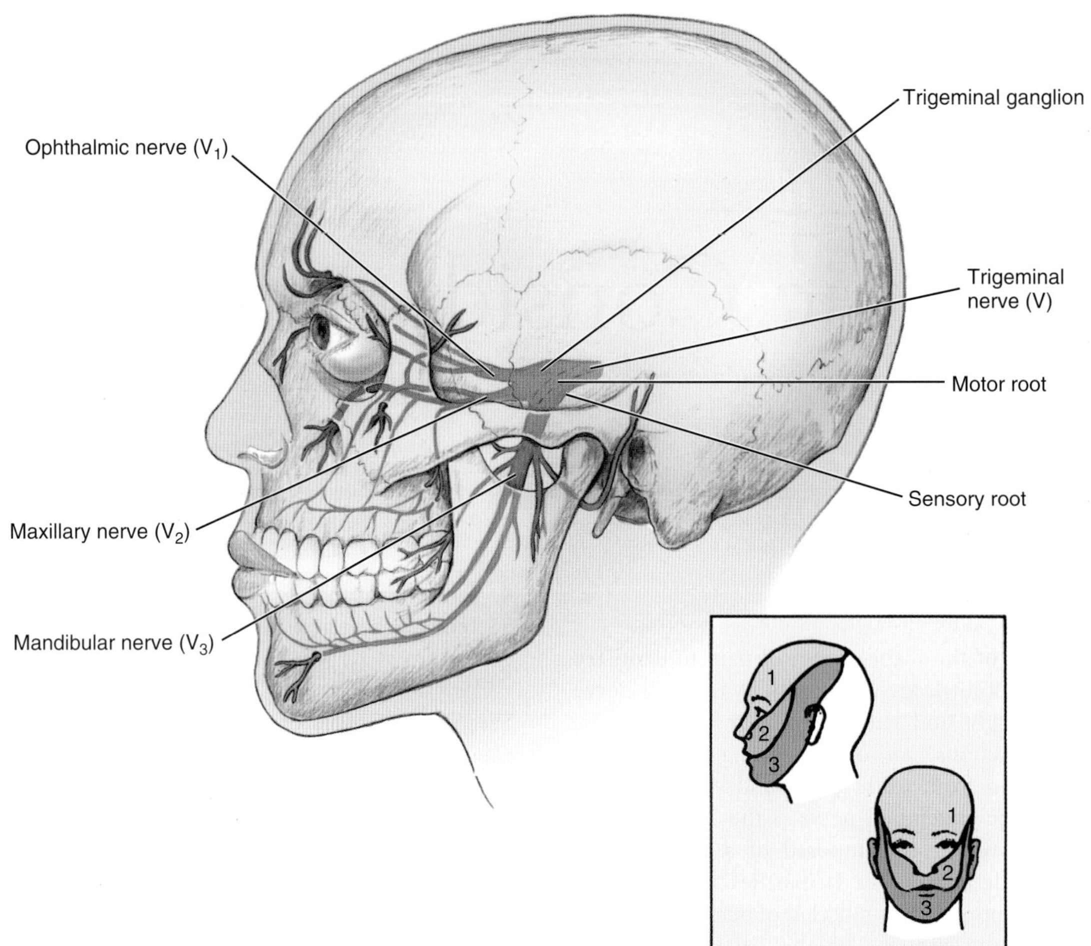

Figure 12-1. The general pathway of the trigeminal or fifth cranial nerve and its motor and sensory roots and three divisions (inset shows the pattern of innervation for each nerve division). (From Fehrenbach MJ, Herring SW: Anatomy of the head and neck, ed 3, St Louis, 2007, Saunders.)

TABLE 12-1
Cranial Nerves

Number	Name	Type	Function
I	Olfactory	Sensory	Smell
II	Optic	Sensory	Vision
III	Oculomotor	Motor	Supplies 4 of the 6 extraocular muscles of the eye and the muscle of the upper eyelid
IV	Trochlear	Motor	Innervates superior oblique muscle (turns eye downward and laterally)
V	Trigeminal	Mixed	
V_1	Ophthalmic	Sensory	V_1 Sensory from muscles of forehead; V_2 Sensory from lower eyelids, zygoma and upper lip; V_3 Sensory from lateral scalp, skin anterior to ears, lower cheeks, lower lips and anterior aspect of mandible; Motor to muscles of mastication (temporalis, masseter, medial and lateral pterygoids, tensor veli palatine and tensor tympani)
V_2	Maxillary	Sensory	
V_3	Mandibular	Sensory & motor	
VI	Abducens	Motor	Innervates lateral rectus muscle of eye
VII	Facial	Motor	Innervates muscles of facial expression; taste sensation from anterior 2/3 of tongue, hard and soft palates; Secretomotor innervation of salivary glands (except parotid) and lacrimal gland
VIII	Auditory (vestibulocochlear)	Sensory	Vestibular branch = equilibrium; Cochlear branch = hearing
IX	Glossopharyngeal	Mixed	Taste from posterior 1/3 of tongue; Secretomotor innervation to parotid gland; Motor to stylopharyngeal muscle
X	Vagus	Mixed	Motor to voluntary muscles of pharynx and larynx (except stylopharyngeal); Parasympathetic to smooth muscle and glands of pharynx and larynx, and viscera of thorax and abdomen; Sensory from stretch receptors of aortic arch and chemoreceptors of aortic bodies; Controls muscles for voice and resonance and the soft palate
XI	Accessory	Motor	Motor to sternocleidomastoid and trapezius muscles; Innervates muscles of larynx and pharynx
XII	Hypoglossal	Motor	Motor to muscles of tongue and other glossal muscles

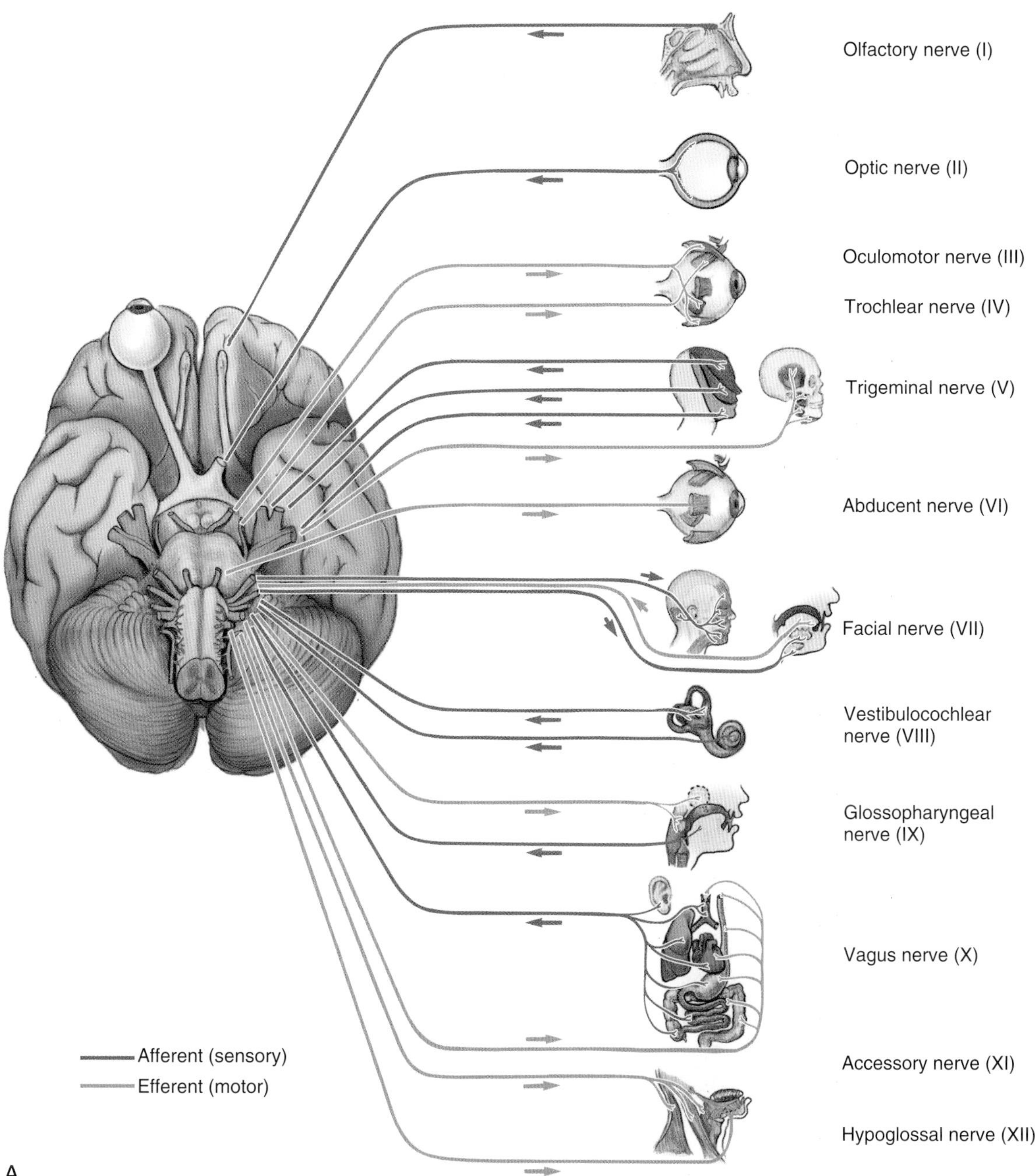

Figure 12-2. A, Inferior view of the brain showing cranial nerves and the organs and tissues they innervate.

Continued

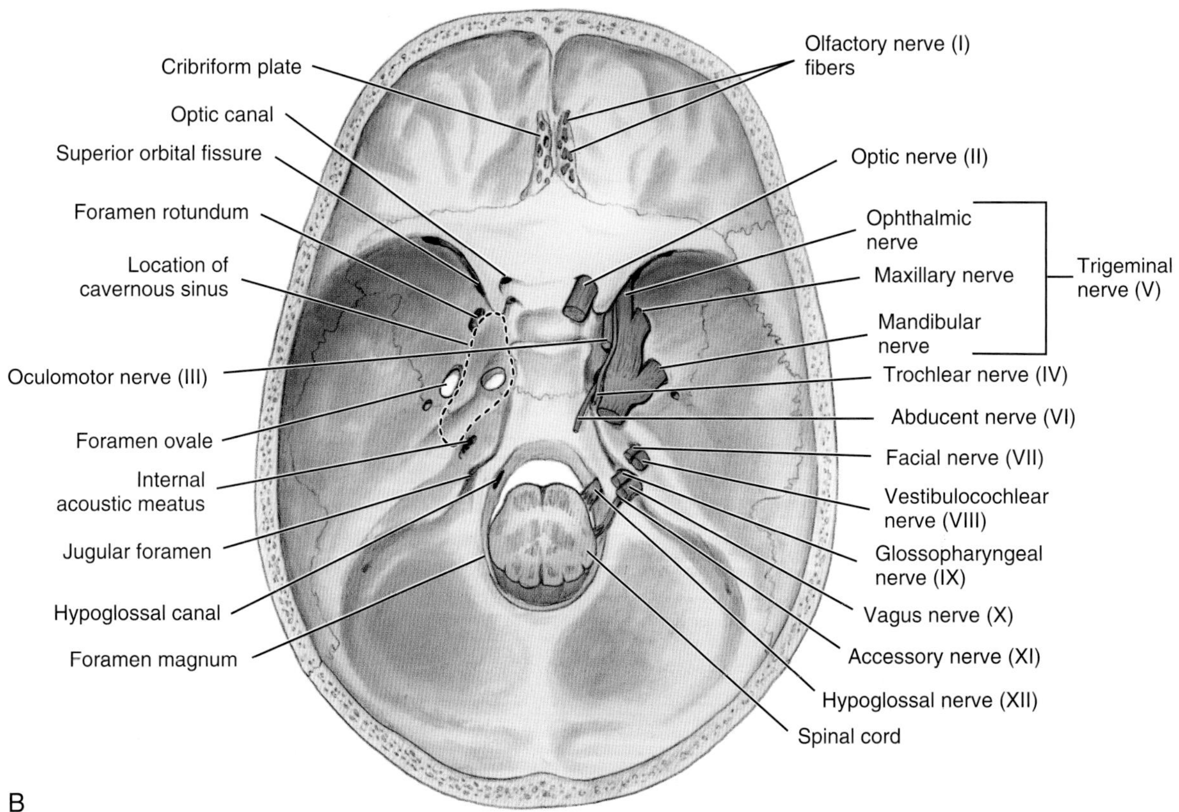

Figure 12-2, cont'd. B, Internal view of the base of the skull showing cranial nerves exiting or entering the skull. (From Fehrenbach MJ, Herring SW: Anatomy of the head and neck, ed 3, St Louis, 2007, Saunders.)

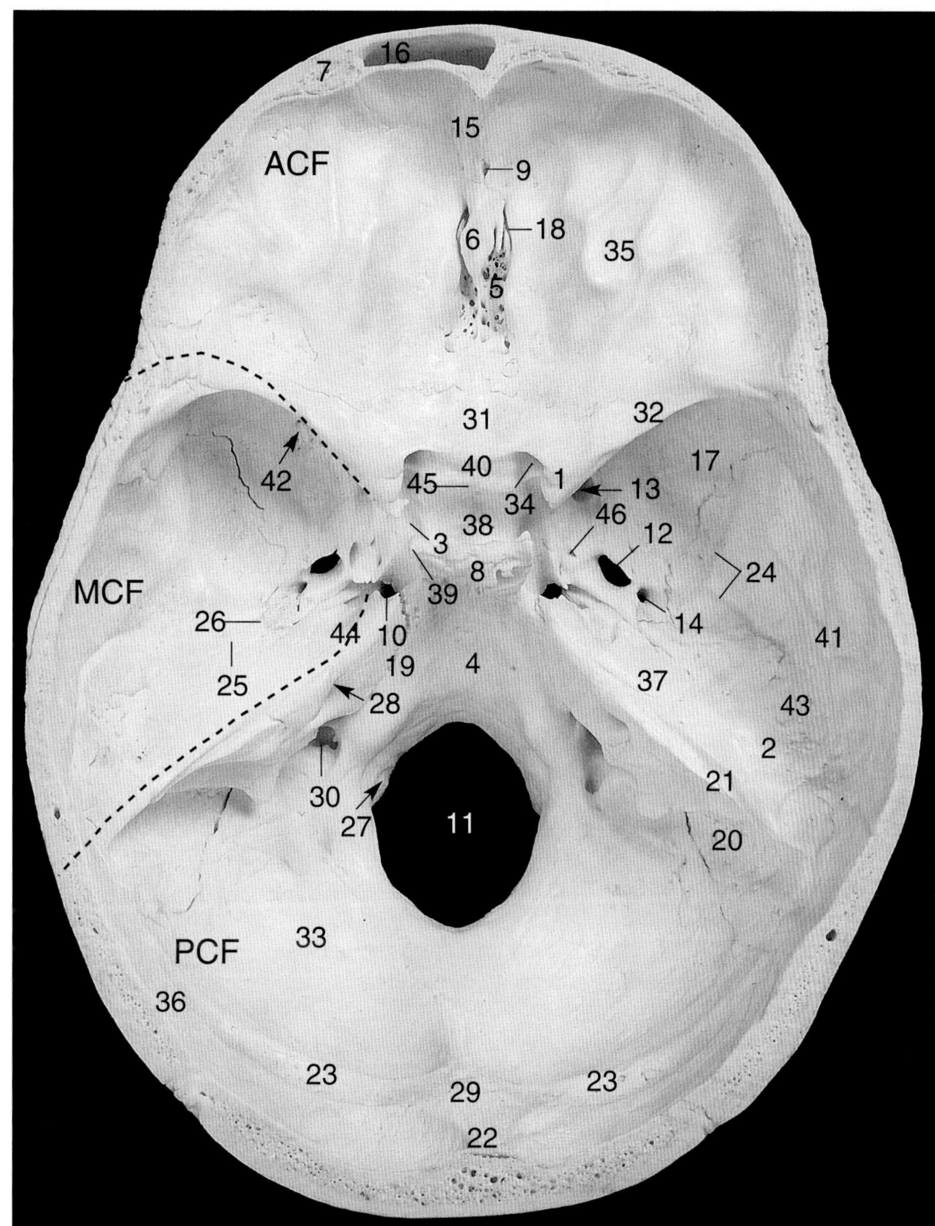

Figure 12-3. Internal surface of the base of the skull (cranial fossa). *ACF,* Anterior cranial fossa; *MCF,* middle cranial fossa; *PCF,* posterior cranial fossa. *1,* Anterior clinoid process; *2,* arcuate eminence; *3,* carotid groove; *4,* clivus; *5,* cribriform plate of ethmoid bone; *6,* crista galli; *7,* diploë; *8,* dorsum sellae; *9,* foramen cecum; *10,* foramen lacerum; *11,* foramen magnum; *12,* foramen ovale; *13,* foramen rotundum; *14,* foramen spinosum; *15,* frontal crest; *16,* frontal sinus; *17,* greater wing of sphenoid bone; *18,* groove for anterior ethmoidal nerve and vessels; *19,* groove for inferior petrosal sinus; *20,* groove for sigmoid sinus; *21,* groove for superior petrosal sinus; *22,* groove for superior sagittal sinus; *23,* groove for transverse sinus; *24,* grooves for middle meningeal vessels; *25,* hiatus and groove for greater petrosal nerve; *26,* hiatus and groove for lesser petrosal nerve; *27,* hypoglossal canal; *28,* internal acoustic meatus; *29,* internal occipital protuberance; *30,* jugular foramen; *31,* jugum of sphenoid bone; *32,* lesser wing of sphenoid bone; *33,* occipital bone; *34,* optic canal; *35,* orbital part of frontal bone; *36,* parietal bone (posteroinferior angle only); *37,* petrous part of temporal bone; *38,* pituitary fossa (sella turcica); *39,* posterior clinoid process; *40,* prechiasmatic groove; *41,* squamous part of temporal bone; *42,* superior orbital fissure; *43,* tegmen tympani; *44,* trigeminal impression; *45,* tuberculum sellae; *46,* venous foramen. (Data from Abrahams PH, Marks SC Jr, Hutchings RT: McMinn's color atlas of human anatomy, ed 5, St Louis, 2003, Mosby.)

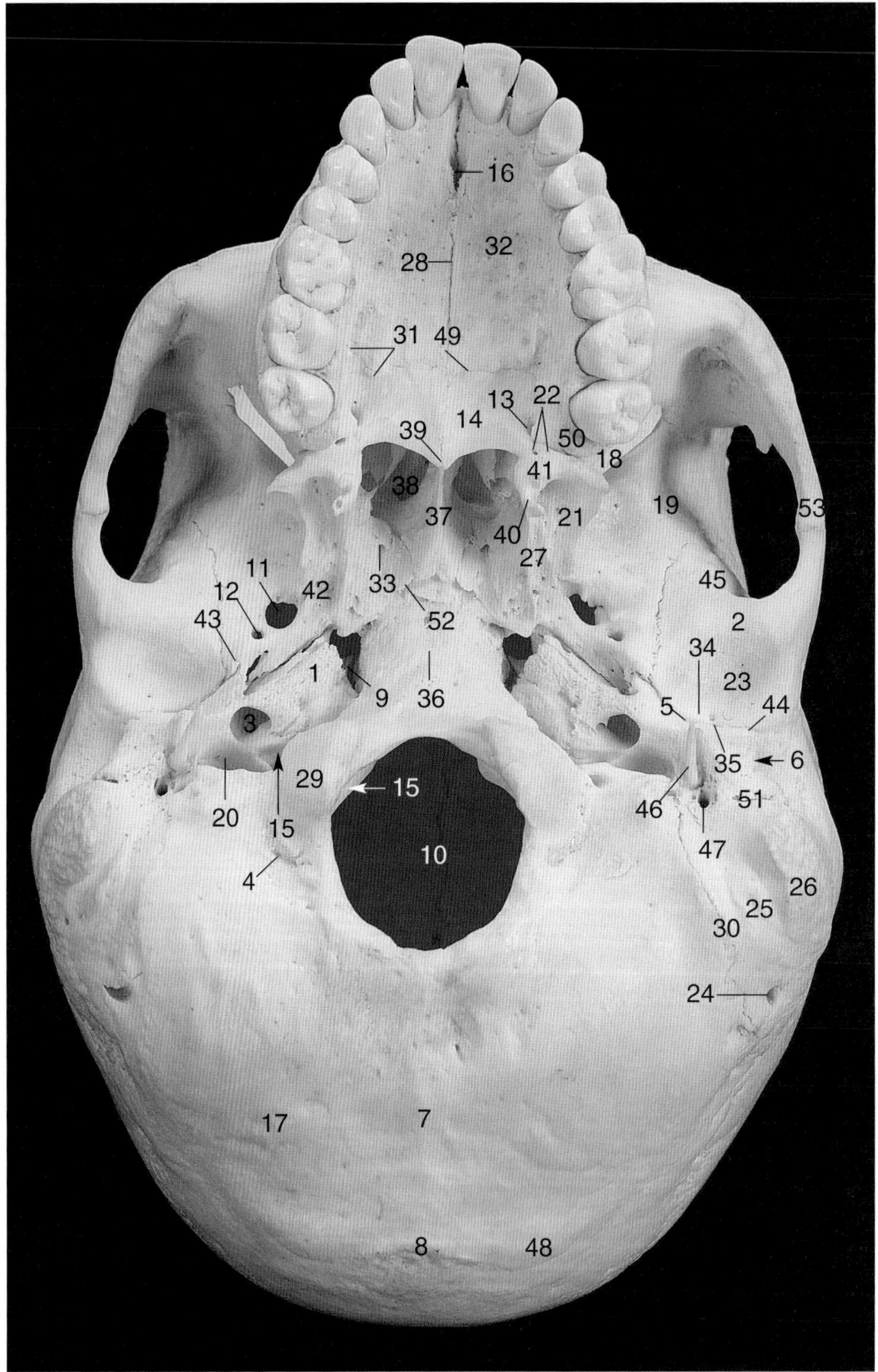

Figure 12-4. External surface of the base of the skull. *1,* Apex of petrous part of temporal bone; *2,* articular tubercle; *3,* carotid canal; *4,* condylar canal (posterior); *5,* edge of tegmen tympani; *6,* external acoustic meatus; *7,* external occipital crest; *8,* external occipital protuberance; *9,* foramen lacerum; *10,* foramen magnum; *11,* foramen ovale; *12,* foramen spinosum; *13,* greater palatine foramen; *14,* horizontal plate of palatine bone; *15,* hypoglossal (anterior condylar) canal; *16,* incisive fossa; *17,* inferior nuchal line; *18,* inferior orbital fissure; *19,* infratemporal crest of greater wing of sphenoid bone; *20,* jugular foramen; *21,* lateral pterygoid plate; *22,* lesser palatine foramina; *23,* mandibular fossa; *24,* mastoid foramen; *25,* mastoid notch; *26,* mastoid process; *27,* medial pterygoid plate; *28,* median palatine (intermaxillary) suture; *29,* occipital condyle; *30,* occipital groove; *31,* palatine grooves and spines; *32,* palatine process of maxilla; *33,* palatinovaginal canal; *34,* petrosquamous fissure; *35,* petrotympanic fissure; *36,* pharyngeal tubercle; *37,* posterior border of vomer; *38,* posterior nasal aperture (choana); *39,* posterior nasal spine; *40,* pterygoid hamulus; *41,* pyramidal process of palatine bone; *42,* scaphoid fossa; *43,* spine of sphenoid bone; *44,* squamotympanic fissure; *45,* squamous part of temporal bone; *46,* styloid process; *47,* stylomastoid foramen; *48,* superior nuchal line; *49,* transverse palatine (palatomaxillary) suture; *50,* tuberosity of maxilla; *51,* tympanic part of temporal bone; *52,* vomerovaginal canal; *53,* zygomatic arch. (Data from Abrahams PH, Marks SC Jr, Hutchings RT: McMinn's color atlas of human anatomy, ed 5, St Louis, 2003, Mosby.)

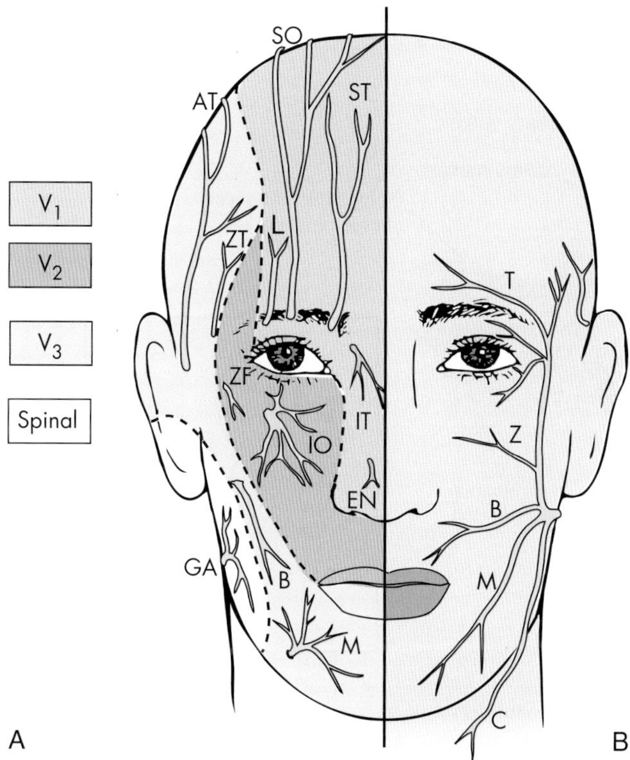

Figure 12-5. **A,** Cutaneous nerves of face. V_1 (ophthalmic nerve): *EN,* External nasal nerve; *IT,* infratrochlear nerve; *L,* lacrimal nerve; *SO,* Supraorbital nerve; *ST,* supratrochlear nerve. V_2 (maxillary nerve): *IO,* Infraorbital nerve; *ZF,* zygomaticofacial nerve; *ZT,* zygomaticotemporal nerve. V_3 (mandibular nerve): *AT,* Auriculotemporal nerve; *B,* buccal nerve; *M,* mental nerve. Spinal nerve: *GA,* Great auricular nerve. **B,** Motor nerves to muscles of facial expression. Facial branches of cranial nerve (CN) VII: *B,* buccal branches; *C,* cervical branches; *M,* mandibular branches; *T,* Temporal branches; *Z,* zygomatic branches. (Data from Liebgott B: The anatomical basis of dentistry, ed 3, St Louis, 2010, Mosby.)

and enters the orbit through the superior orbital fissure (Fig. 12-6). The nerve trunk is approximately 2.5 cm long. It supplies the eyeball, conjunctiva, lacrimal gland, parts of the mucous membrane of the nose and paranasal sinuses, and the skin of the forehead, eyelids, and nose. When the ophthalmic nerve (V_1) is paralyzed, the ocular conjunctiva becomes insensitive to touch.

Just before the ophthalmic nerve passes through the superior orbital fissure, it divides into its three main branches: nasociliary, frontal, and lacrimal nerves.

Nasociliary Nerve. The nasociliary nerve travels along the medial border of the orbital roof, giving off branches to the nasal cavity and ending in the skin at the root of the nose. It then branches into the anterior ethmoidal and external nasal nerves. The internal nasal nerve (from the anterior ethmoidal) supplies the mucous membrane of the anterior part of the nasal septum and the lateral wall of the nasal cavity. The ciliary ganglion contains sensory fibers that travel to the eyeball via the short ciliary nerves. Two or three long ciliary nerves supply the iris and cornea. The infratrochlear nerve supplies the skin of the lacrimal sac and the lacrimal caruncle, the posterior ethmoidal nerve supplies the ethmoidal and sphenoidal sinuses, and the external nasal nerve supplies the skin over the apex (tip) and the ala of the nose.

Frontal Nerve. The frontal nerve travels anteriorly in the orbit, dividing into two branches: supratrochlear and supraorbital. The frontal is the largest branch of the ophthalmic division. The supratrochlear nerve supplies the conjunctiva and skin of the medial aspect of the upper eyelid and the skin over the lower and mesial aspects of the forehead. The supraorbital nerve is sensory to the upper eyelid, the scalp as far back as the parietal bone, and the lambdoidal suture.

Lacrimal Nerve. The lacrimal nerve is the smallest branch of the ophthalmic division. It supplies the lateral part of the upper eyelid and a small adjacent area of skin.

Maxillary Division (V_2). The maxillary division of the trigeminal nerve arises from the middle of the trigeminal ganglion. Intermediate in size between ophthalmic and mandibular divisions, it is purely sensory in function.

Origins. The maxillary nerve passes horizontally forward, leaving the cranium through the foramen rotundum (see Fig. 12-3). The foramen rotundum is located in the greater wing of the sphenoid bone. Once outside the cranium, the maxillary nerve crosses the uppermost part of the pterygopalatine fossa, between the pterygoid plates of the sphenoid bone and the palatine bone. As it crosses the pterygopalatine fossa, it gives off branches to the sphenopalatine ganglion, the posterior superior alveolar nerve, and the zygomatic branches. It then angles laterally in a groove on the posterior surface of the maxilla, entering the orbit through the inferior orbital fissure. Within the orbit, it occupies the infraorbital groove and becomes the infraorbital nerve, which courses anteriorly into the infraorbital canal.

The maxillary division emerges on the anterior surface of the face through the infraorbital foramen, where it divides into its terminal branches, supplying the skin of the face, nose, lower eyelid, and upper lip (Fig. 12-7). The following is a summary of maxillary division innervation:

1. Skin
   a. Middle portion of the face
   b. Lower eyelid
   c. Side of the nose
   d. Upper lip
2. Mucous membrane
   a. Nasopharynx
   b. Maxillary sinus
   c. Soft palate
   d. Tonsil
   e. Hard palate
3. Maxillary teeth and periodontal tissues

Branches. The maxillary division gives off branches in four regions: within the cranium, in the pterygopalatine fossa, in the infraorbital canal, and on the face.

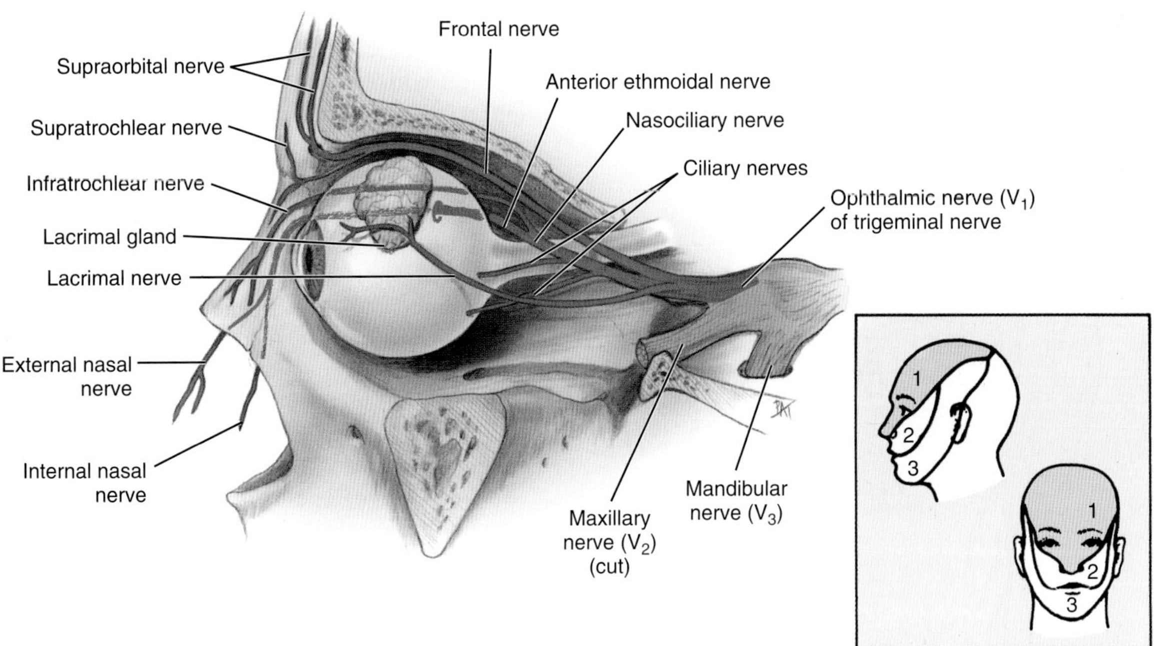

Figure 12-6. Lateral view of the cut-away orbit with the pathway of the ophthalmic nerve of the trigeminal nerve highlighted. (From Fehrenbach MJ, Herring SW: Anatomy of the head and neck, ed 3, St Louis, 2007, Saunders.)

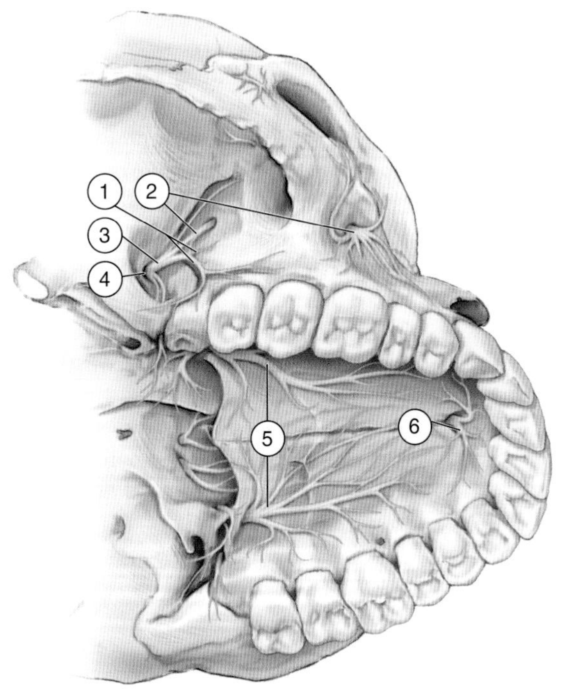

Figure 12-7. Distribution of the maxillary division (V_2). 1, Posterior superior alveolar branches; 2, infraorbital nerve; 3, maxillary nerve; 4, foramen rotundum; 5, greater palatine nerve; 6, nasopalatine nerve. (Data from Haglund J, Evers H: Local anaesthesia in dentistry, ed 2, Södertälje, Sweden, 1975, Astra Läkemedel.)

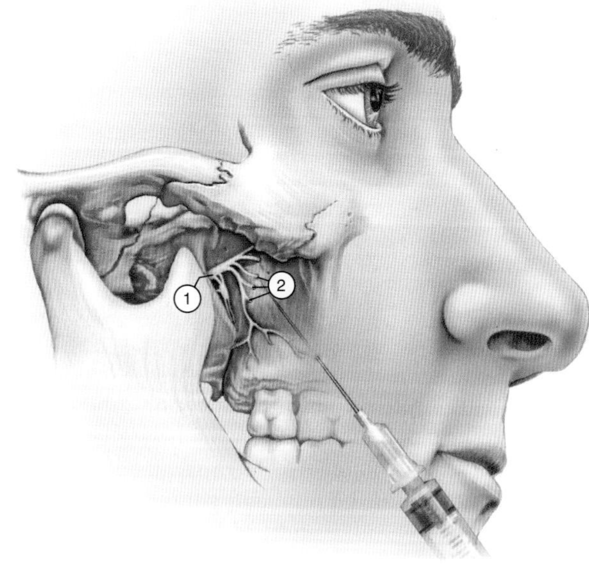

Figure 12-8. Branches of V_2 in the pterygopalatine fossa. 1, Maxillary nerve; 2, posterior superior alveolar branches. (Data from Haglund J, Evers H: Local anaesthesia in dentistry, ed 2, Södertälje, Sweden, 1975, Astra Läkemedel.)

Branch Within the Cranium. Immediately after separating from the trigeminal ganglion, the maxillary division gives off a small branch, the middle meningeal nerve, which travels with the middle meningeal artery to provide sensory innervation to the dura mater.

Branches in the Pterygopalatine Fossa. After exiting the cranium through the foramen rotundum, the maxillary division crosses the pterygopalatine fossa. In this fossa, several branches are given off (Fig. 12-8): the zygomatic nerve, the pterygopalatine nerves, and the posterior superior alveolar nerve.

The zygomatic nerve comes off the maxillary division in the pterygopalatine fossa and travels anteriorly, entering the orbit through the inferior orbital fissure, where it divides into the zygomaticotemporal and zygomaticofacial nerves: the zygomaticotemporal supplying sensory innervation to the skin on the side of the forehead, and the zygomaticofacial supplying the skin on the prominence of the cheek. Just before leaving the orbit, the zygomatic nerve sends a branch that communicates with the lacrimal nerve of the ophthalmic division. This branch carries secretory fibers from the sphenopalatine ganglion to the lacrimal gland.

The pterygopalatine nerves are two short trunks that unite in the pterygopalatine ganglion and are then redistributed into several branches. They also serve as a communication between the pterygopalatine ganglion and the maxillary nerve (V_2). Postganglionic secretomotor fibers from the pterygopalatine ganglion pass through these nerves and back along V_2 to the zygomatic nerve, through which they are routed to the lacrimal nerve and the lacrimal gland.

Branches of the pterygopalatine nerves include those that supply four areas: orbit, nose, palate, and pharynx.

1. The orbital branches supply the periosteum of the orbit.
2. The nasal branches supply the mucous membranes of the superior and middle conchae, the lining of the posterior ethmoidal sinuses, and the posterior portion of the nasal septum. One branch is significant in dentistry, the nasopalatine nerve, which passes across the roof of the nasal cavity downward and forward, where it lies between the mucous membrane and the periosteum of the nasal septum. The nasopalatine nerve continues downward, reaching the floor of the nasal cavity and giving branches to the anterior part of the nasal septum and the floor of the nose. It then enters the incisive canal, through which it passes into the oral cavity via the incisive foramen, located in the midline of the palate about 1 cm posterior to the maxillary central incisors. The right and left nasopalatine nerves emerge together through this foramen and provide sensation to the palatal mucosa in the region of the premaxilla (canines through central incisors) (Fig. 12-9).
3. The palatine branches include the greater (or anterior) palatine nerve and the lesser (middle and posterior) palatine nerves (Fig. 12-10). The greater (or anterior) palatine nerve descends through the pterygopalatine canal, emerging on the hard palate through the greater palatine foramen (which is usually located about 1 cm toward the palatal midline, just distal to the second molar). Sicher and DuBrul have stated that the greater palatine foramen may be located 3 to 4 mm in front of the posterior border of the hard palate.[1] The nerve courses anteriorly between the mucoperiosteum and the osseous hard palate, supplying sensory innervation to the palatal soft tissues and bone as far anterior as the first premolar, where it communicates with terminal fibers of the nasopalatine nerve (see Fig. 12-10). It also provides sensory innervation to some parts of the soft palate. The middle palatine nerve emerges from the lesser palatine foramen, along with the posterior palatine nerve. The middle palatine nerve provides sensory innervation to the mucous membrane of

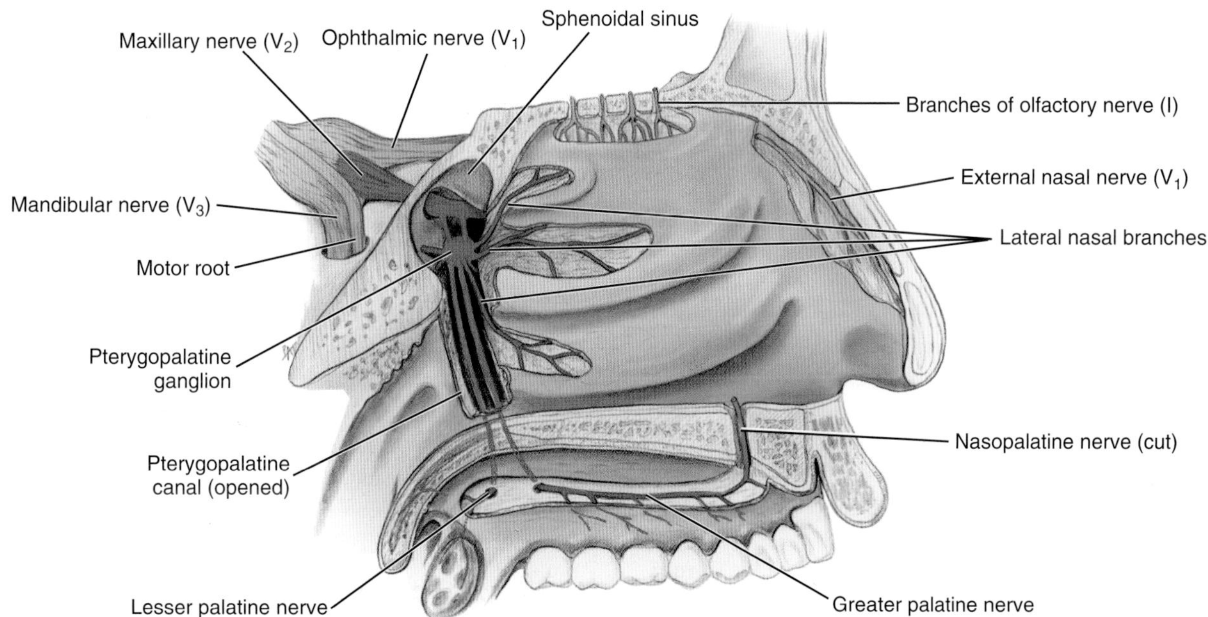

Figure 12-9. Medial view of the lateral nasal wall and the opened pterygopalatine canal highlighting the maxillary nerve and its palatine branches. The nasal septum has been removed, thus severing the nasopalatine nerve. (From Fehrenbach MJ, Herring SW: Anatomy of the head and neck, ed 3, St Louis, 2007, Saunders.)

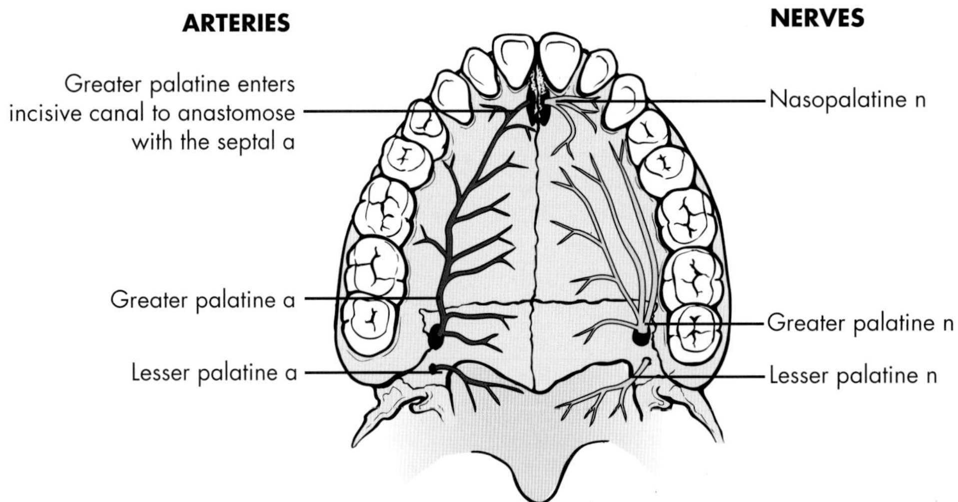

Figure 12-10. Blood and sensory nerve supply to hard and soft palate. *a,* Artery; *n,* nerve. (Data from Liebgott B: The anatomical basis of dentistry, ed 3, St Louis, 2010, Mosby.)

the soft palate; the tonsillar region is innervated, in part, by the posterior palatine nerve.

4. The pharyngeal branch is a small nerve that leaves the posterior part of the pterygopalatine ganglion, passes through the pharyngeal canal, and is distributed to the mucous membrane of the nasal part of the pharynx, posterior to the auditory (eustachian) tube.

The posterior superior alveolar (PSA) nerve descends from the main trunk of the maxillary division in the pterygopalatine fossa just before the maxillary division enters the infraorbital canal (see Fig. 12-7). Commonly there are two PSA branches, but on occasion a single trunk arises. Passing downward through the pterygopalatine fossa, they reach the inferior temporal (posterior) surface of the maxilla. When two trunks are present, one remains external to the bone, continuing downward on the posterior surface of the maxilla to provide sensory innervation to the buccal gingiva in the maxillary molar region and adjacent facial mucosal surfaces, whereas the other branch enters into the maxilla (along with a branch of the internal maxillary artery) through the PSA canal to travel down the posterior or posterolateral wall of the maxillary sinus, providing sensory innervation to the mucous membrane of the sinus. Continuing downward, this second branch of the PSA nerve provides sensory innervation to the alveoli, periodontal ligaments, and pulpal tissues of the maxillary third, second, and first molars (with the exception [in 28% of patients] of the mesiobuccal root of the first molar).

Branches in the Infraorbital Canal. Within the infraorbital canal, the maxillary division (V_2) gives off two branches of significance in dentistry: the middle superior and anterior superior alveolar nerves. While in the infraorbital groove and canal, the maxillary division is known as the *infraorbital nerve.*

The middle superior alveolar (MSA) nerve branches off the main nerve trunk (V_2) within the infraorbital canal to form a part of the superior dental plexus,[1] composed of the posterior, middle, and anterior superior alveolar nerves. The site of origin of the MSA nerve varies, from the posterior portion of the infraorbital canal to the anterior portion, near the infraorbital foramen. The MSA nerve provides sensory innervation to the two maxillary premolars and, perhaps, to the mesiobuccal root of the first molar and periodontal tissues, buccal soft tissue, and bone in the premolar region. Traditionally it has been stated that the MSA nerve is absent in 30%[2] to 54%[3] of individuals. Loetscher and Walton[4] found the MSA nerve to be present in 72% of the specimens examined. In its absence, its usual innervations are provided by either the PSA or the anterior superior alveolar (ASA) nerve, most frequently the latter.[1]

The anterior superior alveolar (ASA) nerve, a relatively large branch, is given off the infraorbital nerve (V_2) approximately 6 to 10 mm before the latter exits from the infraorbital foramen. Descending within the anterior wall of the maxillary sinus, it provides pulpal innervation to the central and lateral incisors and the canine, and sensory innervation to the periodontal tissues, buccal bone, and mucous membranes of these teeth (Fig. 12-11).

The ASA nerve communicates with the MSA nerve and gives off a small nasal branch that innervates the anterior part of the nasal cavity, along with branches of the pterygopalatine nerves. In persons without an MSA nerve, the ASA nerve frequently provides sensory innervation to the premolars and occasionally to the mesiobuccal root of the first molar.

The actual innervation of individual roots of all teeth, bone, and periodontal structures in both the maxilla and the mandible derives from terminal branches of larger nerves in the region. These nerve networks are termed the *dental plexus.*

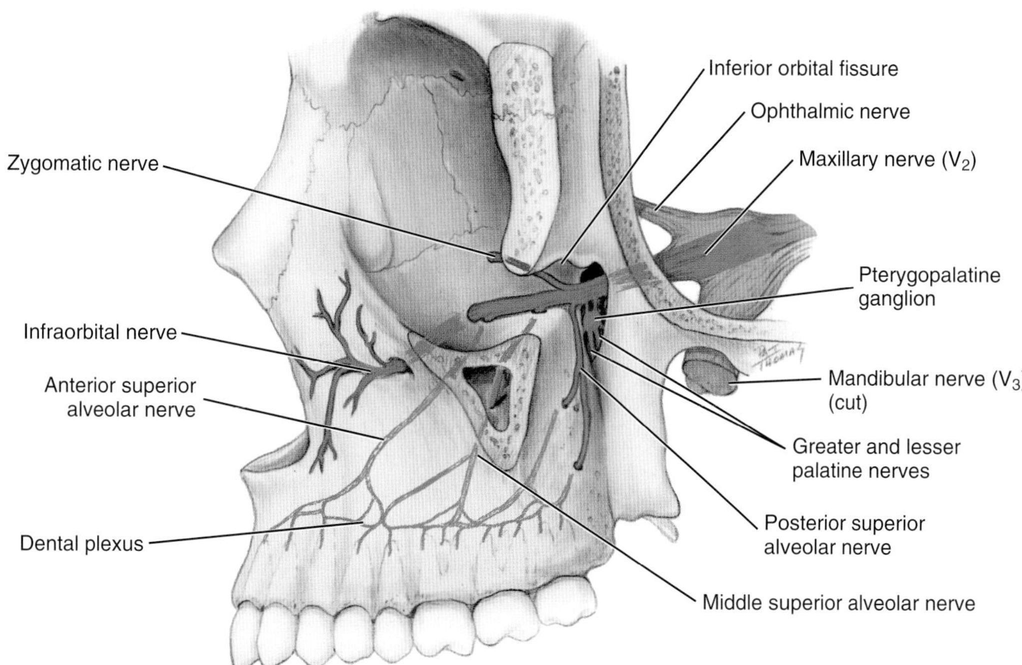

Figure 12-11. Lateral view of the skull (a portion of the lateral wall of the orbit has been removed) with the branches of the maxillary nerve highlighted. (From Fehrenbach MJ, Herring SW: Anatomy of the head and neck, ed 3, St Louis, 2007, Saunders.)

The superior dental plexus is composed of smaller nerve fibers from the three superior alveolar nerves (and in the mandible, from the inferior alveolar nerve). Three types of nerves emerge from these plexuses: dental nerves, interdental branches, and interradicular branches. Each is accompanied along its pathway by a corresponding artery.

The dental nerves are those that enter a tooth through the apical foramen, dividing into many small branches within the pulp. Pulpal innervation of all teeth is derived from dental nerves. Although in most instances one easily identifiable nerve is responsible, in some cases (usually the maxillary first molar) more than one nerve is responsible.

The interdental branches (also termed *perforating branches*) travel through the entire height of the interradicular septum, providing sensory innervation to the periodontal ligaments of adjacent teeth through the alveolar bone. They emerge at the height of the crest of the interalveolar septum and enter the gingiva to innervate the interdental papillae and the buccal gingiva.

The interradicular branches traverse the entire height of the interradicular or interalveolar septum, providing sensory innervation to the periodontal ligaments of adjacent roots. They terminate in the periodontal ligament (PDL) at the root furcations.

Branches on the Face. The infraorbital nerve emerges through the infraorbital foramen onto the face to divide into its terminal branches: inferior palpebral, external nasal, and superior labial. The inferior palpebral branches supply the skin of the lower eyelid with sensory innervation, the external nasal branches provide sensory innervation to the skin on the lateral aspect of the nose, and the superior labial branches provide sensory innervation to the skin and mucous membranes of the upper lip.

Although anesthesia of these nerves is not necessary for adequate pain control during dental treatment, they are frequently blocked in the process of carrying out other anesthetic procedures.

Summary. The following is a summary of the branches of the maxillary division (italicized nerves denote those of special significance in dental pain control):

1. Branches within the cranium
   a. Middle meningeal nerve
2. Branches within the pterygopalatine fossa
   a. Zygomatic nerve:
      Zygomaticotemporal nerve
      Zygomaticofacial nerve
   b. Pterygopalatine nerves
      Orbital branches
      Nasal branches
         Nasopalatine nerve
         Palatine branches
            Greater (anterior) palatine nerve
         Lesser (middle and posterior) palatine nerves
         Pharyngeal branch
   c. *Posterior superior alveolar nerve*
3. Branches within the infraorbital canal
   a. *Middle superior alveolar nerve*
   b. *Anterior superior alveolar nerve* (Fig. 12-12)
4. Branches on the face
   a. Inferior palpebral branches
   b. External nasal branches
   c. Superior labial branches

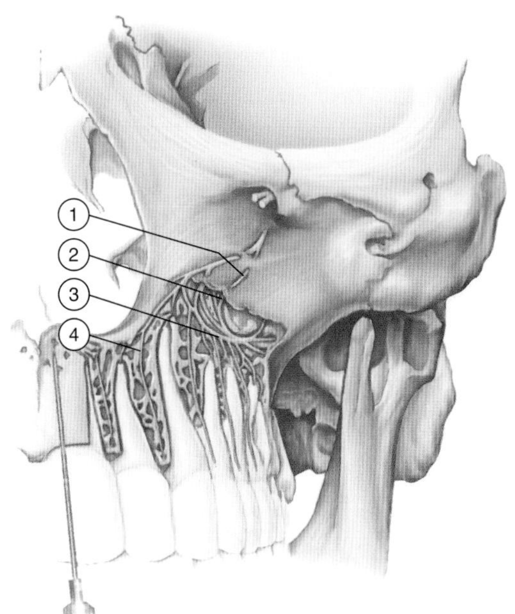

Figure 12-12. Anterior superior alveolar (ASA) nerve (bone over the nerves removed). 1, Branches of the ASA nerve; 2, superior dental plexus; 3, dental branches; 4, interdental and interradicular branches. (Data from Haglund J, Evers H: Local anaesthesia in dentistry, ed 2, Södertälje, Sweden, 1975, Astra Läkemedel.)

Mandibular Division (V_3). The mandibular division is the largest branch of the trigeminal nerve. It is a mixed nerve with two roots: a large sensory root and a smaller motor root (the latter representing the entire motor component of the trigeminal nerve). The sensory root of the mandibular division originates at the inferior angle of the trigeminal ganglion, whereas the motor root arises in motor cells located in the pons and medulla oblongata. The two roots emerge from the cranium separately through the foramen ovale, the motor root lying medial to the sensory. They unite just outside the skull and form the main trunk of the third division. This trunk remains undivided for only 2 to 3 mm before it splits into a small anterior and a large posterior division (Figs. 12-13 and 12-14).

The areas innervated by V_3 are included in the following outline:

1. Sensory root
   a. Skin
      Temporal region
      Auricula
      External auditory meatus
      Cheek
      Lower lip
      Lower part of the face (chin region)
   b. Mucous membrane
      Cheek
      Tongue (anterior two thirds)
      Mastoid cells

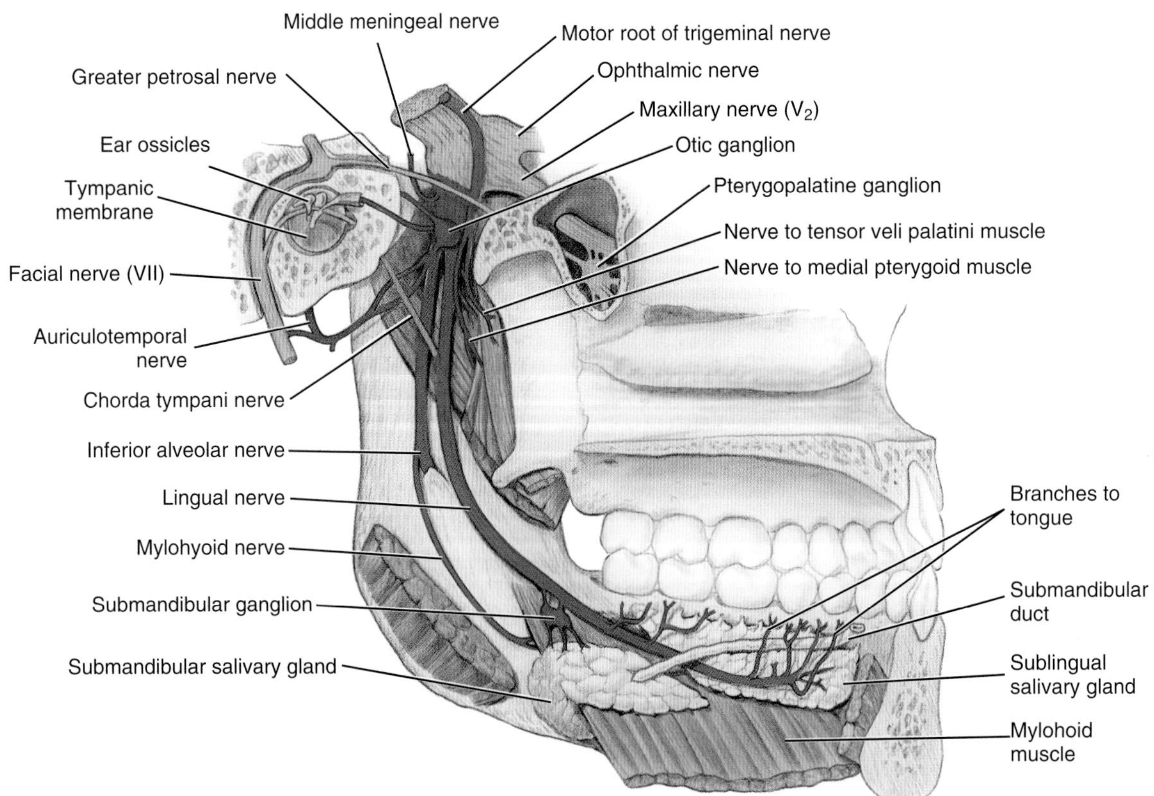

Figure 12-13. Medial view of the mandible with the motor and sensory branches of the mandibular nerve highlighted. (From Fehrenbach MJ, Herring SW: Anatomy of the head and neck, ed 3, St Louis, 2007, Saunders.)

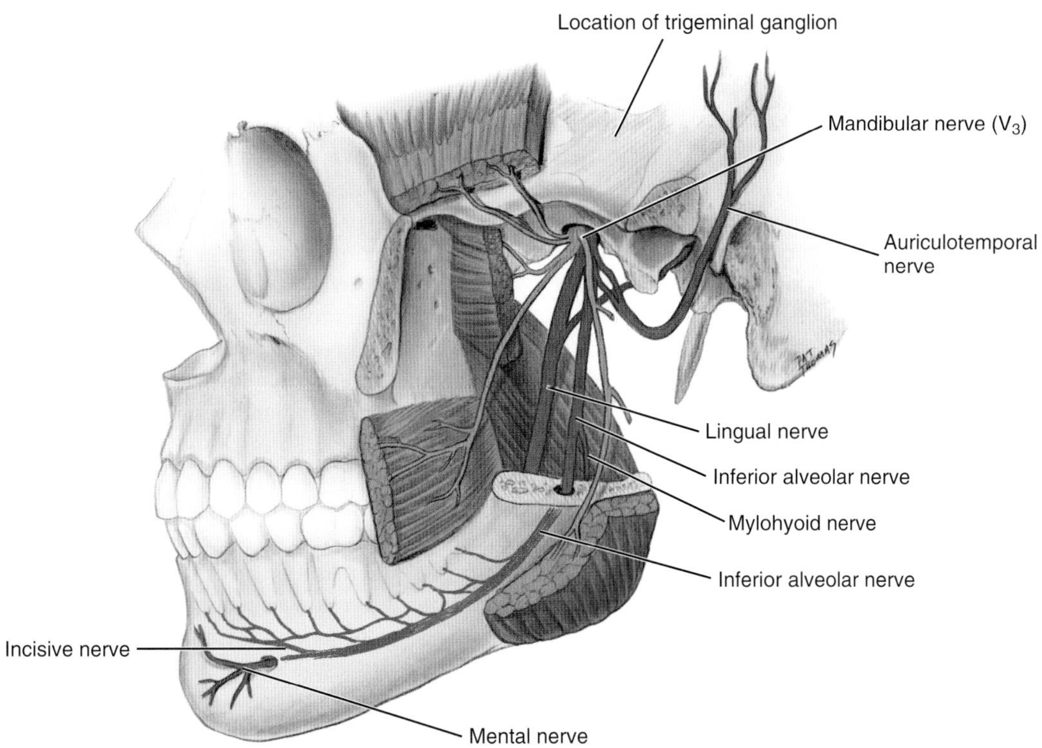

Figure 12-14. The pathway of the posterior trunk of the mandibular nerve of the trigeminal nerve is highlighted. (From Fehrenbach MJ, Herring SW: Anatomy of the head and neck, ed 3, St Louis, 2007, Saunders.)

   c. Mandibular teeth and periodontal tissues
   d. Bone of the mandible
   e. Temporomandibular joint
   f. Parotid gland
2. Motor root
   a. Masticatory muscles
      Masseter
      Temporalis
      Pterygoideus medialis
      Pterygoideus lateralis
   b. Mylohyoid
   c. Anterior belly of the digastric
   d. Tensor tympani
   e. Tensor veli palatini

Branches. The third division of the trigeminal nerve gives off branches in three areas: from the undivided nerve, and from the anterior and posterior divisions.

Branches from the Undivided Nerve. On leaving the foramen ovale, the main undivided nerve trunk gives off two branches during its 2- to 3-mm course. These are the nervus spinosus (meningeal branch of the mandibular nerve) and the medial pterygoid nerve. The nervus spinosus reenters the cranium through the foramen spinosum along with the middle meningeal artery to supply the dura mater and mastoid air cells. The medial pterygoid nerve is a motor nerve to the medial (internal) pterygoid muscle. It gives off small branches that are motor to the tensor veli palatini and the tensor tympani.

Branches from the Anterior Division. Branches from the anterior division of V_3 provide motor innervation to the muscles of mastication and sensory innervation to the mucous membrane of the cheek and the buccal mucous membrane of the mandibular molars.

The anterior division is significantly smaller than the posterior. It runs forward under the lateral (external) pterygoid muscle for a short distance and then reaches the external surface of that muscle by passing between its two heads or, less frequently, by winding over its upper border. From this point, it is known as the *buccal nerve.* Although under the lateral pterygoid muscle, the buccal nerve gives off several branches: the deep temporal nerves (to the temporal muscle) and the masseter and lateral pterygoid nerves (providing motor innervation to the respective muscles).

The buccal nerve, also known as the *buccinator nerve* and the *long buccal nerve,* usually passes between the two heads of the lateral pterygoid to reach the external surface of that muscle. It then follows the inferior part of the temporal muscle and emerges under the anterior border of the masseter muscle, continuing in an anterolateral direction. At the level of the occlusal plane of the mandibular third or second molar, it crosses in front of the anterior border of the ramus and enters the cheek through the buccinator muscle. Sensory fibers are distributed to the skin of the cheek. Other fibers pass into the retromolar triangle, providing sensory innervation to the buccal gingiva of the mandibular molars and the mucobuccal fold in that region. The buccal nerve does not innervate the buccinator muscle; the facial nerve does. Nor does it provide sensory innervation to the lower lip or the corner of the mouth. This is significant because some doctors do not administer the "long" buccal injection immediately after completing the inferior alveolar nerve block until the patient's lower lip has become numb. Their thinking is that the buccal nerve block will provide anesthesia to the lower lip and therefore might lead them to believe that their inferior alveolar nerve block has been successful, when in fact it has been missed. Such concern is unwarranted. *The buccal nerve block may be administered immediately after completion of the inferior alveolar nerve block.*

Anesthesia of the buccal nerve is important for dental procedures requiring soft tissue manipulation on the buccal surface of the mandibular molars.

Branches of the Posterior Division. The posterior division of V_3 is primarily sensory with a small motor component. It descends for a short distance downward and medial to the lateral pterygoid muscle, at which point it branches into the auriculotemporal, lingual, and inferior alveolar nerves.

The auriculotemporal nerve is not profoundly significant in dentistry. It traverses the upper part of the parotid gland and then crosses the posterior portion of the zygomatic arch. It gives off a number of branches, all of which are sensory. These include a communication with the facial nerve, providing sensory fibers to the skin over areas of innervation of the following motor branches of the facial nerve: zygomatic, buccal, and mandibular; a communication with the otic ganglion, providing sensory, secretory, and vasomotor fibers to the parotid gland; the anterior auricular branches, supplying the skin over the helix and tragus of the ear; branches to the external auditory meatus, innervating the skin over the meatus and the tympanic membrane; articular branches to the posterior portion of the temporomandibular joint; and superficial temporal branches, supplying the skin over the temporal region.[1-6]

The lingual nerve is the second branch of the posterior division of V_3. It passes downward medial to the lateral pterygoid muscle and, as it descends, lies between the ramus and the medial pterygoid muscle in the pterygomandibular space. It runs anterior and medial to the inferior alveolar nerve, whose path it parallels. It then continues downward and forward, deep to the pterygomandibular raphe and below the attachment of the superior constrictor of the pharynx, to reach the side of the base of the tongue slightly below and behind the mandibular third molar (see Figs. 12-13 and 12-14). Here it lies just below the mucous membrane in the lateral lingual sulcus, where it is so superficial in some persons that it may be seen just below the mucous membrane. It then proceeds anteriorly across the muscles of the tongue, looping downward and medial to the submandibular (Wharton's) duct to the deep surface of the sublingual gland, where it breaks up into its terminal branches.

The lingual nerve is the sensory tract to the anterior two thirds of the tongue. It provides both general sensation and gustation (taste) for this region. It is the nerve that supplies fibers for general sensation, whereas the chorda tympani (a branch of the facial nerve) supplies fibers for taste. In addition, the lingual nerve provides sensory innervation to the mucous membranes of the floor of the mouth and the gingiva on the lingual of the mandible. The lingual nerve is the nerve most commonly associated with cases of paresthesia (prolonged or permanent sensory nerve damage).

The inferior alveolar nerve is the largest branch of the mandibular division (see Fig. 12-14). It descends medial to the lateral pterygoid muscle and lateroposterior to the lingual nerve, to the region between the sphenomandibular ligament and the medial surface of the mandibular ramus, where it enters the mandibular canal at the level of the mandibular foramen. Throughout its path, it is accompanied by the inferior alveolar artery (a branch of the internal maxillary artery) and the inferior alveolar vein. The artery lies just anterior to the nerve. The nerve, artery, and vein travel anteriorly in the mandibular canal as far forward as the mental foramen, where the nerve divides into its terminal branches: the incisive nerve and the mental nerve.

Bifid (from the Latin meaning "cleft into two parts") inferior alveolar nerves and mandibular canals have been observed radiographically and categorized by Langlais and associates.[5] Among 6000 panoramic radiographs studied, bifid mandibular canals were evident in 0.95%. The bifid mandibular canal is clinically significant in that it increases the difficulty of achieving adequate anesthesia in the mandible through conventional techniques. This is especially so in the type 4 variation (Fig. 12-15), in which two separate mandibular foramina are present on each side of the mouth.

The mylohyoid nerve branches from the inferior alveolar nerve before entry of the latter into the mandibular canal (see Figs. 12-13 and 12-14). It runs downward and forward in the mylohyoid groove on the medial surface of the ramus and along the body of the mandible to reach the mylohyoid muscle. The mylohyoid is a mixed nerve, being motor to the mylohyoid muscle and the anterior belly of the digastric. It is thought to contain sensory fibers that supply the skin on the inferior and anterior surfaces of the mental protuberance. It also may provide sensory innervation to the mandibular incisors. Evidence suggests that the mylohyoid nerve also may be involved in supplying pulpal innervation to portions of the mandibular molars in some persons, usually the mesial root of the mandibular first molar.[6]

Once the inferior alveolar nerve enters the mandibular canal, it travels anteriorly along with the inferior alveolar artery and vein. The dental plexus serves the mandibular posterior teeth, entering through their apices and providing pulpal innervation. Other fibers supply sensory innervation to the buccal periodontal tissues of these same teeth.

The inferior alveolar nerve divides into its two terminal branches: the incisive nerve and the mental nerve at the mental foramen (see Fig. 12-14). The incisive nerve remains within the mandibular canal and forms a nerve plexus that innervates the pulpal tissues of the mandibular first premolar, canine, and incisors via the dental branches. The

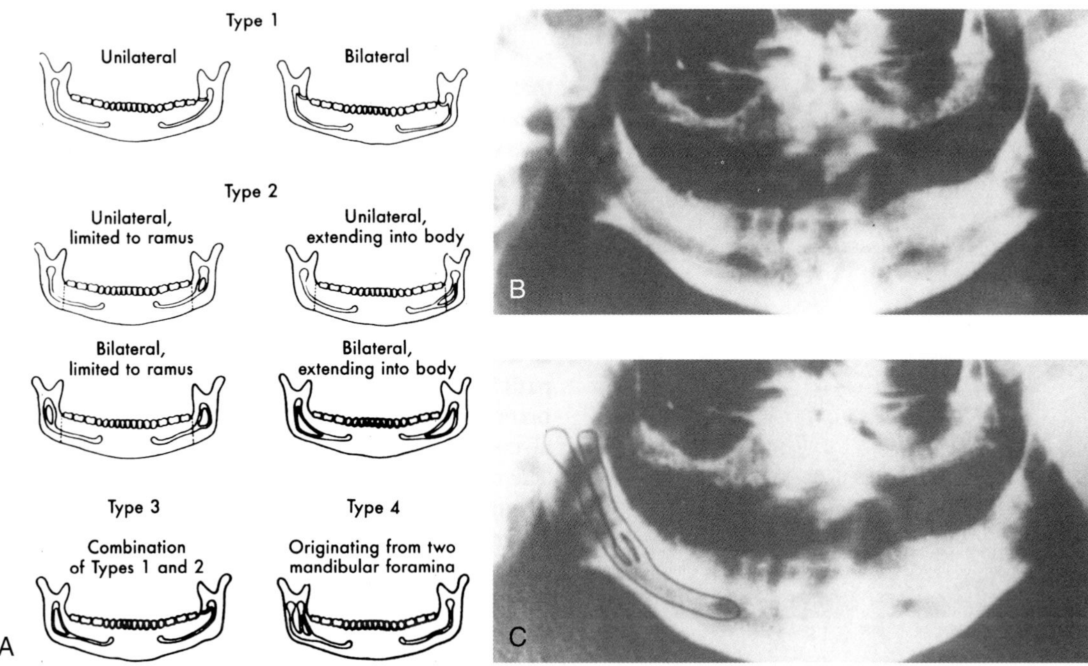

Figure 12-15. **A,** Variations in bifid mandibular canals. **B** and **C,** Radiographs of a type 4 bifid mandibular canal (**B,** on the patient's right; **C,** outlined). (Data from Langlais RP, Broadus R, Glass BJ: Bifid mandibular canals in panoramic radiographs, J Am Dent Assoc 110:923–926, 1985.)

mental nerve exits the canal through the mental foramen and divides into three branches that innervate the skin of the chin and the skin and mucous membrane of the lower lip.

Summary. The following outline summarizes the branches of the mandibular division (italicized nerves denote those especially significant in dental pain control):

1. Undivided nerve
   a. Nervus spinosus
   b. Nerve to the medial pterygoid muscle
2. Divided nerve
   a. Anterior division
      Nerve to the lateral pterygoid muscle
      Nerve to the masseter muscle
      Nerve to the temporal muscle
      Buccal nerve
   b. Posterior division
      Auriculotemporal nerve
      Lingual nerve
      Mylohyoid nerve
      Inferior alveolar nerve: dental branches
      Incisive branch: dental branches
      Mental nerve

OSTEOLOGY: MAXILLA

In addition to the neuroanatomy of pain control in dentistry, one should be aware of the relationship of these nerves to the osseous and soft tissues through which they course.

The maxilla (more properly, the right and left maxillae) is the largest bone of the face, excluding the mandible. Its anterior (or facial) surface (Fig. 12-16) is directed both forward and laterally. At its inferior borders are a series of eminences that correspond to the roots of the maxillary teeth. The most prominent usually is found over the canine tooth and is often referred to as the *canine eminence.* Superior to the canine fossa (located just distal to the canine eminence) is the infraorbital foramen, through which blood vessels and terminal branches of the infraorbital nerve emerge. Bone in the region of the maxillary teeth is commonly of the more porous cancellous variety, leading to a significantly greater incidence of clinically adequate anesthesia than in areas where more dense cortical bone is present, such as in the mandible. In many areas, bone over the apices of the maxillary teeth is tissue-paper thin or shows evidence of dehiscence.

The inferior temporal surface of the maxilla is directed backward and laterally (Fig. 12-17). Its posterior surface is pierced by several alveolar canals that transmit the posterior superior alveolar nerves and blood vessels. The maxillary tuberosity, a rounded eminence, is found on the inferior posterior surface. On the superior surface is a groove, directed laterally and slightly superiorly, through which the maxillary nerve passes. This groove is continuous with the infraorbital groove.

The palatal processes of the maxilla are thick horizontal projections that form a large portion of the floor of the nose and the roof of the mouth. The bone here is considerably thicker anteriorly than posteriorly. Its inferior (or palatal) surface constitutes the anterior three fourths of the hard palate (Fig. 12-18). Many foramina (passages for nutrient blood vessels) perforate it. Along its lateral border, at the junction with the alveolar process, is a groove through which

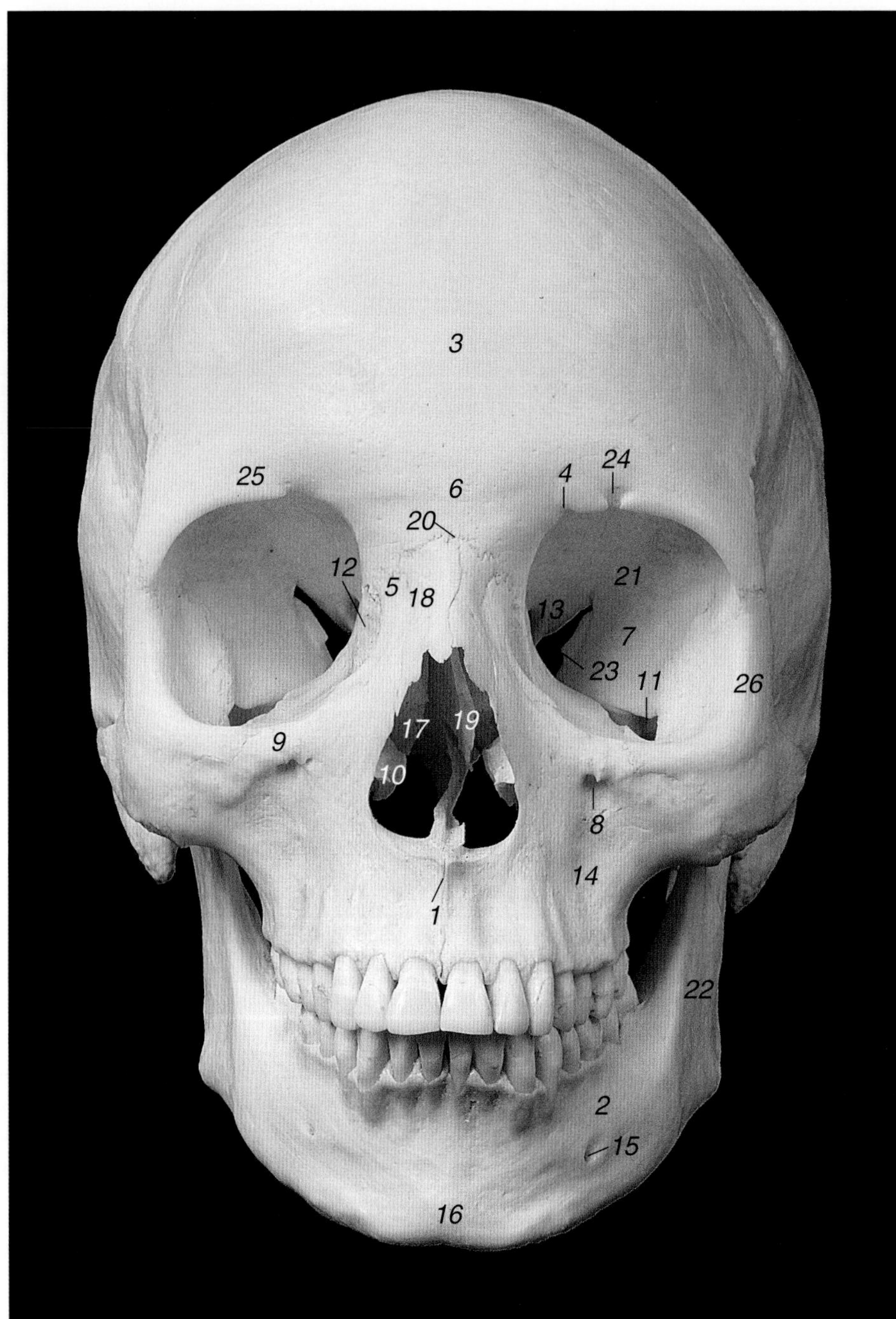

Figure 12-16. Anterior view of the skull. *1,* Anterior nasal spine; *2,* body of mandible; *3,* frontal bone; *4,* frontal notch; *5,* frontal process of maxilla; *6,* glabella; *7,* greater wing of sphenoid bone; *8,* infraorbital foramen; *9,* infraorbital margin; *10,* inferior nasal concha; *11,* inferior orbital fissure; *12,* lacrimal bone; *13,* lesser wing of sphenoid bone; *14,* maxilla; *15,* mental foramen; *16,* mental protuberance; *17,* middle nasal concha; *18,* nasal bone; *19,* nasal septum; *20,* nasion; *21,* orbit (orbital cavity); *22,* ramus of mandible; *23,* superior orbital fissure; *24,* supraorbital foramen; *25,* supraorbital margin; *26,* zygomatic bone. (Data from Abrahams PH, Marks SC Jr, Hutchings RT: McMinn's color atlas of human anatomy, ed 5, St Louis, 2003, Mosby.)

the anterior palatine nerve passes from the greater palatine foramen. In the midline in the anterior region is the funnel-shaped opening of the incisive foramen. Four canals are located in this opening: two for the descending palatine arteries and two for the nasopalatine nerves. In many skulls, especially those of younger persons, a fine suture line extends laterally from the incisive foramen to the border of the palatine process by the canine teeth. The small area anterior to this suture is termed the *premaxilla.*

The horizontal plate of the palatine bone forms the posterior fourth of the hard palate. Its anterior border articulates with the palatine process of the maxilla, and its posterior border serves as the attachment for the soft palate. Foramina are present on its surface, representing the lower end of the

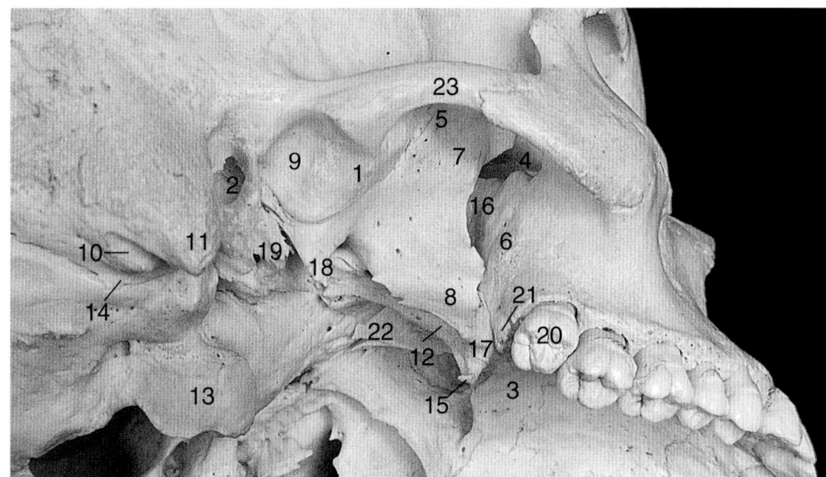

Figure 12-17. Infratemporal aspect of the maxilla. *1,* Articular tubercle; *2,* external acoustic meatus; *3,* horizontal plate of palatine bone; *4,* inferior orbital fissure; *5,* infratemporal crest; *6,* infratemporal (posterior) surface of maxilla; *7,* infratemporal surface of greater wing of sphenoid bone; *8,* lateral pterygoid plate; *9,* mandibular fossa; *10,* mastoid notch; *11,* mastoid process; *12,* medial pterygoid plate; *13,* occipital condyle; *14,* occipital groove; *15,* pterygoid hamulus; *16,* pterygomaxillary fissure and pterygopalatine fossa; *17,* pyramidal process of palatine bone; *18,* spine of sphenoid bone; *19,* styloid process and sheath; *20,* third molar tooth; *21,* tuberosity of maxilla; *22,* vomer; *23,* zygomatic arch. (Data from Abrahams PH, Marks SC Jr, Hutchings RT: McMinn's color atlas of human anatomy, ed 5, St Louis, 2003, Mosby.)

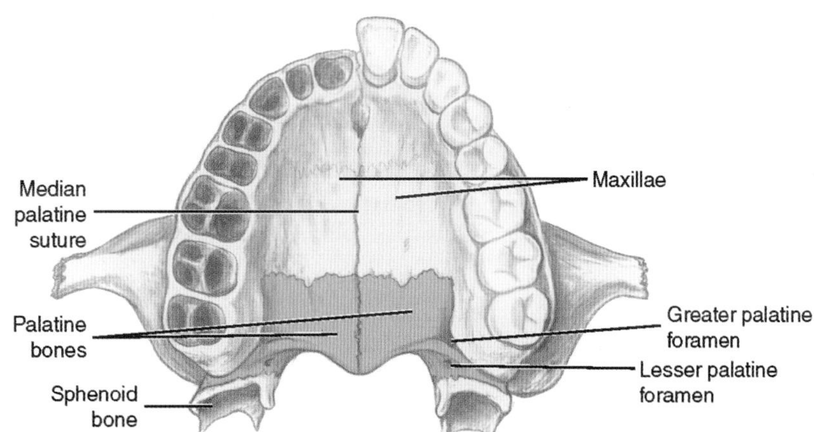

Figure 12-18. Inferior view of the hard palate. (Data from Fehrenbach MJ, Herring SW: Illustrated anatomy of the head and neck, ed 2, Philadelphia, 2002, WB Saunders.)

pterygopalatine canal, through which descending palatine blood vessels and the anterior palatine nerve run.

OSTEOLOGY: MANDIBLE

The mandible is the largest and strongest bone of the face. It consists of a curved horizontal portion (the body) and two perpendicular portions (the rami). The buccal cortical plate of the adult mandible most often is sufficiently dense so as to preclude effective infiltration of anesthesia in its vicinity.[7]

The external (lateral) surface of the body of the mandible is marked in the midline by a faint ridge, an indication of the symphysis of the two pieces of bone from which the mandible is created (Fig. 12-19, *A* and *C*). The bone that forms the buccal and lingual alveolar processes in the anterior region (incisors) is usually less dense than that over the posterior teeth, permitting infiltration (supraperiosteal) anesthesia to be employed with some expectation of success.[8,9] In the region of the second premolar on each side, midway between the upper and lower borders of the body, lies the mental foramen. Phillips and associates, in an evaluation of 75 dry, adult human mandibles, determined that the usual position of the mental foramen is below the crown of the second premolar.[10] The mental nerve, artery, and vein exit the mandibular canal here. Bone along this external surface of the mandible is commonly thick cortical bone.

The lingual border of the body of the mandible is concave from side to side (Fig. 12-19, *B* and *D*). Extending upward and backward is the mylohyoid line, giving origin to the mylohyoid muscle. Bone along the lingual of the mandible is usually quite thick; however, in approximately 68% of

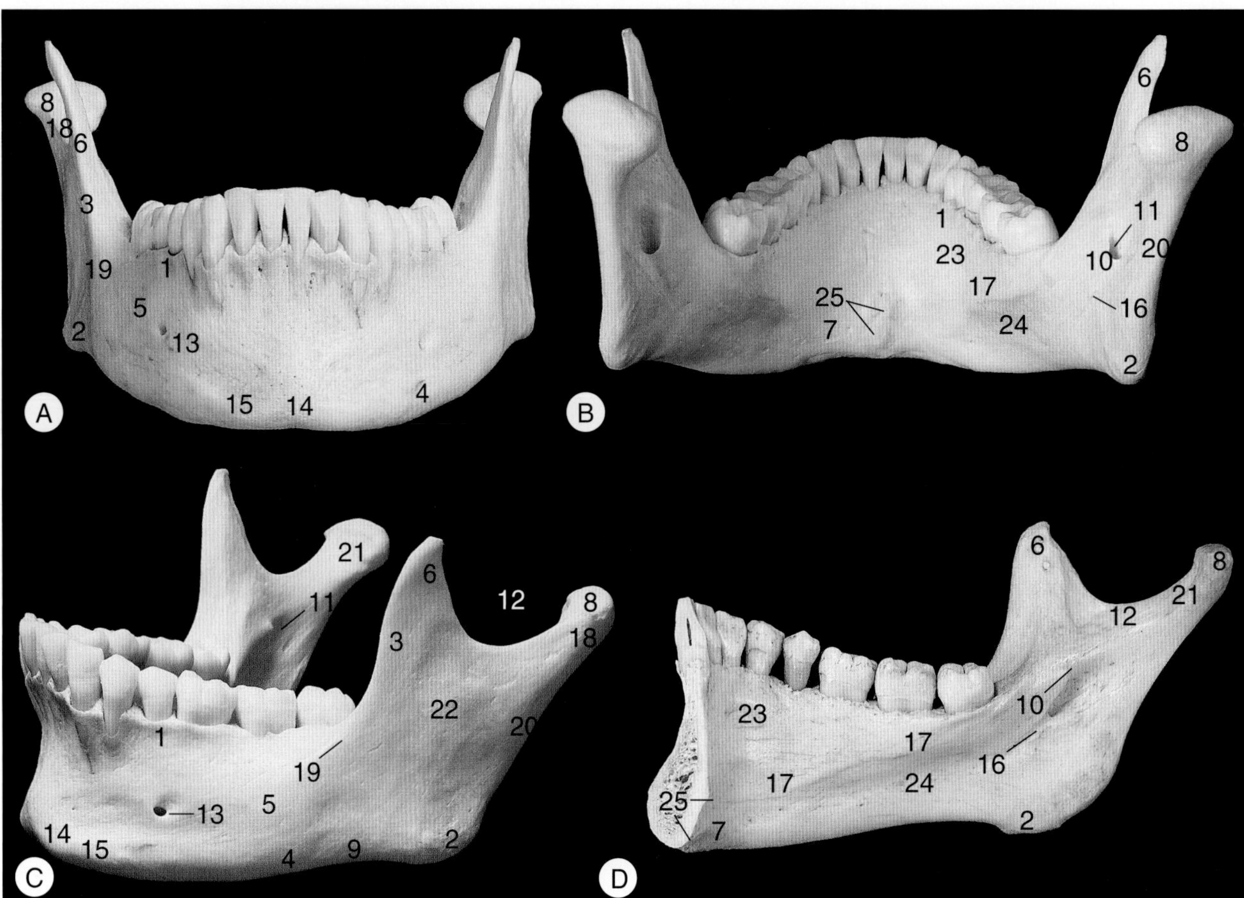

Figure 12-19. The mandible (**A**) from the front, (**B**) from behind and above, and (**C**) from the left and front, and (**D**) internal view from the left. *1,* Alveolar part; *2,* angle; *3,* anterior border of ramus; *4,* base; *5,* body; *6,* coronoid process; *7,* digastric fossa; *8,* head; *9,* inferior border of ramus; *10,* lingula; *11,* mandibular foramen; *12,* mandibular notch; *13,* mental foramen; *14,* mental protuberance; *15,* mental tubercle; *16,* mylohyoid groove; *17,* mylohyoid line; *18,* neck; *19,* oblique line; *20,* posterior border of ramus; *21,* pterygoid fovea; *22,* ramus; *23,* sublingual fossa; *24,* submandibular fossa; *25,* superior and inferior mental spines (genial tubercles). (Data from Abrahams PH, Marks SC Jr, Hutchings RT: McMinn's color atlas of human anatomy, ed 5, St Louis, 2003, Mosby.)

mandibles, lingual foramina are located in the posterior (molar) region.[11] The function of these foramina is as yet unclear, but some may contain sensory fibers from the mylohyoid nerve that innervate portions of mandibular molars.[2] In addition, bone on the lingual surface of the incisor teeth frequently demonstrates multiple small perforations, perhaps explaining recent clinical trials in which mandibular lingual infiltration had significant success rates in providing pulpal anesthesia.[8]

The lateral surface of each ramus is flat, composed of dense cortical bone and providing attachment for the masseter muscle along most of its surface (see Fig. 12-19, *C*). The medial surface (see Fig. 12-19, *D*) contains the mandibular foramen, located roughly halfway between the superior and inferior borders and two thirds to three fourths the distance from the anterior border of the ramus to its posterior border.[12] Other studies of the anteroposterior location of the mandibular foramen have provided differing locations. Hayward and associates[13] found the foramen most often in the third quadrant from the anterior part of the ramus, Monheim[14] found it at the midpoint of the ramus, and Hetson and associates[15] located it 55% distal to the anterior ramus (range, 44.4% to 65.5%). The mandibular canal extends obliquely downward and anteriorly within the ramus. It then courses horizontally forward in the body, distributing small dental branches to the mandibular teeth posterior to the mental foramen. The mandibular foramen is the point of entrance through which the inferior alveolar nerve, artery, and vein enter the mandibular canal. The height of this foramen varies greatly, ranging from 1 to 19 mm or more above the level of the occlusal plane.[13] A prominent ridge, the lingula mandibulae, lies on the anterior margin of the foramen. The lingula serves as an attachment for the sphenomandibular ligament. At the lower end of the mandibular foramen, the mylohyoid groove begins, coursing obliquely downward and anteriorly. In this groove lie the mylohyoid nerve and vessels.

Bone along the lingual surface of the mandible usually is dense (see Fig. 12-19, *D*). On rare occasions, bone over the lingual aspect of the third molar roots is less dense, permitting a greater chance that supraperiosteal anesthesia will be successful. However, the proximity of the lingual nerve to this site leads to cautions against attempting lingual infiltration in the area of the mandibular molars.

The superior border of the ramus has two processes: the coronoid anteriorly and the condylar posteriorly. Between these two processes is a deep concavity, the mandibular (sigmoid) notch. The coronoid process is thinner than the condylar. Its anterior border is concave—the coronoid notch. The coronoid notch represents a landmark for determining the height of needle penetration in the inferior alveolar nerve block technique. The condylar process is thicker than the coronoid. The condylar head, the thickened articular portion of the condyle, sits atop the constricted neck of the condyle. The condylar neck is flattened front to back. The attachment for the external pterygoid muscle is on its anterior surface.

When cut horizontally at the level of the mandibular foramen, the ramus of the mandible can be seen to be thicker in its anterior region than it is posteriorly. This is of clinical importance during the inferior alveolar nerve block. The thickness of soft tissues between needle penetration and the osseous tissues of the ramus at the level of the mandibular foramen averages about 20 to 25 mm. Because of increased thickness of bone in the anterior third of the ramus, the thickness of soft tissue is decreased accordingly (approximately 10 mm). Knowing the depth of penetration of soft tissue before contacting osseous tissues can aid the administrator in determining correct positioning of the needle tip.

References

1. DuBrul EL: Sicher's oral anatomy, ed 7, St Louis, 1980, Mosby.
2. Heasman PA: Clinical anatomy of the superior alveolar nerves, Br J Oral Maxillofac Surg 22:439–447, 1984.
3. McDaniel WL: Variations in nerve distributions of the maxillary teeth, J Dent Res 35:916–921, 1956.
4. Loetscher CA, Walton RE: Patterns of innervation of the maxillary first molar: a dissection study, Oral Surg 65:86–90, 1988.
5. Langlais RP, Broadus R, Glass BJ: Bifid mandibular canals in panoramic radiographs, J Am Dent Assoc 110:923–926, 1985.
6. Frommer J, Mele FA, Monroe CW: The possible role of the mylohyoid nerve in mandibular posterior tooth sensation, J Am Dent Assoc 85:113–117, 1972.
7. Blanton PL, Jeske AH: The key to profound local anesthesia: neuroanatomy, J Am Dent Assoc 134:753–760, 2003.
8. Yonchak T, Reader A, Beck M, et al: Anesthetic efficacy of infiltrations in mandibular anterior teeth, Anesth Prog 48:55–60, 2001.
9. Meechan JG, Ledvinka JI: Pulpal anaesthesia for mandibular central incisor teeth: a comparison of infiltration and intraligamentary injections, Int Endod J 35:629–634, 2002.
10. Phillips JL, Weller N, Kulild JC: The mental foramen. Part III. Size and position on panoramic radiographs, J Endodont 18:383–386, 1992.
11. Shiller WR, Wiswell OB: Lingual foramina of the mandible, Anat Rec 119:387–390, 1954.
12. Bremer G: Measurements of special significance in connection with anesthesia of the inferior alveolar nerve, Oral Surg 5:966–988, 1952.
13. Hayward J, Richardson ER, Malhotra SK: The mandibular foramen: its anteroposterior position, Oral Surg 44:837–843, 1977.
14. Monheim LM: Local anesthesia and pain control in dental practice, ed 4, St Louis, 1969, Mosby.
15. Hetson G, Share J, Frommer J, et al: Statistical evaluation of the position of the mandibular ramus, Oral Surg 65:32–34, 1988.

CHAPTER 13

Techniques of Maxillary Anesthesia

Several general methods of obtaining pain control with local anesthetics are available. The site of deposition of the drug relative to the area of operative intervention determines the type of injection administered. Three major types of local anesthetic injection can be differentiated: local infiltration, field block, and nerve block.

◆ **Local Infiltration** Small terminal nerve endings in the area of the dental treatment are flooded with local anesthetic solution. Incision (or treatment) is then made into the same area in which the local anesthetic has been deposited (Fig. 13-1). An example of local infiltration is the administration of a local anesthetic into an interproximal papilla before root planing. The term *infiltration* has been in common usage in dentistry to define an injection in which the local anesthetic solution is deposited at or above the apex of the tooth to be treated. Although technically incorrect—this technique is a *field block* (see following)—the common term will continue to be used for this type of injection.

◆ **Field Block** Local anesthetic is deposited near the larger terminal nerve branches so the anesthetized area will be circumscribed, preventing the passage of impulses from the tooth to the central nervous system (CNS). Incision (or treatment) is then made into an area away from the site of injection of the anesthetic (Fig. 13-2). Maxillary injections administered above the apex of the tooth to be treated are properly termed *field blocks* (although common usage identifies them as *infiltration* or *supraperiosteal*).

◆ **Nerve Block** Local anesthetic is deposited close to a main nerve trunk, usually at a distance from the site of operative intervention (Fig. 13-3). Posterior superior alveolar, inferior alveolar, and nasopalatine injections are examples of maxillary nerve blocks.

◆ **Discussion** Technically, the injection commonly referred to in dentistry as a local infiltration is a field block because anesthetic solution is deposited at or above the apex of the tooth to be treated. Terminal nerve branches to pulpal and soft tissues distal to the injection site are anesthetized.

Field block and nerve block may be distinguished by the extent of anesthesia achieved. In general, field blocks are more circumscribed, involving tissues in and around one or two teeth, whereas nerve blocks affect a larger area (e.g., that observed after inferior alveolar or anterior superior alveolar nerve block).

The type of injection administered for a given treatment is determined by the extent of the operative area. For management of small, localized areas, as in providing hemostasis for soft tissue procedures, infiltration anesthesia may suffice. When two or three teeth are being restored, field block is indicated, whereas for pain control in quadrant dentistry, regional block anesthesia is recommended.

MAXILLARY INJECTION TECHNIQUES

Numerous injection techniques are available to provide clinically adequate anesthesia of the teeth and soft and hard tissues in the maxilla. Selection of the specific technique to be used is determined, in large part, by the nature of the treatment to be provided. The following techniques are available:

1. Supraperiosteal (infiltration), recommended for limited treatment protocols
2. Periodontal ligament (PDL, intraligamentary) injection, recommended as an adjunct to other techniques or for limited treatment protocols
3. Intraseptal injection, recommended primarily for periodontal surgical techniques
4. Intracrestal injection, recommended for single teeth (primarily mandibular molars) when other techniques have failed
5. Intraosseous (IO) injection, recommended for single teeth (primarily mandibular molars) when other techniques have failed
6. Posterior superior alveolar (PSA) nerve block, recommended for management of several molar teeth in one quadrant

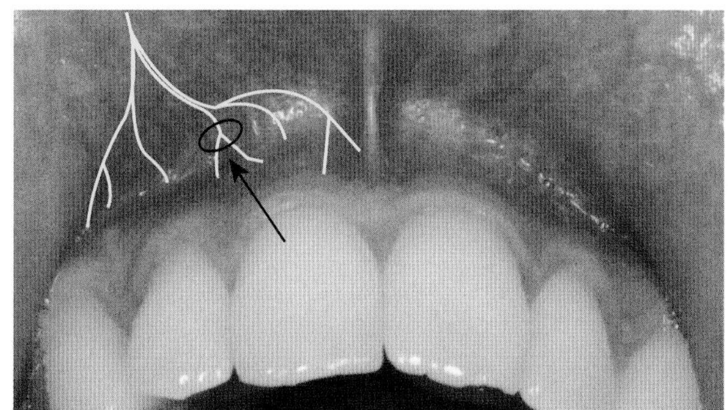

Figure 13-1. Local infiltration. The area of treatment is flooded with local anesthetic. An incision is made into the same area *(arrow)*.

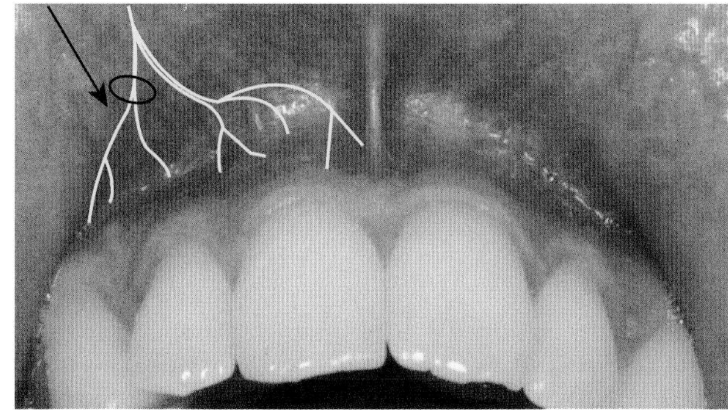

Figure 13-2. Field block. Local anesthetic is deposited near the larger terminal nerve endings *(arrow)*. An incision is made away from the site of injection.

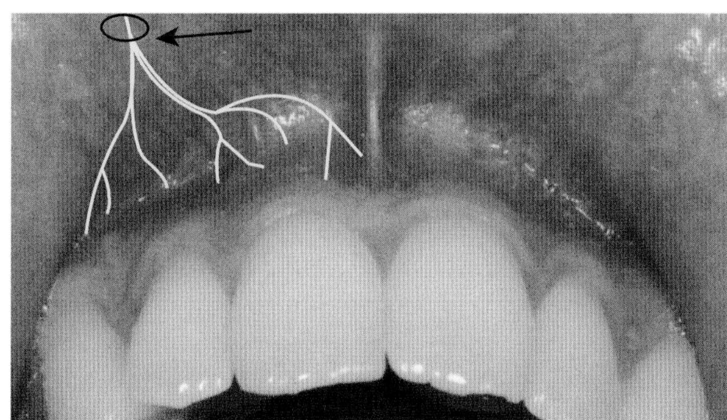

Figure 13-3. Nerve block. Local anesthetic is deposited close to the main nerve trunk, located at a distance from the site of incision *(arrow)*.

7. Middle superior alveolar (MSA) nerve block, recommended for management of premolars in one quadrant
8. Anterior superior alveolar (ASA) nerve block, recommended for management of anterior teeth in one quadrant
9. Maxillary (V_2, second division) nerve block, recommended for extensive buccal, palatal, and pulpal management in one quadrant
10. Greater (anterior) palatine nerve block, recommended for palatal soft and osseous tissue treatment distal to the canine in one quadrant
11. Nasopalatine nerve block, recommended for palatal soft and osseous tissue management from canine to canine bilaterally
12. Anterior middle superior alveolar (AMSA) nerve block, recommended for extensive management of anterior teeth, palatal and buccal soft and hard tissues
13. Palatal approach-anterior superior alveolar (P-ASA) nerve block, recommended for treatment of maxillary anterior teeth and their palatal and facial soft and hard tissues

Supraperiosteal, periodontal ligament, intraseptal, and intraosseous injections are appropriate for administration in the maxilla or the mandible. Because of the great success of supraperiosteal injection in the maxilla, it is discussed in this chapter. Periodontal ligament, intraseptal, intracrestal, and intraosseous injections, supplemental injections of considerably greater importance in the mandible, are described in Chapter 15.

TEETH AND BUCCAL SOFT AND HARD TISSUES

Supraperiosteal Injection

The supraperiosteal injection, more commonly (but incorrectly) called *local infiltration,* is the most frequently used technique for obtaining pulpal anesthesia in maxillary teeth. Although it is a simple procedure with a high success rate, there are several valid reasons for using other techniques (e.g., regional nerve blocks) whenever more than two or three teeth are involved in treatment.

Multiple supraperiosteal injections necessitate multiple needle penetrations, each with the potential to produce pain, either during the procedure or after the anesthetic effect has resolved, or damage, either permanent or transient, to the involved tissues (blood vessels, nerves). In addition, and perhaps even more important, using supraperiosteal injections for pulpal anesthesia on multiple teeth leads to the administration of a larger volume of local anesthetic, with an attendant increase (although usually minor in adults) in the risk of systemic and local complications.

The supraperiosteal injection is indicated whenever dental procedures are confined to a relatively circumscribed area in the maxillary or mandibular incisor region.

Other Common Names. Local infiltration, paraperiosteal injection.

Nerves Anesthetized. Large terminal branches of the dental plexus.

Areas Anesthetized. The entire region innervated by the large terminal branches of this plexus: pulp and root area of the tooth, buccal periosteum, connective tissue, and mucous membrane (Fig. 13-4).

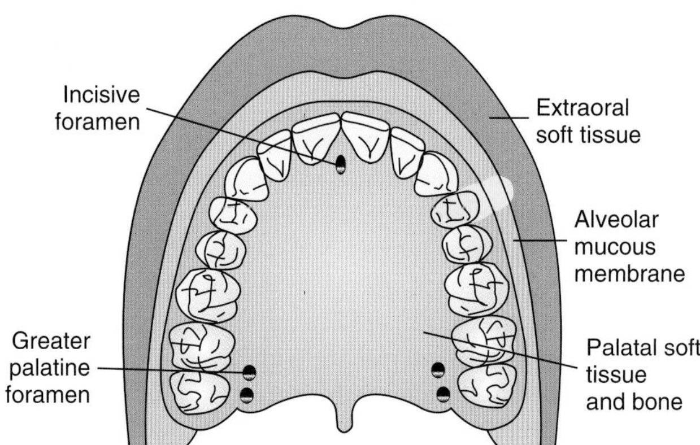

Figure 13-4. Supraperiosteal injection in the anterior region of the maxilla. Note the area anesthetized *(yellow)*.

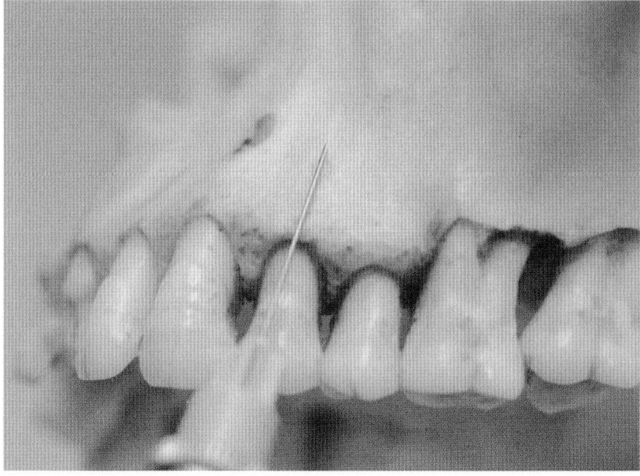

Figure 13-5. The syringe should be held parallel to the long axis of the tooth and inserted at the height of the mucobuccal fold over the tooth.

Indications

1. Pulpal anesthesia of the maxillary teeth when treatment is limited to one or two teeth
2. Soft tissue anesthesia when indicated for surgical procedures in a circumscribed area

Contraindications

1. Infection or acute inflammation in the area of injection.
2. Dense bone covering the apices of teeth (can be determined only by trial and error; most likely over the permanent maxillary first molar in children, as its apex may be located beneath the zygomatic bone, which is relatively dense). The apex of an adult's central incisor may also be located beneath denser bone (e.g., of the nose), thereby increasing the failure rate (although not significantly).

Advantages

1. High success rate (>95%)
2. Technically easy injection
3. Usually entirely atraumatic

Disadvantages. Not recommended for large areas because of the need for multiple needle insertions and the necessity to administer larger total volumes of local anesthetic.

Positive Aspiration. Negligible, but possible (<1%).

Alternatives. PDL, IO, regional nerve block.

Technique

1. A 27-gauge short needle is recommended.
2. Area of insertion: height of the mucobuccal fold above the apex of the tooth being anesthetized
3. Target area: apical region of the tooth to be anesthetized
4. Landmarks:
   a. Mucobuccal fold
   b. Crown of the tooth
   c. Root contour of the tooth
5. Orientation of the bevel*: toward bone
6. Procedure:
   a. Prepare tissue at the injection site.
      (1) Clean with sterile dry gauze.
      (2) Apply topical antiseptic (optional).
      (3) Apply topical anesthetic for minimum of 1 minute.
   b. Orient needle so bevel faces bone.
   c. Lift the lip, pulling the tissue taut.
   d. Hold the syringe parallel with the long axis of the tooth (Fig. 13-5).
   e. Insert the needle into the height of the mucobuccal fold over the target tooth.
   f. Advance the needle until its bevel is at or above the apical region of the tooth (Table 13-1). In most instances, the depth of penetration is only a few millimeters. Because the needle is in soft tissue (not touching bone), there should be no resistance to its advancement, nor should there be any patient discomfort with this injection.
   g. Aspirate ×2.
      (1) If negative, deposit approximately 0.6 mL (one third of a cartridge) slowly over 20 seconds. (Do not allow the tissues to balloon.)
   h. Slowly withdraw the syringe.

*Bevel orientations are specified for all injection techniques in Chapters 13 and 14. The orientation of the needle bevel is not a significant factor in the success or failure of an injection technique, and these recommendations need not be rigidly adhered to; yet there will be a fuller expectation of successful anesthesia if they are followed, provided all other technical and anatomic principles are maintained. In general, whenever possible, the bevel of the needle is to be facing toward bone; then, in the unlikely event that the needle comes into contact with bone, the bevel will slide over the periosteum, provoking minor discomfort but not tearing the periosteum. If the bevel faces away from bone, the sharp point of the needle would contact the periosteum, tearing it and leading to a more painful (subperiosteal) injection. Postinjection discomfort is considerably greater with subperiosteal than with supraperiosteal injections.

i. Make the needle safe.
j. Wait 3 to 5 minutes before commencing the dental procedure.

Signs and Symptoms

1. Subjective: feeling of numbness in the area of administration
2. Objective: use of electrical pulp testing (EPT) with no response from tooth with maximal EPT output (80/80)
3. Absence of pain during treatment

Safety Features

1. Minimal risk of intravascular administration
2. Slow injection of anesthetic; aspiration

Precautions. Supraperiosteal injection is not recommended for larger areas of treatment. The greater number of tissue penetrations increases the possibility of pain both during and after the injection, and the larger volume of solution administered increases the possibility of local anesthetic overdose (in lighter-weight patients) and postinjection pain. Additionally, needle puncture of tissue can lead to permanent or transient damage to structures in the area, such as blood vessels (hematoma) and nerves (paresthesia).

Failures of Anesthesia

1. Needle tip lies below the apex (along the root) of the tooth (see Table 13-1). Depositing anesthetic solution below the apex of a maxillary tooth results in excellent soft tissue anesthesia but poor or absent pulpal anesthesia.
2. Needle tip lies too far from the bone (solution deposited in buccal soft tissues). To correct: Redirect the needle closer to the periosteum.

Complications. Pain on needle insertion with the needle tip against the periosteum. To correct: Withdraw the needle and reinsert it farther from the periosteum.

Posterior Superior Alveolar Nerve Block

The posterior superior alveolar (PSA) nerve block is a commonly used dental nerve block. Although it is a highly successful technique (>95%), several issues should be weighed when its use is considered. These include the extent of anesthesia produced and the potential for hematoma formation.

When used to achieve pulpal anesthesia, the PSA nerve block is effective for the maxillary third, second, and first molars (in 77% to 100% of patients).[1] However, the mesiobuccal root of the maxillary first molar is not consistently innervated by the PSA nerve. In a dissection study by Loetscher and associates,[1] the middle superior alveolar nerve provided sensory innervation to the mesiobuccal root of the maxillary first molar in 28% of specimens examined. Therefore a second injection, usually supraperiosteal, is indicated after the PSA nerve block when effective anesthesia of the first molar does not develop. Loetscher and associates[1] concluded by stating that the PSA nerve usually provides sole pulpal innervation to the maxillary first molar, and that a single PSA nerve block usually provides clinically adequate pulpal anesthesia.

The risk of a potential complication must be considered whenever the PSA block is used. Insertion of the needle too far distally may lead to a temporarily (10 to 14 days) unesthetic hematoma. When the PSA is to be administered, one must always consider the patient's skull size in determining the depth of soft tissue penetration. An "average" depth of penetration in a patient with a smaller than average-sized

TABLE 13-1
Average Tooth Length

	Length of Crown, mm	+	Length of Root, mm	=	Length of Tooth
Maxillary					
Central incisors	11.6		12.4		24.0
Lateral incisors	9.0-10.2		12.3-13.5		22.5
Canines	10.9		16.1		27.0
First premolars	8.7		13.0		21.7
Second premolars	7.9		13.6		21.5
First molars	7.7		13.6		21.3
Second molars	7.7		13.4		21.1
Third molars	Extremely variable		Extremely variable		Extremely variable
Mandibular					
Central incisors	9.4		12.0		21.4
Lateral incisors	9.9		13.3		23.2
Canines	11.4		14.0		25.4
First premolars	7.5-11.0		11.0-16.0		18.5-27.0
Second premolars	8.5		14.7		23.2
First molars	8.3		14.5		22.8
Second molars	8.1		14.7		22.8
Third molars	Extremely variable		Extremely variable		Extremely variable

skull may produce a hematoma, whereas a needle inserted "just right" in a larger-skulled patient might not provide anesthesia to any teeth. As a means of decreasing the risk of hematoma formation after a PSA nerve block, use of a "short" dental needle is recommended for all but the largest of patients. Because the average depth of soft tissue penetration from the insertion site (the mucobuccal fold over the maxillary second molar) to the area of the PSA nerves is 16 mm, the short dental needle (≈20 mm) can be successfully and safely used. Overinsertion of the needle is less likely to occur, thereby minimizing the risk of hematoma. A 27-gauge short needle is recommended as long as aspiration is performed carefully and the local anesthetic is injected slowly. One must remember to aspirate several times before and during drug deposition during PSA nerve block to avoid inadvertent intravascular injection.

Other Common Names. Tuberosity block, zygomatic block.

Nerves Anesthetized. Posterior superior alveolar and branches.

Areas Anesthetized

1. Pulps of the maxillary third, second, and first molars (entire tooth = 72%; mesiobuccal root of the maxillary first molar not anesthetized = 28%)
2. Buccal periodontium and bone overlying these teeth (Fig. 13-6)

Indications

1. When treatment involves two or more maxillary molars
2. When supraperiosteal injection is contraindicated (e.g., with infection or acute inflammation)
3. When supraperiosteal injection has proved ineffective

Contraindication. When the risk of hemorrhage is too great (as with a hemophiliac), in which case a supraperiosteal or PDL injection is recommended.

Advantages

1. Atraumatic; when administered properly, no pain is experienced by the patient receiving the PSA because of the relatively large area of soft tissue into which the local anesthetic is deposited and the fact that bone is not contacted
2. High success rate (>95%)
3. Minimum number of necessary injections
   a. One injection compared with option of three infiltrations
4. Minimizes the total volume of local anesthetic solution administered
   a. Equivalent volume of anesthetic solution necessary for three supraperiosteal injections = 1.8 mL

Disadvantages

1. Risk of hematoma, which is usually diffuse; also discomfiting and visually embarrassing to the patient
2. Technique somewhat arbitrary: no bony landmarks during insertion
3. Second injection necessary for treatment of the first molar (mesiobuccal root) in 28% of patients

Positive Aspiration. Approximately 3.1%.

Alternatives

1. Supraperiosteal or PDL injections for pulpal and root anesthesia
2. Infiltrations for the buccal periodontium and hard tissues
3. Maxillary nerve block

Technique

1. A 27-gauge short needle recommended
2. Area of insertion: height of the mucobuccal fold above the maxillary second molar
3. Target area: PSA nerve—posterior, superior, and medial to the posterior border of the maxilla (Fig. 13-7)

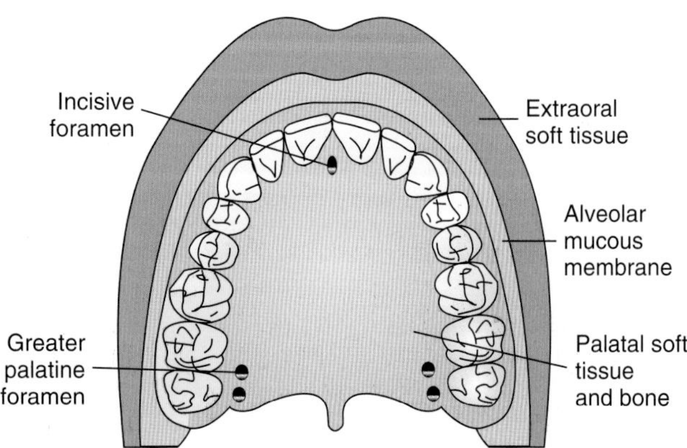

Figure 13-6. Area anesthetized by a posterior superior alveolar (PSA) nerve block. Infratemporal surface of maxilla; maxillary tuberosity.

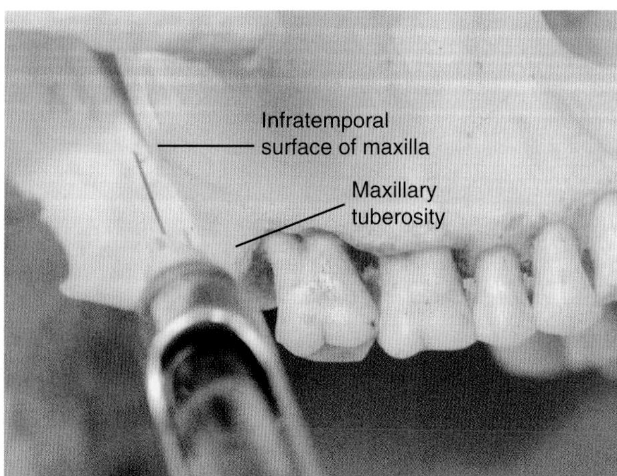

Figure 13-7. Needle at the target area for a posterior superior alveolar (PSA) nerve block.

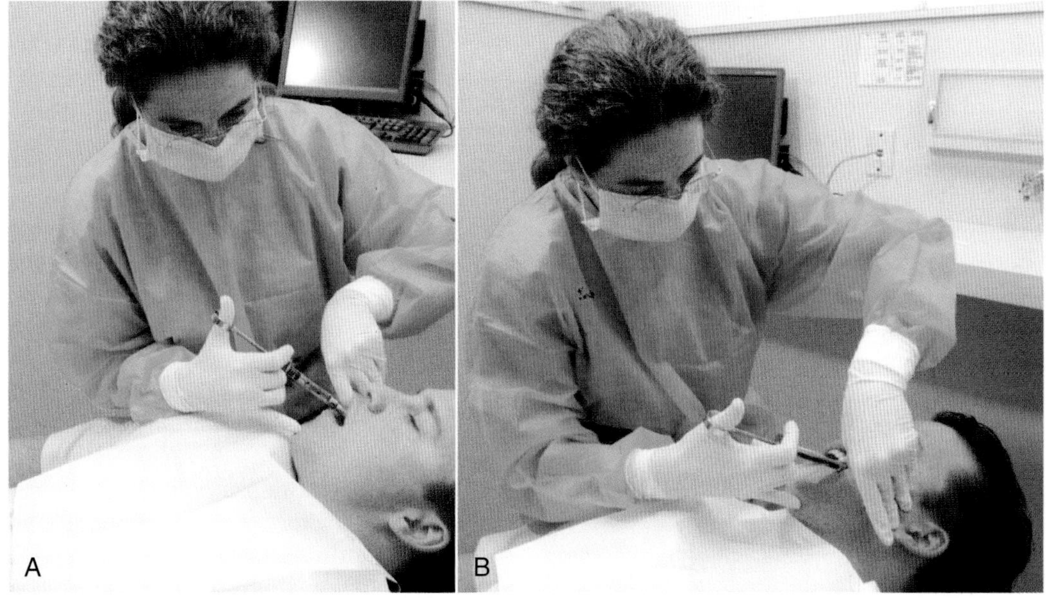

Figure 13-8. Position of the administrator for (**A**) right and (**B**) left posterior superior alveolar (PSA) nerve block.

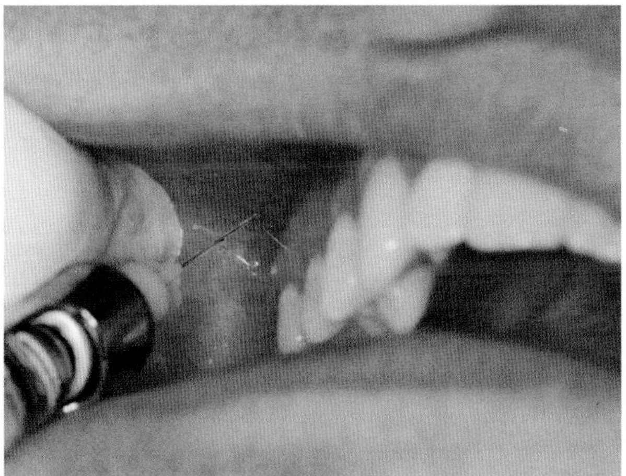

Figure 13-9. Posterior superior alveolar (PSA) nerve block. Tissue retracted at the site of penetration. Note the orientation of the needle: inward, upward, backward.

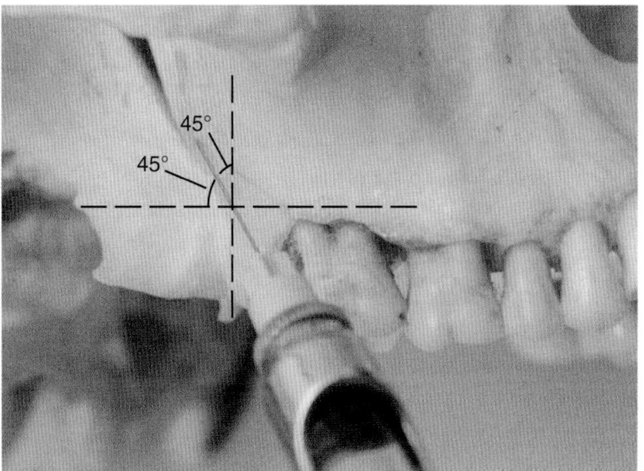

Figure 13-10. Advance the needle upward, inward, and backward.

4. Landmarks:
   a. Mucobuccal fold
   b. Maxillary tuberosity
   c. Zygomatic process of the maxilla
5. Orientation of the bevel: toward bone during the injection. If bone is accidentally touched, the sensation is less unpleasant.
6. Procedure:
   a. Assume the correct position (Fig. 13-8).
      (1) For a left PSA nerve block, a right-handed administrator should sit at the 10 o'clock position facing the patient.
      (2) For a right PSA block, a right-handed administrator should sit at the 8 o'clock position facing the patient.
   b. Prepare the tissues at the height of the mucobuccal fold for penetration.
      (1) Dry with a sterile gauze.
      (2) Apply a topical antiseptic (optional).
      (3) Apply topical anesthetic for a minimum of 1 minute.
   c. Orient the bevel of the needle toward bone.
   d. Partially open the patient's mouth, pulling the mandible to the side of injection.
   e. Retract the patient's cheek with your finger (for visibility).
   f. Pull the tissues at the injection site taut.
   g. Insert the needle into the height of the mucobuccal fold over the second molar (Fig. 13-9).
   h. Advance the needle slowly in an upward, inward, and backward direction (Fig. 13-10) in one movement (not three).
      (1) Upward: superiorly at a 45-degree angle to the occlusal plane

(2) Inward: medially toward the midline at a 45-degree angle to the occlusal plane (Fig. 13-11)

(3) Backward: posteriorly at a 45-degree angle to the long axis of the second molar

i. Slowly advance the needle through soft tissue.

(1) There should be no resistance and therefore no discomfort to the patient.

(2) If resistance (bone) is felt, the angle of the needle in toward the midline is too great.

(a) Withdraw the needle slightly (but do not remove it entirely from the tissues) and bring the syringe barrel closer to the occlusal plane.

(b) Readvance the needle.

j. Advance the needle to the desired depth (see Fig. 13-11).

(1) In an adult of normal size, penetration to a depth of 16 mm places the needle tip in the immediate vicinity of the foramina through which the PSA nerves enter the posterior surface of the maxilla. When a long needle is used (average length, 32 mm), it is inserted half its length into the tissue. With a short needle (average length, 20 mm), approximately 4 mm should remain visible.

(2) For smaller adults and children, it is prudent to halt the advance of the needle short of its usual depth of penetration to avoid a possible hematoma caused by overpenetration. Penetrating to a depth of 10 to 14 mm places the needle tip in the target area in most smaller-skulled patients.

Note: The goal is to deposit local anesthetic close to the PSA nerves, located posterosuperior and medial to the maxillary tuberosity.

k. Aspirate in two planes.

(1) Rotate the syringe barrel (needle bevel) one fourth turn and reaspirate.

l. If both aspirations are negative:

(1) Slowly, over 30 to 60 seconds, deposit 0.9 to 1.8 mL of anesthetic solution.

(2) Aspirate several additional times (in one plane) during drug administration.

(3) The PSA injection is normally atraumatic because of the large tissue space available to accommodate the anesthetic solution and the fact that bone is not touched.

m. Slowly withdraw the syringe.

n. Make the needle safe.

o. Wait minimally 3 to 5 minutes before commencing the dental procedure.

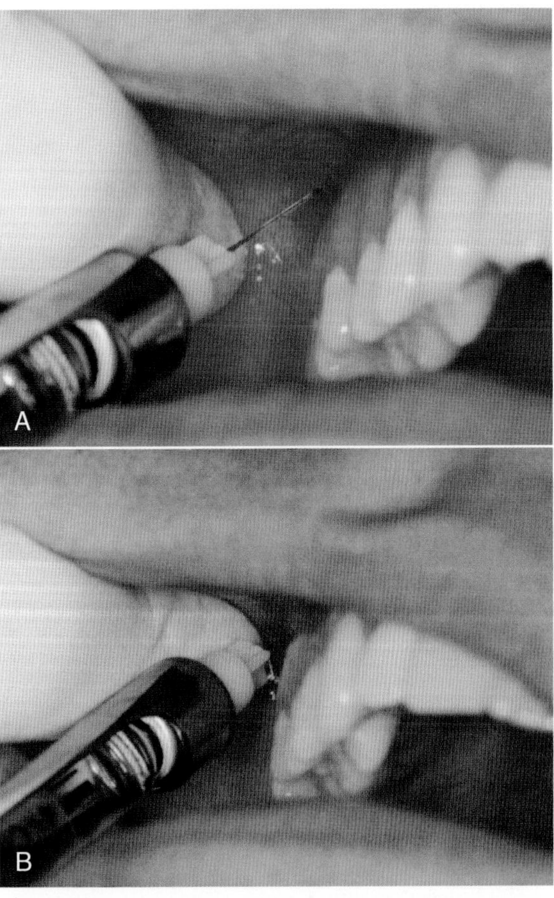

Figure 13-11. **A,** With a "long" dental needle (>32 mm in length) in an average-sized adult, the depth of penetration is half its length. Use of "long" needle on posterior superior alveolar (PSA) nerve block increases risks of overinsertion and hematoma. **B,** PSA nerve block using a "short" dental needle (≈20 mm in length). Overinsertion is less likely.

Signs and Symptoms

1. Subjective: usually none; the patient has difficulty reaching this region to determine the extent of anesthesia
2. Objective: use of electrical pulp testing with no response from tooth with maximal EPT output (80/80)
3. Absence of pain during treatment

Safety Features

1. Slow injection, repeated aspirations
2. No anatomic safety features to prevent overinsertion of the needle; therefore careful observation is necessary

Precaution. The depth of needle penetration should be checked: overinsertion (too deep) increases the risk of hematoma; too shallow might still provide adequate anesthesia.

Failures of Anesthesia

1. Needle too lateral. To correct: Redirect the needle tip medially (see complication 2).
2. Needle not high enough. To correct: Redirect the needle tip superiorly.
3. Needle too far posterior. To correct: Withdraw the needle to the proper depth.

Complications

1. Hematoma:
   a. This is commonly produced by inserting the needle too far posteriorly into the pterygoid plexus of veins. In addition, the maxillary artery may be perforated. Use of a short needle minimizes the risk of pterygoid plexus puncture.
   b. A visible intraoral hematoma develops within several minutes, usually noted in the buccal tissues of the mandibular region (see Chapter 17).
      (1) There is no easily accessible intraoral area to which pressure can be applied to stop the hemorrhage.
      (2) Bleeding continues until the pressure of extravascular blood is equal to or greater than that of intravascular blood.
2. Mandibular anesthesia:
   a. The mandibular division of the fifth cranial nerve (V_3) is located lateral to the PSA nerves. Deposition of local anesthetic lateral to the desired location may produce varying degrees of mandibular anesthesia. Most often, when this occurs, patients mention that their tongue and perhaps their lower lip are anesthetized.

Middle Superior Alveolar Nerve Block

The middle superior alveolar (MSA) nerve is present in only about 28% of the population, thereby limiting the clinical usefulness of this block. However, when the ASA nerve block fails to provide pulpal anesthesia distal to the maxillary canine, the MSA block is indicated for procedures on premolars and on the mesiobuccal root of the maxillary first molar. The success rate of the MSA nerve block is high.

Nerves Anesthetized. Middle superior alveolar and terminal branches.

Areas Anesthetized

1. Pulps of the maxillary first and second premolars, mesiobuccal root of the first molar
2. Buccal periodontal tissues and bone over these same teeth (Fig. 13-12)

Indications

1. Where the ASA nerve block fails to provide pulpal anesthesia distal to the maxillary canine
2. Dental procedures involving both maxillary premolars only

Contraindications

1. Infection or inflammation in the area of injection or needle insertion or drug deposition
2. Where the MSA nerve is absent, innervation is through the anterior superior alveolar (ASA) nerve; branches of the ASA innervating the premolars and the mesiobuccal root of the first molar can be anesthetized by means of the MSA technique.

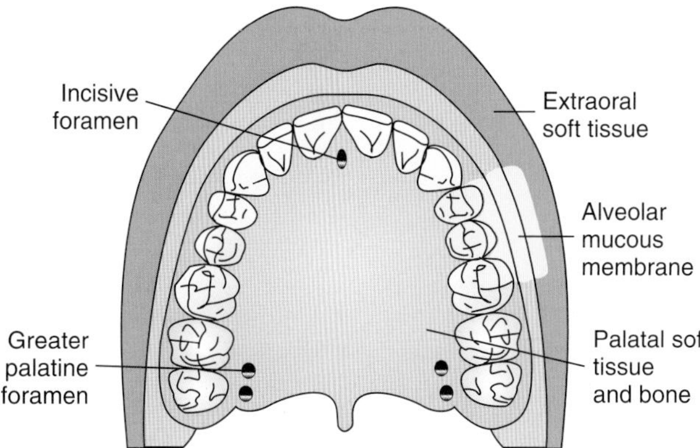

Figure 13-12. Area anesthetized by a middle superior alveolar (MSA) nerve block.

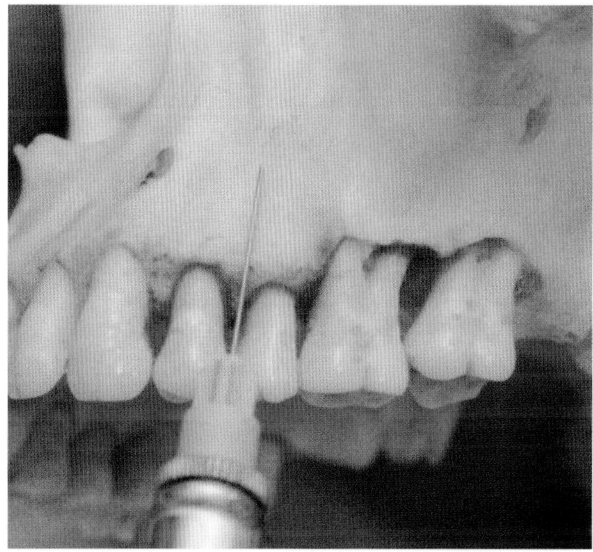

Figure 13-13. Position of needle between maxillary premolars for a middle superior alveolar (MSA) nerve block.

Advantages. Minimizes the number of injections and the volume of solution.

Disadvantages. None.

Positive Aspiration. Negligible (<3%).

Alternatives

1. Local infiltration (supraperiosteal), PDL, IO injections
2. ASA nerve block for the first and second premolar and the mesiobuccal root of the first molar

Technique

1. A 27-gauge short or long needle is recommended.
2. Area of insertion: height of the mucobuccal fold above the maxillary second premolar
3. Target area: maxillary bone above the apex of the maxillary second premolar (Fig. 13-13)
4. Landmark: mucobuccal fold above the maxillary second premolar

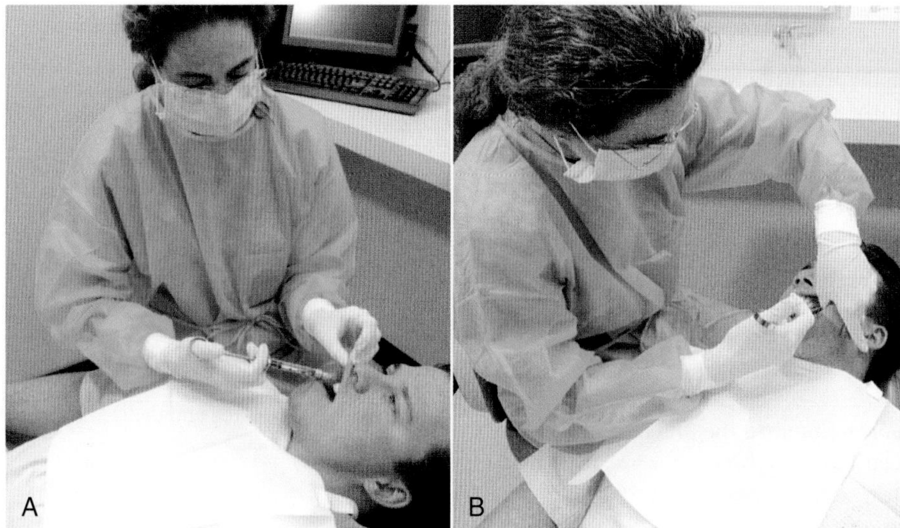

Figure 13-14. Position of the administrator for a **(A)** right and **(B)** left middle superior alveolar (MSA) nerve block.

5. Orientation of the bevel: toward bone
6. Procedure:
   a. Assume the correct position (Fig. 13-14).
      (1) For a right MSA nerve block, a right-handed administrator should face the patient from the 10 o'clock position.
      (2) For a left MSA nerve block, a right-handed administrator should face the patient directly from the 8 or 9 o'clock position.
   b. Prepare the tissues at the site of injection.
      (1) Dry with sterile gauze.
      (2) Apply topical antiseptic (optional).
      (3) Apply topical anesthetic for a minimum of 1 minute.
   c. Stretch the patient's upper lip to make the tissues taut and to gain visibility.
   d. Insert the needle into the height of the mucobuccal fold above the second premolar with the bevel directed toward bone.
   e. Penetrate the mucous membrane and slowly advance the needle until its tip is located well above the apex of the second premolar (Fig. 13-15).
   f. Aspirate.
   g. Slowly deposit 0.9 to 1.2 mL (one half to two thirds cartridge) of solution (approximately 30 to 40 seconds).
   h. Withdraw the syringe and make the needle safe.
   i. Wait a minimum of 3 to 5 minutes before commencing dental therapy.

Signs and Symptoms

1. Subjective: upper lip numb
2. Objective: use of electrical pulp testing with no response from tooth with maximal EPT output (80/80)
3. Absence of pain during treatment

Safety Feature. Relatively avascular area, anatomically safe.

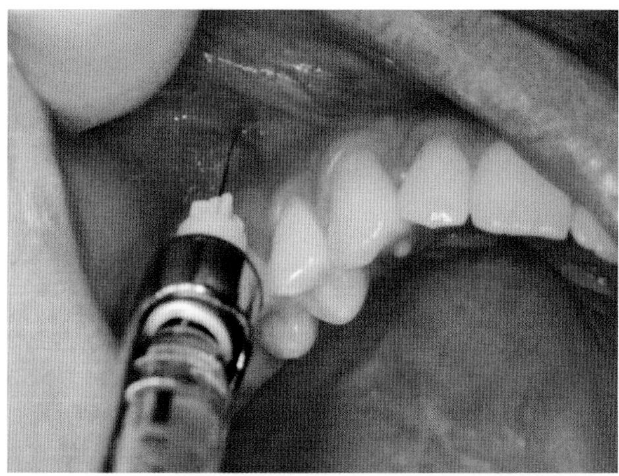

Figure 13-15. Needle penetration for a middle superior alveolar (MSA) nerve block.

Precautions. To prevent pain, do not insert too close to the periosteum and do not inject too rapidly; the MSA should be an atraumatic injection.

Failures of Anesthesia

1. Anesthetic solution not deposited high above the apex of the second premolar
   a. To correct: Check radiographs and increase the depth of penetration.
2. Deposition of solution too far from the maxillary bone with the needle placed in tissues lateral to the height of the mucobuccal fold
   a. To correct: Reinsert at the height of the mucobuccal fold.
3. Bone of the zygomatic arch at the site of injection preventing the diffusion of anesthetic
   a. To correct: Use the supraperiosteal, ASA, or PSA injection in place of the MSA.

Complications (rare). A hematoma may develop at the site of injection. Apply pressure with sterile gauze over the site of swelling and discoloration for a minimum of 60 seconds.

Anterior Superior Alveolar Nerve Block (Infraorbital Nerve Block)

The ASA nerve block does not enjoy the popularity of the PSA block, primarily because there is a general lack of experience with this highly successful and extremely safe technique. It provides profound pulpal and buccal soft tissue anesthesia from the maxillary central incisor through the premolars in about 72% of patients.

Used in place of supraperiosteal injection, the ASA nerve block necessitates a smaller volume of local anesthetic solution to achieve equivalent anesthesia: 0.9 to 1.2 mL versus 3.0 mL for supraperiosteal injections of the same teeth.

Generally speaking, the major factor inhibiting dentists from using the ASA nerve block is fear of injury to the patient's eye. Fortunately this fear is unfounded. Adherence to the following protocol produces a high success rate devoid of complications and adverse side effects.

Other Common Name. Infraorbital nerve block (technically, the infraorbital nerve provides anesthesia to the soft tissues of the anterior portion of the face, not to the teeth or intraoral soft and hard tissues; therefore it is inaccurate to call the ASA nerve block the infraorbital nerve block).

Nerves Anesthetized

1. Anterior superior alveolar
2. Middle superior alveolar
3. Infraorbital nerve
   a. Inferior palpebral
   b. Lateral nasal
   c. Superior labial

Areas Anesthetized

1. Pulps of the maxillary central incisor through the canine on the injected side
2. In about 72% of patients, pulps of the maxillary premolars and mesiobuccal root of the first molar
3. Buccal (labial) periodontium and bone of these same teeth
4. Lower eyelid, lateral aspect of the nose, upper lip (Fig. 13-16)

Indications

1. Dental procedures involving more than two maxillary teeth and their overlying buccal tissues
2. Inflammation or infection (which contraindicates supraperiosteal injection): If a cellulitis is present, the maxillary nerve block may be indicated in lieu of the ASA nerve block.
3. When supraperiosteal injections have been ineffective because of dense cortical bone

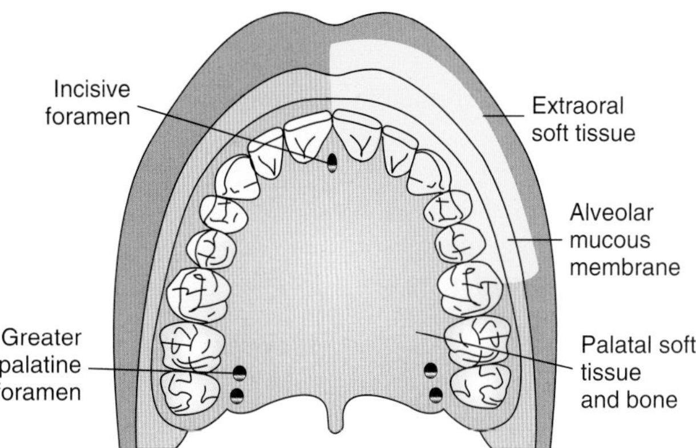

Figure 13-16. Anterior superior alveolar (ASA) nerve block, showing area anesthetized in 72% of patients.

Contraindications

1. Discrete treatment areas (one or two teeth only; supraperiosteal preferred)
2. Hemostasis of localized areas, when desirable, cannot be adequately achieved with this injection; local infiltration into the treatment area is indicated.

Advantages

1. Comparatively simple technique
2. Comparatively safe; minimizes the volume of solution used and the number of needle punctures necessary to achieve anesthesia

Disadvantages

1. Psychological:
   a. Administrator: There may be an initial fear of injury to the patient's eye (experience with the technique leads to confidence).
   b. Patient: An extraoral approach to the infraorbital nerve may prove disturbing; however, intraoral techniques are rarely a problem.
2. Anatomic: difficulty defining landmarks (rare)

Positive Aspiration. 0.7%.

Alternatives

1. Supraperiosteal, PDL, or IO injection for each tooth
2. Infiltration for the periodontium and hard tissues
3. Maxillary nerve block

Technique

1. A 25- or 27-gauge long needle is recommended, although the 27-gauge short also may be used, especially for children and smaller adults.
2. Area of insertion: height of the mucobuccal fold directly over the first premolar

Note: The needle may be inserted into the height of the mucobuccal fold over any tooth from the second premolar anteriorly to the central incisor. The ensuing path of penetration is toward the target area, the infraorbital foramen. The first premolar usually provides the shortest route to this target area.

3. Target area: infraorbital foramen (below the infraorbital notch).
4. Landmarks:
   a. Mucobuccal fold
   b. Infraorbital notch
   c. Infraorbital foramen
5. Orientation of the bevel: toward bone
6. Procedure:
   a. Assume the correct position (Fig. 13-17). For a right or left infraorbital nerve block, a right-handed administrator should sit at the 10 o'clock position, directly facing the patient or facing in the same direction as the patient.

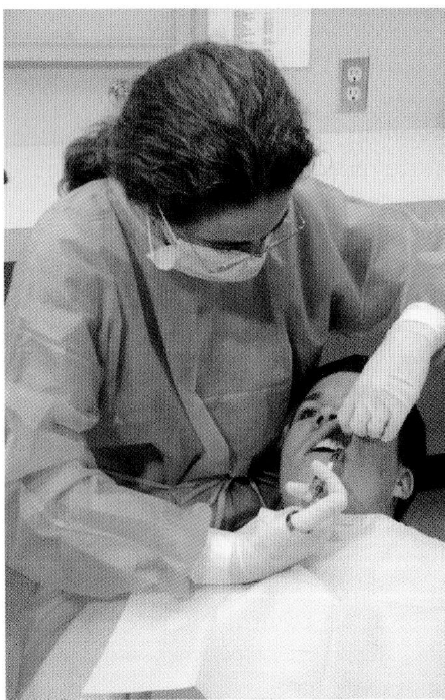

Figure 13-17. Position of the administrator for a right or left anterior superior alveolar (ASA) nerve block. The patient's head should be turned slightly to improve visibility.

   b. Position the patient supine (much preferred) or semisupine with the neck extended slightly. If the patient's neck is not extended, the patient's chest may interfere with the syringe barrel.
   c. Prepare the tissues at the injection site (height of the mucobuccal fold) for penetration.
      (1) Dry with sterile gauze.
      (2) Apply topical antiseptic (optional).
      (3) Apply topical anesthetic for a minimum of 1 minute.
   d. Locate the infraorbital foramen (Fig. 13-18).
      (1) Feel the infraorbital notch.
      (2) Move your finger downward from the notch, applying gentle pressure to the tissues.
      (3) The bone immediately inferior to the notch is convex (felt as an outward bulge). This represents the lower border of the orbit and the roof of the infraorbital foramen (Fig. 13-18, *B*).
      (4) As your finger continues inferiorly, a concavity is felt; this is the infraorbital foramen.
      (5) While applying pressure, feel the outlines of the infraorbital foramen at this site. The patient senses a mild soreness when the foramen is palpated as the infraorbital nerve is pressed against bone.
   e. Maintain your finger on the foramen or mark the skin at the site (Fig. 13-19).
   f. Retract the lip, pulling the tissues in the mucobuccal fold taut and increasing visibility. A 2 × 2-inch sterile gauze placed beneath your gloved finger aids in retraction of the lip during the ASA injection.
   g. Insert the needle into the height of the mucobuccal fold over the first premolar with the bevel facing bone (Fig. 13-20).
   h. Orient the syringe toward the infraorbital foramen.

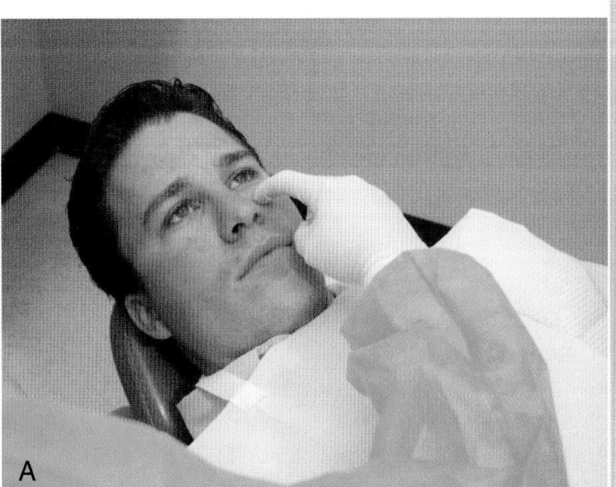

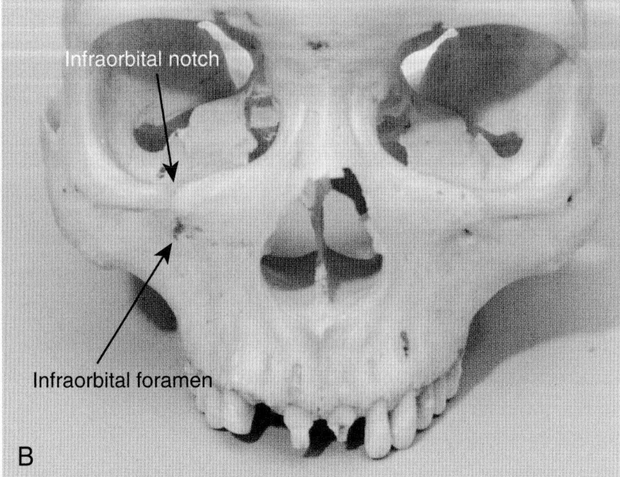

Figure 13-18. **A,** Palpate the infraorbital notch. **B,** Location of the infraorbital foramen in relation to the infraorbital notch.

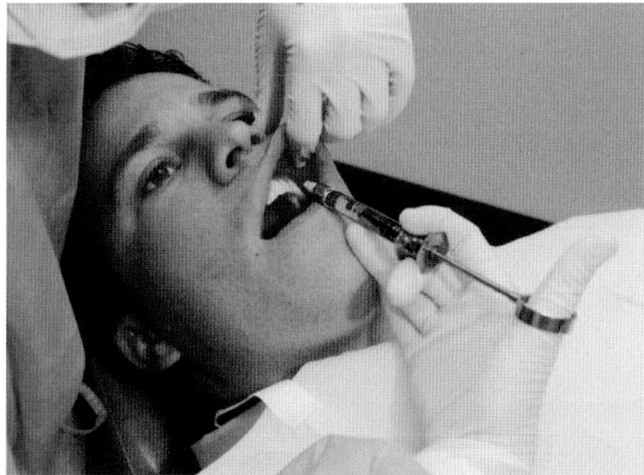

Figure 13-19. Using a finger over the foramen, lift the lip, and hold the tissues in the mucobuccal fold taut.

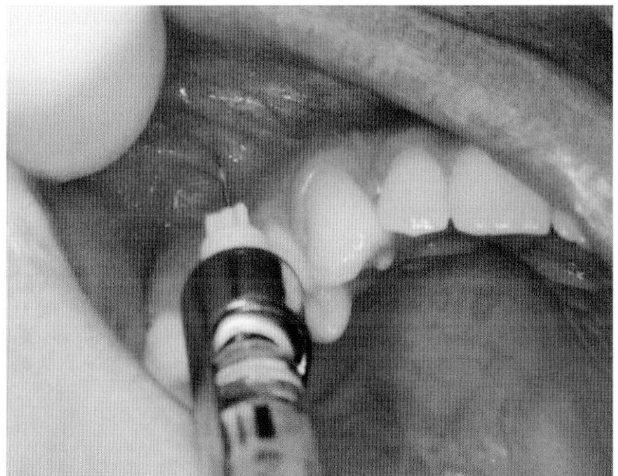

Figure 13-20. Insert the needle for anterior superior alveolar (ASA) nerve block in the mucobuccal fold over the maxillary first premolar.

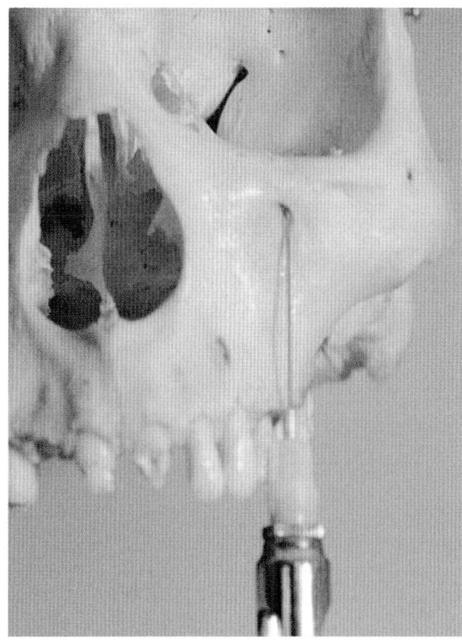

Figure 13-21. Advance the needle parallel to the long axis of the tooth to preclude prematurely contacting bone. Note how the bone of the maxilla becomes concave between the root eminence and the infraorbital foramen (note shadow).

i. The needle should be held parallel with the long axis of the tooth as it is advanced, to avoid premature contact with bone (Fig. 13-21).
j. Advance the needle slowly until bone is gently contacted.
   (1) The point of contact should be the upper rim of the infraorbital foramen.
   (2) The general depth of needle penetration is 16 mm for an adult of average height (equivalent to about half the length of a long needle).
   (3) The depth of penetration varies, of course. In a patient with a high (deep) mucobuccal fold or a low infraorbital foramen, less tissue penetration is necessary than in one with a shallow mucobuccal fold or a high infraorbital foramen.
   (4) A preinjection approximation of the depth of penetration can be made by placing one finger on the infraorbital foramen and another on the injection site in the mucobuccal fold and estimating the distance between them.
k. Before injecting the anesthetic solution, check for the following:
   (1) Depth of needle penetration (adequate to reach the foramen)
   (2) Any lateral deviation of the needle from the infraorbital foramen; correct before injecting solution
   (3) Orientation of the bevel (facing bone)
l. Position the needle tip during injection with the bevel facing into the infraorbital foramen and the needle tip touching the roof of the foramen (Fig. 13-22).
m. Aspirate in two planes.
n. Slowly deposit 0.9 to 1.2 mL (over 30 to 40 seconds). Little or no swelling should be visible as the solution is deposited. If the needle tip is properly inserted at the opening of the foramen, solution is directed toward the foramen.
   (1) The administrator is able to "feel" the anesthetic solution as it is deposited beneath the finger on the foramen if the needle tip is in the correct position. At the conclusion of the injection, the foramen should no longer be palpable (because of the volume of anesthetic in this position).

At this point, the infraorbital nerve block (providing anesthesia to the soft tissues on the anterior portion of the face and the lateral aspect of the nose) is complete. To transform it into the anterior superior alveolar nerve block

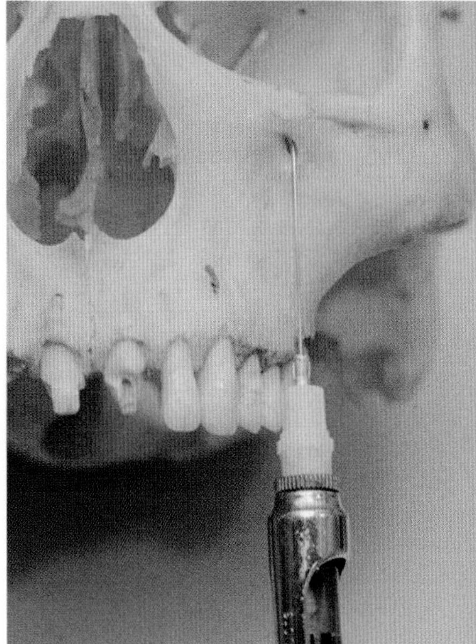

Figure 13-22. Position of the needle tip before deposition of local anesthetic at the infraorbital foramen.

(providing anesthesia to the teeth and their supporting structures), do the following:

o. Maintain firm pressure with your finger over the injection site both during and for at least 1 minute after the injection (to increase the diffusion of local anesthetic solution into the infraorbital foramen).
p. Withdraw the syringe slowly and immediately make the needle safe.
q. Maintain direct finger pressure over the injection site for a minimum of 1 minute, preferably 2 minutes, after injection.
r. Wait a minimum of 3 to 5 minutes after completion of the injection before commencing the dental procedure.

Signs and Symptoms

1. Subjective: Tingling and numbness of the lower eyelid, side of the nose, and upper lip indicate anesthesia of the infraorbital nerve, not the ASA or MSA nerve (soft tissue anesthesia develops almost instantly as the anesthetic is being administered).
2. Subjective and objective: numbness in the teeth and soft tissues along the distribution of the ASA and MSA nerves (developing within 3 to 5 minutes if pressure is maintained over the injection site)
3. Objective: use of electrical pulp testing with no response from tooth with maximal EPT output (80/80)
4. Absence of pain during treatment

Safety Features

1. Needle contact with bone at the roof of the infraorbital foramen prevents inadvertent overinsertion and possible puncture of the orbit.
2. A finger positioned over the infraorbital foramen helps direct the needle toward the foramen.
   a. The needle should not be palpable. If it is felt, then its path is too superficial (away from the bone). If this occurs, withdraw the needle slightly and redirect it toward the target area.
   b. In most patients, it is not possible to palpate the needle through soft tissues over the foramen unless it is too superficial. However, in some patients with less well-developed facial musculature, a properly positioned needle may be palpable.

Precautions

1. For pain on insertion of the needle and tearing of the periosteum, reinsert the needle in a more lateral (away from bone) position, or deposit solution as the needle advances through soft tissue.
2. To prevent overinsertion of the needle, estimate the depth of penetration before injection (review procedure), and exert finger pressure over the infraorbital foramen.
   a. Overinsertion is unlikely because of the rim of bone that forms the superior rim of the infraorbital foramen. The needle tip contacts this rim.

Failures of Anesthesia

1. Needle contacting bone below (inferior to) the infraorbital foramen: Anesthesia of the lower eyelid, lateral side of the nose, and upper lip may develop with little or no dental anesthesia; a bolus of solution may be felt beneath the skin in the area of deposition, which lies at a distance from the infraorbital foramen (which is still palpable after the local anesthetic solution has been injected). These are, by far, the most common causes of anesthetic failure within the distribution of the ASA nerve. In essence, a failed ASA is a supraperiosteal injection over the first premolar. To correct:
   a. Keep the needle in line with the infraorbital foramen during penetration. Do not direct the needle toward bone.
   b. Estimate the depth of penetration before injecting.
2. Needle deviation medial or lateral to the infraorbital foramen. To correct:
   a. Direct the needle toward the foramen immediately after inserting and before advancing through the tissue.
   b. Recheck needle placement before aspirating and depositing the anesthetic solution.

Complications. Hematoma (rare) may develop across the lower eyelid and the tissues between it and the infraorbital foramen. To manage, apply pressure on the soft tissue over the foramen for 2 to 3 minutes. Hematoma is extremely rare because pressure is routinely applied to the injection site both during and after administration of the ASA nerve block.

PALATAL ANESTHESIA

Anesthesia of the hard palate is necessary for dental procedures involving manipulation of palatal soft or hard tissues. For many dental patients, palatal injections prove to be a very traumatic experience. For many dentists, administration of palatal anesthesia is one of the most traumatic procedures they perform in dentistry.[2] Indeed, many dentists and dental hygienists advise their patients that they expect them to feel pain (dental professionals usually use the term *discomfort* rather than *pain* when describing painful procedures) during palatal injections! Forewarning the patient about procedural pain permits the patient to become more prepared psychologically ("psych themselves up") and relieves the administrator of responsibility when the pain occurs. When the patient acknowledges the existence of pain, the administrator can console the patient with a shrug of the shoulders and a kind word, once again confirming to both the patient and the administrator that palatal injections always hurt.

However, palatal anesthesia can be achieved atraumatically. At best, patients are unaware of the needle penetration of soft tissues and deposition of the local anesthetic solution (they won't even feel it). At worst, when the following techniques are adhered to, patients state that although they still were somewhat uncomfortable, this palatal injection was the least painful they had ever received.

With the introduction of computer-controlled local anesthetic delivery (C-CLAD) systems (The Wand, Comfort Control Syringe, and STA [see Chapter 5]), delivery of atraumatic palatal injections has become even more simplified.[3-5]

The steps in the atraumatic administration of palatal anesthesia are as follows:

1. Provide adequate topical anesthesia at the site of needle penetration.
2. Use pressure anesthesia at the site both before and during needle insertion and the deposition of solution.
3. Maintain control over the needle.
4. Deposit the anesthetic solution slowly.
5. Trust yourself…that you can complete the procedure atraumatically.

Adequate topical anesthesia at the injection site can be provided by allowing topical anesthetic to remain in contact with the soft tissues for at least 2 minutes. The palate is the one area in the mouth where the cotton swab must be held in position by the administrator the entire time.

Pressure anesthesia can be produced at the site of injection by applying considerable pressure to tissues adjacent to the injection site with a firm object, such as the cotton applicator stick previously used to apply the topical anesthetic. Other objects, such as the handle of a mouth mirror, are used by some, but because these objects are metal or plastic, they are more likely to hurt the patient. The goal is to produce anesthesia of the soft tissues through use of the gate control theory of pain.[6] The applicator stick should be pressed firmly enough to produce ischemia (blanching) of the normally pink tissues at the penetration site and a feeling of intense pressure (dull and tolerable, not sharp and painful) (Fig. 13-23). Pressure anesthesia should be maintained during penetration of the soft tissues with the needle and must be maintained throughout the time the needle remains in the palatal soft tissues.

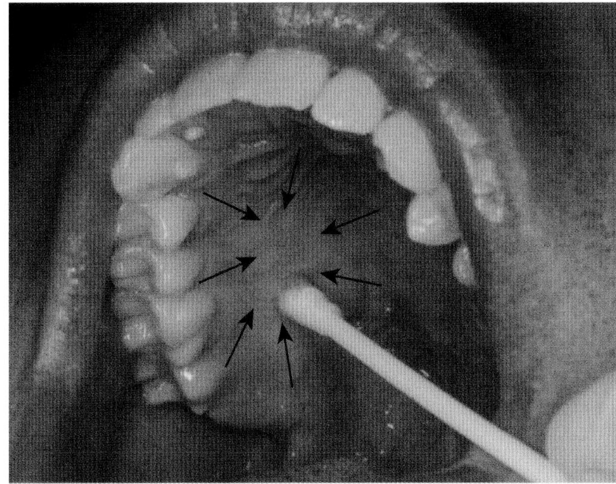

Figure 13-23. Note ischemia *(arrows)* of palatal tissues produced by pressure from the applicator stick.

Control over the needle is probably of greater importance in palatal anesthesia than in other intraoral injections. To achieve this control, the administrator must secure a firm hand rest. Several positions are illustrated in Chapter 11. When palatal anesthesia is administered, it is possible on occasion to stabilize the needle with both hands (Fig. 13-24). Perfection of this technique is attained only with experience.

The 27-gauge short needle is recommended for palatal injection techniques because patients are unable to distinguish the "feel" between a 27- and a 30-gauge needle.[7]

Slow deposition of the local anesthetic is important in all injection techniques, not only as a safety feature but also as a means of providing an atraumatic injection. Because of the density of the palatal soft tissues and their firm adherence to underlying bone, slow deposition is of even greater importance here. Rapid injection of the solution produces high tissue pressure, which tears the palatal soft tissues and leads to both pain on injection and localized soreness when the anesthetic actions are terminated. Slow injection of the local anesthetic is not uncomfortable for the patient.

Probably the most important factor in providing an atraumatic palatal injection is the belief by the administrator that it can be done painlessly; from this belief, special care is then taken to minimize discomfort to the patient; this generally results in a more atraumatic palatal injection.

Five palatal injections are described. Three—the anterior (or greater) palatine nerve block, providing anesthesia of the posterior portions of the hard palate; the nasopalatine nerve block, producing anesthesia of the anterior hard palate; and local infiltration of the hard palate—are used primarily to achieve soft tissue anesthesia and hemostasis before surgical procedures. None provides any pulpal anesthesia to the

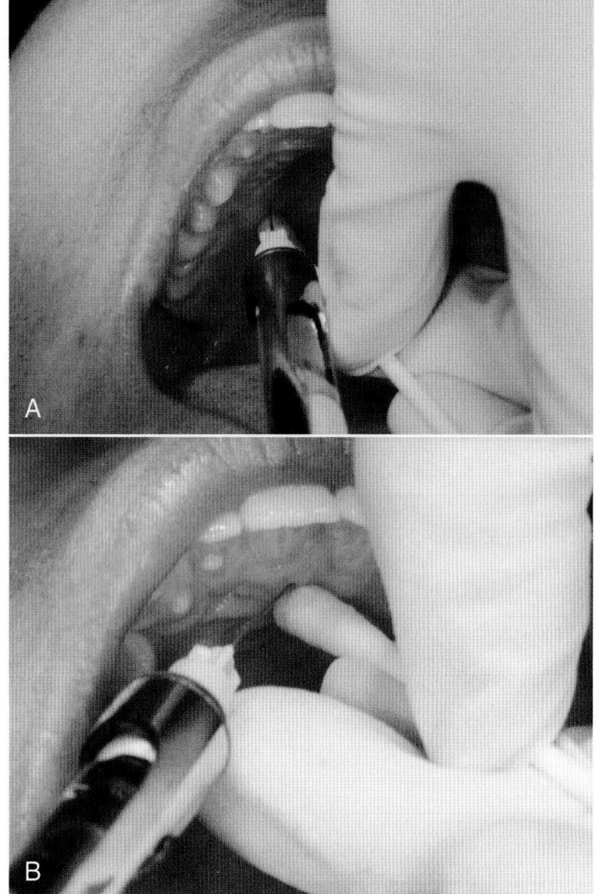

Figure 13-24. Stabilization of the needle for (**A**) greater palatine and (**B**) nasopalatine nerve block. With both injections, the barrel of the syringe should rest against the patient's lower lip.

maxillary teeth. AMSA and P-ASA are recently introduced techniques that provide extensive areas of pulpal and palatal anesthesia.[5,8]

Greater Palatine Nerve Block

The greater palatine nerve block is useful for dental procedures involving the palatal soft tissues distal to the canine. Minimum volumes of solution (0.45 to 0.6 mL) provide profound hard and soft tissue anesthesia. Although potentially traumatic, the greater palatine nerve block is less so than the nasopalatine nerve block because tissues surrounding the greater palatine foramen are not as firmly adherent to bone and therefore are better able to accommodate the volume of solution deposited.

Other Common Name. Anterior palatine nerve block.

Nerve Anesthetized. Greater palatine.

Areas Anesthetized. The posterior portion of the hard palate and its overlying soft tissues, anteriorly as far as the first premolar and medially to the midline (Fig. 13-25).

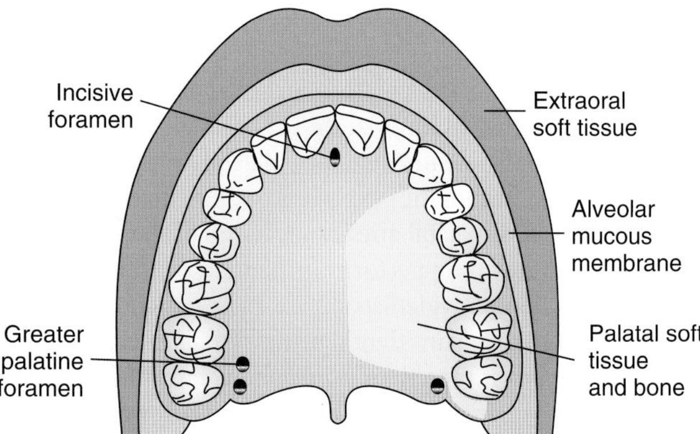

Figure 13-25. Area anesthetized by greater palatine nerve block.

Indications

1. When palatal soft tissue anesthesia is necessary for restorative therapy on more than two teeth (e.g., with subgingival restorations, with insertion of matrix bands subgingivally)
2. For pain control during periodontal or oral surgical procedures involving the palatal soft and hard tissues

Contraindications

1. Inflammation or infection at the injection site
2. Smaller areas of therapy (one or two teeth)

Advantages

1. Minimizes needle penetrations and volume of solution
2. Minimizes patient discomfort

Disadvantages

1. No hemostasis except in the immediate area of injection
2. Potentially traumatic

Positive Aspiration. Less than 1%.

Alternatives

1. Local infiltration into specific regions
2. Maxillary nerve block

Technique

1. A 27-gauge short needle is recommended.
2. Area of insertion: soft tissue slightly anterior to the greater palatine foramen
3. Target area: greater (anterior) palatine nerve as it passes anteriorly between soft tissues and bone of the hard palate (Fig. 13-26)
4. Landmarks: greater palatine foramen and junction of the maxillary alveolar process and palatine bone
5. Path of insertion: advance the syringe from the opposite side of the mouth at a right angle to the target area
6. Orientation of the bevel: toward the palatal soft tissues (See steps g and h, p. 204.)
7. Procedure:
   a. Assume the correct position (Fig. 13-27).

(1) For a right greater palatine nerve block, a right-handed administrator should sit facing the patient at the 7 or 8 o'clock position.
(2) For a left greater palatine nerve block, a right-handed administrator should sit facing in the same direction as the patient at the 11 o'clock position.

b. Ask the patient, who is in a supine position (Fig. 13-28, *A*), to do the following:
(1) Open wide.
(2) Extend the neck.
(3) Turn the head to the left or right (for improved visibility).

c. Locate the greater palatine foramen (Fig. 13-28, *B*, and Table 13-2).

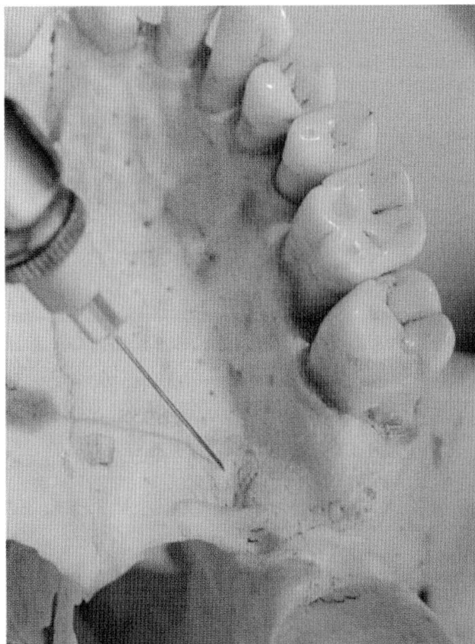

Figure 13-26. Target area for a greater palatine nerve block.

(1) Place a cotton swab at the junction of the maxillary alveolar process and the hard palate.
(2) Start in the region of the maxillary first molar and palpate posteriorly by pressing firmly into the tissues with the swab.
(3) The swab "falls" into the depression created by the greater palatine foramen (Fig. 13-29).
(4) The foramen is most frequently located distal to the maxillary second molar, but it may be located anterior or posterior to its usual position. (See "Maxillary Nerve Block," p. 220.)

d. Prepare the tissue at the injection site, just 1 to 2 mm anterior to the greater palatine foramen.
(1) Clean and dry with sterile gauze.
(2) Apply topical antiseptic (optional).
(3) Apply topical anesthetic for 2 minutes.

e. After 2 minutes of topical anesthetic application, move the swab posteriorly so it is directly over the greater palatine foramen.
(1) Apply considerable pressure at the area of the foramen with the swab in the left hand (if right-handed).
(2) Note the ischemia (whitening of the soft tissues) at the injection site.

TABLE 13-2
Location of the Greater Palatine Foramen*

Location	No.	Percent
Anterior half second molar	0	0
Posterior half second molar	63	39.87
Anterior half third molar	80	50.63
Posterior half third molar	15	9.49

From Malamed SF, Trieger N: Intraoral maxillary nerve block: an anatomical and clinical study, Anesth Prog 30:44–48, 1983.
*Measurements from 158 skulls with the maxillary second and third molars present.

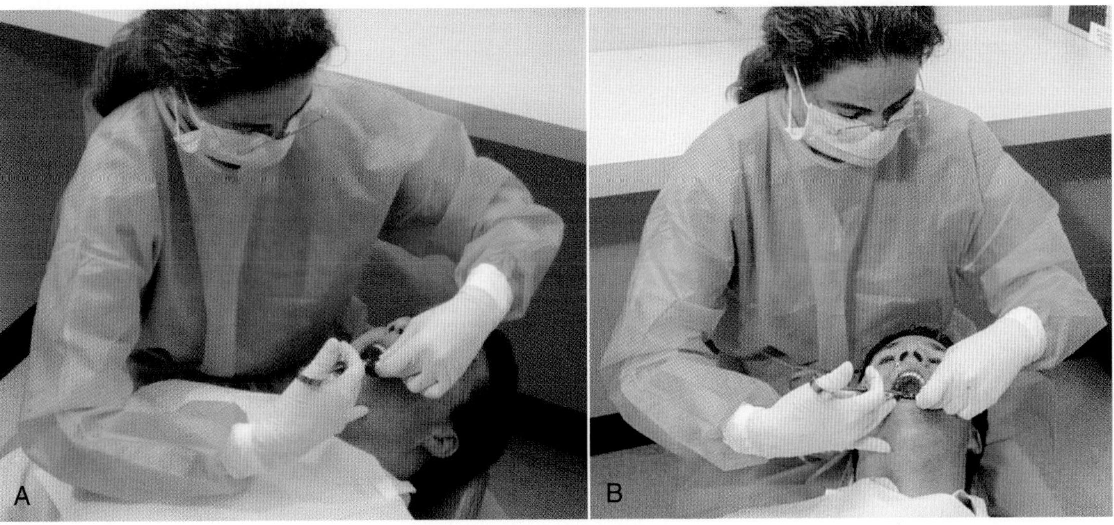

Figure 13-27. Position of the administrator for **(A)** right and **(B)** left greater palatine nerve block.

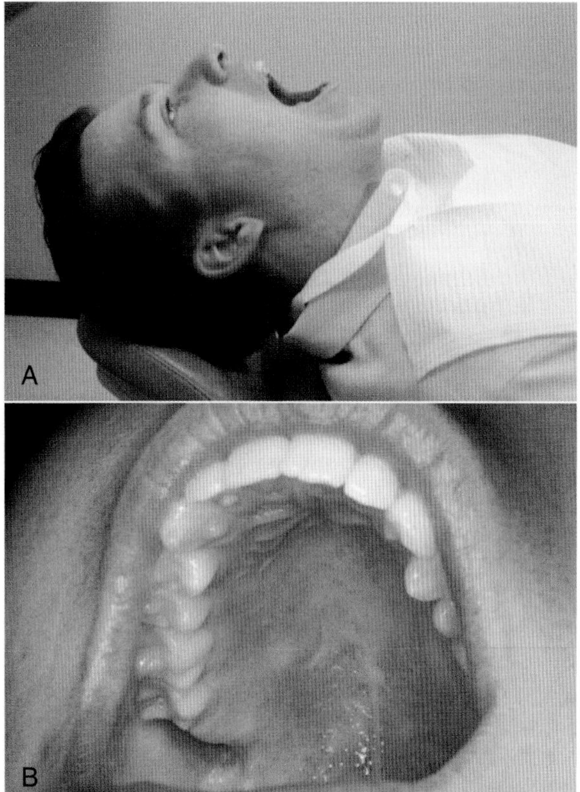

Figure 13-28. **A,** Patient position for a greater palatine nerve block. **B,** Administrator's view of hard palate when patient is properly positioned.

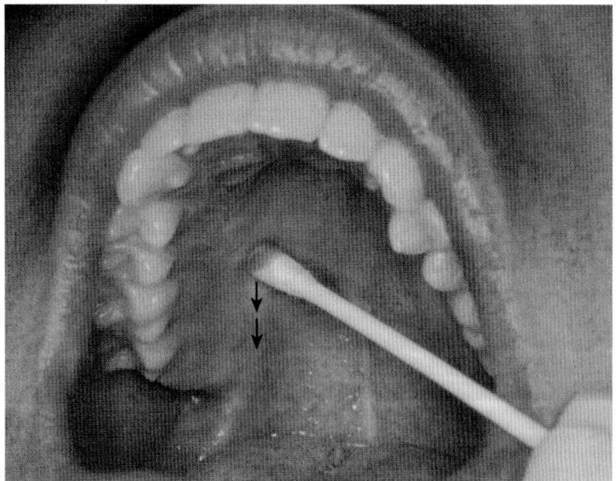

Figure 13-29. A cotton swab is pressed against the hard palate at the junction of the maxillary alveolar process and palatal bone. The swab is slowly moved distally *(arrows)* until a depression in the tissue is felt. This is the greater (anterior) palatine foramen.

(3) Apply pressure for a minimum of 30 seconds, and while doing this proceed to the following steps.

f. Direct the syringe into the mouth from the opposite side with the needle approaching the injection site at a right angle (Fig. 13-30).

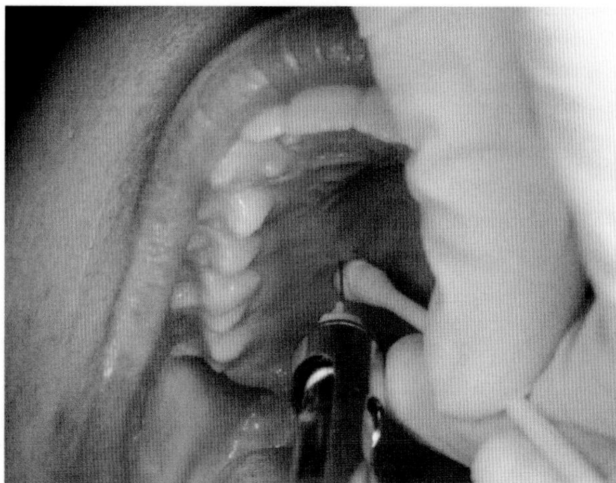

Figure 13-30. Note the angle of needle entry into the mouth. The insertion is into ischemic tissues slightly anterior to the applicator stick. The barrel of the syringe is stabilized by the corner of the mouth and the teeth.

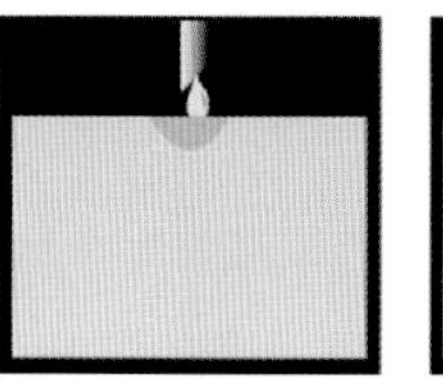
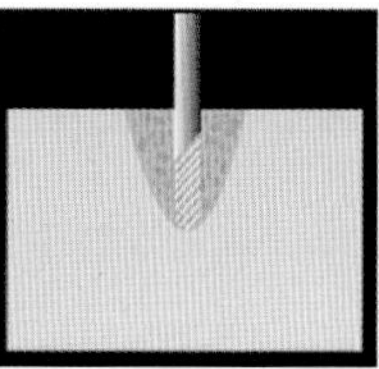
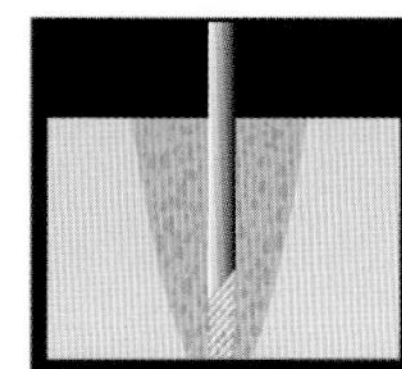

Figure 13-31. Prepuncture technique: bevel of needle placed on soft tissue; pressure exerted by cotton applicator stick. Local anesthetic solution deposited before needle enters tissues.

g. Place the bevel (not the point) of the needle gently against the previously blanched (ischemic) soft tissue at the injection site. It must be well stabilized to prevent accidental penetration of the tissues.

h. With the bevel lying against the tissue:
   (1) Apply enough pressure to bow the needle slightly.
   (2) Deposit a small volume of anesthetic. The solution is forced against the mucous membrane, and a droplet forms (Fig. 13-31).

i. Straighten the needle and permit the bevel to penetrate mucosa.
   (1) Continue to deposit small volumes of anesthetic throughout the procedure.
   (2) Ischemia spreads into adjacent tissues as the anesthetic (usually with a vasoconstrictor) is deposited (Figs. 13-32 and 13-33).

j. Continue to apply pressure anesthesia throughout the deposition of the anesthetic solution (see Fig. 13-32). Ischemia spreads as the vasoconstrictor decreases tissue perfusion.

k. Slowly advance the needle until palatine bone is gently contacted.
   (1) The depth of penetration is usually about 5 mm.

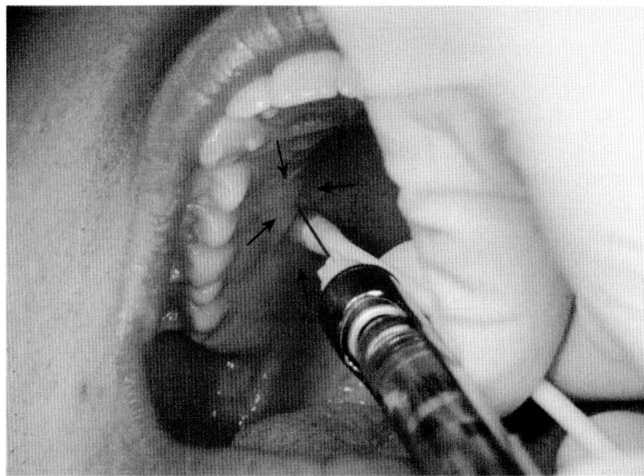

Figure 13-32. Note the spread of ischemia *(arrows)* as the anesthetic is deposited.

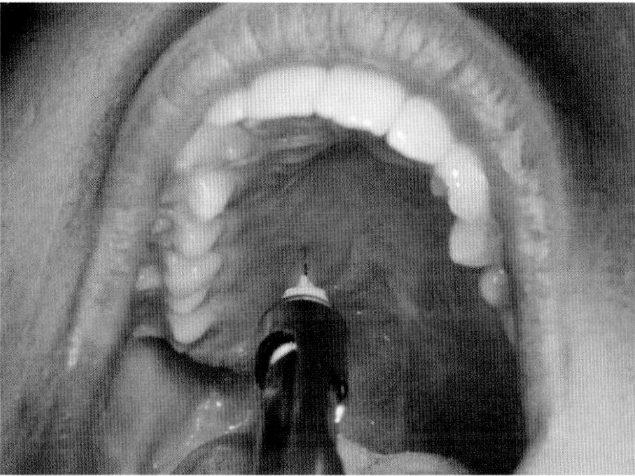

Figure 13-33. The cotton swab is removed when the deposition of solution ceases.

(2) Continue to deposit small volumes of anesthetic. As the tissue is entered, a slight increase in resistance to the deposition of solution may be noted; this is entirely normal in the greater palatine nerve block.

l. Aspirate in two planes.
m. If negative, slowly deposit (30 second minimum) not more than one fourth to one third of a cartridge (0.45 to 0.6 mL).
n. Withdraw the syringe.
o. Make the needle safe.
p. Wait 2 to 3 minutes before commencing the procedure.

Signs and Symptoms

1. Subjective: numbness in the posterior portion of the palate
2. Objective: no pain during dental therapy

Safety Features

1. Contact with bone
2. Aspiration

Precautions. Do not enter the greater palatine canal. Although this is not hazardous, there is no reason to enter the canal for this technique to be successful.

Failures of Anesthesia

1. The greater palatine nerve block is not a technically difficult injection to administer. The incidence of success is well above 95%.
2. If local anesthetic is deposited too far anterior to the foramen, adequate soft tissue anesthesia may not occur in the palatal tissues posterior to the site of injection (partial success).
3. Anesthesia on the palate in the area of the maxillary first premolar may prove inadequate because of overlapping fibers from the nasopalatine nerve (partial success).
   a. To correct: Local infiltration may be necessary as a supplement in the area of inadequate anesthesia.

Complications

1. Few of significance
2. Ischemia and necrosis of soft tissues when highly concentrated vasoconstricting solution used for hemostasis over a prolonged period
   a. Norepinephrine should never be used for hemostasis on the palatal soft tissues (norepinephrine is not available in dental local anesthetics in the United States or Canada).
3. Hematoma is possible but rare because of the density and firm adherence of palatal tissues to underlying bone.
4. Some patients may be uncomfortable if their soft palate becomes anesthetized; this is a distinct possibility when the middle palatine nerve exits near the injection site.

Nasopalatine Nerve Block

Nasopalatine nerve block is an invaluable technique for palatal pain control in that, with administration of a minimum volume of anesthetic solution (maximally, one quarter of a cartridge), a wide area of palatal soft tissue anesthesia is achieved, thereby minimizing the need for multiple palatal injections. Unfortunately, the nasopalatine nerve block has the distinction of being a potentially highly traumatic (e.g., painful) injection. With no other injection technique is the need for strict adherence to the protocol of atraumatic injection more important than with the nasopalatine nerve block. Two approaches to this injection are presented. Readers should become familiar with both techniques and then should use the one with which they feel more comfortable (e.g., that works best in their hands).

The first approach involves only one tissue penetration, lateral to the incisive papilla on the palatal aspect of the maxillary central incisors. The soft tissue in this area is dense, firmly adherent to underlying bone, and quite sensitive; these three factors combine to increase patient discomfort during injection. The second approach was recommended by a number of readers of earlier editions of this book. It involves three needle punctures but, when carried out properly, is significantly less traumatic than the more direct one-puncture technique. In it, the labial soft tissues between maxillary central incisors are anesthetized (injection #1), then the needle is directed from the labial aspect through the interproximal papilla between the central incisors toward the incisive papilla on the palate to anesthetize the superficial tissues in this area (injection #2). A third injection, directly into the now partially anesthetized palatal soft tissues overlying the nasopalatine nerve, is necessary. Although the single-needle puncture technique may be preferred whenever possible, the second approach can produce effective nasopalatine anesthesia with a minimum of discomfort.

Other Common Names. Incisive nerve block, sphenopalatine nerve block.

Nerves Anesthetized. Nasopalatine nerves bilaterally.

Areas Anesthetized. Anterior portion of the hard palate (soft and hard tissues) bilaterally from the mesial of the right first premolar to the mesial of the left first premolar (Fig. 13-34).

Indications

1. When palatal soft tissue anesthesia is necessary for restorative treatment on more than two teeth (e.g., subgingival restorations, insertion of matrix bands subgingivally)
2. For pain control during periodontal or oral surgical procedures involving palatal soft and hard tissues

Contraindications

1. Inflammation or infection at the injection site
2. Smaller area of therapy (one or two teeth)

Advantages

1. Minimizes needle penetrations and volume of solution
2. Minimal patient discomfort from multiple needle penetrations

Disadvantages

1. No hemostasis except in the immediate area of injection
2. Potentially the most traumatic intraoral injection; however, the protocol for an atraumatic injection or use of a C-CLAD system or a buffered local anesthetic solution can minimize or entirely eliminate discomfort

Positive Aspiration. Less than 1%.

Alternatives

1. Local infiltration into specific regions
2. Maxillary nerve block (unilateral only)
3. Anterior middle superior alveolar (AMSA) nerve block (unilateral only)

Technique (Single-Needle Penetration of the Palate)

1. A 27-gauge short needle is recommended.
2. Area of insertion: palatal mucosa just lateral to the incisive papilla (located in the midline behind the central incisors); the tissue here is more sensitive than other palatal mucosa
3. Target area: incisive foramen, beneath the incisive papilla (Fig. 13-35)
4. Landmarks: central incisors and incisive papilla
5. Path of insertion: Approach the injection site at a 45-degree angle toward the incisive papilla.
6. Orientation of the bevel: toward the palatal soft tissues (review procedure for the basic palatal injection)
7. Procedure:
   a. Sit at the 9 or 10 o'clock position facing in the same direction as the patient (Fig. 13-36).
   b. Request the patient to do the following:
      (1) Open wide.
      (2) Extend the neck.

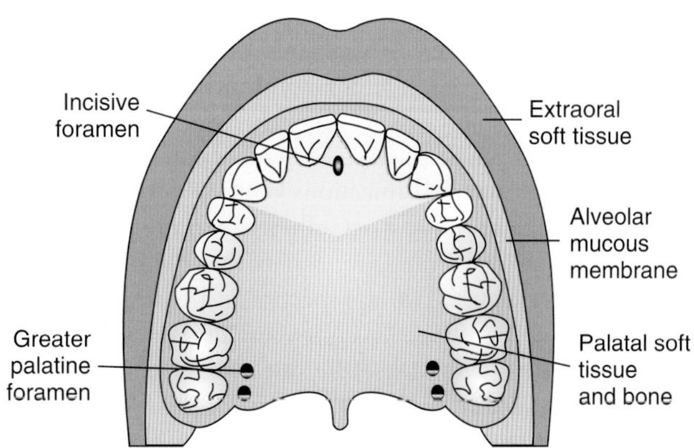

Figure 13-34. Area anesthetized by a nasopalatine nerve block.

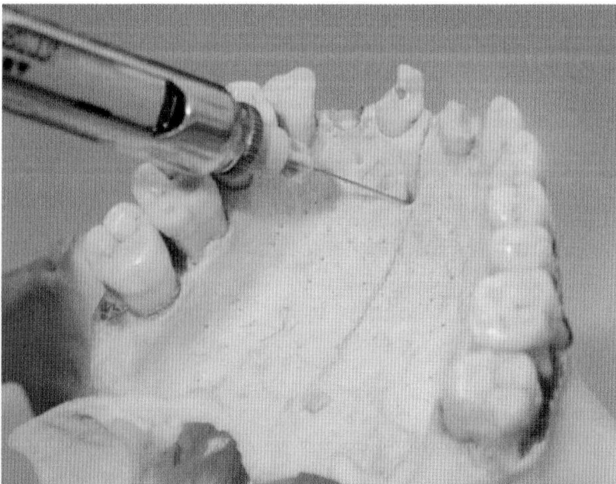

Figure 13-35. Target area for a nasopalatine nerve block.

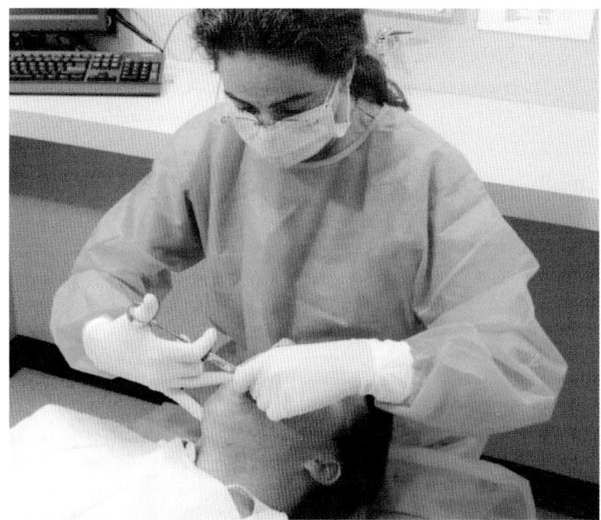

Figure 13-36. Position of the administrator for a nasopalatine nerve block.

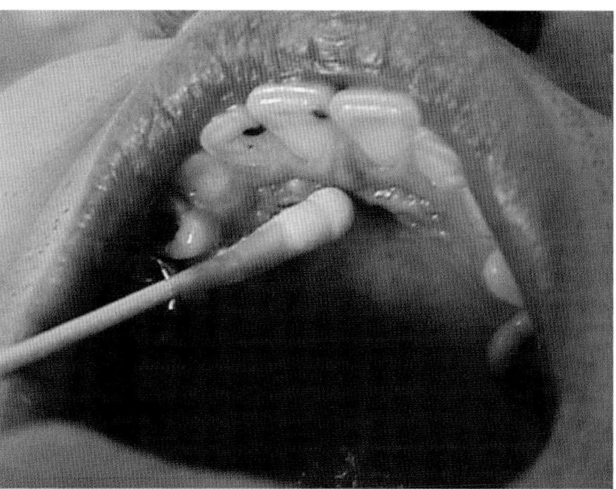

Figure 13-38. Topical anesthetic is applied lateral to the incisive papilla for 2 minutes, and then pressure is applied directly to the incisive papilla.

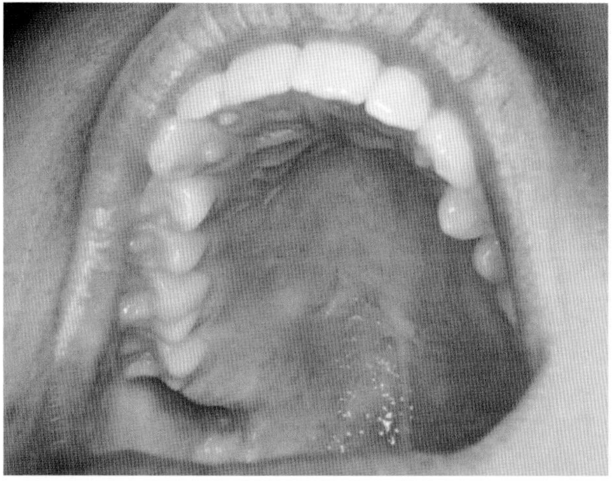

Figure 13-37. Palate when the patient is positioned properly.

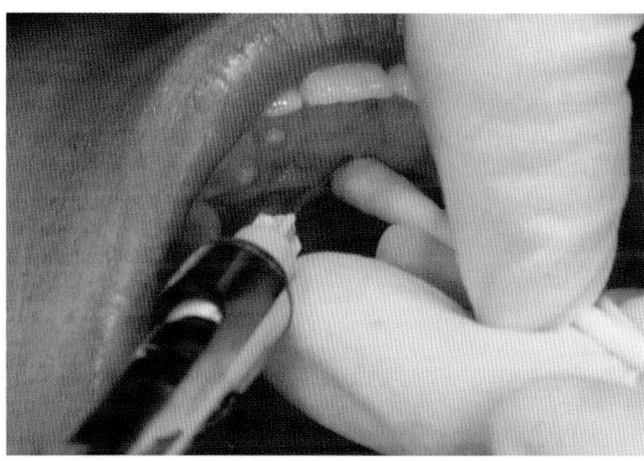

Figure 13-39. Pressure is maintained until the deposition of solution is completed. Needle penetration is just lateral to the incisive papilla.

(3) Turn the head to the left or right for improved visibility (Fig. 13-37).

c. Prepare the tissue just lateral to the incisive papilla (Fig. 13-38).
   (1) Clean and dry with sterile gauze.
   (2) Apply topical antiseptic (optional).
   (3) Apply topical anesthetic for 2 minutes.

d. After 2 minutes of topical anesthetic application, move the swab directly onto the incisive papilla (see Figs. 13-38 and 13-39).
   (1) With the swab in your left hand (if right-handed), apply pressure to the area of the papilla.
   (2) Note ischemia at the injection site.

e. Place the bevel against the ischemic soft tissues at the injection site. The needle must be well stabilized to prevent accidental penetration of tissues (see Fig. 13-39).

f. With the bevel lying against the tissue:
   (1) Apply enough pressure to bow the needle slightly.
   (2) Deposit a small volume of anesthetic. The solution will be forced against the mucous membrane.

g. Straighten the needle and permit the bevel to penetrate the mucosa.
   (1) Continue to deposit small volumes of anesthetic throughout the procedure.
   (2) Observe ischemia spreading into adjacent tissues as solution is deposited.

h. Continue to apply pressure with the cotton applicator stick while injecting the anesthetic.

i. Slowly advance the needle toward the incisive foramen until bone is gently contacted (see Fig. 13-35).
   (1) The depth of penetration normally is not greater than 5 mm.

(2) Deposit small volumes of anesthetic while advancing the needle. As the tissue is entered, resistance to the deposition of solution is significantly increased; this is normal with the nasopalatine nerve block.

j. Withdraw the needle 1 mm (to prevent subperiosteal injection). The bevel now lies over the center of the incisive foramen.

k. Aspirate in two planes.

l. If negative, slowly deposit (15- to 30-second minimum) not more than one fourth of a cartridge (0.45 mL).

(1) In some patients, it is difficult to deposit 0.45 mL of anesthetic solution in this injection. Injection of anesthetic can cease when the area of ischemia noted at the injection site has expanded from that produced by the application of pressure alone.

m. Slowly withdraw the syringe.

n. Make the needle safe.

o. Wait 2 to 3 minutes before commencing the dental procedure.

Signs and Symptoms

1. Subjective: numbness in the anterior portion of the palate
2. Objective: no pain during dental therapy

Safety Features

1. Contact with bone
2. Aspiration

Precautions

1. Against pain:
   a. Do not insert directly into the incisive papilla (quite painful).
   b. Do not deposit solution too rapidly.
   c. Do not deposit too much solution.
2. Against infection:
   a. If the needle is advanced more than 5 mm into the incisive canal and the floor of the nose is entered accidentally, infection may result. There is no reason for the needle to enter the incisive canal during a nasopalatine nerve block.

Failures of Anesthesia

1. Highly successful injection (>95% incidence of success)
2. Unilateral anesthesia:
   a. If solution is deposited to one side of the incisive canal, unilateral anesthesia may develop.
   b. To correct: Reinsert the needle into the already anesthetized tissue and reinject solution into the unanesthetized area.
3. Inadequate palatal soft tissue anesthesia in the area of the maxillary canine and first premolar:
   a. If fibers from the greater palatine nerve overlap those of the nasopalatine nerve, anesthesia of the soft tissues palatal to the canine and the first premolar could be inadequate.
   b. To correct: Local infiltration may be necessary as a supplement in the area inadequately anesthetized.

Complications

1. Few of significance
2. Hematoma is possible but extremely rare because of the density and firm adherence of palatal soft tissues to bone.
3. Necrosis of soft tissues is possible when highly concentrated vasoconstricting solution (e.g., norepinephrine) is used for hemostasis over a prolonged period (norepinephrine is not available in dental local anesthetics in the United States or Canada).
4. Because of the density of soft tissues, anesthetic solution may "squirt" back out the needle puncture site during administration or after needle withdrawal. (This is of no clinical significance. However, do not let it surprise you into uttering a statement such as "Whoops!" that might frighten the patient.)

Technique (Multiple Needle Penetrations)

1. A 27-gauge short needle is recommended.
2. Areas of insertion:
   a. Labial frenum in the midline between the maxillary central incisors (Fig. 13-40, *B*)
   b. Interdental papilla between the maxillary central incisors (Fig. 13-40, *C*)
   c. If needed, palatal soft tissues lateral to the incisive papilla (Fig. 13-40, *D*)
3. Target area: incisive foramen, beneath the incisive papilla
4. Landmarks: central incisors and incisive papilla
5. Path of insertion:
   a. First injection: infiltration into the labial frenum
   b. Second injection: needle held at a right angle to the interdental papilla
   c. Third injection: needle held at a 45-degree angle to the incisive papilla
6. Orientation of the bevel:
   a. First injection: bevel toward bone
   b. Second injection: not relevant
   c. Third injection: not relevant
7. Procedure:
   a. ***First injection:*** infiltration of 0.3 mL into the labial frenum (see Fig. 13-40, *B*)
      (1) Prepare the tissue at the injection site.
         (a) Clean and dry with sterile gauze.
         (b) Apply topical antiseptic (optional).
         (c) Apply topical anesthetic for 1 minute (Fig. 13-40, *A*).
      (2) Retract the upper lip to stretch tissues and improve visibility. (Be careful not to overstretch the frenum.)
      (3) Gently insert the needle into the frenum and deposit 0.3 mL of anesthetic in approximately 15

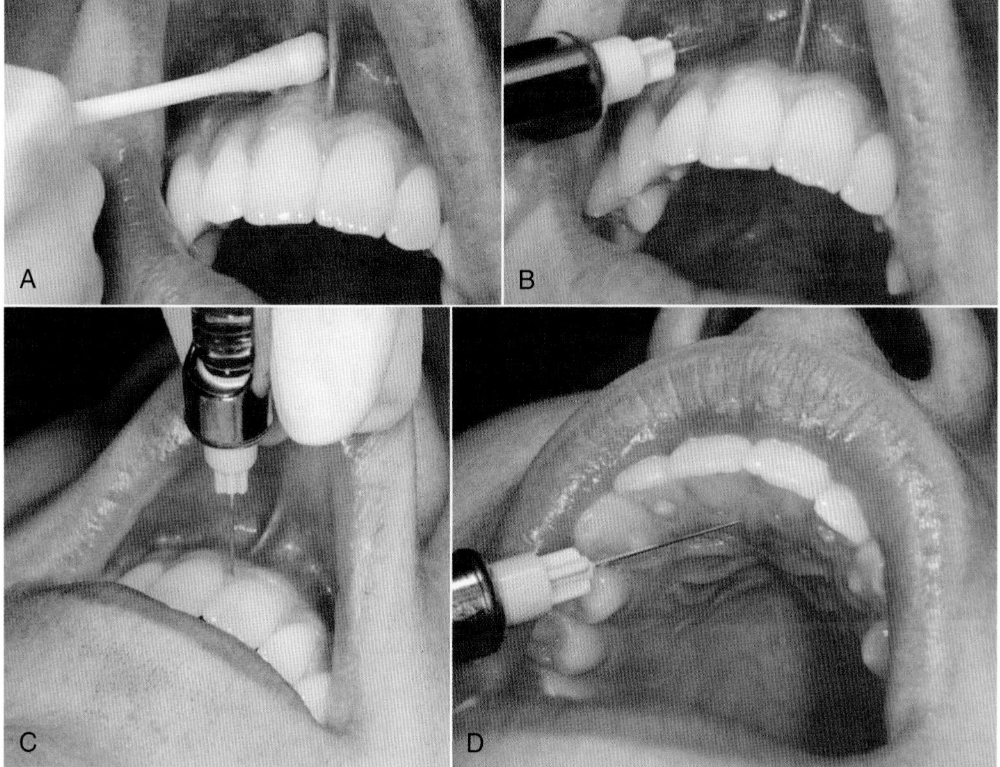

Figure 13-40. **A,** Topical anesthetic is applied to the mucosa of the frenum. **B,** First injection, into the labial frenum. **C,** Second injection, into the interdental papilla between the central incisors. **D,** Third injection, when anesthesia of the nasopalatine area is inadequate after the first two injections.

seconds. (The tissue may balloon as solution is injected.)

(4) Anesthesia of soft tissue develops immediately. The aim of this first injection is to anesthetize the interdental papilla between the two central incisors.

b. ***Second injection:*** penetration through the labial aspect of the papilla between the maxillary central incisors toward the incisive papilla (see Fig. 13-40, *C*)

(1) Retract the upper lip gently to increase visibility. (Do not overstretch the labial frenum.)

(2) If a right-handed administrator, sit at 11 or 12 o'clock facing in the same direction as the patient. Tilt the patient's head toward the right to provide a proper angle for needle penetration.

(3) Holding the needle at a right angle to the interdental papilla, insert it into the papilla just above the level of crestal bone.

(a) Direct it toward the incisive papilla (on the palatal side of the interdental papilla).

(b) Soft tissues on the labial surface have been anesthetized by the first injection, so there is no discomfort. However, as the needle penetrates toward the unanesthetized palatal side, it becomes necessary to administer minute amounts of local anesthetic to prevent discomfort.

(c) With the patient's head extended backward, you can see the ischemia produced by the local anesthetic and (on occasion) can see the needle tip as it nears the palatal aspect of the incisive papilla. Care must be taken to avoid needle puncturing through the papilla into the oral cavity on the palatal side.

(4) Aspirate in two planes when ischemia is noted in the incisive papilla or when the needle tip becomes visible just beneath the tissue surface. If negative, administer no more than 0.3 mL of anesthetic solution in approximately 15 seconds. There is considerable resistance to the deposition of solution but no patient discomfort.

(5) Stabilization of the syringe in this second injection is somewhat awkward, but critical. Use of a finger from the other hand to stabilize the needle is recommended (Fig. 13-41). However, the syringe barrel must be held such that it remains within the patient's line of sight; this is potentially disconcerting to some patients.

(6) Slowly withdraw the syringe.

(7) Make the needle safe.

(8) Anesthesia within the distribution of the right and left nasopalatine nerves usually develops in a minimum of 2 to 3 minutes.

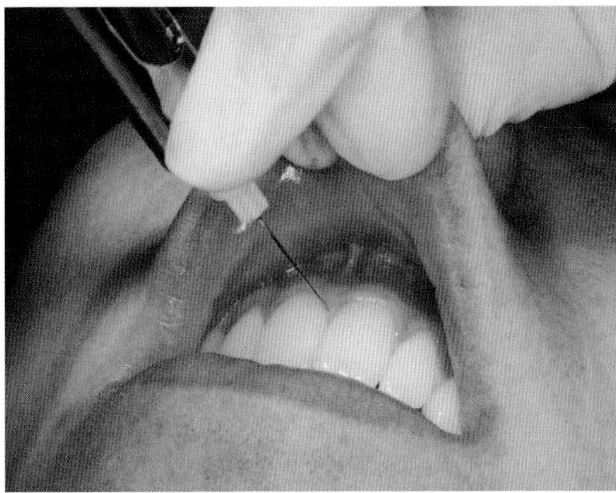

Figure 13-41. Use a finger of the opposite hand to stabilize the syringe during the second injection.

(9) If the area of clinically effective anesthesia proves to be less than adequate (as frequently happens), proceed to the third injection.

c. ***Third injection:***
   (1) Dry the tissue just lateral to the incisive papilla.
   (2) Ask the patient to open wide.
   (3) Extend the patient's neck.
   (4) Place the needle into soft tissue adjacent to the (diamond-shaped) incisive papilla, aiming toward the most distal portion of the papilla.
   (5) Advance the needle until contact is made with bone.
   (6) Withdraw the needle 1 mm to avoid subperiosteal injection.
   (7) Aspirate in two planes.
   (8) If negative, slowly deposit not more than 0.3 mL of anesthetic in approximately 15 seconds.
   Note: Use of topical and pressure anesthesia is unnecessary in the second and third injections because the tissues being penetrated by the needle are already anesthetized (by the first and second injections, respectively).
   (9) Withdraw the syringe.
   (10) Make the needle safe.
   (11) Wait a minimum of 2 to 3 minutes for the onset of anesthesia before beginning dental treatment.

Signs and Symptoms
1. Subjective: numbness of the upper lip (in the midline) and the anterior portion of the palate
2. Objective: no pain during dental therapy

Safety Features
1. Aspiration
2. Contact with bone (third injection)

Advantage. Entirely or relatively atraumatic

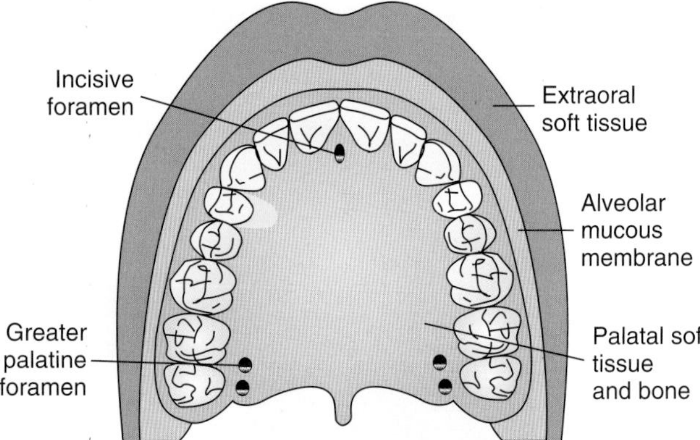

Figure 13-42. Area anesthetized by a palatal infiltration.

Disadvantages
1. Requires multiple injections (three)
2. Difficult to stabilize the syringe during the second injection
3. Syringe barrel usually within the patient's line of sight during the second injection

Precautions
1. Against pain: If each injection is performed as recommended, the entire technique should be atraumatic.
2. Against infection: On the third injection, do not advance the needle into the incisive canal. With accidental penetration of the nasal floor, the risk of infection is increased.

Failures of Anesthesia
1. A highly successful (>95%) injection
2. Inadequate anesthesia of soft tissues around the canine and first premolar because of overlapping fibers from the greater palatine nerve
   a. To correct: Local infiltration may be necessary as a supplement in the area.

Complications
1. Few of significance
2. Necrosis of soft tissues is possible when a highly concentrated vasoconstrictor solution, such as norepinephrine, is used for hemostasis over a prolonged period (norepinephrine is not available in dental local anesthetics in the United States or Canada).
3. Interdental papillae between the maxillary incisors sometimes are tender for several days after injection.

Local Infiltration of the Palate

Other Common Names. None.

Nerves Anesthetized. Terminal branches of the nasopalatine and greater palatine.

Areas Anesthetized. Soft tissues in the immediate vicinity of injection (Fig. 13-42).

Indications
1. Primarily for achieving hemostasis during surgical procedures
2. Palatogingival pain control when limited areas of anesthesia are necessary for application of a rubber dam clamp, packing of retraction cord in the gingival sulcus, or operative procedures on not more than two teeth

Contraindications
1. Inflammation or infection at the injection site
2. Pain control in soft tissue areas involving more than two teeth

Advantages
1. Provides acceptable hemostasis when a vasoconstrictor is used
2. Provides a minimum area of numbness

Disadvantage. Potentially traumatic injection.

Positive Aspiration. Negligible.

Alternatives
1. For hemostasis: none
2. For pain control: nasopalatine or greater palatine nerve block, AMSA, maxillary nerve block

Technique
1. A 27-gauge short needle is recommended.
2. Area of insertion: the attached gingiva 5 to 10 mm from the free gingival margin (Fig. 13-43)
3. Target area: gingival tissues 5 to 10 mm from the free gingival margin
4. Landmark: gingival tissue in the estimated center of the treatment area
5. Pathway of insertion: approaching the injection site at a 45-degree angle
6. Orientation of the bevel: toward palatal soft tissues

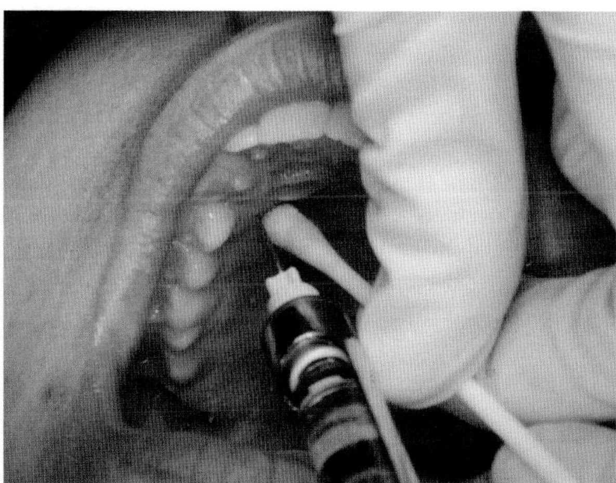

Figure 13-43. Area of insertion and target area for a palatal infiltration.

7. Procedure:
   a. If a right-handed administrator, sit at the 10 o'clock position.
      (1) Face toward the patient for palatal infiltration on the right side.
      (2) Face in the same direction as the patient for palatal infiltration on the left side.
   b. Ask the patient to do the following:
      (1) Open wide.
      (2) Extend the neck.
      (3) Turn the head to the left or right for improved visibility.
   c. Prepare the tissue at the site of injection.
      (1) Clean and dry with sterile gauze.
      (2) Apply topical antiseptic (optional).
      (3) Apply topical anesthetic for 2 minutes.
   d. After 2 minutes of topical anesthetic application, place the swab on the tissue immediately adjacent to the injection site.
      (1) With the swab in your left hand (if right-handed), apply pressure to the palatal soft tissues.
      (2) Observe the ischemia at the injection site.
   e. Place the bevel of the needle against the ischemic soft tissue at the injection site. The needle must be well stabilized to prevent accidental penetration of tissues.
   f. With the bevel lying against tissue:
      (1) Apply enough pressure to bow the needle slightly.
      (2) Deposit a small volume of local anesthetic. The solution is forced against the mucous membrane, forming a droplet.
   g. Straighten the needle and permit the bevel to penetrate mucosa.
      (1) Continue to deposit small volumes of local anesthetic throughout this procedure.
      (2) Ischemia of the tissues spreads as additional anesthetic is deposited. (When this injection is used for hemostasis, the vasoconstrictor in the local anesthetic produces intense ischemia of tissues.)
   h. Continue to apply pressure with the cotton applicator stick throughout the injection.
   i. Continue to advance the needle and deposit anesthetic until bone is gently contacted. Tissue thickness is only 3 to 5 mm in most patients.
   j. If hemostasis is the goal in this technique, continue to administer solution until ischemia encompasses the surgical site. In usual practice, 0.2 to 0.3 mL of solution is adequate.
   k. For hemostasis of larger surgical sites:
      (1) Remove the needle from the first injection site.
      (2) Place it in the new injection site at the periphery of the previously anesthetized tissue (Fig. 13-44).
      (3) Penetrate the tissues and deposit anesthetic as in Step j. Topical anesthetic may be omitted for

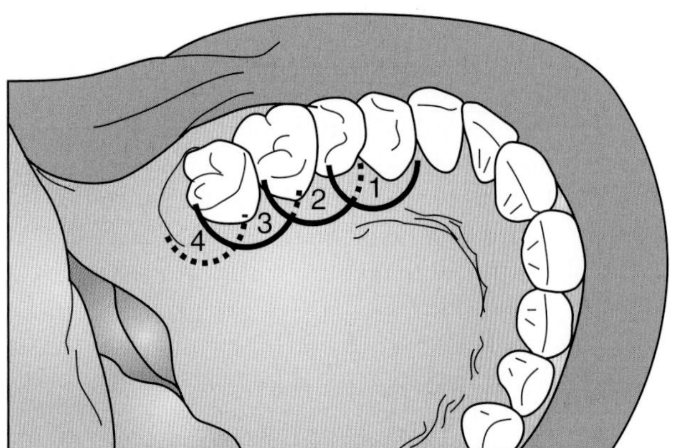

Figure 13-44. Overlapping of sequential palatal infiltrations and needle penetration sites.

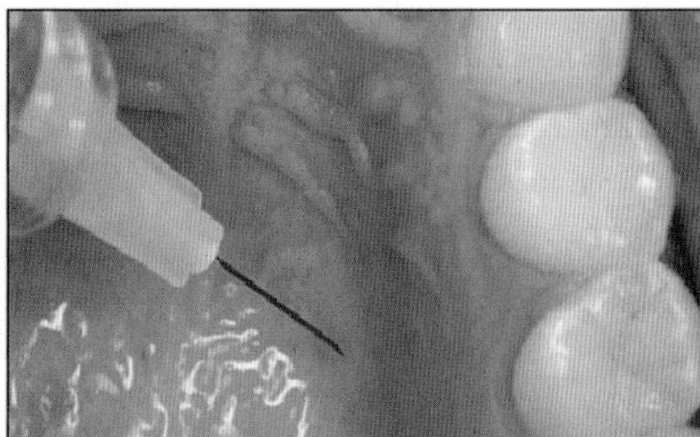

Figure 13-45. Location of injection site for anterior middle superior alveolar (AMSA) nerve block.

subsequent injections because the tissue penetrated is already anesthetized.

(4) Continue this overlapping procedure until adequate hemostasis develops over the entire surgical area.

l. Withdraw the syringe.
m. Make the needle safe.
n. Commence the dental procedure immediately.

Signs and Symptoms

1. Subjective: numbness, ischemia of the palatal soft tissues
2. Objective: no pain during dental therapy

Safety Features. Anatomically safe area for injection.

Precaution. Highly traumatic procedure if performed improperly.

Failure of Hemostasis

1. The percentage of success is higher if vasoconstrictor is included in the anesthetic solution; however, inflamed tissues may continue to hemorrhage despite the use of vasoconstrictor.

Complications

1. Few of significance
2. Necrosis of soft tissues may be observed when a highly concentrated vasoconstricting solution is used for hemostasis over a prolonged period (e.g., norepinephrine, repeated injections of epinephrine in a 1:50,000 concentration). (Norepinephrine is not available in dental local anesthetics in the United States or Canada.)

Anterior Middle Superior Alveolar Nerve Block

The anterior middle superior alveolar nerve block (AMSA) injection represents a recently described maxillary nerve block injection. It was first reported by Friedman and Hochman during development of a C-CLAD system.[5,9] This technique provides pulpal anesthesia to multiple maxillary teeth (incisors, canine, and premolars) from a single injection site on the hard palate about halfway along an imaginary line connecting the midpalatal suture to the free gingival margin. The line is located at the contact point between the first and second premolars (Fig. 13-45).

Because the local anesthetic is deposited on the palate, the muscles of facial expression and the upper lip are not anesthetized. A minimal volume of local anesthetic is necessary to provide pulpal anesthesia from the central incisor to the second premolar on the side of the injection. The AMSA nerve block can be administered with little to no pain following the basic atraumatic palatal injection techniques previously described. Use of a C-CLAD system definitely aids in atraumatic administration of this injection.

The AMSA injection is most accurately described as a field block of the terminal branches (subneural dental plexus) of the ASA nerve that innervates the incisors to the premolar teeth. In spite of the fact that studies suggest that the MSA nerve may be absent in a high percentage of individuals, a complete subneural dental plexus must be present to provide innervation to the premolars and incisor teeth on all patients. It is this subneural dental plexus of the ASA nerve that is anesthetized in the AMSA injection. Two anatomic structures, the nasal aperture and the maxillary sinus, cause the convergence of branches of the anterior and middle superior alveolar nerves and associated subneural dental plexus in the region of the apices of the premolars (Fig. 13-46). The injection site is at this region of convergence of these neural structures. Depositing a sufficient volume of local anesthetic allows it to diffuse through nutrient canals and porous cortical bone on the palate to envelop the concentrated subneural dental plexus at this location.

The AMSA injection may be particularly useful for esthetic-restorative (cosmetic) dental procedures in which the dentist wishes to evaluate the smile line during treatment.[5] In addition, this injection has been found to be very useful for periodontal scaling and root planing of the maxillary region.[10] It provides profound soft tissue anesthesia and

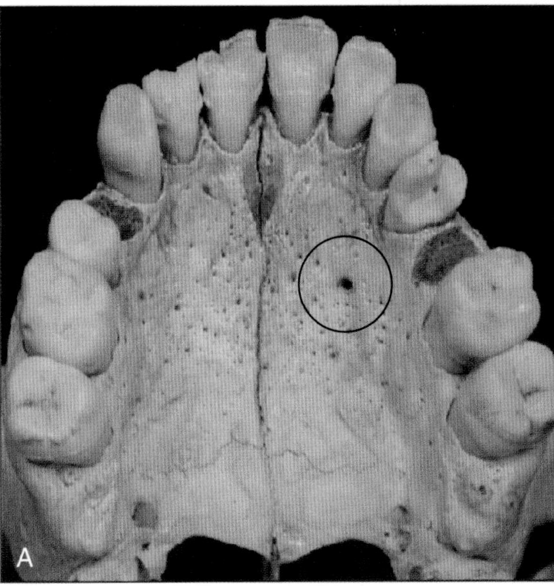

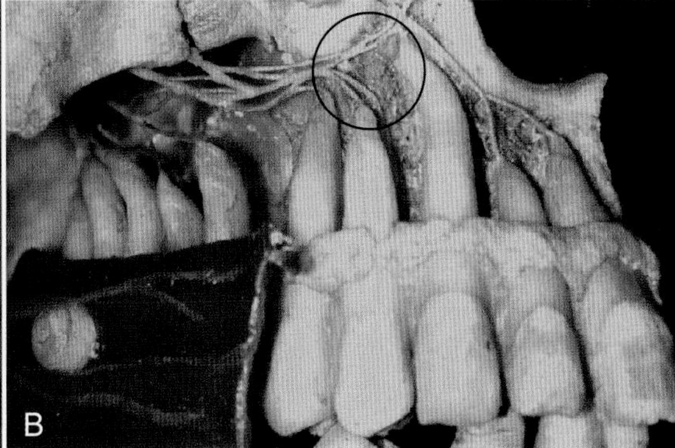

Figure 13-46. Anatomy of anterior middle superior alveolar (AMSA) nerve block. **A,** Palatal aspect: local anesthetic injected in area of circle. **B,** Buccal aspect: local anesthetic injected on palatal side in area of circle.

anesthesia of the attached gingiva of associated teeth. Perry and Loomer demonstrated a patient preference for AMSA compared with supraperiosteal infiltration injection.[10] Subjects found the AMSA to be as effective as multiple maxillary infiltrations in the maxilla.

Several important procedures should be followed in performing this injection comfortably. These techniques are most easily accomplished when performed with a C-CLAD system; however, this injection also has been successful when a standard aspirating dental syringe is used.

Other Common Name. Palatal approach anterior middle superior alveolar (AMSA).

Nerves Anesthetized
1. ASA nerve
2. MSA nerve, when present
3. Subneural dental nerve plexus of the anterior and middle superior alveolar nerves

Areas Anesthetized. (Fig. 13-47)
1. Pulpal anesthesia of the maxillary incisors, canines, and premolars
2. Buccal attached gingiva of these same teeth
3. Attached palatal tissues from midline to free gingival margin on associated teeth

Indications
1. Is more easily performed with a C-CLAD system
2. When dental procedures involving multiple maxillary anterior teeth or soft tissues are to be performed
3. When anesthesia to multiple maxillary anterior teeth is desired from a single-site injection
4. When scaling and root planing of the anterior teeth are to be performed

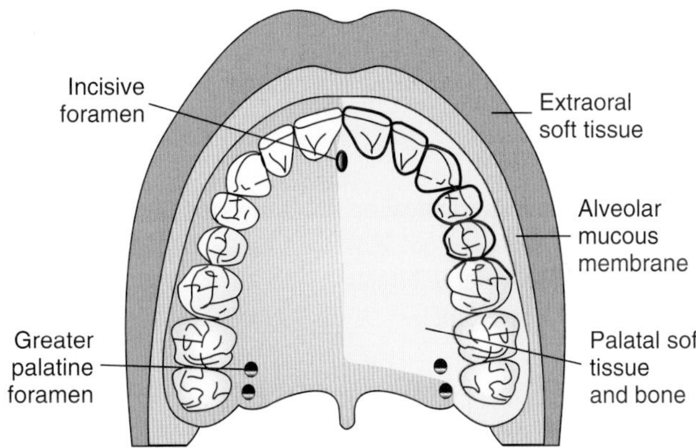

Figure 13-47. Anterior middle superior alveolar (AMSA) extent of anesthesia.

5. When anterior cosmetic procedures are to be performed and a smile-line assessment is important for a successful outcome
6. When a facial approach supraperiosteal injection has been ineffective because of dense cortical bone

Contraindications
1. Patients with unusually thin palatal tissues
2. Patients unable to tolerate the 3- to 4-minute administration time
3. Procedures requiring longer than 90 minutes

Advantages
1. Provides anesthesia of multiple maxillary teeth with a single injection
2. Comparatively simple technique
3. Comparatively safe; minimizes the volume of anesthetic and the number of punctures required compared with traditional maxillary infiltrations of these teeth

4. Allows effective soft tissue and pulpal anesthesia for periodontal scaling and root planing of associated maxillary teeth
5. Allows an accurate smile-line assessment to be performed after anesthesia has occurred, which may be helpful during cosmetic dentistry procedures
6. Eliminates the postoperative inconvenience of numbness to the upper lip and muscles of facial expression
7. Can be performed comfortably with a C-CLAD system

Disadvantages
1. Requires a slow administration (0.5 mL/min) time
2. Can cause operator fatigue with a manual syringe because of extended injection time
3. May be uncomfortable for the patient if administered improperly
4. May need supplemental anesthesia for central and lateral incisor teeth
5. May cause excessive ischemia if administered too rapidly
6. Use of local anesthetic containing epinephrine with a concentration of 1:50,000 is contraindicated.

Positive Aspirations. Less than 1%.

Alternatives
1. Multiple supraperiosteal or PDL injections for each tooth
2. ASA and MSA nerve blocks
3. Maxillary nerve block

Technique
1. A 27-gauge short needle is recommended.
2. Area of insertion: on the hard palate about halfway along an imaginary line connecting the midpalatal suture to the free gingival margin; the location of the line is at the contact point between the first and second premolars
3. Target area: palatal bone at injection site
4. Landmarks: the intersecting point midway along a line from the midpalatine suture to the free gingival margin intersecting the contact point between the first and second premolars
5. Orientation of the bevel: The bevel of the needle is placed "face down" against the epithelium. The needle is typically held at a 45-degree angle to the palate.
6. Procedure:
   a. Sit at the 9 or 10 o'clock position facing same direction as the patient.
   b. Position the patient supine with slight hyperextension of the head and neck so you can visualize the nasopalatine papilla more easily.
   c. Use preparatory communication to inform the patient that the injection may take several minutes to administer, and that it may produce a sensation of firm pressure in the palate.

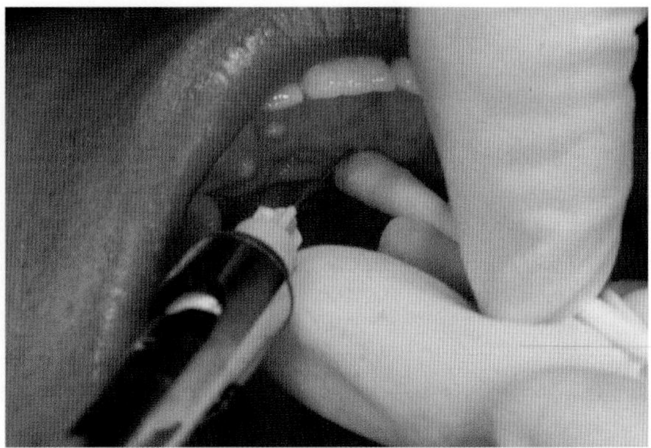

Figure 13-48. Prepuncture technique.

   d. Use comfortable arm and finger rests to avoid fatigue during the extended administration time.
   e. Use of a C-CLAD system is suggested because it makes this injection easier to administer.
   f. Initial orientation of bevel is "face down" toward the epithelium, while the needle is held at approximately a 45-degree angle with a tangent to the palate.
   g. The final target is the bevel in contact with the palatal bone.
   h. A prepuncture technique can be utilized. Apply the bevel of the needle toward the palatal tissue. Place a sterile cotton applicator on top of the needle tip (Fig. 13-48). Apply light pressure on the cotton applicator to create a "seal" of the needle bevel against the outer surface. Initiate delivery of the local anesthetic to the surface of the epithelium. The objective is to force the solution through the outer epithelium into the surface tissue. The cotton applicator provides stabilization of the needle and prevents any excess local anesthetic solution from dripping into the patient's mouth. When a C-CLAD system is used, a slow rate of delivery (approximately 0.5 mL/min) is maintained during the entire injection. Maintain this position and pressure on the surface of the epithelium for 8 to 10 seconds.
   i. An "anesthetic pathway technique" can be utilized. Very slowly advance the needle tip into the tissue. Rotating the needle allows the needle to penetrate the tissue more efficiently.[11] Advance the needle 1 to 2 mm every 4 to 6 seconds while administering the anesthetic solution at the recommended slow rate. Attempt to not expand the tissue or advance the needle too rapidly if performing this with a manual syringe. Use of a C-CLAD system makes this process considerably easier to perform.
   j. After initial blanching is observed (approximately 30 seconds), pause for several seconds to allow for onset of superficial anesthesia.
   k. Continue the slow insertion technique into the palatal tissue. Orientation of the handpiece should

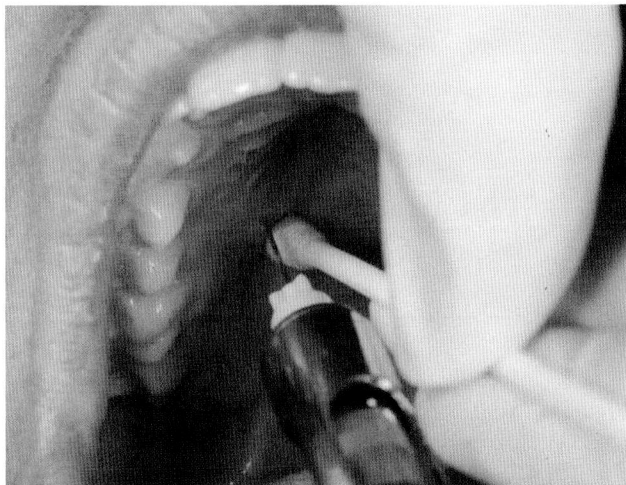

Figure 13-49. Anterior middle superior alveolar (AMSA) nerve block. Note syringe angulation from opposite side of mouth.

be from the contralateral premolars (Fig. 13-49). The needle is advanced until contact with bone occurs.

l. Ensure that needle contact is maintained with the bony surface of the palate. The bevel of the needle should face the surface of the bone.
m. Aspirate in two planes.
n. Anesthetic is delivered at a rate of approximately 0.5 mL per minute during the injection for a total dosage of approximately 1.4 to 1.8 mL.
o. Advise the patient that he or she will experience a sensation of firm pressure.

Signs and Symptoms

1. Subjective: A sensation of firmness and numbness is experienced immediately on the palatal tissues.
2. Subjective: Numbness of the teeth and associated soft tissues extends from the central incisor to the second premolar on the side of the injection.
3. Objective: Blanching of the soft tissues (if a vasoconstrictor is used) of the palatal and facial attached gingiva is evident, extending from the central incisor to the premolar region.
4. Objective: Use of electrical pulp testing with no response from teeth with maximal EPT output (80/80)
5. Objective: Absence of pain during treatment
6. Objective: No anesthesia of the face and upper lip occurs. *Note: In some patients, additional anesthetic may be necessary to supplement the incisor teeth. This can be provided from a palatal approach or as individual PDL injections.*

Safety Features

1. Contact with bone
2. Low risk of positive aspiration
3. Slow insertion of needle (1 to 2 mm every 4 to 6 seconds)
4. Slow administration of local anesthetic (0.5 mL/min)
5. Less anesthetic required than if traditional injections are used.

Precautions

1. Against pain:
   a. Extremely slow insertion of needle
   b. Slow administration during insertion with simultaneous administration of anesthetic solution
   c. C-CLAD device recommended
2. Against tissue damage:
   a. Avoid excessive ischemia by avoiding local anesthetics containing vasoconstrictors with a concentration of 1:50,000.
   b. Avoid multiple infiltrations of local anesthetic with vasoconstrictor in the same area at a single appointment.

Failure of Anesthesia

1. May need supplemental anesthesia for central and lateral incisors
   a. Adequate volume of anesthetic may not reach dental branches.
   b. To correct: Add more anesthetic or supplement in proximity to these teeth from the palatal approach.

Complications

1. Palatal ulcer at injection site developing 1 to 2 days postoperatively
   a. Self-limiting
   b. Heals in 5 to 10 days
   c. Prevention includes slow administration to avoid excessive ischemia.
   d. Avoid excessive concentrations of vasoconstrictor (e.g., 1:50,000).
   e. Avoid multiple infiltrations of local anesthetic with vasoconstrictor in the same area at a single appointment.
2. Unexpected contact with the nasopalatine nerve
3. Density of tissues at injection site causing squirt-back of anesthetic and bitter taste
   a. Aspirate while withdrawing syringe from tissue.
   b. Pause 3 to 4 seconds before withdrawing the needle to allow pressure to dissipate.
   c. Instruct assistant to suction any excess anesthetic that escapes during administration.

Palatal Approach-Anterior Superior Alveolar

The palatal approach-anterior superior alveolar (P-ASA) injection, as with the AMSA injection, was defined by Friedman and Hochman in conjunction with the clinical use and development of a C-CLAD system in the mid-1990s.[4,5,8] The P-ASA injection shares several common elements with the nasopalatine nerve block but differs sufficiently to be considered a distinct identity. The P-ASA uses a similar tissue point of entry (lateral aspect of the incisive papilla) as the nasopalatine but differs in its final target, that is, the needle positioned within the incisive canal. The volume of anesthetic recommended for the P-ASA is 1.4 to 1.8 mL, administered at a rate of 0.5 mL per minute.

The distribution of anesthesia differs between these injections as well. Nasopalatine nerve block provides anesthesia to the anterior palatal gingiva and mucoperiosteum and is recommended for surgical procedures on the anterior palate. It also may serve as a supplemental technique for achieving pulpal anesthesia to the incisor teeth. In contrast, the P-ASA is recommended as a primary method for achieving bilateral pulpal anesthesia of the anterior six maxillary teeth (incisors and canines). The P-ASA provides profound soft tissue anesthesia of the gingiva and mucoperiosteum in the region of the anterior palatal one third innervated by the nasopalatine nerve. In addition, soft tissue anesthesia of the facial attached gingiva of the six anterior teeth is noted. Therefore, the P-ASA is an attractive alternative for pain control before scaling and root planing, esthetic-restorative (dental) cosmetic procedures, and minor surgical procedures involving the premaxilla region. The P-ASA can be noted as the first dental injection to produce bilateral pulpal anesthesia from a single injection as its primary objective, making this a unique characteristic of this injection technique.

It is well documented in the dental literature that subjective pain associated with injections into the nasopalatine region is typically associated with a significant degree of discomfort when performed with a manual syringe.[12-14] The introduction of C-CLAD systems has demonstrated that injections even into the dense, highly innervated tissues of the palate can be performed predictably with little or no pain.[15] The P-ASA injection may be performed with a traditional syringe; however, a comfortable injection is more easily achieved with a C-CLAD system.[10,16-18]

The P-ASA is useful when anesthesia to the maxillary anterior teeth is desired, without collateral anesthesia to the lips and muscles of facial expression. It has been shown to be desirable during scaling and root planing of the anterior teeth. It is also beneficial when anterior esthetic dentistry procedures are to be performed. The smile line and the interrelationships between lips, teeth, and soft tissues cannot be accurately assessed when a traditional (mucobuccal fold) approach to anesthesia is utilized, because of paralysis of the muscles of the upper lip. The palatal approach allows anesthesia to be limited to the subneural plexus for the maxillary anterior teeth and the nasopalatine nerve. The minimum volume for this injection is 1.8 mL delivered at a slow rate of 0.5 mL per minute.

Other Common Name. Palatal approach ASA or palatal approach maxillary anterior field block.

Nerves Anesthetized
1. Nasopalatine
2. Anterior branches of the ASA

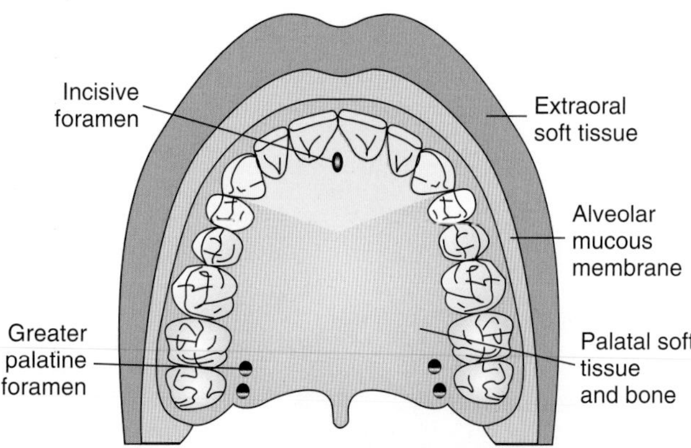

Figure 13-50. Palatal approach-anterior superior alveolar (P-ASA) extent of anesthesia.

Areas Anesthetized. (Fig. 13-50)
1. Pulps of the maxillary central incisors, the lateral incisors, and (to a lesser degree) the canines
2. Facial periodontal tissue associated with these same teeth
3. Palatal periodontal tissue associated with these same teeth

Indications
1. When dental procedures involving the maxillary anterior teeth and soft tissues are to be performed.
2. When bilateral anesthesia of the maxillary anterior teeth is desired from a single site injection
3. When scaling and root planing of the anterior teeth are to be performed.
4. When anterior cosmetic procedures are to be performed and a smile-line assessment is important to a successful outcome
5. When a facial approach supraperiosteal injection has been ineffective because of dense cortical bone

Contraindications
1. Patients with extremely long canine roots may not achieve profound anesthesia of these teeth from a palatal approach alone.
2. Patients who cannot tolerate the 3- to 4-minute administration time
3. Procedures requiring longer than 90 minutes

Advantages
1. Provides bilateral maxillary anesthesia from a single injection site.
2. Comparatively simple technique to perform
3. Comparatively safe; minimizes the volume of anesthetic and the number of punctures necessary compared with traditional maxillary infiltrations of these teeth
4. Allows for accurate smile-line assessment to be performed after anesthesia has occurred, which may be useful during cosmetic dentistry procedures

5. Eliminates the postoperative inconvenience of numbness to the upper lip and muscles of facial expression
6. Can be performed comfortably with a C-CLAD system

Disadvantages
1. Requires slow administration (0.5 mL/min)
2. Operator fatigue with a manual syringe because of extended injection time
3. May be uncomfortable for the patient if administered improperly
4. May require supplemental anesthesia for canine teeth
5. May cause excessive ischemia if administered too rapidly
6. Use of local anesthetic containing epinephrine with a concentration of 1:50,000 is contraindicated.

Positive Aspiration. Less than 1% (assumed from data on nasopalatine block).

Alternatives
1. Supraperiosteal or PDL injections for each tooth
2. Right and left (bilateral) ASA nerve blocks
3. Right and left (bilateral) maxillary nerve blocks

Technique
1. A 27-gauge short needle is recommended.
2. Area of insertion: just lateral to the incisive papilla in the papillary groove (Fig. 13-51)
3. Target area: nasopalatine foramen
4. Landmarks: nasopalatine papilla
5. Orientation of the bevel: The bevel of the needle is placed "face down" against the epithelium. The needle is typically held at a 45-degree angle to the palate.
6. Procedure:
   a. Sit at the 9 or 10 o'clock position facing in the same direction as the patient.

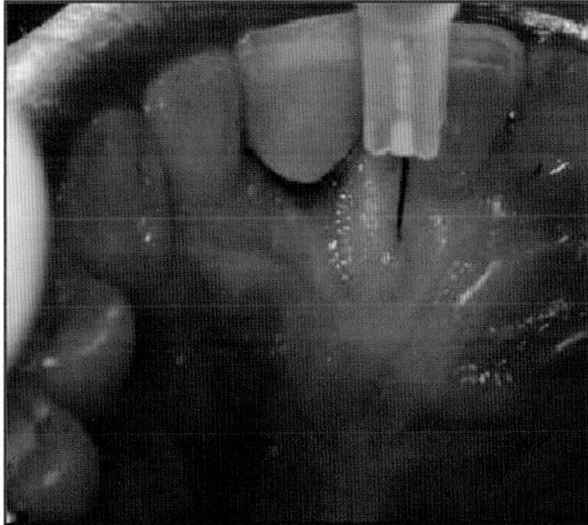

Figure 13-51. Palatal approach-anterior superior alveolar (P-ASA) area of needle insertion.

   b. Position the patient supine with slight hyperextension of the head and neck so you can visualize the nasopalatine papilla more easily.
   c. Use preparatory communication to inform the patient that the injection may take several minutes to administer and may produce a sensation of firm pressure in the palate.
   d. Use comfortable arm and finger rests to prevent fatigue during the extended administration time.
   e. Use of a C-CLAD system makes this injection easier to administer.
   f. Initial orientation of bevel is "face down" against the epithelium, while the needle is held at approximately a 45-degree angle with a tangent to the palate.
   g. A prepuncture technique can be utilized. Place the bevel of the needle against the palatal tissue. Place a sterile cotton applicator on top of the needle tip (see Fig. 13-48). Apply light pressure on the cotton applicator to create a "seal" of the needle bevel against the outer surface. Initiate delivery of the anesthetic solution to the surface of the epithelium. The objective is to force the solution through the outer epithelium into the tissue. Allow anesthetic solution to be delivered through the layer of the outer epithelium. The cotton applicator provides stabilization of the needle and prevents any excess dripping of anesthetic solution into the patient's mouth. When a C-CLAD device is used, a slow rate of delivery (approximately 0.5 mL/min) is maintained throughout injection. Maintain this position and pressure on the surface of the epithelium for 8 to 10 seconds.
   h. An anesthetic pathway technique can be utilized. Very slowly advance the needle into the tissue. Rotating the needle allows the needle to penetrate the tissue more efficiently. Advance the needle 1 to 2 mm every 4 to 6 seconds while administering the anesthetic solution at the recommended (slow) rate. Avoid expanding the tissue or advancing the needle too rapidly if performing the P-ASA with a traditional syringe. It is at this step where a C-CLAD system makes the process easier to achieve.
   i. After initial blanching is observed (approximately 30 seconds), pause for several seconds to permit onset of superficial anesthesia.
   j. Continue the slow insertion technique into the nasopalatine canal. Orientation of the needle should be parallel to the long axis of the central incisors. The needle is advanced to a depth of 6 to 10 mm (Fig. 13-52). *Note: If resistance is encountered before the final depth of penetration is reached, do not force the needle forward. Withdraw it slightly and reorient it to minimize the risk of penetration of the floor of the nose.*
   k. Ensure that the needle is in contact with the inner bony wall of the canal. (A well-defined nasopalatine canal may not be present in some patients.)

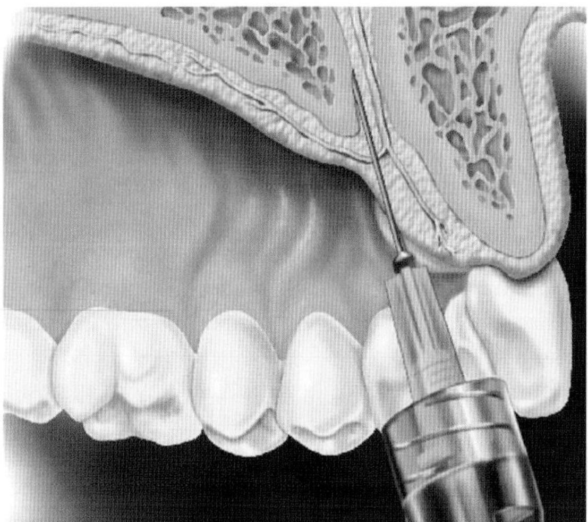

Figure 13-52. Palatal approach-anterior superior alveolar (P-ASA) orientation of syringe.

l. Aspirate in two planes within the canal space to avoid intravascular injection.
m. Anesthetic is delivered at a rate of approximately 0.5 mL during the injection to a total volume of 1.4 to 1.8 mL. Advise the patient that he or she will experience a sensation of firm pressure. *Note: It has been reported that in a small percentage of cases, needle insertion can stimulate the nasopalatine nerve (similar to contacting a nerve during an inferior alveolar block). This may be an unsettling surprise to the patient (and the operator) if it occurs. Reassure the patient with verbal support that this is not uncommon and is not a problem. If this should occur, reposition the needle and continue to administer the anesthetic before advancing farther.*

Signs and Symptoms

1. Subjective: A sensation of firmness and anesthesia is immediately experienced in the anterior palate.
2. Subjective: Numbness of the teeth and associated soft tissues extends from the right to the left canine.
3. Objective: Ischemia (blanching) of the soft tissues (if a vasoconstrictor is used) of the palatal and the facial attached gingiva is evident extending from the right to the left canine region.
4. Objective: Use of electrical pulp testing with no response from teeth with maximal EPT output (80/80)
5. Objective: Absence of pain during treatment
6. Objective: No anesthesia of the face and upper lip occurs. *Note: In patients with long canine roots, additional local anesthetic may be needed. This can be provided through a palatal approach at a point that approximates the canine root tips.*
   a. In rare instances, a facial approach (traditional) supraperiosteal injection may be necessary for the canine teeth.

Safety Features

1. Contact with bone
2. Minimal aspiration rate
3. Slow needle insertion (1 to 2 mm every 4 to 6 seconds)
4. Slow administration (0.5 mL/min) of local anesthetic
5. Less anesthetic volume than necessary if administered via traditional injections

Precautions

1. Against pain:
   a. Extremely slow insertion
   b. Slow administration during insertion with simultaneous administration of anesthetic solution (creating an anesthetic pathway)
   c. Consider use of a C-CLAD system.
2. Against tissue damage
   a. Avoid excessive ischemia by not using drugs containing epinephrine in a concentration of 1:50,000.
   b. Avoid multiple infiltrations of local anesthetic with vasoconstrictor in the same area at a single appointment.

Failure of Anesthesia

1. Highly successful injection for maxillary incisors
2. May need supplemental anesthesia for canines in patients with long roots
   a. Adequate volume of anesthetic may not reach dental branches.
   b. To correct: Add more anesthetic or supplement in proximity to the canine teeth from the palatal approach.
3. Unilateral anesthesia
   a. Look for bilateral blanching.
   b. To correct: Administer additional anesthetic.

Complications

1. Palatal ulcer at injection site developing 1 to 2 days postoperatively
   a. Self-limiting
   b. Heals in 5 to 10 days
   c. Prevention includes slow administration to avoid excessive ischemia.
   d. Avoid excessive concentrations of vasoconstrictor (e.g., 1:50,000)
2. Unexpected contact with the nasopalatine nerve
3. Density of soft tissues at injection site causing squirt-back of anesthetic and bitter taste
   a. Aspirate while withdrawing syringe from tissue.
   b. Pause 3 to 4 seconds before withdrawing the needle to allow pressure to dissipate.
   c. Instruct assistant to suction any excess anesthetic that escapes during administration.

Maxillary Nerve Block

The maxillary (second division or V_2) nerve block is an effective method of achieving profound anesthesia of a hemimaxilla. It is useful in procedures involving quadrant dentistry

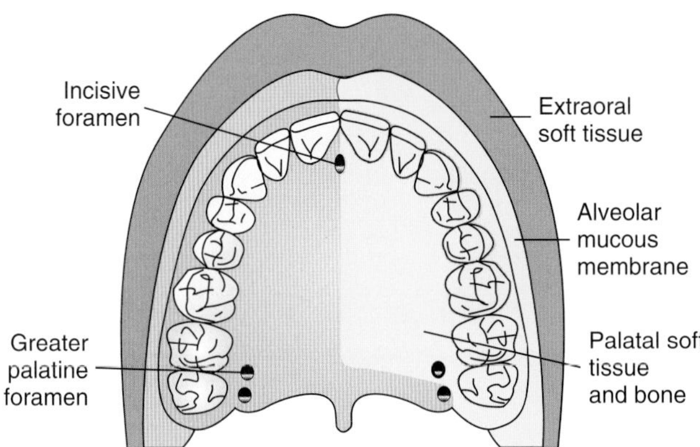

Figure 13-53. Areas anesthetized by a maxillary nerve block.

and in extensive surgical procedures. Two approaches are presented here. Both are effective, and the author does not maintain a preference for either one. Major difficulties with the greater palatine canal approach involve locating the canal and negotiating it successfully. The major difficulty in the high-tuberosity approach is the higher incidence of hematoma.

Other Common Names. Second division block, V_2 nerve block.

Nerve Anesthetized. Maxillary division of the trigeminal nerve.

Areas Anesthetized. (Fig. 13-53)
1. Pulpal anesthesia of the maxillary teeth on the side of the block
2. Buccal periodontium and bone overlying these teeth
3. Soft tissues and bone of the hard palate and part of the soft palate, medial to midline
4. Skin of the lower eyelid, side of the nose, cheek, and upper lip

Indications
1. Pain control before extensive oral surgical, periodontal, or restorative procedures requiring anesthesia of the entire maxillary division
2. When tissue inflammation or infection precludes the use of other regional nerve blocks (e.g., PSA, ASA, AMSA, P-ASA) or supraperiosteal injection
3. Diagnostic or therapeutic procedures for neuralgias or tics of the second division of the trigeminal nerve

Contraindications
1. Inexperienced administrator
2. Pediatric patients
   a. More difficult because of smaller anatomic dimensions
   b. A cooperative patient is needed.
   c. Usually unnecessary in children because of the high success rate of other regional block techniques
3. Uncooperative patients
4. Inflammation or infection of tissues overlying the injection site
5. When hemorrhage is risky (e.g., in a hemophiliac)
6. In the greater palatine canal approach: inability to gain access to the canal; bony obstructions may be present in 5% to 15% of canals

Advantages
1. Atraumatic injection via the high-tuberosity approach
2. High success rate (>95%)
3. Positive aspiration is less than 1% (greater palatine canal approach).
4. Minimizes the number of needle penetrations necessary for successful anesthesia of the hemimaxilla (minimum of four via PSA, infraorbital, greater palatine, and nasopalatine)
5. Minimizes total volume of local anesthetic solution injected to 1.8 versus 2.7 mL
6. Neither high-tuberosity nor greater palatine canal approach is usually traumatic.

Disadvantages
1. Risk of hematoma, primarily with the high-tuberosity approach.
2. High-tuberosity approach is relatively arbitrary. Overinsertion is possible because of the absence of bony landmarks if proper technique is not followed.
3. Lack of hemostasis: If necessary, this necessitates infiltration with vasoconstrictor-containing local anesthetic at the surgical site.
4. Pain: The greater palatine canal approach is potentially (although not usually) traumatic.

Alternatives. To achieve the same distribution of anesthesia present with a maxillary nerve block, *all* of the following must be administered:
1. PSA nerve block
2. ASA nerve block
3. Greater palatine nerve block
4. Nasopalatine nerve block

Technique (High-Tuberosity Approach). (Fig. 13-54)
1. A 25-gauge long needle is recommended. A 27-gauge long is acceptable.
2. Area of insertion: height of the mucobuccal fold above the distal aspect of the maxillary second molar
3. Target area:
   a. Maxillary nerve as it passes through the pterygopalatine fossa
   b. Superior and medial to the target area of the PSA nerve block
4. Landmarks:
   a. Mucobuccal fold at the distal aspect of the maxillary second molar
   b. Maxillary tuberosity
   c. Zygomatic process of the maxilla
5. Orientation of the bevel: toward bone

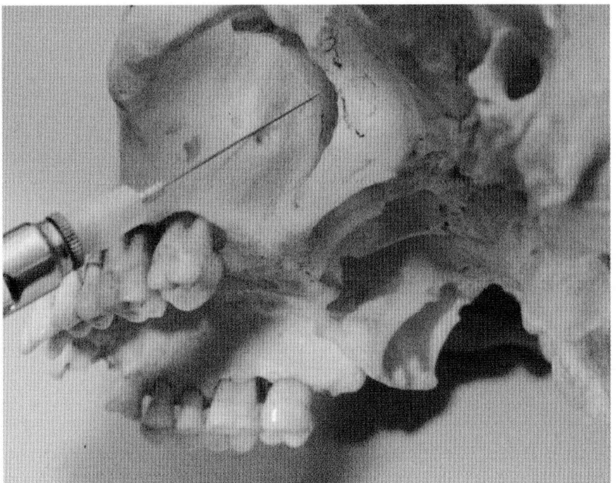

Figure 13-54. Maxillary nerve block, high-tuberosity approach.

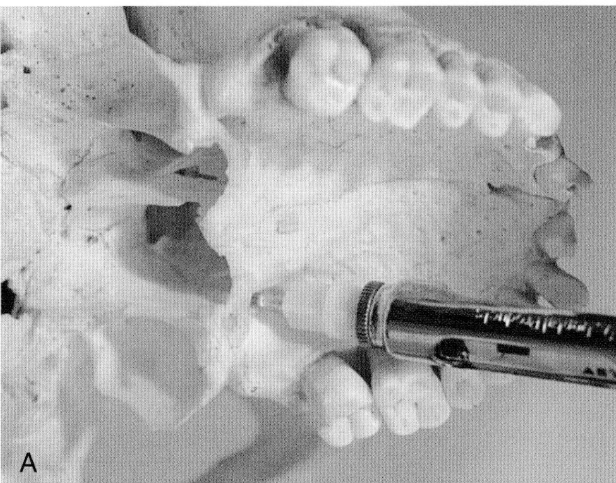

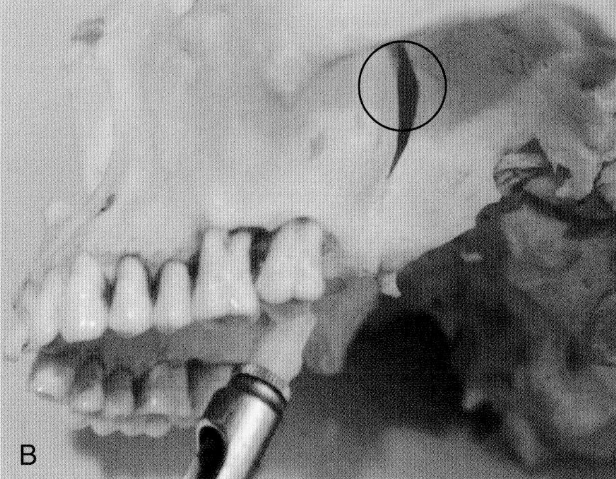

Figure 13-55. **A,** Maxillary nerve block, greater palatine canal approach. Note the direction of the needle and the syringe barrel into the canal. **B,** Second division nerve block (V_2), greater palatine canal approach. Note the location of the needle tip in the pterygopalatine fossa *(circle)*.

6. Procedure:
   a. Measure the length of a long needle from the tip to the hub (average, 32 mm, but varies by manufacturer).
   b. Assume the correct position.
      (1) For a left high-tuberosity injection, a right-handed administrator should sit at the 10 o'clock position facing the patient (see Figure 13-8, *A*).
      (2) For a right high-tuberosity injection, a right-handed administrator should sit at the 8 o'clock position facing the patient (see Figure 13-8, *B*).
   c. Position the patient supine or semisupine for the right or left block.
   d. Prepare the tissue in the height of the mucobuccal fold at the distal of the maxillary second molar.
      (1) Dry with sterile gauze.
      (2) Apply topical antiseptic (optional).
      (3) Apply topical anesthetic.
   e. Partially open the patient's mouth; pull the mandible toward the side of injection.
   f. Retract the cheek in the injection area with your index finger to increase visibility.
   g. Pull the tissues taut with this finger.
   h. Place the needle into the height of the mucobuccal fold over the maxillary second molar.
   i. Advance the needle slowly in an upward, inward, and backward direction as described for the PSA nerve block (p. 191).
   j. Advance the needle to a depth of 30 mm.
      (1) No resistance to needle penetration should be felt. If resistance is felt, the angle of the needle in toward the midline is too great.
      (2) At this depth (30 mm), the needle tip should lie in the pterygopalatine fossa in proximity to the maxillary division of the trigeminal nerve.
   k. Aspirate in two planes.
      (1) Rotate the syringe (needle bevel) one fourth turn and reaspirate.
      (2) If negative:
         (a) Slowly (more than 60 seconds) deposit 1.8 mL.
         (b) Aspirate several times during injection.
   l. Withdraw the syringe.
   m. Make the needle safe.
   n. Wait a minimum of 3 to 5 minutes before commencing the dental procedure.

Technique (Greater Palatine Canal Approach). (Fig. 13-55)

1. A 25-gauge long needle is recommended. A 27-gauge long needle is also acceptable.
2. Area of insertion: palatal soft tissue directly over the greater palatine foramen
3. Target area: the maxillary nerve as it passes through the pterygopalatine fossa; the needle passes through the greater palatine canal to reach the pterygopalatine fossa
4. Landmark: greater palatine foramen, junction of the maxillary alveolar process and the palatine bone
5. Orientation of the bevel: toward palatal soft tissues

6. Procedure:
   a. Measure the length of a long needle from the tip to the hub (average, 32 mm, but varies by manufacturer).
   b. Assume the correct position.
      (1) For a right greater palatine canal V_2 block, sit facing toward the patient at the 7 or 8 o'clock position.
      (2) For a left greater palatine canal V_2 block, sit facing in the same direction as the patient at the 10 or 11 o'clock position.
   c. Ask the patient, who is supine, to do the following:
      (1) Open wide.
      (2) Extend the neck.
      (3) Turn the head to the left or right (to improve visibility).
   d. Locate the greater palatine foramen.
      (1) Place a cotton swab at the junction of the maxillary alveolar process and the hard palate.
      (2) Start in the region of the second molar and palpate by pressing posteriorly into the tissues with the swab.
      (3) The swab "falls" into the depression created by the greater palatine foramen.
      (4) The foramen is most frequently located at the distal aspect of the maxillary second molar (see Table 13-2).
   e. Prepare the tissues directly over the greater palatine foramen.
      (1) Clean and dry with sterile gauze.
      (2) Apply topical antiseptic (optional).
      (3) Apply topical anesthetic for 2 minutes.
   f. After 2 minutes of topical anesthetic application, move the swab posteriorly so it lies just behind the greater palatine foramen.
      (1) Apply pressure to the tissue with the cotton swab, held in the left hand (if right-handed).
      (2) Note ischemia at the injection site.
   g. Direct the syringe into the mouth from the opposite side with the needle approaching the injection site at a right angle (Fig. 13-56).
   h. Place the bevel against the ischemic soft tissue at the injection site. The needle must be well stabilized to prevent accidental penetration of the tissues.
   i. With the bevel lying against the tissue:
      (1) Apply enough pressure to bow the needle slightly.
      (2) Deposit a small volume of local anesthetic. The solution is forced against the mucous membrane, forming a droplet.
   j. Straighten the needle and permit the bevel to penetrate the mucosa.
      (1) Continue to deposit small volumes of anesthetic throughout the procedure.
      (2) Ischemia spreads into adjacent tissues as the anesthetic is deposited.

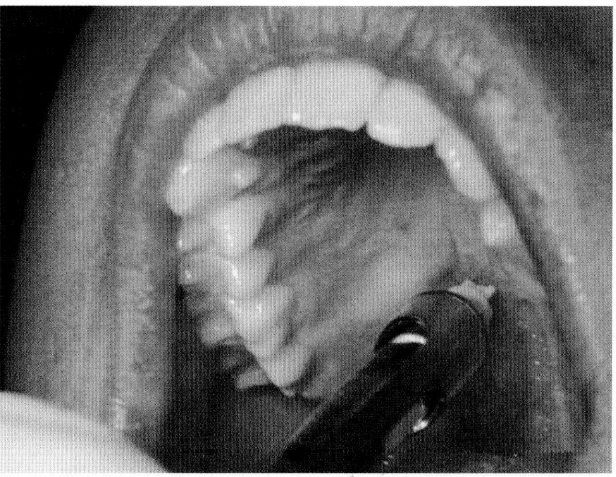

Figure 13-56. Maxillary nerve block, greater palatine canal approach.

TABLE 13-3
Angle of the Greater Palatine Foramen to the Hard Palate

Angle, degrees	n = 199	Percent
20-22.5	2	1.005
25-27.5	4	2.01
30-32.5	18	9.045
35-37.5	28	14.07
40-42.5	25	12.56
45-47.5	34	17.08
50-52.5	34	17.08
55-57.5	29	14.57
60-62.5	17	8.54
65-67.5	7	3.51
70	1	0.50

From Malamed SF, Trieger N: Intraoral maxillary nerve block: an anatomical and clinical study, Anesth Prog 30:44–48, 1983.

   k. Continue to apply pressure with the cotton applicator stick during this part of the procedure. **The greater palatine nerve block is now complete.**
   l. Probe gently for the greater palatine foramen.
      (1) The patient feels no discomfort because of the previously deposited anesthetic solution.
      (2) The angle of the needle and syringe may be changed if needed.
      (3) The needle usually must be held at a 45-degree angle to facilitate entry into the greater palatine foramen (Table 13-3).
   m. After locating the foramen, very slowly advance the needle into the greater palatine canal to a depth of 30 mm. Approximately 5% to 15% of greater palatine canals have bony obstructions that prevent passage of the needle.
      (1) Never attempt to force the needle against resistance.

   (2) If resistance is felt, withdraw the needle slightly and slowly attempt to advance it at a different angle.
   (3) If the needle cannot be advanced farther and the depth of penetration is almost adequate, continue with the next steps; however, if the depth is considerably deficient, withdraw the needle and discontinue the attempt.
n. Aspirate in two planes.
   (1) Rotate the needle one fourth turn and reaspirate.
   (2) If negative, slowly deposit 1.8 mL of solution over a minimum of 1 minute.
o. Withdraw the syringe.
p. Make the needle safe.
q. Wait a minimum of 3 to 5 minutes before commencing the dental procedure.

Signs and Symptoms
1. Subjective: Pressure behind the upper jaw on the side being injected; this usually subsides rapidly, progressing to tingling and numbness of the lower eyelid, side of the nose, and upper lip
2. Subjective: Sensation of numbness in the teeth and buccal and palatal soft tissues on the side of injection
3. Objective: Use of electrical pulp testing with no response from teeth with maximal EPT output (80/80)
4. Objective: Absence of pain during treatment

Safety Feature. Careful adherence to technique.

Precautions
1. Pain on insertion of the needle, primarily with the greater palatine canal approach; prevent by using atraumatic palatal injection protocol
2. Overinsertion of the needle; can occur with both approaches (although much less likely with the greater palatine canal approach); prevent through careful adherence to protocol
3. Resistance to needle insertion in the greater palatine canal approach; never try to advance a needle against resistance

Failures of Anesthesia
1. Partial anesthesia; may result from underpenetration by needle. To correct: Reinsert the needle to proper depth, and reinject.
2. Inability to negotiate the greater palatine canal. To correct:
   a. Withdraw the needle slightly and reangulate it.
   b. Reinsert carefully to the proper depth.
   c. If unable to bypass the obstruction easily, withdraw the needle and terminate the injection.
      (1) The high-tuberosity approach may prove more successful in this situation.
   d. The greater palatine canal approach usually is successful if the long dental needle has been advanced at least two thirds of its length into the canal.

Complications
1. Hematoma develops rapidly if the maxillary artery is punctured during maxillary nerve block via the high-tuberosity approach. (Refer to discussion of PSA nerve block, complications, p. 195.)
2. Penetration of the orbit may occur during a greater palatine foramen approach if the needle goes in too far; more likely to occur in the smaller-than-average skull
3. Complications produced by injection of local anesthetic into the orbit include the following*:
   a. Volume displacement of the orbital structures, producing periorbital swelling and proptosis
   b. Regional block of the sixth cranial nerve (abducens), producing diplopia
   c. Classic retrobulbar block, producing mydriasis, corneal anesthesia, and ophthalmoplegia
   d. Possible optic nerve block with transient loss of vision (Amaurosis)
   e. Possible retrobulbar hemorrhage
   f. To prevent intraorbital injection: Strictly adhere to protocol and modify your technique for the smaller patient.
4. Penetration of the nasal cavity
   a. If the needle deviates medially during insertion through the greater palatine canal, the paper-thin medial wall of the pterygopalatine fossa is penetrated and the needle enters the nasal cavity.
      (1) On aspiration, large amounts of air appear in the cartridge.
      (2) On injection, the patient complains that local anesthetic solution is running down his or her throat.
      (3) To prevent: Keep the patient's mouth wide open and take care during penetration that the advancing needle stays in the correct plane.
      (4) To prevent: Do not force needle if resistance is encountered.

Table 13-4 summarizes the indications for maxillary local anesthesia. Table 13-5 includes volumes of solutions recommended for maxillary injections.

SUMMARY

Providing clinically adequate anesthesia in the maxilla is rarely a problem. The thin and porous bone of the maxilla permits the ready diffusion of local anesthetic to the apex of the tooth to be treated. For this reason, many dentists rely

*It has been reported that complications a, b, and c were most common after intraorbital injection; complications d and e were never encountered.[19,20]

TABLE 13-4
Maxillary Teeth and Available Local Anesthetic Techniques

Teeth	Pulpal Anesthesia	SOFT TISSUE Buccal	SOFT TISSUE Palatal
Incisors	Infraorbital (IO)	Infraorbital (IO)	Nasopalatine
	Infiltration	Infiltration	Infiltration
	AMSA	AMSA	AMSA
	P-ASA	P-ASA	P-ASA
	V_2	V_2	V_2
Canines	Infraorbital	Infraorbital	Nasopalatine
	Infiltration	Infiltration	Infiltration
	AMSA	AMSA	AMSA
	P-ASA	P-ASA	P-ASA
	V_2	V_2	V_2
Premolars	Infraorbital	Infraorbital	Greater palatine
	Infiltration	Infiltration	Infiltration
	MSA	MSA	AMSA
	AMSA	AMSA	V_2
	V_2	V_2	
Molars	PSA	PSA	Greater palatine
	Infiltration	Infiltration	Infiltration
	V_2	V_2	V_2

AMSA, Anterior middle superior alveolar; *MSA,* middle superior alveolar; *P-ASA,* palatal approach-anterior superior alveolar; *PSA,* posterior superior alveolar.

TABLE 13-5
Recommended Volumes of Local Anesthetic for Maxillary Techniques

Technique	Volume, mL
Supraperiosteal (infiltration)	0.6
Posterior superior alveolar (PSA)	0.9-1.8
Middle superior alveolar (MSA)	0.9-1.2
Anterior superior alveolar (ASA, infraorbital)	0.9-1.2
Anterior middle superior alveolar (AMSA)	1.4-1.8
Palatal approach-anterior superior alveolar (P-ASA)	1.4-1.8
Greater (anterior) palatine	0.45-0.6
Nasopalatine	0.45 (maximum)
Palatal infiltration	0.2-0.3
Maxillary (V2) nerve block	1.8

solely on supraperiosteal (or "infiltration") anesthesia for most treatment in the maxilla.

It is only on rare occasions that difficulty arises with maxillary pain control. Most notable, of course, is the pulpally involved tooth; because of infection or inflammation, the use of supraperiosteal anesthesia is contraindicated or ineffective in treating this tooth. In nonpulpally involved teeth, the most often observed problems in attaining adequate pulpal anesthesia via supraperiosteal injection develop in the central incisor (whose apex may lie beneath the denser bone and cartilage of the nose), the canine (whose root length may be considerable, with local anesthetic deposited below the apex), and the maxillary molars (whose buccal root apices may be covered by denser bone of the zygomatic arch—a problem more often noted in patients 6 to 8 years of age whose palatal root may flare toward the palate, making the distance that local anesthetic must diffuse too great). In such situations, the use of regional nerve block anesthesia is essential for clinical success in pain control. In reality, two safe and simple nerve blocks—posterior superior alveolar (PSA) and anterior superior alveolar (ASA)—enable dental care to be provided painlessly in virtually all patients.

Palatal anesthesia, although commonly thought of as being highly traumatic, can be provided in most cases with little or no discomfort to the patient.

References

1. Loetscher CA, Melton DC, Walton RE: Injection regimen for anesthesia of the maxillary first molar, J Am Dent Assoc 117:337–340, 1988.
2. Frazer M: Contributing factors and symptoms of stress in dental practice, Br Dent J 173:211, 1992.
3. Friedman MJ, Hochman MN: A 21(st) century computerized injection system for local pain control, Compend Contin Educ Dent 18:995–1000, 1002–1004, 1997.
4. Friedman MJ, Hochman MN: The AMSA injection: a new concept for local anesthesia of maxillary teeth using a computer-controlled injection system, Quint Int 29:297–303, 1998.
5. Lee S, Reader A, Nusstein J, et al: Anesthetic efficacy of the anterior middle superior alveolar (AMSA) injection, Anesth Prog 51:80–89, 2004.
6. Melzack R: The puzzle of pain, New York, 1973, Basic Books.
7. Jeske AH, Blanton PL: Misconception involving dental local anesthesia. Part 2. Pharmacology, Tex Dent J 119:296–300, 302–304, 306–307, 2002.
8. Friedman MJ, Hochman MN: P-ASA block injection: a new palatal technique to anesthetize maxillary anterior teeth, J Esthet Dent 11:63–71, 1999.
9. Friedman MJ, Hochman MN: 21(st) century computerized injection for local pain control, Compend Contin Educ Dent 18:995–1003, 1997.
10. Perry DA, Loomer PM: Maximizing pain control: the AMSA injection can provide anesthesia with few injections and less pain, Dimens Dent Hyg 49:28–33, 2003.
11. Hochman MN, Friedman MJ: In vitro study of needle deflection: a linear insertion technique versus a bidirectional rotation insertion technique, Quint Int 31:33–39, 2000.
12. Malamed SF: Handbook of local anesthesia, ed 5, St Louis, 2004, Mosby.
13. Jastak JT, Yagiela JA, Donaldson D: Local anesthesia of the oral cavity, Philadelphia, 1995, WB Saunders.
14. McArdle BF: Painless palatal anesthesia, J Am Dent Assoc 128:647, 1997.

15. Nicholson JW, Berry TG, Summitt JB, et al: Pain perception and utility: a comparison of the syringe and computerized local injection techniques, Gen Dent 49:167–172, 2001.
16. Hochman MN, Chiiarello D, Hochman C, et al: Computerized local anesthesia vs traditional syringe technique: subjective pain response, NYSDJ 63:24–29, 1997.
17. Nicholson JW, Berry TG, Summitt JB, et al: Pain perception and utility: a comparison of the syringe and computerized local injection techniques, Gen Dent 49:167–172, 2001.
18. Fukayama H, Yoshikawa F, Kohase H, et al: Efficacy of AMSA anesthesia using a new injection system, the Wand, Quint Int 34:537–541, 2003.
19. Malamed SF, Trieger N: Intraoral maxillary nerve block: an anatomical and clinical study, Anesth Prog 30:44–48, 1983.
20. Poore TE, Carney FMT: Maxillary nerve block: a useful technique, J Oral Surg 31:749–755, 1973.

CHAPTER 14

Techniques of Mandibular Anesthesia

Providing effective pain control is one of the most important aspects of dental care. Indeed, patients rate a dentist "who does not hurt" and one who can "give painless injections" as meeting the second and first most important criteria used in evaluating dentists.[1] Unfortunately, the ability to obtain consistently profound anesthesia for dental procedures in the mandible has proved extremely elusive. This is even more of a problem when infected teeth are involved, primarily mandibular molars. Anesthesia of maxillary teeth on the other hand, although on occasion difficult to achieve, is rarely an insurmountable problem. Reasons for this include the fact that the cortical plate of bone overlying maxillary teeth is normally quite thin, thus allowing the local anesthetic drug to diffuse when administered by supraperiosteal injection (infiltration). Additionally, relatively simple nerve blocks, such as the posterior superior alveolar (PSA), middle superior alveolar (MSA), anterior superior alveolar (ASA, infraorbital), and anterior middle superior alveolar (AMSA),[2] are available as alternatives to infiltration.

It is commonly stated that the significantly higher failure rate for mandibular anesthesia is related to the thickness of the cortical plate of bone in the adult mandible. Indeed it is generally acknowledged that mandibular infiltration is successful in cases where the patient has a full primary dentition.[3,4] Once a mixed dentition develops, it is a general rule of teaching that the mandibular cortical plate of bone has thickened to the degree that infiltration might not be effective, leading to the recommendation that "mandibular block" techniques should now be employed.[5]

A second difficulty with the traditional Halsted approach to the inferior alveolar nerve (IAN) (i.e., "mandibular block," or IANB) is the absence of consistent landmarks. Multiple authors have described numerous approaches to this oftentimes elusive nerve.[6-8] Indeed, reported failure rates for the IANB are commonly high, ranging from 31% and 41% in mandibular second and first molars to 42%, 38%, and 46% in second and first premolars and canines, respectively,[9] and 81% in lateral incisors.[10]

Not only is the inferior alveolar nerve elusive, studies using ultrasound[11] and radiography[12,13] to accurately locate the inferior alveolar neurovascular bundle or the mandibular foramen revealed that accurate needle location did not guarantee successful pain control.[14] The central core theory best explains this problem.[15,16] Nerves on the outside of the nerve bundle supply the molar teeth, while nerves on the inside (core fibers) supply incisor teeth. Therefore the local anesthetic solution deposited near the IAN may diffuse and block the outermost fibers but not those located more centrally, leading to incomplete mandibular anesthesia.

This difficulty in achieving mandibular anesthesia has over the years led to the development of alternative techniques to the traditional (Halsted approach) inferior alveolar nerve block. These have included the Gow-Gates mandibular nerve block,[17] the Akinosi-Vazirani closed-mouth mandibular nerve block,[18] the periodontal ligament (PDL, intraligamentary) injection,[19] intraosseous anesthesia,[20] and, most recently, buffered local anesthetics.[21] Although all maintain some advantages over the traditional Halsted approach, none is without its own faults and contraindications.

Six nerve blocks are described in this chapter. Two of these—involving the mental and buccal nerves—provide regional anesthesia to soft tissues only and have exceedingly high success rates. In both instances, the nerve anesthetized lies directly beneath the soft tissues, not encased in bone. The four remaining blocks—inferior alveolar, incisive, Gow-Gates mandibular, and Vazirani-Akinosi (closed-mouth) mandibular—provide regional anesthesia to the pulps of some or all of the mandibular teeth in a quadrant. Three other injections of importance in mandibular anesthesia—periodontal ligament, intraosseous, and intraseptal—are described in Chapter 15. Although these supplemental techniques can be used successfully in the maxilla or the mandible, their greatest utility lies in the mandible, because in the mandible, they can provide pulpal anesthesia of a single tooth without providing the accompanying lingual and facial soft tissue anesthesia that occurs with other mandibular nerve block techniques.

The success rate of the inferior alveolar nerve block is considerably lower than that of most other nerve blocks.

Because of anatomic considerations in the mandible (primarily the density of bone), the administrator must accurately deposit local anesthetic solution to within 1 mm of the target nerve. The inferior alveolar nerve block has a significantly lower success rate because of two factors—anatomic variation in the height of the mandibular foramen on the lingual aspect of the ramus, and the greater depth of soft tissue penetration necessary—that lead to greater inaccuracy. Fortunately, the incisive nerve block can provide pulpal anesthesia to the teeth anterior to the mental foramen (e.g., incisors, canines, first premolars, and [in most instances] second premolars). The incisive nerve block is a valuable alternative to the inferior alveolar nerve block when treatment is limited to these teeth. To achieve anesthesia of the mandibular molars, however, the inferior alveolar nerve must be anesthetized, and this frequently entails (with all its attendant disadvantages) a lower incidence of successful anesthesia.

The third injection technique that provides pulpal anesthesia to mandibular teeth, the Gow-Gates mandibular nerve block, is a true mandibular block injection, providing regional anesthesia to virtually all sensory branches of V_3. In actual fact, the Gow-Gates may be thought of as a (very) high inferior alveolar nerve block. When used, two benefits are seen: (1) the problems associated with anatomic variations in the height of the mandibular foramen are obviated, and (2) anesthesia of the other sensory branches of V_3 (e.g., the lingual, buccal, and mylohyoid nerves) is usually attained along with that of the inferior alveolar nerve. With proper adherence to protocol (and experience using this technique), a success rate in excess of 95% can be achieved.

Another V_3 nerve block, the closed-mouth mandibular nerve block, is included in this discussion, primarily because it allows the doctor to achieve clinically adequate anesthesia in an extremely difficult situation—one in which a patient has limited mandibular opening as a result of infection, trauma, or postinjection trismus. It is also known as the Vazirani-Akinosi technique (after the two doctors who developed it independent of each other). Some practitioners use it routinely for anesthesia in the mandibular arch. The closed-mouth technique is described mainly because with experience it can provide a success rate of better than 80% in situations (extreme trismus) in which the inferior alveolar and Gow-Gates nerve blocks have little or no likelihood of success.

In ideal circumstances, the individual who is to administer the local anesthetic should be familiar with each of these techniques. The greater the number of techniques at one's disposal with which to attain mandibular anesthesia, the less likely it is that a patient will be dismissed from an office as a result of inadequate pain control. More realistically, however, the administrator should become proficient with at least one of these procedures and should have a working knowledge of the others to be able to use them with a good expectation of success should the appropriate situation arise.

Recent work with mandibular infiltration in adult patients with the local anesthetic drug articaine HCl has demonstrated significant rates of success in mandibular anterior teeth in lieu of block injection.[22-24] When articaine HCl is administered by buccal infiltration in the adult mandible following IANB, success rates are even greater.[25,26] The concept of mandibular infiltration in adult patients will be discussed in depth in Chapter 20.

INFERIOR ALVEOLAR NERVE BLOCK

The inferior alveolar nerve block (IANB), commonly (but inaccurately) referred to as the *mandibular nerve block*, is the second most frequently used (after infiltration) and possibly the most important injection technique in dentistry. Unfortunately, it also proves to be the most frustrating, with the highest percentage of clinical failures even when properly administered.[6-10]

It is an especially useful technique for quadrant dentistry. A supplemental block (buccal nerve) is needed only when soft tissue anesthesia in the buccal posterior region is necessary. On rare occasions, a supraperiosteal injection (infiltration) may be needed in the lower incisor region to correct partial anesthesia caused by the overlap of sensory fibers from the contralateral side. A periodontal ligament (PDL) injection might be necessary when isolated portions of mandibular teeth (usually the mesial root of a first mandibular molar) remain sensitive after an otherwise successful inferior alveolar nerve block. Intraosseous anesthesia (IO) is a supplemental technique employed, usually on molars, when the IANB has proven ineffective, primarily when the tooth is pulpally involved.

Administration of bilateral IANBs is rarely indicated in dental treatments other than bilateral mandibular surgeries. They produce considerable discomfort, primarily from the lingual soft tissue anesthesia, which usually persists for several hours after injection (the duration is dependent on the particular local anesthetic used). The patient feels unable to swallow and, because of the absence of all sensation, is more likely to self-injure the anesthetized soft tissues. Additional residual soft tissue anesthesia affects the patient's ability to speak and to swallow. When possible, it is preferable to treat the entire right or left side of a patient's oral cavity (maxillary and mandibular) at one appointment rather than administer a bilateral IANB. Patients are much more capable of handling the posttreatment discomfort (e.g., feeling of anesthesia) associated with bilateral maxillary than with bilateral mandibular anesthesia.

One situation in which bilateral mandibular anesthesia is frequently used involves the patient who presents with six, eight, or ten lower anterior teeth (e.g., canine to canine; premolar to premolar) requiring restorative or soft tissue procedures. Two excellent alternatives to bilateral IANBs are bilateral incisive nerve blocks (where lingual soft tissue anesthesia is not necessary) and unilateral inferior alveolar blocks on the side that has the greater number of teeth requiring restoration or that requires the greater degree of lingual

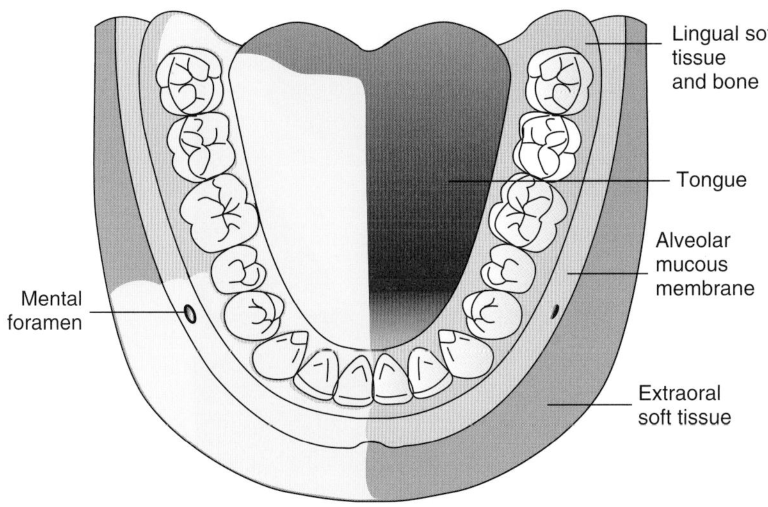

Figure 14-1. Area anesthetized by an inferior alveolar nerve block.

intervention, combined with an incisive nerve block on the opposite side. It must be remembered that the incisive nerve block does not provide lingual soft tissue anesthesia; thus lingual infiltration may be necessary. Infiltration of articaine HCl in the mandibular incisor region on both the buccal and lingual aspects of the tooth has been associated with considerable success in providing pulpal anesthesia.[22]

In the following description of the inferior alveolar nerve block, the injection site is noted to be slightly higher than that usually depicted.

Other Common Names. Mandibular block.

Nerves Anesthetized
1. Inferior alveolar, a branch of the posterior division of the mandibular division of the trigeminal nerve (V_3)
2. Incisive
3. Mental
4. Lingual (commonly)

Areas Anesthetized. (Fig. 14-1)
1. Mandibular teeth to the midline
2. Body of the mandible, inferior portion of the ramus
3. Buccal mucoperiosteum, mucous membrane anterior to the mental foramen (mental nerve)
4. Anterior two thirds of the tongue and floor of the oral cavity (lingual nerve)
5. Lingual soft tissues and periosteum (lingual nerve)

Indications
1. Procedures on multiple mandibular teeth in one quadrant
2. When buccal soft tissue anesthesia (anterior to the mental foramen) is necessary
3. When lingual soft tissue anesthesia is necessary

Contraindications
1. Infection or acute inflammation in the area of injection (rare)
2. Patients who are more likely to bite their lip or tongue, for instance, a very young child or a physically or mentally handicapped adult or child

Advantages. One injection provides a wide area of anesthesia (useful for quadrant dentistry).

Disadvantages
1. Wide area of anesthesia (not indicated for localized procedures)
2. Rate of inadequate anesthesia (31% to 81%)
3. Intraoral landmarks not consistently reliable
4. Positive aspiration (10% to 15%, highest of all intraoral injection techniques)
5. Lingual and lower lip anesthesia, discomfiting to many patients and possibly dangerous (self-inflicted soft tissue trauma) for certain individuals
6. Partial anesthesia possible where a bifid inferior alveolar nerve and bifid mandibular canals are present; cross-innervation in lower anterior region

Positive Aspiration. 10% to 15%.

Alternatives
1. Mental nerve block, for buccal soft tissue anesthesia anterior to the first molar
2. Incisive nerve block, for pulpal and buccal soft tissue anesthesia of teeth anterior to the mental foramen (usually second premolar to central incisor)
3. Supraperiosteal injection, for pulpal anesthesia of the central and lateral incisors, and sometimes the premolars and molars (discussed fully in Chapter 20)
4. Gow-Gates mandibular nerve block
5. Vazirani-Akinosi mandibular nerve block
6. PDL injection for pulpal anesthesia of any mandibular tooth
7. IO injection for pulpal and soft tissue anesthesia of any mandibular tooth, but especially molars

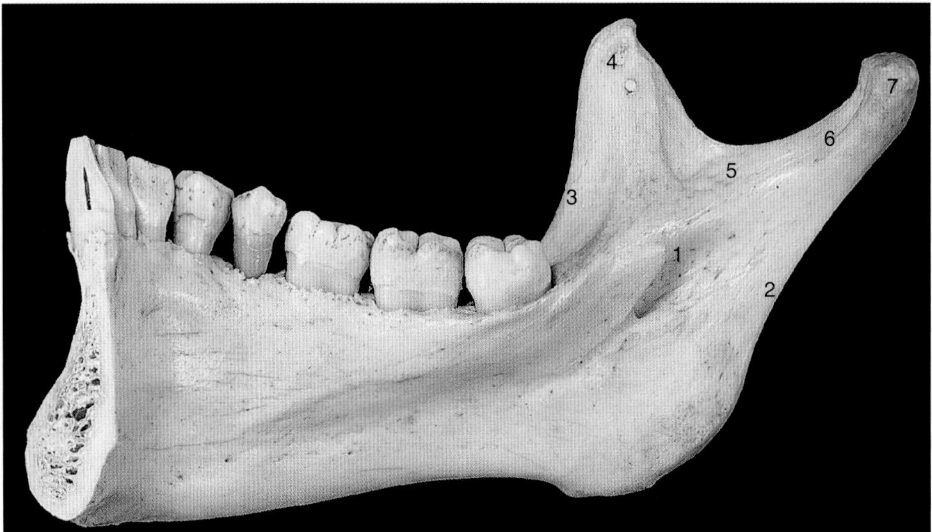

Figure 14-2. Osseous landmarks for inferior alveolar nerve block. 1, Lingula; 2, distal border of ramus; 3, coronoid notch; 4, coronoid process; 5, sigmoid (mandibular) notch; 6, neck of condyle; 7, head of condyle.

8. Intraseptal injection for pulpal and soft tissue anesthesia of any mandibular tooth

Technique

1. A long dental needle is recommended for the adult patient. A 25-gauge long needle is preferred; a 27-gauge long is acceptable.
2. *Area of insertion:* Mucous membrane on the medial (lingual) side of the mandibular ramus, at the intersection of two lines—one horizontal, representing the height of needle insertion, the other vertical, representing the anteroposterior plane of injection
3. *Target area:* Inferior alveolar nerve as it passes downward toward the mandibular foramen but before it enters into the foramen
4. Landmarks (Figs. 14-2 and 14-3)
   a. Coronoid notch (greatest concavity on the anterior border of the ramus)
   b. Pterygomandibular raphe (vertical portion)
   c. Occlusal plane of the mandibular posterior teeth
5. *Orientation of the needle bevel:* Less critical than with other nerve blocks, because the needle approaches the inferior alveolar nerve at roughly a right angle
6. Procedure
   a. Assume the correct position.
      (1) For a right IANB, a right-handed administrator should sit at the 8 o'clock position facing the patient (Fig. 14-4, *A*).
      (2) For a left IANB, a right-handed administrator should sit at the 10 o'clock position facing in the same direction as the patient (Fig. 14-4, *B*).
   b. Position the patient supine (recommended) or semisupine (if necessary). The mouth should be opened wide to allow greater visibility of, and access to, the injection site.
   c. Locate the needle penetration (injection) site.

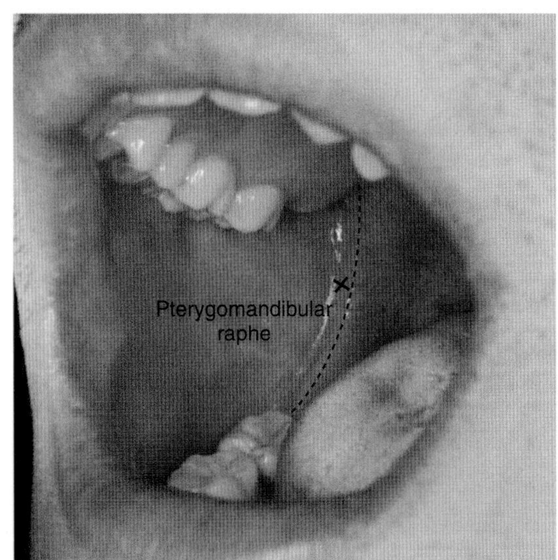

Figure 14-3. The posterior border of the mandibular ramus can be approximated intraorally by using the pterygomandibular raphe as it turns superiorly toward the maxilla.

Three parameters must be considered during administration of IANB: (1) the height of the injection, (2) the anteroposterior placement of the needle (which helps to locate a precise needle entry point), and (3) the depth of penetration (which determines the location of the inferior alveolar nerve).

(1) *Height of injection:* Place the index finger or the thumb of your left hand in the coronoid notch.
   (a) An imaginary line extends posteriorly from the fingertip in the coronoid notch to the deepest part of the pterygomandibular raphe (as it turns vertically upward toward the maxilla), determining the height of injection. This imaginary line should be parallel to the

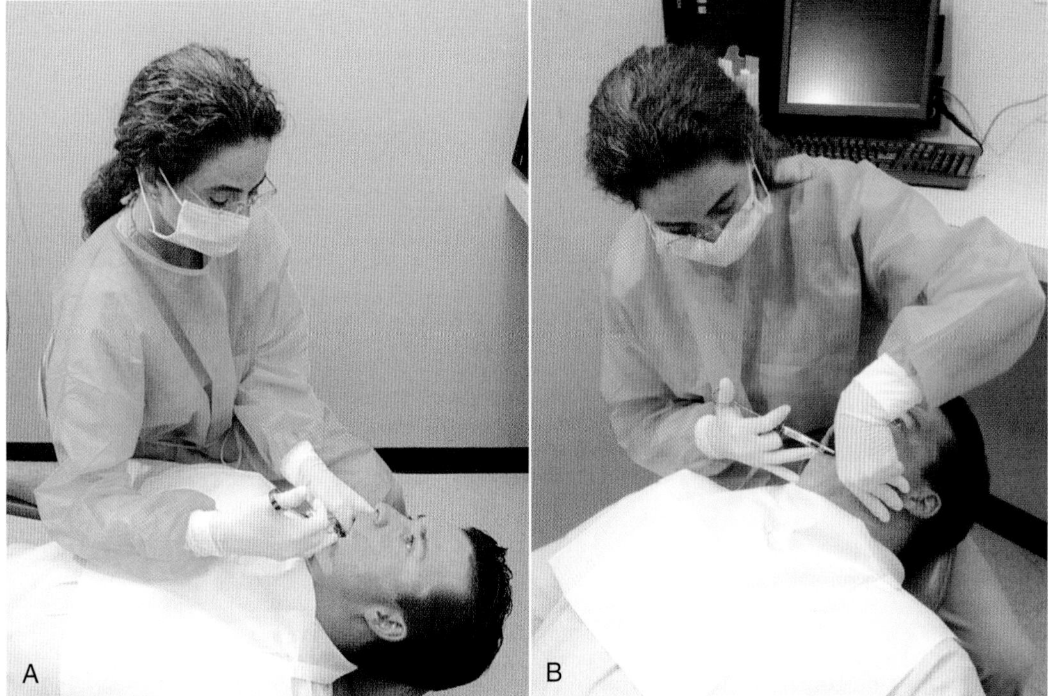

Figure 14-4. Position of the administrator for a (**A**) right and (**B**) left inferior alveolar nerve block.

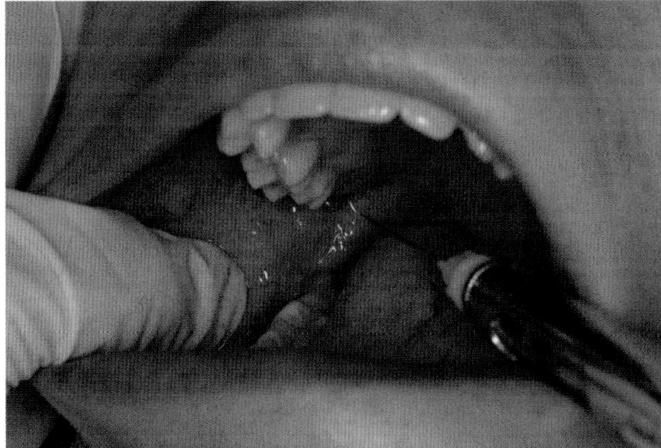

Figure 14-5. Note the placement of the syringe barrel at the corner of the mouth, usually corresponding to the premolars. The needle tip gently touches the most distal end of the pterygomandibular raphe.

occlusal plane of the mandibular molar teeth. In most patients, this line lies 6 to 10 mm above the occlusal plane.

(b) The finger on the coronoid notch is used to pull the tissues laterally, stretching them over the injection site, making them taut, and enabling needle insertion to be less traumatic, while providing better visibility.

(c) The needle insertion point lies three fourths of the anteroposterior distance from the coronoid notch back to the deepest part of the pterygomandibular raphe (Fig. 14-5).

Note: The line should begin at the midpoint of the notch and terminate at the deepest (most posterior) portion of the pterygomandibular raphe as the raphe bends vertically upward toward the palate.

(d) The posterior border of the mandibular ramus can be approximated intraorally by using the pterygomandibular raphe as it bends vertically upward toward the maxilla* (see Fig. 14-3).

(e) An alternative method of approximating the length of the ramus is to place your thumb on the coronoid notch and your index finger extraorally on the posterior border of the ramus and estimate the distance between these points. However, many practitioners (including this author) have difficulty envisioning the width of the ramus in this manner.

(f) Prepare tissue at the injection site:
   (1) Dry with sterile gauze.
   (2) Apply topical antiseptic (optional).
   (3) Apply topical anesthetic for 1 to 2 minutes.

Place the barrel of the syringe in the corner of the mouth on the contralateral side (Figs. 14-5 and 14-6).

---

*The pterygomandibular raphe continues posteriorly in a horizontal plane from the retromolar pad before turning vertically toward the palate; only the vertical portion of the pterygomandibular raphe is used as an indicator of the posterior border of the ramus.

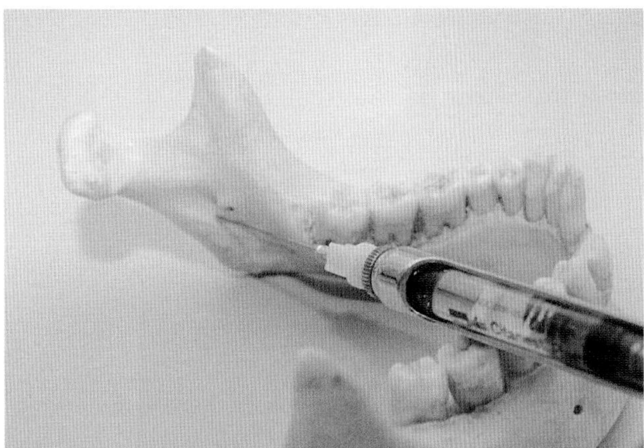

Figure 14-6. Placement of the needle and syringe for an inferior alveolar nerve block.

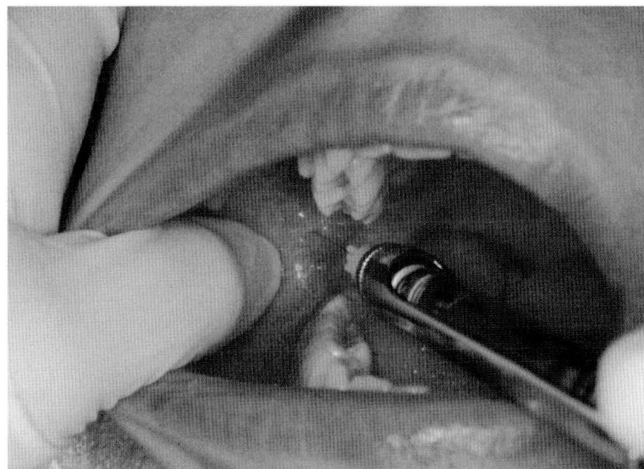

Figure 14-7. Inferior alveolar nerve block. The depth of penetration is 20 to 25 mm (two thirds to three fourths the length of a long needle).

(2) *Anteroposterior site of injection:* Needle penetration occurs at the intersection of two points.
   (a) Point 1 falls along the horizontal line from the coronoid notch to the deepest part of the pterygomandibular raphe as it ascends vertically toward the palate as just described.
   (b) Point 2 is on a vertical line through point 1 about three fourths of the distance from the anterior border of the ramus. This determines the anteroposterior site of the injection.

(3) *Penetration depth:* In the third parameter of the IANB, bone should be contacted. Slowly advance the needle until you can feel it meet bony resistance.
   (a) For most patients, it is not necessary to inject any local anesthetic solution as soft tissue is penetrated.
   (b) For anxious or sensitive patients, it may be advisable to deposit small volumes as the needle is advanced. Buffered LA solution decreases the patient's sensitivity during needle advancement.
   (c) The average depth of penetration to bony contact will be 20 to 25 mm, approximately two thirds to three fourths the length of a long dental needle (Fig. 14-7).
   (d) The needle tip should now be located slightly superior to the mandibular foramen (where the inferior alveolar nerve enters [disappears] into bone). The foramen can neither be seen nor palpated clinically.
   (e) If bone is contacted too soon (less than half the length of a long dental needle), the needle tip is usually located too far anteriorly (laterally) on the ramus (Fig. 14-8). To correct:

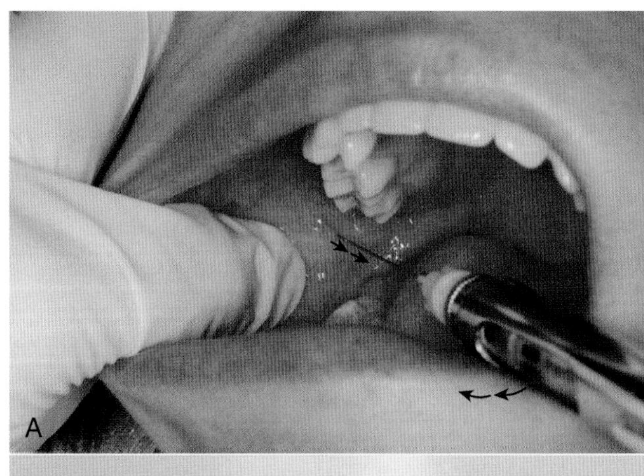

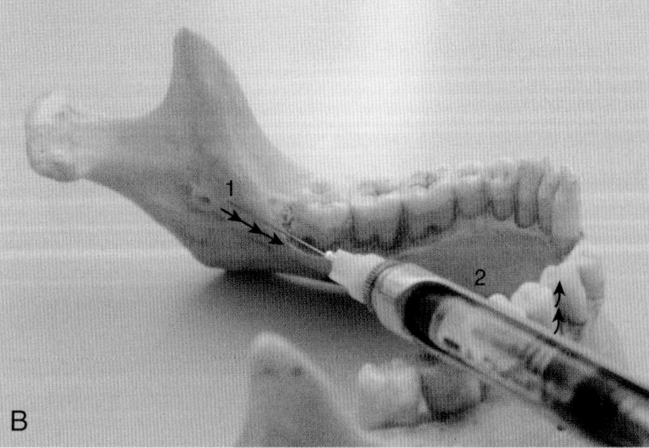

Figure 14-8. **A,** The needle is located too far anteriorly (laterally) on the ramus. **B,** To correct: Withdraw it slightly from the tissues (1) and bring the syringe barrel anteriorly toward the lateral incisor or canine (2); reinsert to proper depth.

(i) Withdraw the needle slightly but do not remove it from the tissue.
(ii) Bring the syringe barrel more toward the front of the mouth, over the canine or lateral incisor on the contralateral side.
(iii) Redirect the needle until a more appropriate depth of insertion is obtained. The needle tip is now located more posteriorly in the mandibular sulcus.

(f) If bone is not contacted, the needle tip usually is located too far posterior (medial) (Fig. 14-9). To correct:
(i) Withdraw it slightly in tissue (leaving approximately one fourth its length in tissue) and reposition the syringe barrel more posteriorly (over the mandibular molars).
(ii) Continue needle insertion until contact with bone is made at an appropriate depth (20 to 25 mm).

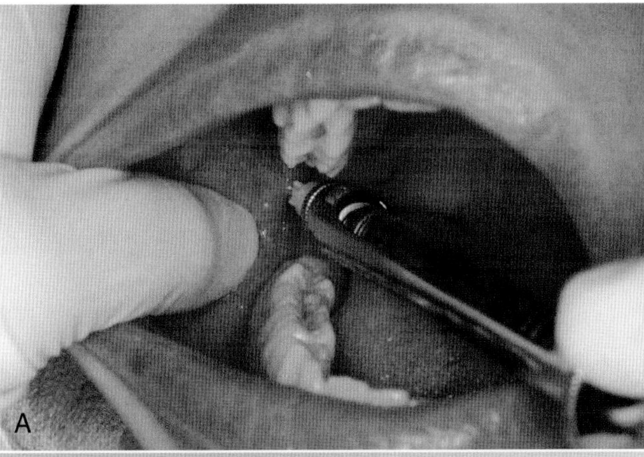

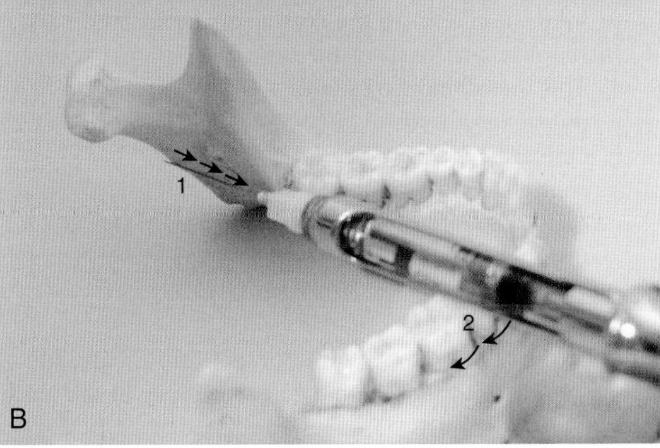

Figure 14-9. **A,** Overinsertion with no contact of bone. The needle is usually posterior (medial) to the ramus. **B,** To correct: Withdraw it slightly from the tissues (1) and reposition the syringe barrel over the premolars (2); reinsert.

d. Insert the needle. When bone is contacted, withdraw approximately 1 mm to prevent subperiosteal injection.
e. Aspirate in two planes. If negative, slowly deposit 1.5 mL of anesthetic over a minimum of 60 seconds. (Because of the high incidence of positive aspiration and the natural tendency to deposit solution too rapidly, the sequence of slow injection, reaspiration, slow injection, reaspiration is strongly recommended.)
f. Slowly withdraw the syringe, and when approximately half its length remains within tissues, reaspirate. If negative, deposit a portion of the remaining solution (0.2 mL) to anesthetize the lingual nerve.
  (1) In most patients, this deliberate injection for lingual nerve anesthesia is not necessary, because local anesthetic from the IANB anesthetizes the lingual nerve.
g. Withdraw the syringe slowly and make the needle safe.
h. After approximately 20 seconds, return the patient to the upright or semiupright position.
i. Wait 3 to 5 minutes before testing for pulpal anesthesia.

Signs and Symptoms

1. *Subjective:* Tingling or numbness of the lower lip indicates anesthesia of the mental nerve, a terminal branch of the inferior alveolar nerve. This is a good indication that the inferior alveolar nerve is anesthetized, although it is not a reliable indicator of the depth of anesthesia.
2. *Subjective:* Tingling or numbness of the tongue indicates anesthesia of the lingual nerve, a branch of the posterior division of V_3. It usually accompanies IANB but may be present without anesthesia of the inferior alveolar nerve.
3. *Objective:* Using an electrical pulp tester (EPT) and eliciting no response to maximal output (80/80) on two consecutive tests at least 2 minutes apart serves as a "guarantee" of successful pulpal anesthesia in nonpulpitic teeth.[24,27,28]
4. *Objective:* No pain is felt during dental therapy.

Safety Feature. The needle contacts bone, preventing over-insertion with its attendant complications.

Precautions

1. Do not deposit local anesthetic if bone is not contacted. The needle tip may be resting within the parotid gland near the facial nerve (cranial nerve VII), and a transient blockade (paralysis) of the facial nerve may develop if local anesthetic solution is deposited.
2. Avoid pain by not contacting bone too forcefully.

Failures of Anesthesia. The most common causes of absent or incomplete IANB follow:

1. Deposition of anesthetic too low (below the mandibular foramen). To correct: Reinject at a higher site (approximately 5 to 10 mm above the previous site).
2. Deposition of the anesthetic too far anteriorly (laterally) on the ramus. This is diagnosed by lack of anesthesia except at the injection site and by the minimum depth of needle penetration before contact with bone (e.g., the [long] needle is usually less than halfway into tissue). To correct: Redirect the needle tip posteriorly.
3. Accessory innervation to the mandibular teeth
   a. The primary symptom is isolated areas of incomplete pulpal anesthesia encountered in the mandibular molars (most commonly the mesial portion of the mandibular first molar).
   b. Although it has been postulated that several nerves provide the mandibular teeth with accessory sensory innervation (e.g., the cervical accessory and mylohyoid nerves), current thinking supports the mylohyoid nerve as the prime candidate.[29-31] The Gow-Gates mandibular nerve block, which routinely blocks the mylohyoid nerve, is not associated with problems of accessory innervation (unlike the IANB, which normally does not block the mylohyoid nerve).
   c. To correct:
      (1) Technique #1
         (a) Use a 25-gauge (or 27-gauge) long needle.
         (b) Retract the tongue toward the midline with a mirror handle or tongue depressor to provide access and visibility to the lingual border of the body of the mandible (Fig. 14-10).
         (c) Place the syringe in the corner of mouth on the opposite side and direct the needle tip to the apical region of the tooth immediately posterior to the tooth in question (e.g., the apex of the second molar if the first molar is the problem).
         (d) Penetrate the soft tissues and advance the needle until bone (e.g., the lingual border of the body of the mandible) is contacted. Topical anesthesia is unnecessary if lingual anesthesia is already present. The depth of penetration to bone is 3 to 5 mm.
         (e) Aspirate in two planes. If negative, slowly deposit approximately 0.6 mL (one third cartridge) of anesthetic (in about 20 seconds).
         (f) Withdraw the syringe and make the needle safe.
      (2) Technique #2. In any situation in which partial anesthesia of a tooth occurs, the PDL or IO injection may be administered; both techniques have a high expectation of success. (See Chapter 15 for discussion of PDL and IO techniques.)

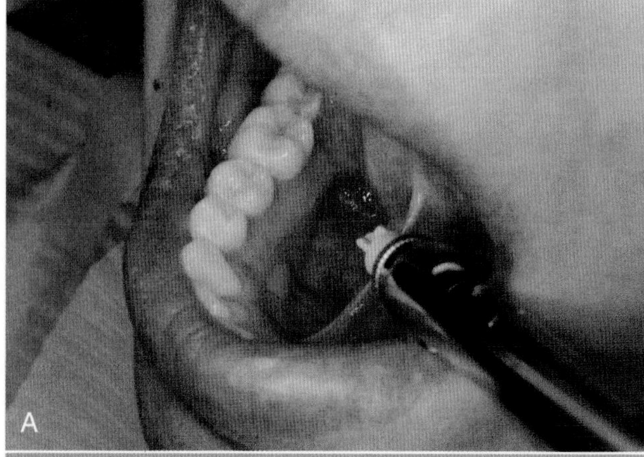

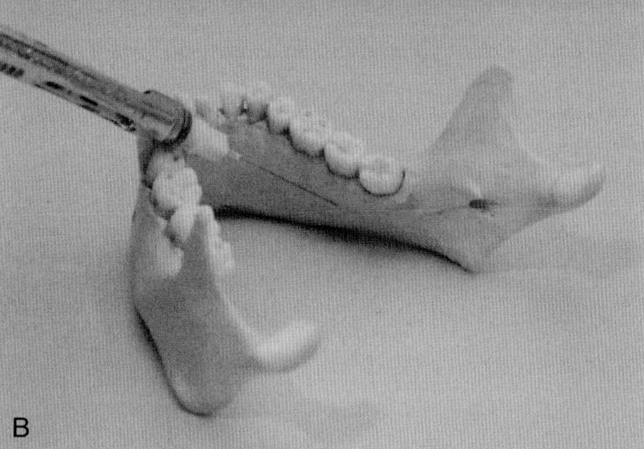

Figure 14-10. **A,** Retract the tongue to gain access to, and increase the visibility of, the lingual border of the mandible. **B,** Direct the needle tip below the apical region of the tooth immediately posterior to the tooth in question.

   d. Whenever a bifid inferior alveolar nerve is detected on the radiograph, incomplete anesthesia of the mandible may develop after IANB. In many such cases, a second mandibular foramen, located more inferiorly, exists. To correct: Deposit a volume of solution inferior to the normal anatomic landmark.
4. Incomplete anesthesia of the central or lateral incisors
   a. This may comprise isolated areas of incomplete pulpal anesthesia.
   b. Often this is due to overlapping fibers of the contralateral inferior alveolar nerve, although it may also arise (rarely) from innervation from the mylohyoid nerve.
   c. To correct:
      (1) Technique #1
         (a) Infiltrate 0.9 mL supraperiosteally into the mucobuccal fold below the apex of the tooth in question, followed immediately by injection of 0.9 mL onto the lingual aspect of the same tooth (Fig. 14-11). This generally is highly effective in the central and lateral incisor teeth because of the many small nutrient canals in the cortical bone near the

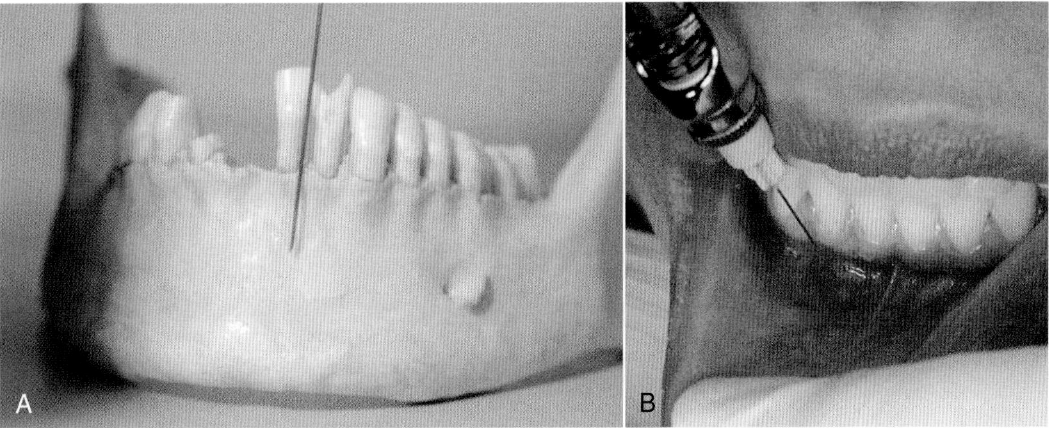

Figure 14-11. With supraperiosteal injection, the needle tip is directed toward the apical region of the tooth in question. **A,** On a skull. **B,** In the mouth.

region of the incisive fossa. The local anesthetic articaine HCl appears to have the greatest success.[22,32]

(b) A 27-gauge short needle is recommended.
(c) Direct the needle tip toward the apical region of the tooth in question. Topical anesthesia is not necessary if mental nerve anesthesia is present.
(d) Aspirate.
(e) If negative, slowly deposit 0.9 mL of local anesthetic solution in approximately 30 seconds.
(f) Administer 0.9 mL on the lingual aspect of the same tooth
(g) Wait about 5 minutes before starting the dental procedure.

(2) As an alternative, the PDL injection may be used. The PDL has great success in the mandibular anterior region.

Complications

1. Hematoma (rare)
   a. Swelling of tissues on the medial side of the mandibular ramus after the deposition of anesthetic
   b. *Management:* Pressure and cold (e.g., ice) to the area for a minimum of 3 to 5 minutes
2. Trismus
   a. Muscle soreness or limited movement
      (1) A slight degree of soreness when opening the mandible is extremely common after IANB (after anesthesia has dissipated).
      (2) More severe soreness associated with limited mandibular opening is rare.
   b. Causes and management of limited mandibular opening after injection are discussed in Chapter 17.
3. Transient facial paralysis (facial nerve anesthesia)
   a. Produced by the deposition of local anesthetic into the body of the parotid gland, blocking the VII cranial nerve (facial n.), a motor nerve to the muscles of facial expression. Signs and symptoms include an inability to close the lower eyelid and drooping of the upper lip on the affected side.
   b. Management of transient facial nerve paralysis is discussed in Chapter 17.

BUCCAL NERVE BLOCK

The buccal nerve is a branch of the anterior division of V_3 and consequently is not anesthetized during IANB. Nor is anesthesia of the buccal nerve necessary for most restorative dental procedures. The buccal nerve provides sensory innervation to the buccal soft tissues adjacent to the mandibular molars only. The sole indication for administration of a buccal nerve block therefore is when manipulation of these tissues is contemplated (e.g., with scaling or curettage, the placement of a rubber dam clamp on soft tissues, the removal of subgingival caries, subgingival tooth preparation, placement of gingival retraction cord, or the placement of matrix bands).

It is common for the buccal nerve block to be routinely administered after IANB, even when buccal soft tissue anesthesia in the molar region is not required. There is absolutely no indication for this injection in such a situation.

The buccal nerve block, commonly referred to as the *long buccal nerve block,* has a success rate approaching 100%. The reason for this is that the buccal nerve is readily accessible to the local anesthetic as it lies immediately beneath the mucous membrane, not buried within bone.

Other Common Names. Long buccal nerve block, buccinator nerve block.

Nerve Anesthetized. Buccal (a branch of the anterior division of the V_3).

Area Anesthetized. Soft tissues and periosteum buccal to the mandibular molar teeth (Fig. 14-12).

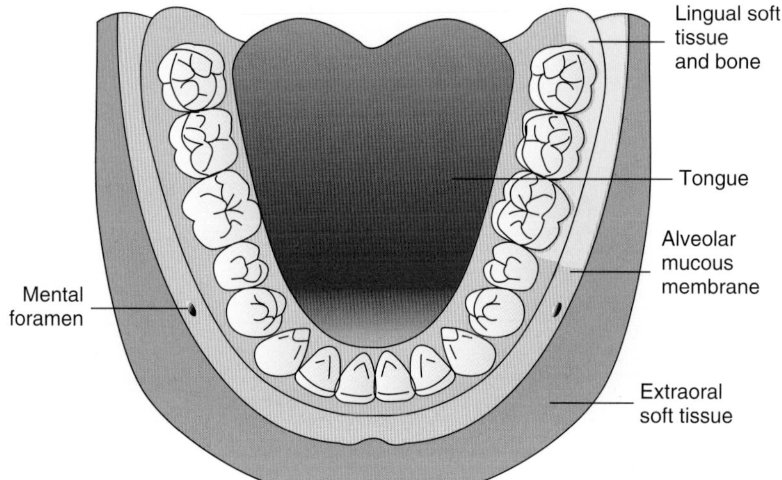

Figure 14-12. Area anesthetized by a buccal nerve block.

Indication. When buccal soft tissue anesthesia is necessary for dental procedures in the mandibular molar region.

Contraindication. Infection or acute inflammation in the area of injection.

Advantages
1. High success rate
2. Technically easy

Disadvantages. Potential for pain if the needle contacts the periosteum during injection.

Positive Aspiration. 0.7%.

Alternatives
1. Buccal infiltration
2. Gow-Gates mandibular nerve block
3. Vazirani-Akinosi mandibular nerve block
4. PDL injection
5. Intraosseous injection
6. Intraseptal injection

Technique
1. A 25- or 27-gauge long needle is recommended. This is most often used because the buccal nerve block is usually administered immediately after an IANB. A long needle is recommended because of the posterior deposition site, not the depth of tissue insertion (which is minimal).
2. *Area of insertion:* Mucous membrane distal and buccal to the most distal molar tooth in the arch
3. *Target area:* Buccal nerve as it passes over the anterior border of the ramus
4. *Landmarks:* Mandibular molars, mucobuccal fold
5. *Orientation of the bevel:* Toward bone during the injection
6. Procedure
   a. Assume the correct position.
      (1) For a right buccal nerve block, a right-handed operator should sit at the 8 o'clock position directly facing the patient (Fig. 14-13, *A*).
      (2) For a left buccal nerve block, a right-handed operator should sit at 10 o'clock facing in the same direction as the patient (Fig. 14-13, *B*).
   b. Position the patient supine (recommended) or semisupine.
   c. Prepare the tissues for penetration distal and buccal to the most posterior molar. *
      (1) Dry with sterile gauze.
      (2) Apply topical antiseptic (optional).
      (3) Apply topical anesthetic for 1 to 2 minutes.
   d. With your left index finger (if right-handed), pull the buccal soft tissues in the area of injection laterally so that visibility will be improved. Taut tissues permit an atraumatic needle penetration.
   e. Direct the syringe toward the injection site with the bevel facing down toward bone and the syringe aligned parallel to the occlusal plane on the side of injection but buccal to the teeth (Fig. 14-14, *A*).
   f. Penetrate mucous membrane at the injection site, distal and buccal to the last molar (Fig. 14-14, *B*).
   g. Advance the needle slowly until mucoperiosteum is gently contacted.
      (1) To prevent pain when the needle contacts mucoperiosteum, deposit a few drops of local anesthetic just before contact.
      (2) The depth of penetration is seldom more than 2 to 4 mm, and usually only 1 or 2 mm.
   h. Aspirate.
   i. If negative, slowly deposit 0.3 mL (approximately one eighth of a cartridge) over 10 seconds.

*Because the buccal nerve block most often immediately follows an inferior alveolar nerve block, steps (1), (2), and (3) of tissue preparation usually are completed before the inferior alveolar block.

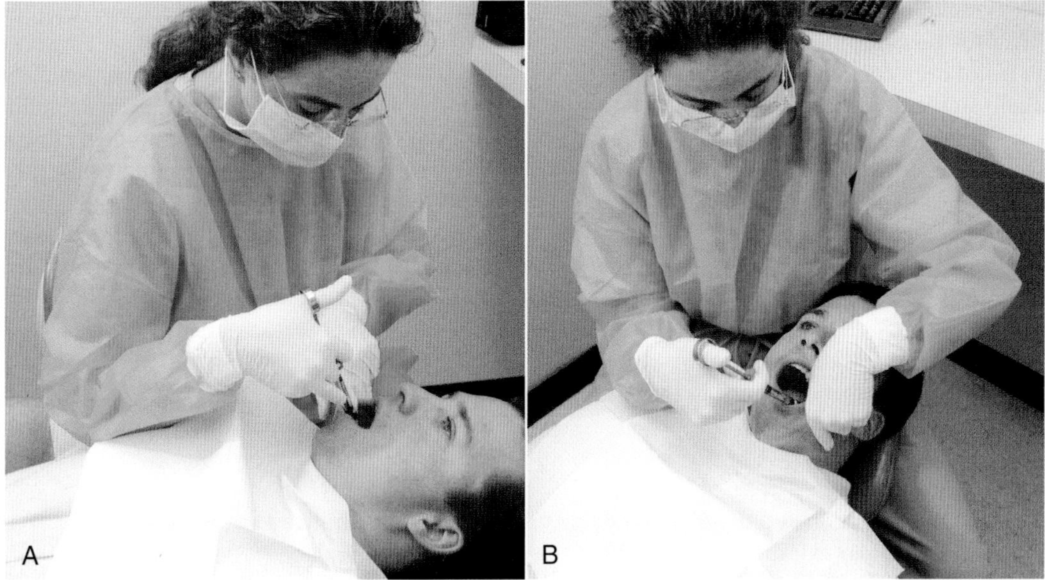

Figure 14-13. Position of the administrator for a (**A**) right and (**B**) left buccal nerve block.

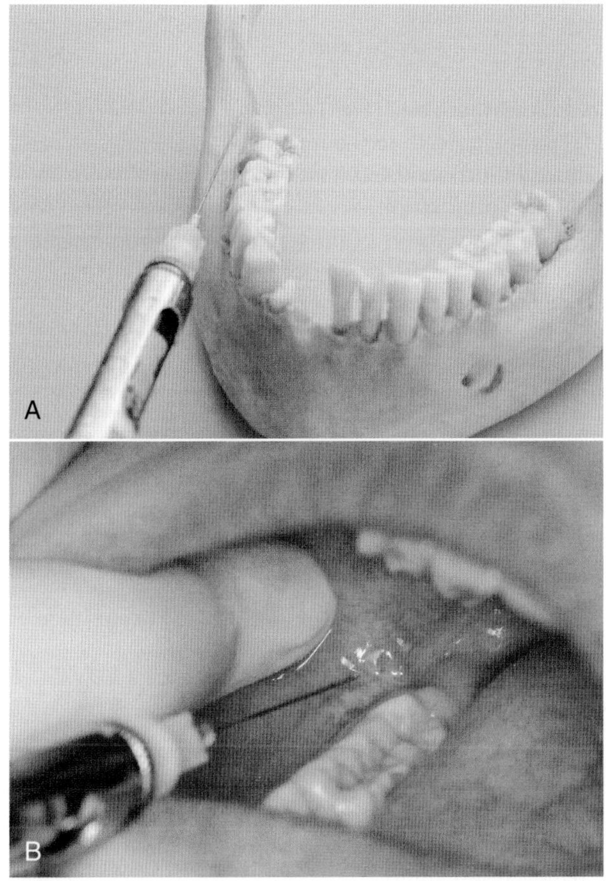

Figure 14-14. Syringe alignment. **A,** Parallel to the occlusal plane on the side of injection but buccal to it. **B,** Distal and buccal to the last molar.

(1) If tissue at the injection site balloons (becomes swollen during injection), stop depositing solution.
(2) If solution runs out the injection site (back into the patient's mouth) during deposition:
 (a) Stop the injection.
 (b) Advance the needle tip deeper into the tissue.*
 (c) Reaspirate.
 (d) Continue the injection.

j. Withdraw the syringe slowly and immediately make the needle safe.
k. Wait approximately 3 to 5 minutes before commencing the planned dental procedure.

Signs and Symptoms

1. Because of the location and small size of the anesthetized area, the patient rarely experiences any subjective symptoms.
2. *Objective:* Instrumentation in the anesthetized area without pain indicates satisfactory pain control.

Safety Features

1. Needle contacts bone, therein preventing overinsertion.
2. Minimum positive aspiration rate

Precautions

1. Pain on insertion from contacting unanesthetized periosteum. This can be prevented by depositing a few drops of local anesthetic before touching the periosteum.

*If an inadequate volume of solution remains in the cartridge, it may be necessary to remove the syringe from the patient's mouth and reload it with a new cartridge.

2. Local anesthetic solution not being retained at the injection site. This generally means that needle penetration is not deep enough, the bevel of the needle is only partially in the tissues, and solution is escaping during the injection.
   a. To correct:
      (1) Stop the injection.
      (2) Insert the needle to a greater depth.
      (3) Reaspirate.
      (4) Continue the injection.

Failures of Anesthesia. Rare with the buccal nerve block:
1. Inadequate volume of anesthetic retained in the tissues

Complications
1. Few of any consequence
2. Hematoma (bluish discoloration and tissue swelling at the injection site). Blood may exit the needle puncture point into the buccal vestibule. To treat: Apply pressure with gauze directly to the area of bleeding for a minimum of 3 to 5 minutes.

MANDIBULAR NERVE BLOCK: THE GOW-GATES TECHNIQUE

Successful anesthesia of the mandibular teeth and soft tissues is more difficult to achieve than anesthesia of maxillary structures. Primary factors for this failure rate are the greater anatomic variation in the mandible and the need for deeper soft tissue penetration. In 1973, George Albert Edwards Gow-Gates (1910-2001),[33] a general practitioner of dentistry in Australia, described a new approach to mandibular anesthesia. He had used this technique in his practice for approximately 30 years, with an astonishingly high success rate (approximately 99% in his experienced hands).

The Gow-Gates technique is a true mandibular nerve block because it provides sensory anesthesia to virtually the entire distribution of V_3. The inferior alveolar, lingual, mylohyoid, mental, incisive, auriculotemporal, and buccal nerves all are blocked in the Gow-Gates injection.

Significant advantages of the Gow-Gates technique over IANB include its higher success rate, its lower incidence of positive aspiration (approximately 2% vs. 10% to 15% with the IANB),[33,34] and the absence of problems with accessory sensory innervation to the mandibular teeth.

The only apparent disadvantage is a relatively minor one: An administrator experienced with the IANB may feel uncomfortable while learning the Gow-Gates mandibular nerve block (GGMNB). Indeed, the incidence of unsuccessful anesthesia with GGMNB may be as high as (if not higher than) that for the IANB until the administrator gains clinical experience with it. Following this "learning curve," success rates greater than 95% are common. A new student of local anesthesia usually does not encounter as much difficulty with the GGMNB as the more experienced administrator. This is a result of the strong bias of the experienced administrator to deposit the anesthetic drug "lower" (e.g., in the "usual" place). Two approaches are suggested for becoming accustomed to the GGMNB. The first is to begin to use the technique on all patients requiring mandibular anesthesia. Allow at least 1 to 2 weeks to gain clinical experience. The second approach is to continue using the conventional IANB, but to use the GGMNB technique whenever clinically inadequate anesthesia occurs. Reanesthetize the patient using the GGMNB. Although experience is accumulated more slowly with this latter approach, its effectiveness is more dramatic because patients who were previously difficult to anesthetize now may be more easily managed.

Other Common Names. Gow-Gates technique, third division nerve block, V_3 nerve block.

Nerves Anesthetized
1. Inferior alveolar
2. Mental
3. Incisive
4. Lingual
5. Mylohyoid
6. Auriculotemporal
7. Buccal (in 75% of patients)

Areas Anesthetized. (Fig. 14-15)
1. Mandibular teeth to the midline
2. Buccal mucoperiosteum and mucous membranes on the side of injection
3. Anterior two thirds of the tongue and floor of the oral cavity
4. Lingual soft tissues and periosteum
5. Body of the mandible, inferior portion of the ramus
6. Skin over the zygoma, posterior portion of the cheek, and temporal regions

Indications
1. Multiple procedures on mandibular teeth
2. When buccal soft tissue anesthesia, from the third molar to the midline, is necessary
3. When lingual soft tissue anesthesia is necessary
4. When a conventional inferior alveolar nerve block is unsuccessful

Contraindications
1. Infection or acute inflammation in the area of injection (rare)
2. Patients who might bite their lip or their tongue, such as young children and physically or mentally handicapped adults
3. Patients who are unable to open their mouth wide (e.g., trismus)

Advantages
1. Requires only one injection; a buccal nerve block is usually unnecessary (accessory innervation has been blocked)

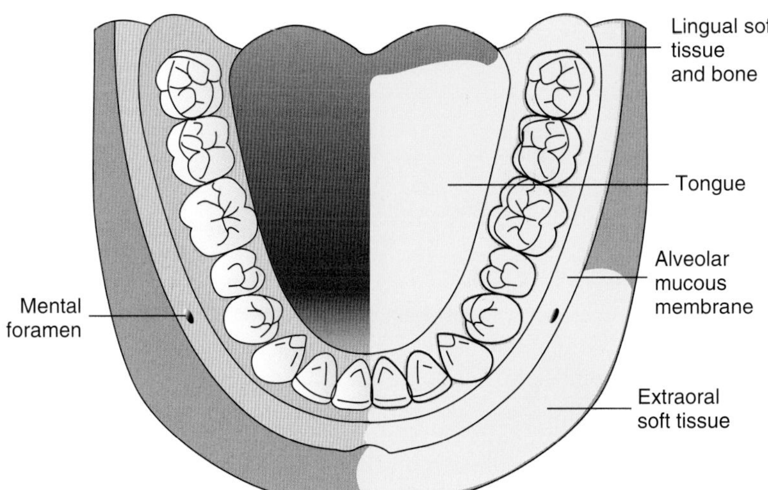

Figure 14-15. Area anesthetized by a mandibular nerve block (Gow-Gates).

2. High success rate (>95%), with experience
3. Minimum aspiration rate
4. Few postinjection complications (e.g., trismus)
5. Provides successful anesthesia where a bifid inferior alveolar nerve and bifid mandibular canals are present

Disadvantages
1. Lingual and lower lip anesthesia is uncomfortable for many patients and is possibly dangerous for certain individuals.
2. The time to onset of anesthesia is somewhat longer (5 minutes) than with an IANB (3 to 5 minutes), primarily because of the size of the nerve trunk being anesthetized and the distance of the nerve trunk from the deposition site (approximately 5 to 10 mm).
3. There is a learning curve with the Gow-Gates technique. Clinical experience is necessary to truly learn the technique and to fully take advantage of its greater success rate. This learning curve may prove frustrating for some persons.

Positive Aspiration. 2%.

Alternatives
1. IANB and buccal nerve block
2. Vazirani-Akinosi closed-mouth mandibular block
3. *Incisive nerve block:* Pulpal and buccal soft tissue anterior to the mental foramen
4. *Mental nerve block:* Buccal soft tissue anterior to the first molar
5. *Buccal nerve block:* Buccal soft tissue from the third to the mental foramen region
6. *Supraperiosteal injection:* For pulpal anesthesia of the central and lateral incisors, and in some instances the canine
7. Intraosseous technique (see Chapter 15 for discussion)
8. PDL injection technique (see Chapter 15 for discussion)

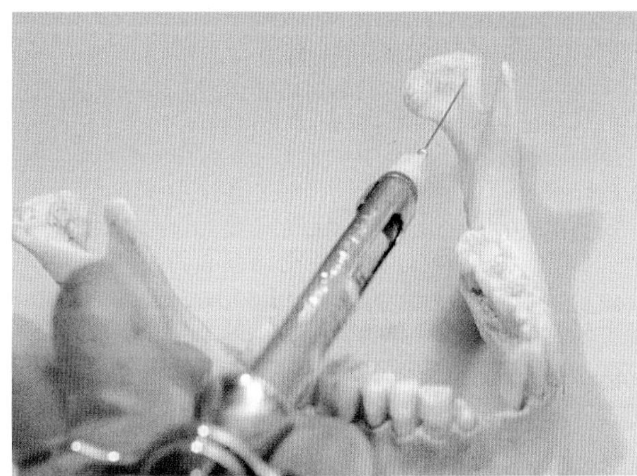

Figure 14-16. Target area for a Gow-Gates mandibular nerve block—neck of the condyle.

Technique
1. 25- or 27-gauge long needle recommended
2. *Area of insertion:* Mucous membrane on the mesial of the mandibular ramus, on a line from the intertragic notch to the corner of the mouth, just distal to the maxillary second molar
3. *Target area:* Lateral side of the condylar neck, just below the insertion of the lateral pterygoid muscle (Fig. 14-16)
4. Landmarks
   a. Extraoral
      (1) Lower border of the tragus (intertragic notch). The correct landmark is the center of the external auditory meatus, which is concealed by the tragus; therefore its lower border is adopted as a visual aid (Fig. 14-17).
      (2) Corner of the mouth
   b. Intraoral
      (1) Height of injection established by placement of the needle tip just below the mesiolingual

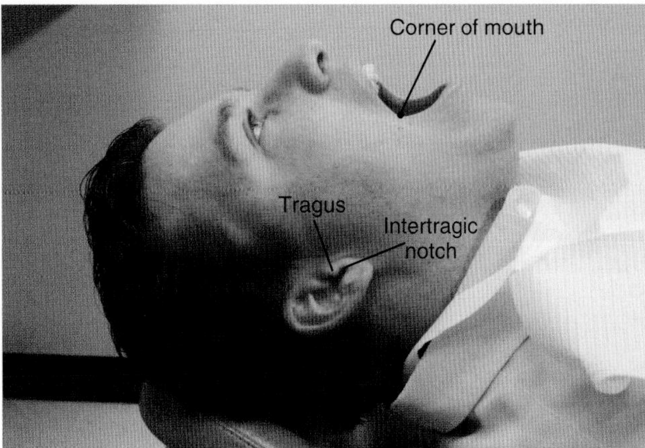

Figure 14-17. Extraoral landmarks for a Gow-Gates mandibular nerve block.

(mesiopalatal) cusp of the maxillary second molar (Fig. 14-18, *A*)
   (2) Penetration of soft tissues just distal to the maxillary second molar at the height established in the preceding step (Fig. 14-18, *B*)
5. *Orientation of the bevel:* Not critical
6. Procedure
   a. Assume the correct position.
      (1) For a right GGMNB, a right-handed administrator should sit in the 8 o'clock position facing the patient.
      (2) For a left GGMNB, a right-handed administrator should sit in the 10 o'clock position facing the same direction as the patient.
      (3) These are the same positions used for a right and a left IANB (see Fig. 14-4).
   b. Position the patient (Fig. 14-19).
      (1) Supine is recommended, although semisupine also may be used.
      (2) Ask the patient to extend his or her neck and to open wide for the duration of the technique. The condyle then assumes a more frontal position and is closer to the mandibular nerve trunk.
   c. Locate the extraoral landmarks:
      (1) Intertragic notch
      (2) Corner of the mouth
   d. Place your left index finger or thumb on the coronoid notch; determination of the coronoid notch is not essential to the success of Gow-Gates, but in the author's experience, palpation of this familiar intraoral landmark provides a sense of security, enables the soft tissues to be retracted, and aids in determination of the site of needle penetration.
   e. Visualize the intraoral landmarks.
      (1) Mesiolingual (mesiopalatal) cusp of the maxillary second molar
      (2) Needle penetration site is just distal to the maxillary second molar at the height of the tip of its mesiolingual cusp.

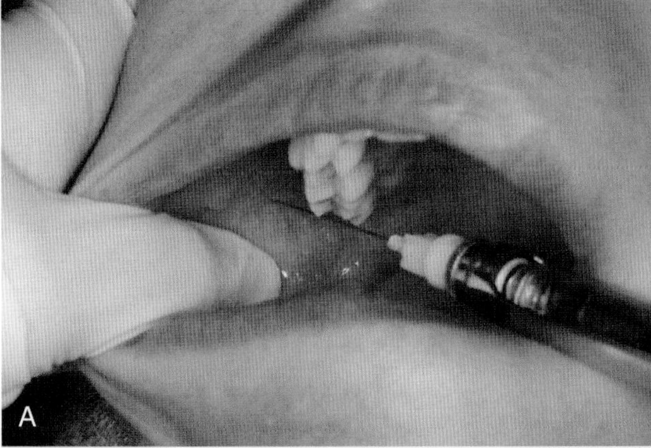

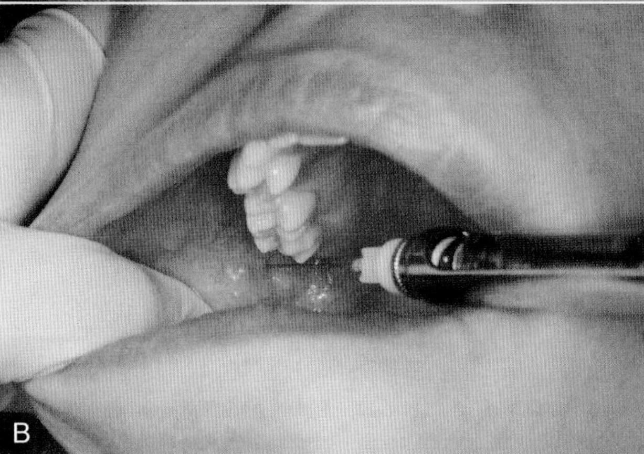

Figure 14-18. Intraoral landmarks for a Gow-Gates mandibular block. The tip of the needle is placed just below the mesiolingual cusp of the maxillary second molar (**A**) and is moved to a point just distal to the molar (**B**), maintaining the height established in the preceding step. This is the insertion point for the Gow-Gates mandibular nerve block.

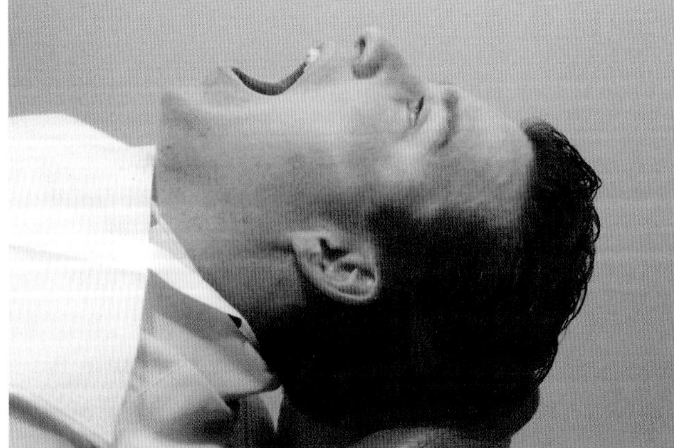

Figure 14-19. Position of the patient for a Gow-Gates mandibular nerve block.

   f. Prepare tissues at the site of penetration.
      (1) Dry tissue with sterile gauze.
      (2) Apply topical antiseptic (optional).
      (3) Apply topical anesthetic for minimum of 1 minute.

g. Direct the syringe (held in your right hand) toward the site of injection from the corner of the mouth on the opposite side (as in IANB).
h. Insert the needle gently into tissues at the injection site just distal to the maxillary second molar at the height of its mesiolingual (mesiopalatal) cusp.
i. Align the needle with the plane extending from the corner of the mouth on the opposite side to the intertragic notch on the side of injection. It should be parallel with the angle between the ear and the face (Fig. 14-20).
j. Direct the syringe toward the target area on the tragus.
   (1) The syringe barrel lies in the corner of the mouth over the premolars, but its position may vary from molars to incisors, depending on the divergence of the ramus as assessed by the angle of the ear to the side of the face (Fig. 14-21).
   (2) The height of insertion above the mandibular occlusal plane is considerably greater (10 to 25 mm, depending on the patient's size) than that of the IANB.
   (3) When a maxillary third molar is present in a normal occlusion, the site of needle penetration is just distal to that tooth.
k. Slowly advance the needle until bone is contacted.
   (1) Bone contacted is the neck of the condyle.
   (2) The average depth of soft tissue penetration to bone is 25 mm, although some variation is observed. For a given patient, the depth of soft tissue penetration with the GGMNB approximates that with the IANB.
   (3) If bone is not contacted, withdraw the needle slightly and redirect. (Experience with the Gow-Gates technique has demonstrated that medial deflection of the needle is the most common cause of failure to contact bone.) Move the barrel of the syringe somewhat more distally, thereby angulating the needle tip anteriorly, and readvance the needle until bony contact is made.

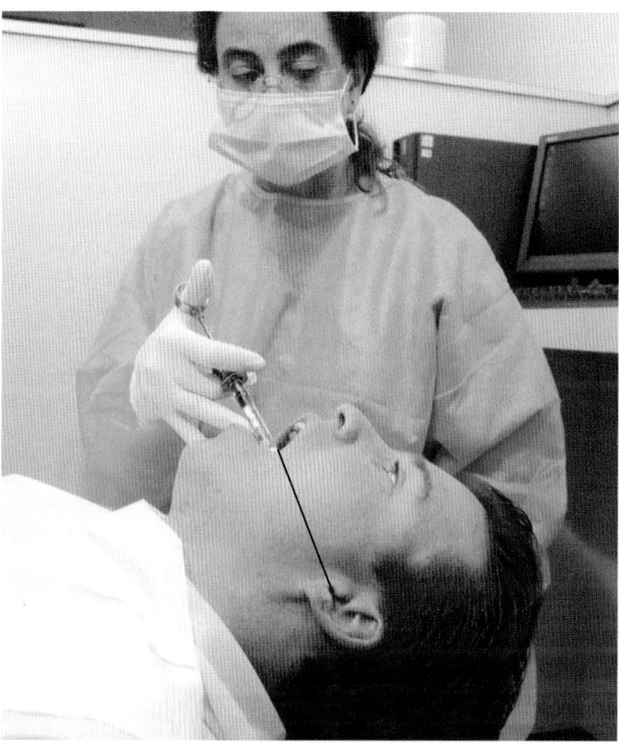

Figure 14-20. The barrel of the syringe and the needle are held parallel to a line connecting the corner of the mouth and the intertragic notch.

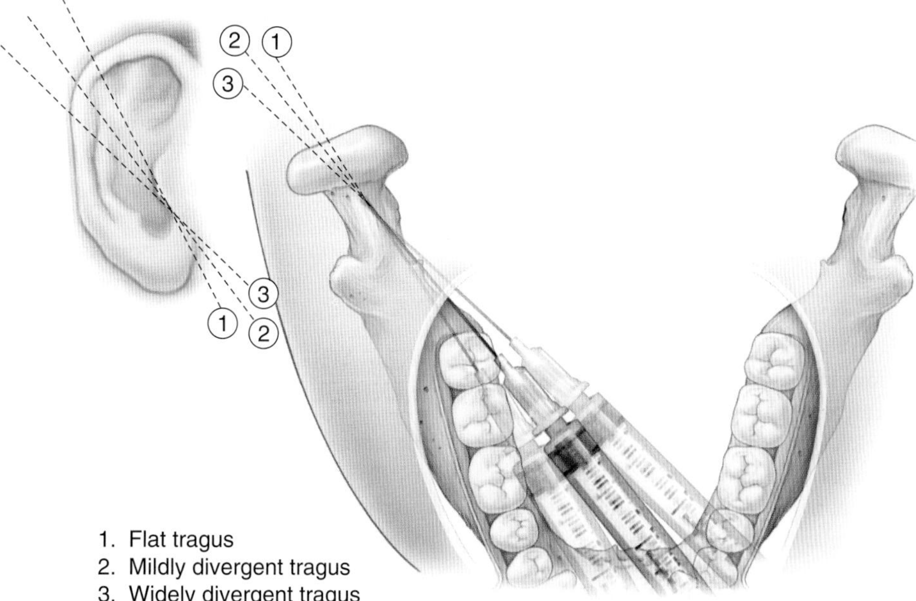

Figure 14-21. The location of the syringe barrel depends on the divergence of the tragus.

(a) A second cause of failure to contact bone is partial closure of the patient's mouth (see step 6, b[2]). Once the patient closes even slightly, two negatives occur: (1) The thickness of soft tissue increases, and (2) the condyle moves in a distal direction. Both of these make it more difficult to locate the condylar neck with the needle.

(4) If bone is not contacted, do not deposit any local anesthetic.

l. Withdraw the needle 1 mm.

m. Aspirate in 2 planes.

n. If positive, withdraw the needle slightly, angle it superiorly, reinsert, reaspirate, and, if now negative, deposit the solution. Positive aspiration usually occurs in the internal maxillary artery, which is located inferior to the target area. The positive aspiration rate with the GGMNB technique is approximately 2%.[33,34]

o. If negative, slowly deposit 1.8 mL of solution over 60 to 90 seconds. Gow-Gates originally recommended that 3 mL of anesthetic be deposited.[33] However, experience with the GGMNB shows that 1.8 mL is usually adequate to provide clinically acceptable anesthesia in virtually all cases. When partial anesthesia develops after administration of 1.8 mL, a second injection of approximately 1.2 mL is recommended.

p. Withdraw the syringe and make the needle safe.

q. Request that the patient keep his or her mouth open for 1 to 2 minutes after the injection to permit diffusion of the anesthetic solution.

(1) Use of a rubber bite block may assist the patient in keeping the mouth open.

r. After completion of the injection, return the patient to the upright or semiupright position.

s. Wait at least 3 to 5 minutes before commencing the dental procedure. Onset of anesthesia with the GGMNB may be somewhat slower, requiring 5 minutes or longer for the following reasons:

(1) Greater diameter of the nerve trunk at the site of injection

(2) Distance (5 to 10 mm) from the anesthetic deposition site to the nerve trunk

Signs and Symptoms

1. *Subjective:* Tingling or numbness of the lower lip indicates anesthesia of the mental nerve, a terminal branch of the inferior alveolar nerve. It is also a good indication that the inferior alveolar nerve may be anesthetized.
2. *Subjective:* Tingling or numbness of the tongue indicates anesthesia of the lingual nerve, a branch of the posterior division of the mandibular nerve. It is always present in a successful Gow-Gates mandibular block.
3. *Objective:* Using an electrical pulp tester (EPT) and eliciting no response to maximal output (80/80) on two consecutive tests at least 2 minutes apart serves as a "guarantee" of successful pulpal anesthesia in nonpulpitic teeth.[24,27,28]
4. *Objective:* No pain is felt during dental therapy.

Safety Features

1. Needle contacting bone, thereby preventing overinsertion
2. Very low positive aspiration rate; minimizes the risk of intravascular injection (the internal maxillary artery lies inferior to the injection site)

Precautions. Do not deposit local anesthetic if bone is not contacted; the needle tip usually is distal and medial to the desired site:

1. Withdraw slightly.
2. Redirect the needle laterally.
3. Reinsert the needle. Make gentle contact with bone.
4. Withdraw 1 mm and aspirate in two planes.
5. Inject if aspiration is negative.

Failures of Anesthesia. Rare with the Gow-Gates mandibular block once the administrator becomes familiar with the technique:

1. Too little volume. The greater diameter of the mandibular nerve may require a larger volume of anesthetic solution. Deposit up to 1.2 mL in a second injection if the depth of anesthesia is inadequate after the initial 1.8 mL.
2. Anatomic difficulties. Do not deposit anesthetic unless bone is contacted.

Complications

1. Hematoma (<2% incidence of positive aspiration)
2. Trismus (extremely rare)
3. Temporary paralysis of cranial nerves III, IV, and VI. In a case of cranial nerve paralysis after a right Gow-Gates mandibular block, diplopia, right-sided blepharoptosis, and complete paralysis of the right eye persisted for 20 minutes after the injection. This has occurred after the accidental rapid intravenous administration of local anesthetic.[35] The recommendations of Dr. Gow-Gates include placing the needle on the lateral side of the anterior surface of the condyle, aspirating carefully, and depositing slowly.[33,34] If bone is not contacted, anesthetic solution should not be administered.

VAZIRANI-AKINOSI CLOSED-MOUTH MANDIBULAR BLOCK

The introduction of the Gow-Gates mandibular nerve block in 1973 spurred interest in alternative methods of achieving anesthesia in the lower jaw. In 1977, Dr. Joseph Akinosi reported on a closed-mouth approach to mandibular anesthesia.[36] Although this technique can be used whenever mandibular anesthesia is desired, its primary indication remains those situations where limited mandibular opening

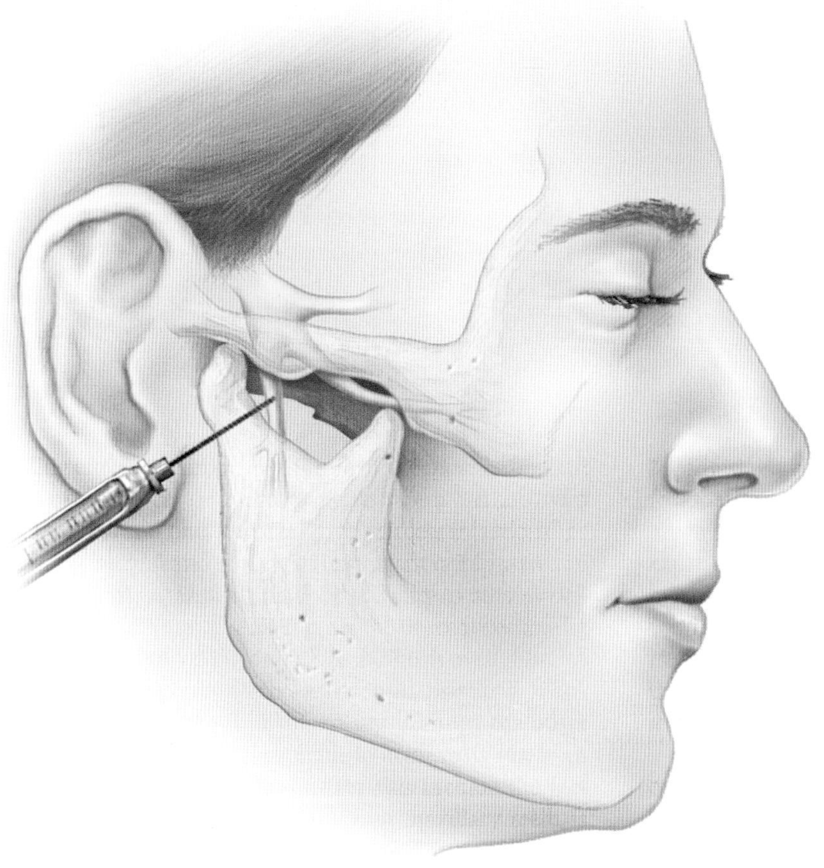

Figure 14-22. Extraoral mandibular block using lateral approach through the sigmoid notch. (Redrawn from Bennett CR: Monheim's local anesthesia and pain control in dental practice, ed 6, St Louis, 1978, Mosby.)

precludes the use of other mandibular injection techniques. Such situations include the presence of spasm of the muscles of mastication (trismus) on one side of the mandible after numerous attempts at IANB, as might occur with a "hot" mandibular molar. In this instance, multiple injections have been necessary to provide anesthesia adequate to extirpate the pulpal tissues of the involved mandibular molar. When the anesthetic effect resolves hours later, the muscles into which the anesthetic solution was deposited become tender, producing some discomfort on opening the jaw. During a period of sleep, when the muscles are not in use, the muscles go into spasm (the same way one's leg muscles might go into spasm after strenuous exercise, making it difficult to stand or walk the next morning), leaving the patient with significantly reduced occlusal opening in the morning.

The management of trismus is reviewed in Chapter 17.

If it is necessary to continue dental care in the patient with significant trismus, the options for providing mandibular anesthesia are extremely limited. Inferior alveolar and Gow-Gates mandibular nerve blocks cannot be attempted when significant trismus is present. Extraoral mandibular nerve blocks can be attempted and, indeed, possess a significantly high success rate in experienced hands. Extraoral mandibular blocks can be administered through the sigmoid notch or inferiorly from the chin (Fig. 14-22).[37,38] Because the mandibular division of the trigeminal nerve provides motor innervation to the muscles of mastication, a third division (V_3) block will relieve trismus that is produced secondary to muscle spasm (trismus may also result from other causes). Although dentists are permitted to administer extraoral nerve blocks, few in clinical practice actually do so. The Vazirani-Akinosi technique is an intraoral approach to providing both anesthesia and motor blockade in cases of severe unilateral trismus.

In early editions of this textbook, the technique described in the following section was termed the *Akinosi closed-mouth mandibular block.* However, a very similar technique was described in 1960 by Vazirani.[39] The name *Vazirani-Akinosi closed-mouth mandibular block* was adopted for the fourth edition, giving recognition to both of the doctors who devised and publicized this closed-mouth approach to mandibular anesthesia.

In 1992, Wolfe described a modification of the original Vazirani-Akinosi technique.[40] The technique described was identical to the original technique, except that the author recommended bending the needle at a 45-degree angle to enable it to remain in close proximity to the medial (lingual)

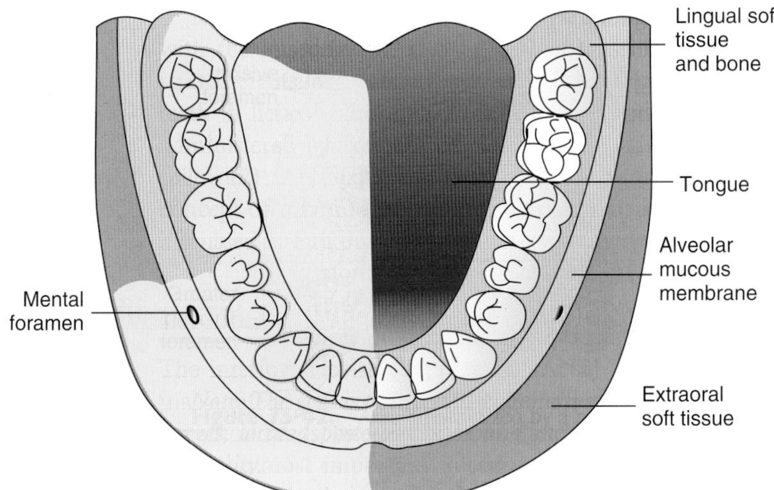

Figure 14-23. Area anesthetized by a Vazirani-Akinosi closed-mouth mandibular nerve block.

side of the mandibular ramus as the needle is advanced through the tissues. Because the potential for needle breakage is increased when it is bent, bending any needle that is to be inserted into tissues to any significant depth cannot be recommended. The Vazirani-Akinosi closed-mouth mandibular block can be administered successfully without bending the needle.

Other Common Names. Akinosi technique, closed-mouth mandibular nerve block, tuberosity technique.

Nerves Anesthetized
1. Inferior alveolar
2. Incisive
3. Mental
4. Lingual
5. Mylohyoid

Areas Anesthetized. (Fig. 14-23)
1. Mandibular teeth to the midline
2. Body of the mandible and inferior portion of the ramus
3. Buccal mucoperiosteum and mucous membrane anterior to the mental foramen
4. Anterior two thirds of the tongue and floor of the oral cavity (lingual nerve)
5. Lingual soft tissues and periosteum (lingual nerve)

Indications
1. Limited mandibular opening
2. Multiple procedures on mandibular teeth
3. Inability to visualize landmarks for IANB (e.g., because of large tongue)

Contraindications
1. Infection or acute inflammation in the area of injection (rare)
2. Patients who might bite their lip or their tongue, such as young children and physically or mentally handicapped adults
3. Inability to visualize or gain access to the lingual aspect of the ramus

Advantages
1. Relatively atraumatic
2. Patient need not be able to open the mouth.
3. Fewer postoperative complications (e.g., trismus)
4. Lower aspiration rate (<10%) than with the inferior alveolar nerve block
5. Provides successful anesthesia where a bifid inferior alveolar nerve and bifid mandibular canals are present

Disadvantages
1. Difficult to visualize the path of the needle and the depth of insertion
2. No bony contact; depth of penetration somewhat arbitrary
3. Potentially traumatic if the needle is too close to the periosteum

Alternatives. No intraoral nerve blocks are available. If a patient is unable to open his or her mouth because of trauma, infection, or postinjection trismus, no other suitable intraoral techniques are available. The extraoral mandibular nerve block may be used when the doctor is well versed in the procedure.

Technique
1. A 25-gauge long needle is recommended (although a 27-gauge long may be preferred in patients whose ramus flares laterally more than usual).
2. *Area of insertion:* Soft tissue overlying the medial (lingual) border of the mandibular ramus directly adjacent to the maxillary tuberosity at the height of the mucogingival junction adjacent to the maxillary third molar (Fig. 14-24)
3. *Target area:* Soft tissue on the medial (lingual) border of the ramus in the region of the inferior alveolar, lingual, and mylohyoid nerves as they run inferiorly

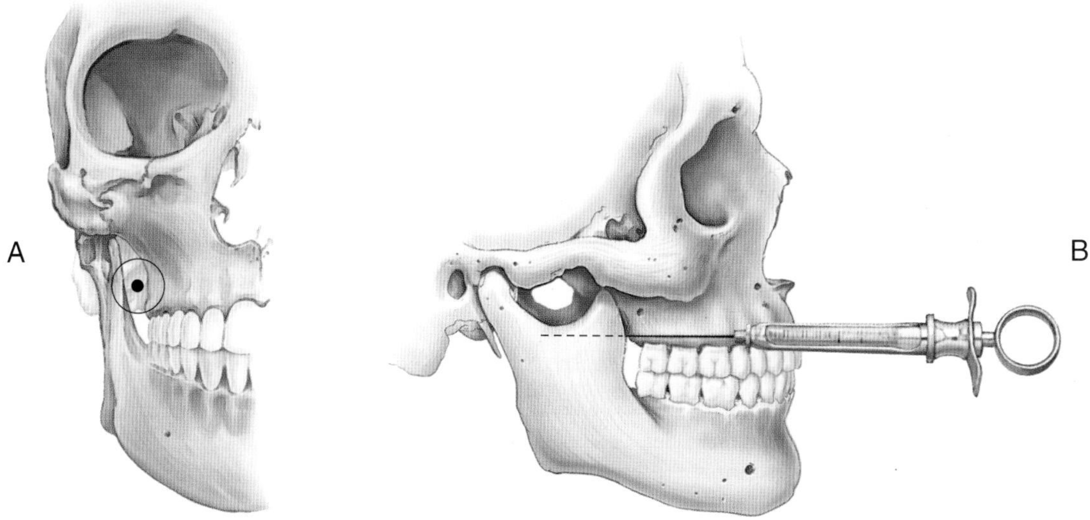

Figure 14-24. **A,** Area of needle insertion for a Vazirani-Akinosi block. **B,** Hold the syringe and needle at the height of the mucogingival junction above the maxillary third molar. (Redrawn from Gustainis JF, Peterson LJ: An alternative method of mandibular nerve block, J Am Dent Assoc 103:33–36, 1981.)

from the foramen ovale toward the mandibular foramen (the height of injection with the Vazirani-Akinosi being below that of the GGMNB but above that of the IANB)

4. Landmarks:
   a. Mucogingival junction of the maxillary third (or second) molar
   b. Maxillary tuberosity
   c. Coronoid notch on the mandibular ramus
5. *Orientation of the bevel* (bevel orientation in the closed-mouth mandibular block is very important): The bevel must be oriented away from the bone of the mandibular ramus (e.g., bevel faces toward the midline).
6. Procedure:
   a. Assume the correct position. For a right or a left Vazirani-Akinosi, a right-handed administrator should sit in the 8 o'clock position facing the patient.
   b. Position the patient supine (recommended) or semisupine.
   c. Place your left index finger or thumb on the coronoid notch, reflecting the tissues on the medial aspect of the ramus laterally. Reflecting the soft tissues aids in visualization of the injection site and decreases trauma during needle insertion.
   d. Visualize landmarks:
      (1) Mucogingival junction of the maxillary third or second molar
      (2) Maxillary tuberosity
   e. Prepare the tissues at the site of penetration:
      (1) Dry with sterile gauze.
      (2) Apply topical antiseptic (optional).
      (3) Apply topical anesthetic for minimum of 1 minute.
   f. Ask the patient to occlude gently with the cheeks and muscles of mastication relaxed.
   g. Reflect the soft tissues on the medial border of the ramus laterally.
   h. The barrel of the syringe is held parallel to the maxillary occlusal plane, with the needle at the level of the mucogingival junction of the maxillary third (or second) molar (Fig. 14-24).
   i. Direct the needle posteriorly and slightly laterally, so it advances at a tangent to the posterior maxillary alveolar process and parallel to the maxillary occlusal plane.
   j. Orient the bevel away from the mandibular ramus; thus as the needle advances through tissues, needle deflection occurs toward the ramus and the needle remains in close proximity to the inferior alveolar nerve (Fig. 14-25).
   k. Advance the needle 25 mm into tissue (for an average-sized adult). This distance is measured from the maxillary tuberosity. The tip of the needle should lie in the midportion of the pterygomandibular space, close to the branches of V_3 (Fig. 14-26).
   l. Aspirate in two planes.
   m. If negative, deposit 1.5 to 1.8 mL of anesthetic solution in approximately 60 seconds.
   n. Withdraw the syringe slowly and immediately make the needle safe.
   o. After the injection, return the patient to an upright or semiupright position.
   p. Motor nerve paralysis develops as quickly as or more quickly than sensory anesthesia. The patient with trismus begins to notice increased ability to open the jaws shortly after the deposition of anesthetic.

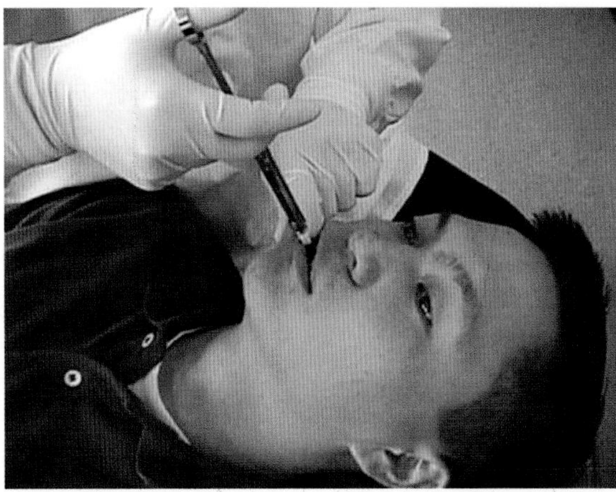

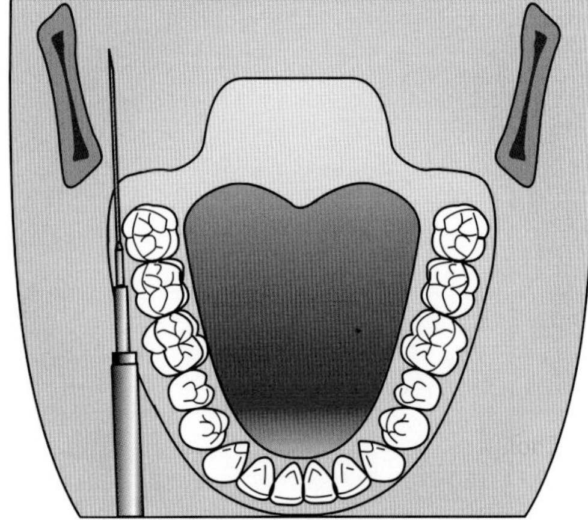

Figure 14-25. Vazirani-Akinosi closed-mouth mandibular nerve block. Barrel of syringe is held parallel to maxillary occlusal plane with the needle at the level of the mucogingival junction of the second or third maxillary molar.

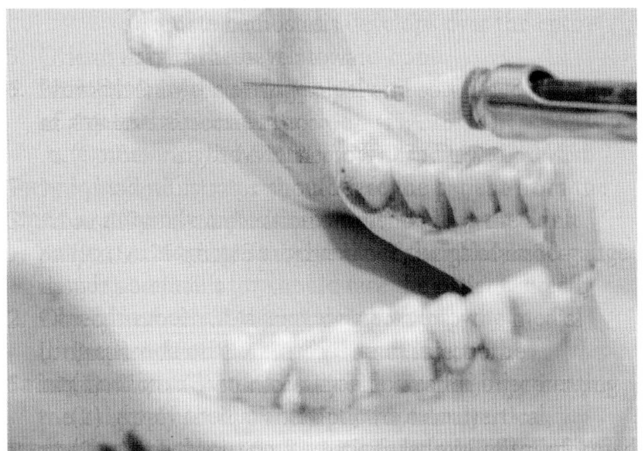

Figure 14-26. Advance the needle posteriorly into tissues on the medial side of the mandibular ramus.

q. Anesthesia of the lip and tongue is noted to start in about in 1 to 1½ minutes; the dental procedure usually can start within 5 minutes.

r. When motor paralysis is present but sensory anesthesia is inadequate to permit the dental procedure to begin, readminister the Vazirani-Akinosi block, or, because the patient can now open his or her jaws, perform a standard inferior alveolar, Gow-Gates, or incisive nerve block, or a PDL or intraosseous injection.

Signs and Symptoms

1. *Subjective:* Tingling or numbness of the lower lip indicates anesthesia of the mental nerve, a terminal branch of the inferior alveolar nerve, which is a good sign that the inferior alveolar nerve has been anesthetized.
2. *Subjective:* Tingling or numbness of the tongue indicates anesthesia of the lingual nerve, a branch of the posterior division of the mandibular nerve.
3. *Objective:* Using an electrical pulp tester (EPT) and eliciting no response to maximal output (80/80) on two consecutive tests at least 2 minutes apart serves as a "guarantee" of successful pulpal anesthesia in nonpulpitic teeth.[24,27,28]
4. *Objective:* No pain is felt during dental therapy.

Safety Feature. Decreased risk of positive aspiration (compared with the IANB).

Precaution. Do not overinsert the needle (>25 mm). Decrease the depth of penetration in smaller patients; the depth of insertion will vary with the anteroposterior size of the patient's ramus.

Failures of Anesthesia

1. Almost always because of failure to appreciate the flaring nature of the ramus. If the needle is directed medially, it rests medial to the sphenomandibular ligament in the pterygomandibular space, and the injection fails. This occurs more commonly when a right-handed administrator uses the left-side Vazirani-Akinosi injection (or a left-handed administrator uses the right-side Vazirani-Akinosi injection). It may be prevented by directing the needle tip parallel to the lateral flare of the ramus and by using a 27-gauge needle in place of a 25-gauge.
2. Needle insertion point too low. To correct: Insert the needle at or slightly above the level of the mucogingival junction of the last maxillary molar. The needle also must remain parallel to the occlusal plane as it advances through the soft tissues.
3. Underinsertion or overinsertion of the needle. Because no bone is contacted in the Vazirani-Akinosi technique, the depth of soft tissue penetration is somewhat arbitrary. Akinosi recommended a penetration depth of 25 mm in the average-sized adult, measuring from the maxillary tuberosity. In smaller or larger patients, this depth of penetration should be altered.

Complications
1. Hematoma (<10%)
2. Trismus (rare)
3. Transient facial nerve (VII) paralysis
   a. This is caused by overinsertion and injection of the local anesthetic solution into the body of the parotid gland.
   b. It can be prevented by modifying the depth of needle penetration based on the length of the mandibular ramus. The 25-mm depth of penetration is average for a normal-sized adult.

MENTAL NERVE BLOCK

The mental nerve is a terminal branch of the inferior alveolar nerve. Exiting the mental foramen at or near the apices of the mandibular premolars, it provides sensory innervation to the buccal soft tissues lying anterior to the foramen and the soft tissues of the lower lip and chin on the side of injection.

For most dental procedures, there is very little indication for use of the mental nerve block. Indeed, of the techniques described in this section, the mental nerve block is the least frequently employed. It is used primarily for buccal soft tissue procedures, such as suturing of lacerations or biopsies. Its success rate approaches 100% because of the ease of accessibility to the nerve.

Other Common Names. None.

Nerve Anesthetized. Mental, a terminal branch of the inferior alveolar.

Areas Anesthetized. Buccal mucous membranes anterior to the mental foramen (around the second premolar) to the midline and skin of the lower lip (Fig. 14-27) and chin.

Indication. When buccal soft tissue anesthesia is necessary for procedures in the mandible anterior to the mental foramen, such as the following:
1. Soft tissue biopsies
2. Suturing of soft tissues

Contraindication. Infection or acute inflammation in the area of injection.

Advantages
1. High success rate
2. Technically easy
3. Usually entirely atraumatic

Disadvantage. Hematoma.

Positive Aspiration. 5.7%.

Alternatives
1. Local infiltration
2. Inferior alveolar nerve block
3. Gow-Gates mandibular nerve block
4. Vazirani-Akinosi nerve block

Technique
1. A 25- or 27-gauge short needle is recommended.
2. *Area of insertion:* Mucobuccal fold at or just anterior to the mental foramen
3. *Target area:* Mental nerve as it exits the mental foramen (usually located between the apices of the first and second premolars)
4. *Landmarks:* Mandibular premolars and mucobuccal fold
5. *Orientation of the bevel:* Toward bone during the injection
   a. Assume the correct position.
      (1) For a right or left mental nerve block. a right-handed administrator should sit comfortably in front of the patient so that the syringe may be placed into the mouth below the patient's line of sight (Fig. 14-28).
   b. Position the patient.
      (1) Supine is recommended, but semisupine is acceptable.

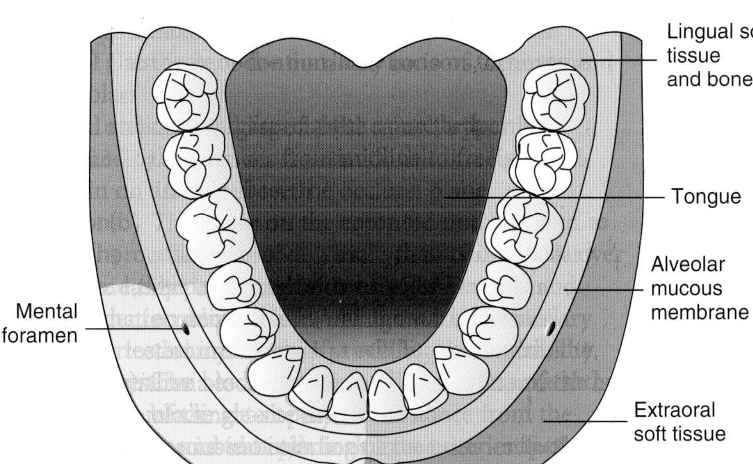

Figure 14-27. Area anesthetized by mental nerve block.

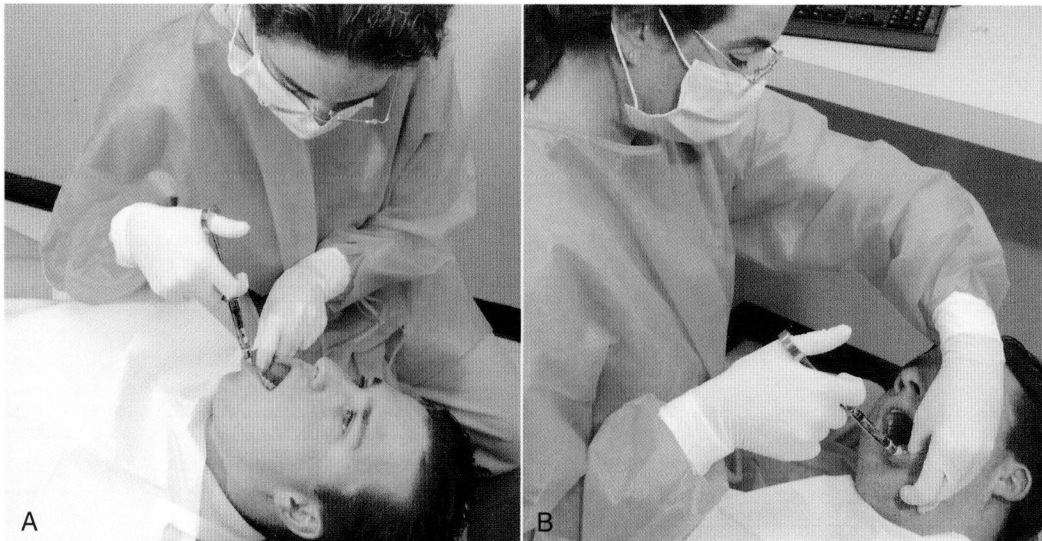

Figure 14-28. Position of the administrator for a (**A**) right and (**B**) left mental/incisive nerve block.

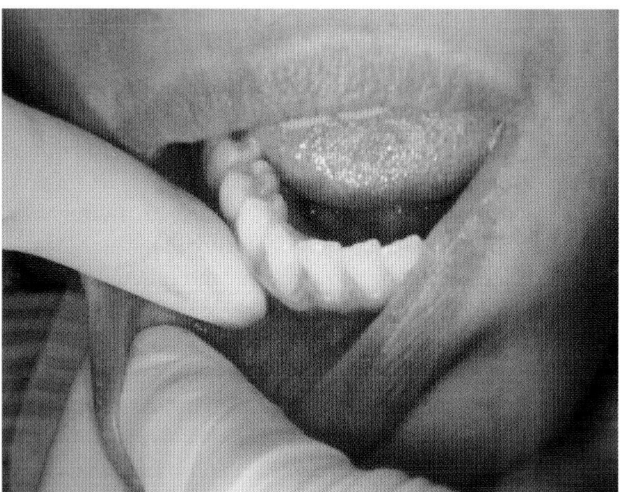

Figure 14-29. Locate the mental foramen by moving the fleshy pad of your finger anteriorly until the bone beneath becomes irregular and somewhat concave.

(2) Have the patient partially close. This permits greater access to the injection site.

c. Locate the mental foramen.
   (1) Place your index finger in the mucobuccal fold and press against the body of the mandible in the first molar area.
   (2) Move your finger slowly anteriorly until the bone beneath your finger feels irregular and somewhat concave (Fig. 14-29).
      (a) The bone posterior and anterior to the mental foramen is smooth; however, the bone immediately around the foramen is rougher to the touch.
      (b) The mental foramen usually is found around the apex of the second premolar. However, it may be found anterior or posterior to this site.
      (c) The patient may comment that finger pressure in this area produces soreness as the mental nerve is compressed against bone.
   (3) If radiographs are available, the mental foramen may be located easily (Fig. 14-30).

d. Prepare tissue at the site of penetration.
   (1) Dry with sterile gauze.
   (2) Apply topical antiseptic (optional).
   (3) Apply topical anesthetic for minimum of 1 minute.

e. With your left index finger, pull the lower lip and buccal soft tissues laterally.
   (1) Visibility is improved.
   (2) Taut tissues permit an atraumatic penetration.

f. Orient the syringe with the bevel directed toward bone.

g. Penetrate the mucous membrane at the injection site, at the canine or first premolar, directing the syringe toward the mental foramen (Fig. 14-31).

h. Advance the needle slowly until the foramen is reached. The depth of penetration is 5 to 6 mm. For the mental nerve block to be successful, there is no need to enter the mental foramen or to contact bone.

i. Aspirate in two planes.

j. If negative, slowly deposit 0.6 mL (approximately one third cartridge) over 20 seconds. If tissue at the injection site balloons (swells as the anesthetic is injected), stop the deposition and remove the syringe.

k. Withdraw the syringe and immediately make the needle safe.
   (1) Wait 2 to 3 minutes before commencing the procedure.

Signs and Symptoms

1. *Subjective:* Tingling or numbness of the lower lip
2. *Objective:* No pain during treatment

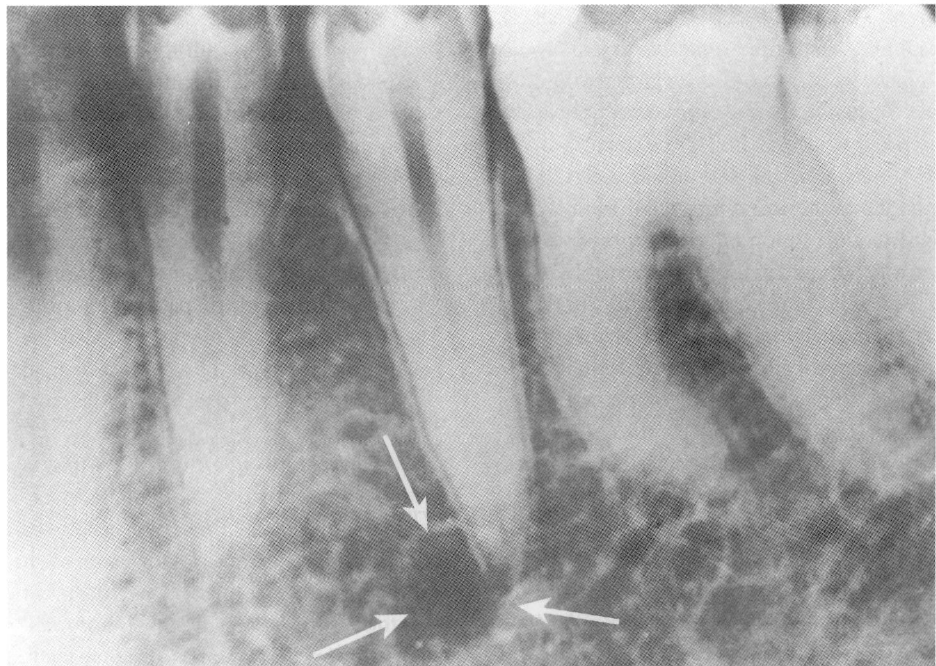

Figure 14-30. Radiographs can assist in locating the mental foramen *(arrows)*. (Courtesy Dr. Robert Ziehm.)

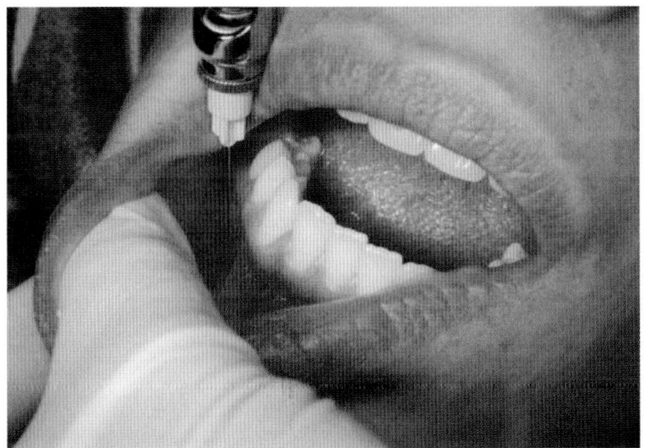

Figure 14-31. Mental nerve block—needle penetration site.

Safety Feature. The region is anatomically "safe."

Precautions. Striking the periosteum produces discomfort. To prevent: Avoid contact with the periosteum or deposit a small amount of solution before contacting the periosteum.

Failures of Anesthesia. Rare with the mental nerve block.

Complications

1. Few of consequence
2. Hematoma (bluish discoloration and tissue swelling at the injection site). Blood may exit the needle puncture point into the buccal fold. To treat: Apply pressure with gauze directly to the area of bleeding for at least 2 minutes (see Fig. 17-2).
3. Paresthesia of lip and/or chin. Contact of the needle with the mental nerve as it exits the mental foramen may lead to the sensation of an "electric shock" or to varying degrees of paresthesia (rare)

INCISIVE NERVE BLOCK

The incisive nerve is a terminal branch of the inferior alveolar nerve. Originating as a direct continuation of the inferior alveolar nerve at the mental foramen, the incisive nerve travels anteriorly in the incisive canal, providing sensory innervation to those teeth located anterior to the mental foramen. The nerve is always anesthetized when an inferior alveolar or mandibular nerve block is successful; therefore the incisive nerve block is not necessary when these blocks are administered.

The premolars, canine, and lateral and central incisors, including their buccal soft tissues and bone, are anesthetized when the incisive nerve block is administered.* An important indication for the incisive nerve block is when the contemplated procedure involves both the right and left sides of the mandible. It is this author's belief that bilateral inferior alveolar or mandibular nerve blocks are seldom needed (except in the case of bilateral surgical procedures in the mandible) because of the degree of discomfort and the inconvenience experienced by the patient both during and after the procedure. Where dental treatment involves bilateral procedures on mandibular premolars and anterior teeth, bilateral incisive nerve blocks can be administered. Pulpal, buccal soft tissue, and bone anesthesia is readily obtained.

*The second premolar may not be anesthetized with this technique if the mental foramen lies beneath the first premolar.

Lingual soft tissues are not anesthetized with this block. If lingual soft tissues in very isolated areas require anesthesia, local infiltration can be readily accomplished by advancing a 27-gauge short needle through the interdental papillae on both mesial and distal aspects of the tooth being treated. Because the buccal soft tissues are already anesthetized (incisive nerve block), the penetration is atraumatic. Local anesthetic solution should be deposited as the needle is advanced through the tissue toward the lingual (Fig. 14-32). This technique provides lingual soft tissue anesthesia adequate for deep curettage, root planing, and subgingival preparations. Where there is a significant requirement for lingual soft tissue anesthesia, an inferior alveolar or mandibular nerve block should be administered on that side, with the incisive nerve block administered on the contralateral side. In this manner, the patient does not have to endure bilateral anesthesia of the tongue, which is a very disconcerting experience for many patients.

Another method of obtaining lingual anesthesia after the incisive nerve block is to administer a partial lingual nerve block (Fig. 14-33). Using a 25-gauge long needle, deposit 0.3 to 0.6 mL of local anesthetic under the lingual mucosa just distal to the last tooth to be treated. This provides lingual soft tissue anesthesia adequate for any dental procedure in this area. The danger in this procedure is that the lingual nerve may be contacted by the needle provoking a sensation of an "electric shock" or varying degrees of paresthesia.

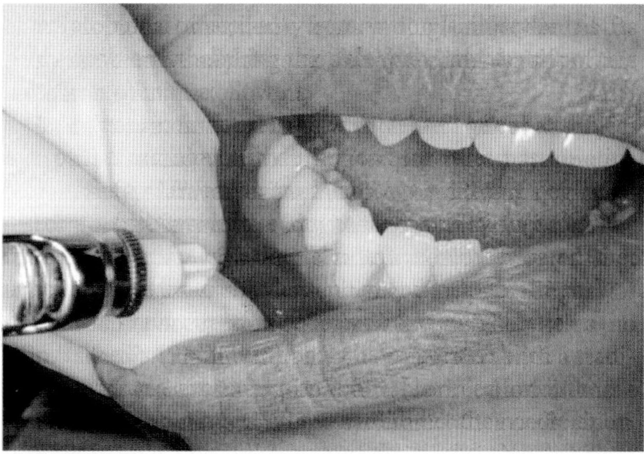

Figure 14-32. To obtain lingual anesthesia, after the incisive nerve block, insert the needle interproximally from buccal, and deposit anesthetic as the needle is advanced toward lingual.

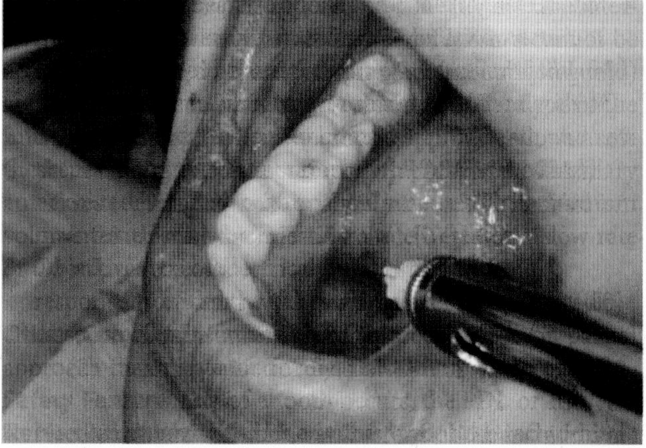

Figure 14-33. Retract the tongue to gain access to, and increase the visibility of, the lingual border of the mandible.

It is not necessary for the needle to enter into the mental foramen for an incisive nerve block to be successful. The first edition of this book and other textbooks of local anesthesia for dentistry recommended insertion of the needle into the foramen.[38,41,42] At least two disadvantages are associated with the needle entering into the mental foramen: (1) The administration of an incisive nerve block becomes technically more difficult, and (2) the risk of traumatizing the mental or incisive nerves and their associated blood vessels is increased. As described in the following sections, for the incisive nerve block to be successful, the anesthetic should be deposited just outside the mental foramen and, under pressure, directed into the foramen. Indeed, the incisive nerve block may be considered the mandibular equivalent of the anterior superior alveolar nerve block, with the mental nerve block the equivalent of the infraorbital nerve block. Both of the disadvantages just mentioned are minimized by not entering into the mental foramen.

Other Common Name. Mental nerve block (inappropriate).

Nerves Anesthetized. Mental and incisive.

Areas Anesthetized. (Fig. 14-34)
1. Buccal mucous membrane anterior to the mental foramen, usually from the second premolar to the midline
2. Lower lip and skin of the chin
3. Pulpal nerve fibers to the premolars, canine, and incisors

Indications
1. Dental procedures requiring pulpal anesthesia on mandibular teeth anterior to the mental foramen
2. When IANB is not indicated:
   a. When six, eight, or ten anterior teeth (e.g., canine to canine or premolar to premolar) are treated, the incisive nerve block is recommended in place of bilateral IANBs.

Contraindication. Infection or acute inflammation in the area of injection.

Advantages
1. Provides pulpal and hard tissue anesthesia without lingual anesthesia (which is uncomfortable and unnecessary for many patients); useful in place of bilateral IANBs
2. High success rate

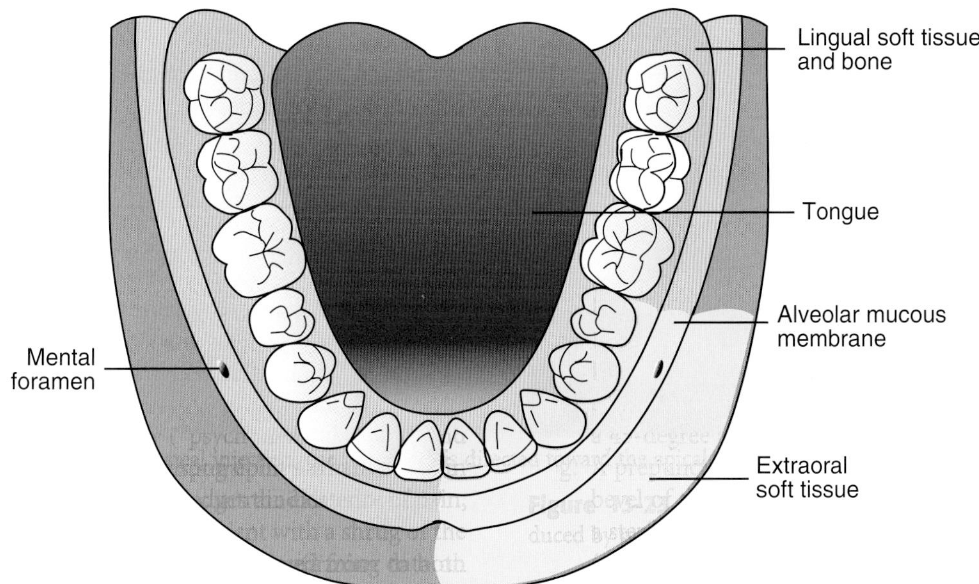

Figure 14-34. Area anesthetized by an incisive nerve block.

Disadvantages

1. Does not provide lingual anesthesia. The lingual tissues must be injected as described earlier if anesthesia is desired.
2. Partial anesthesia may develop at the midline because of nerve fiber overlap with the opposite side (extremely rare). Local infiltration of 0.9 mL of local anesthetic on both the buccal and lingual of the mandibular central incisors may be necessary for complete pulpal anesthesia to be obtained.

Positive Aspiration. 5.7%.

Alternatives

1. Local infiltration for buccal soft tissues and pulpal anesthesia of the central and lateral incisors
2. Inferior alveolar nerve block
3. Gow-Gates mandibular nerve block
4. Vazirani-Akinosi mandibular nerve block
5. Periodontal ligament injection

Technique

1. A 27-gauge short needle is recommended.
2. *Area of insertion:* Mucobuccal fold at or just anterior to the mental foramen
3. *Target area:* Mental foramen, through which the mental nerve exits and inside of which the incisive nerve is located
4. *Landmarks:* Mandibular premolars and mucobuccal fold
5. *Orientation of the bevel:* Toward bone during the injection
6. Procedure
   a. Assume the correct position.
      (1) For a right or left incisive nerve block and a right-handed administrator, sit comfortably in front of the patient so that the syringe may be placed into the mouth below the patient's line of sight (see Fig. 14-28).
   b. Position the patient.
      (1) Supine is recommended, but semisupine is acceptable.
      (2) Request that the patient partially close; this allows for easier access to the injection site.
   c. Locate the mental foramen.
      (1) Place your thumb or index finger in the mucobuccal fold against the body of the mandible in the first molar area.
      (2) Move it slowly anteriorly until you feel the bone become irregular and somewhat concave.
         (a) The bone posterior and anterior to the mental foramen feels smooth; however, the bone immediately around the foramen feels rougher to the touch.
         (b) The mental foramen is usually found at the apex of the second premolar. However, it may be found anterior or posterior to this site.
         (c) The patient may comment that finger pressure in this area produces soreness as the mental nerve is compressed against bone.
      (3) If radiographs are available, the mental foramen may be located easily (see Fig. 14-30).
   d. Prepare tissues at the site of penetration.
      (1) Dry with sterile gauze.
      (2) Apply topical antiseptic (optional).
      (3) Apply topical anesthetic for minimum of 1 minute.
   e. With your left index finger, pull the lower lip and buccal soft tissue laterally (Fig. 14-35).
      (1) Visibility is improved.
      (2) Taut tissues permit atraumatic penetration.
   f. Orient the syringe with the bevel toward bone.

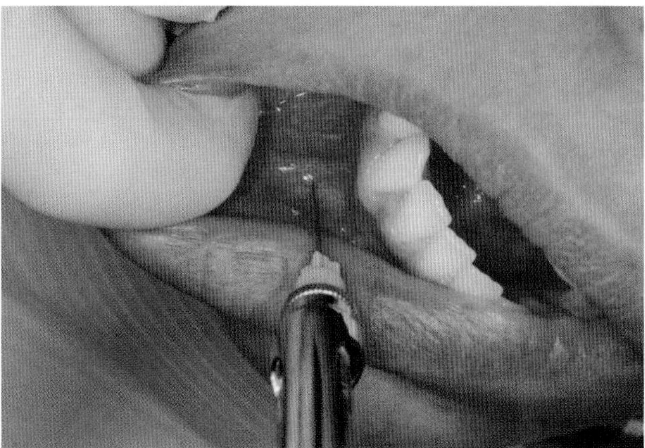

Figure 14-35. Retract the lip to improve access and permit atraumatic needle insertion.

g. Penetrate mucous membrane at the canine or first premolar, directing the needle toward the mental foramen.
h. Advance the needle slowly until the mental foramen is reached. The depth of penetration is 5 to 6 mm. There is no need to enter the mental foramen for the incisive nerve block to be successful.
i. Aspirate in two planes.
j. If negative, slowly deposit 0.6 mL (approximately one third of a cartridge) over 20 seconds.
   (1) During the injection, maintain gentle finger pressure directly over the injection site to increase the volume of solution entering into the mental foramen. This may be accomplished with intraoral or extraoral pressure.
   (2) Tissues at the injection site should balloon, but very slightly.
k. Withdraw the syringe and immediately make the needle safe.
l. Continue to apply pressure at the injection site for 2 minutes.
m. Wait 3 to 5 minutes before commencing the dental procedure.
   (1) Anesthesia of the mental nerve (lower lip, buccal soft tissues) is observed within seconds of the deposition.
   (2) Anesthesia of the incisive nerve requires additional time.

Signs and Symptoms

1. *Subjective:* Tingling or numbness of the lower lip
2. *Objective:* Using an electrical pulp tester (EPT) and eliciting no response to maximal output (80/80) on two consecutive tests at least 2 minutes apart serves as a "guarantee" of successful pulpal anesthesia in nonpulpitic teeth.[24,27,28]
3. *Objective:* No pain is felt during dental therapy.

Safety Feature. Anatomically "safe" region.

TABLE 14-1
Mandibular Teeth and Available Local Anesthetic Techniques

		SOFT TISSUE	
Teeth	**Pulpal**	**Buccal**	**Lingual**
Incisors	Incisive (Inc)	IANB	IANB
	Inferior alveolar (IANB)	GG	GG
	Gow-Gates (GG)	VA	VA
	Vazirani-Akinosi (VA)	Inc	PDL
	Periodontal ligament (PDL) injection	IS	IS
	Intraseptal (IS)	Mental	Inf
	Intraosseous (IO)	PDL	IO
	Infiltration (buccal and lingual infiltration)	Inf	Inf
		IO	
Canines	Inferior alveolar	IANB	IANB
	Gow-Gates	GG	GG
	Vazirani-Akinosi	VA	VA
	Incisive	Inc	PDL
	Periodontal ligament injection	PDL	IS
	Intraseptal	IS	Inf
	Intraosseous	IO	IO
		Inf	
		Mental	
Premolars	Inferior alveolar	IANB	IANB
	Gow-Gates	GG	GG
	Vazirani-Akinosi	VA	VA
	Incisive	Inc	PDL
	Periodontal ligament injection	PDL	IS
	Intraseptal	IS	IO
	Intraosseous	IO	Inf
		Mental	
		Inf	
Molars	Inferior alveolar	IANB	IANB
	Gow-Gates	GG	GG
	Vazirani-Akinosi	VA	VA
	Periodontal ligament injection	PDL	PDL
	Intraseptal	IS	IS
	Intraosseous	IO	IO
		Inf	Inf

TABLE 14-2
Recommended Volumes of Local Anesthetic Solution for Mandibular Injection Techniques

Technique	Volume, mL
Inferior alveolar	1.5
Buccal	0.3
Gow-Gates	1.8-3.0
Vazirani-Akinosi	1.5-1.8
Mental	0.6
Incisive	0.6-0.9

Precaution. Usually an atraumatic injection unless the needle contacts periosteum or solution is deposited too rapidly.

Failures of Anesthesia

1. Inadequate volume of anesthetic solution in the mental foramen, with subsequent lack of pulpal anesthesia. To correct: Reinject into the proper region and apply pressure to the injection site.
2. Inadequate duration of pressure after injection. It is necessary to apply firm pressure over the injection site for a minimum of 2 minutes to force the local anesthetic into the mental foramen and provide anesthesia of the second premolar, which may be distal to the foramen. Failure to achieve anesthesia of the second premolar is usually caused by inadequate application of pressure after the injection.

Complications

1. Few of any consequence
2. Hematoma (bluish discoloration and tissue swelling at injection site). Blood may exit the needle puncture site into the buccal fold. To treat: Apply pressure with gauze directly to the area for 2 minutes. This is rarely a problem because proper incisive nerve block protocol includes the application of pressure at the injection site for 2 minutes.
3. Paresthesia of lip and/or chin. Contact of the needle with the mental nerve as it exits the mental foramen may lead to the sensation of an "electric shock" or to varying degrees of paresthesia (rare).

Table 14-1 summarizes the various injection techniques applicable for mandibular teeth. Table 14-2 summarizes the recommended volumes for the various injection techniques.

References

1. De St Georges J: How dentists are judged by patients, Dent Today 23:96, 98–99, 2004.
2. Friedman MJ, Hochman MN: The AMSA injection: a new concept for local anesthesia of maxillary teeth using a computer-controlled injection system, Quintessence Int 29:297–303, 1998.
3. Oulis CJ, Vadiakis GP, Vasilopoulou A: The effectiveness of mandibular infiltration compared to mandibular block anesthesia in treating primary molars in children, Pediatr Dent 18:301–305, 1996.
4. Sharaf AA: Evaluation of mandibular infiltration versus block anesthesia in pediatric dentistry, J Dent Child 64:276–281, 1997.
5. Malamed SF: Local anesthetic considerations in dental specialties. In Malamed SF, editor: Handbook of local anesthesia, ed 5, St Louis, 2004, CV Mosby.
6. Bennett CR: Techniques of regional anesthesia and analgesia. In Bennett CR, editor: Monheim's local anesthesia and pain control in dental practice, ed 7, St Louis, 1984, CV Mosby.
7. Evers H, Haegerstam G: Anaesthesia of the lower jaw. In Evers H, Haegerstam G, editors: Introduction to dental local anaesthesia, Fribourg, Switzerland, 1990, Mediglobe SA.
8. Trieger N: New approaches to local anesthesia. In Pain control, ed 2, St Louis, 1994, CV Mosby.
9. OnPharma Inc: Results of 38 studies on LA success rates, unpublished. Available at: www.onpharma.com.
10. Kanaa MD, Whitworth JM, Corbett IP, et al: Articaine buccal infiltration enhances the effectiveness of lidocaine inferior alveolar nerve block, Int Endod J 42:238–246, 2009.
11. Hannan L, Reader A, Nist R, et al: The use of ultrasound for guiding needle placement for inferior alveolar nerve blocks, Oral Surg Oral Med Oral Pathol Oral Radiol Endod 87:658–665, 1999.
12. Berns JM, Sadove MS: Mandibular block injection: a method of study using an injected radiopaque material, J Am Dent Assoc 65:736–745, 1962.
13. Galbreath JC: Tracing the course of the mandibular block injection, Oral Surg Oral Med Oral Pathol 30:571–582, 1970.
14. Reader A, American Association of Endodontists: Taking the pain out of restorative dentistry and endodontics: current thoughts and treatment options to help patients achieve profound anesthesia, Endodontics: Colleagues for Excellence. Winter 2009.
15. DeJong RH: Local anesthetics, St Louis, 1994, CV Mosby, pp 110–111.
16. Strichartz G: Molecular mechanisms of nerve block by local anesthetics, Anesthesiology 45:421–444, 1976.
17. Gow-Gates GA: Mandibular conduction anesthesia: a new technique using extraoral landmarks, Oral Surg Oral Med Oral Pathol 36:321–328, 1973.
18. Akinosi JO: A new approach to the mandibular nerve block, Br J Oral Surg 15:83–87, 1977.
19. Malamed SF: The periodontal ligament (PDL) injection: an alternative to inferior alveolar nerve block, Oral Surg 53:117–121, 1982.
20. Coggins R, Reader A, Nist R, et al: Anesthetic efficacy of the intraosseous injection in maxillary and mandibular teeth, Oral Surg Oral Med Oral Pathol 81:634–641, 1996.
21. Whitcomb M, Drum M, Reader A, et al: A prospective, randomized, double-blind study of the anesthetic efficacy of sodium bicarbonate buffered 2% lidocaine with 1:100,000 epinephrine in inferior alveolar nerve blocks, Anesth Prog 57:59–66, 2010.
22. Meechan JG, Ledvinka JI: Pulpal anaesthesia for mandibular central incisor teeth: a comparison of infiltration and intraligamentary injections, Int Endod J 35:629–634, 2002.
23. Kanaa MD, Whitworth JM, Corbett IP, et al: Articaine and lidocaine mandibular buccal infiltration anesthesia: a prospective randomized double-blind cross-over study, J Endod 32:296–298, 2006.
24. Robertson D, Nusstein J, Reader A, et al: The anesthetic efficacy of articaine in buccal infiltration of mandibular posterior teeth, J Am Dent Assoc 138:1104–1112, 2007.
25. Haase A, Reader A, Nusstein J, et al: Comparing anesthetic efficacy of articaine versus lidocaine as a supplemental buccal infiltration of the mandibular first molar after an inferior alveolar nerve block, J Am Dent Assoc 139:1228–1235, 2008.
26. Kanaa MD, Whitworth JM, Corbett IP, et al: Articaine buccal infiltration enhances the effectiveness of lidocaine inferior alveolar nerve block, Int Endod J 42:238–246, 2009.

27. Dreven LJ, Reader A, Beck M, et al: An evaluation of the electric pulp tester as a measure of analgesia in human vital teeth, J Endod 13:233–238, 1987.
28. Certosimo AJ, Archer RD: A clinical evaluation of the electric pulp tester as an indicator of local anesthesia, Oper Dent 21:25–30, 1996.
29. Wilson S, Johns PI, Fuller PM: The inferior alveolar and mylohyoid nerves: an anatomic study and relationship to local anesthesia of the anterior mandibular teeth, J Am Dent Assoc 108:350–352, 1984.
30. Frommer J, Mele FA, Monroe CW: The possible role of the mylohyoid nerve in mandibular posterior tooth sensation, J Am Dent Assoc 85:113–117, 1972.
31. Roda RS, Blanton PL: The anatomy of local anesthesia, Quintessence Int 25:27–38, 1994.
32. Meechan JG: Infiltration anesthesia in the mandible, Dent Clin N Am 54:621–629, 2010.
33. Gow-Gates GAE: Mandibular conduction anesthesia: a new technique using extraoral landmarks, Oral Surg 36:321–328, 1973.
34. Malamed SF: The Gow-Gates mandibular block: evaluation after 4275 cases, Oral Surg 51:463, 1981.
35. Fish LR, McIntire DN, Johnson L: Temporary paralysis of cranial nerves III, IV, and VI after a Gow-Gates injection, J Am Dent Assoc 119:127–130, 1989.
36. Akinosi JO: A new approach to the mandibular nerve block, Br J Oral Surg 15:83–87, 1977.
37. Murphy TM: Somatic blockade. In Cousins MJ, Bridenbaugh PO, editors: Neural blockade in clinical anesthesia and management of pain, Philadelphia, 1980, JB Lippincott.
38. Bennett CR: Monheim's local anesthesia and pain control in dental practice, ed 6, St Louis, 1978, Mosby.
39. Vazirani SJ: Closed mouth mandibular nerve block: a new technique, Dent Dig 66:10–13, 1960.
40. Wolfe SH: The Wolfe nerve block: a modified high mandibular nerve block, Dent Today 11:34–37, 1992.
41. Malamed SF: Handbook of local anesthesia, St Louis, 1980, Mosby.
42. Jastak JT, Yagiela JA, Donaldson D: Local anesthesia of the oral cavity, Philadelphia, 1995, WB Saunders.

CHAPTER 15

Supplemental Injection Techniques

In this chapter, a number of injections are described that are used in specialized clinical situations. Some may be used as the sole technique for pain control for certain types of dental treatment. For example, the periodontal ligament (PDL) injection and intraosseous (IO) and intraseptal techniques provide effective pulpal anesthesia for a single tooth without the need for other injections. On the other hand, use of the intrapulpal injection is almost always reserved for situations in which other injection techniques have failed or are contraindicated for use. The PDL, IO, and intraseptal techniques also are frequently used to supplement failed or only partially successful traditional injection techniques.

Since the previous edition of this textbook was published (2004), considerable interest has arisen in the effectiveness of mandibular infiltration in the adult mandible with the local anesthetic articaine HCl. The ability to provide pulpal anesthesia in circumscribed areas of the mandible without the need for nerve blocks (e.g., inferior alveolar nerve block [IANB], Gow-Gates) is valuable when these nerve blocks fail to provide the depth of anesthesia required for painless dentistry.

INTRAOSSEOUS ANESTHESIA

IO anesthesia involves the deposition of local anesthetic solution into the cancellous bone that supports the teeth. Although not new (IO anesthesia dates back to the early 1900s), a resurgence of interest in this technique in dentistry has occurred over the past 15 years.[1-5] Three techniques are discussed here, two of which—the PDL injection and the intraseptal injection—are modifications of traditional IO anesthesia.

Periodontal Ligament Injection

Because of the thickness of the cortical plate of bone in most patients and in most areas of the mandible, it is not possible to achieve profound pulpal anesthesia on a solitary tooth in the adult mandible with the techniques described in Chapter 14. An exception to this is the mandibular incisor region, where Certosimo demonstrated a 97% success rate for pulpal anesthesia with infiltration of 0.9 mL of articaine HCl (with epinephrine 1 : 100,000) on BOTH the buccal and lingual aspects of the teeth.[6] Some success is achievable in the posterior teeth as well.[7,8] Mandibular infiltration is reviewed later in this chapter.

An old technique has been repopularized. The PDL injection (also known as the intraligamentary injection [ILI]) was originally described as the *peridental injection* in local anesthesia textbooks dating from 1912 to 1923.[9,10]

The peridental injection was not well received in those early years because it was claimed that the risk of producing blood-borne infection and septicemia was too great to warrant its use in patients. The technique never became popular but was used clinically by many doctors, although it was not referred to as the *peridental technique.* In clinical situations in which an inferior alveolar nerve block failed to provide adequate pulpal anesthesia to the first molar (usually its mesial root), the doctor inserted a needle along the long axis of the mesial root as far apically as possible and deposited a small volume of local anesthetic solution under pressure. This invariably provided effective pain control.

It was not until the early 1980s that the intraligamentary or PDL injection regained popularity. Credit for increased interest in this approach must go to the manufacturers of syringe devices designed to make the injection easier to administer. The original devices—the Peripress (Universal Dental, Boyerstown, Pa) and the Ligmaject (IMA Associates, Largo, Fla) (Fig. 15-1)—provide a mechanical advantage that allows the administrator to deposit the anesthetic more easily (and sometimes too easily). They appear similar to the Wilcox-Jewett Obtunder (Fig. 15-2), which was widely advertised to the dental profession in a 1905 catalog, *Dental Furniture, Instruments, and Materials,* perhaps reconfirming the adage that there is "nothing new under the sun."[11]

Why has the PDL (née peridental) injection enjoyed a renewal of popularity? Perhaps it is because the primary thrust of advertising for the new syringes focused on being able to "avoid the mandibular block" injection with the PDL or intraligamentary technique, a concept to which the dental profession is receptive, given the fact that virtually all

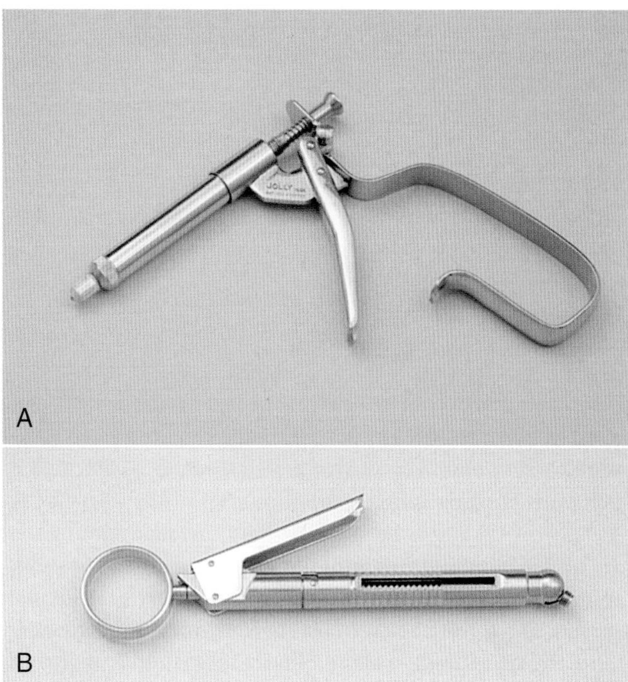

Figure 15-1. **A,** Original pressure syringe designed for a periodontal ligament or intraligamentary injection. **B,** Second-generation syringe for a periodontal ligament injection.

THE WILCOX-JEWETT OBTUNDER.

LEE S. SMITH & SON, PITTSBURG.

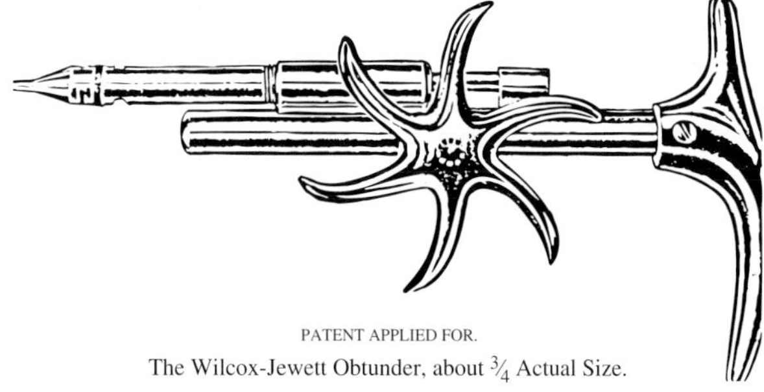

PATENT APPLIED FOR.
The Wilcox-Jewett Obtunder, about ¾ Actual Size.

Figure 15-2. Pressure syringe (1905) designed for a peridental injection.

dentists have experienced periods when they have been unable to achieve adequate anesthesia with the inferior alveolar nerve block (a "mandibular slump").

The PDL injection also may be used successfully in the maxillary arch; however, with the ready availability of other highly effective and atraumatic techniques, such as the supraperiosteal (infiltration) injection, and drugs such as articaine HCl to provide single-tooth pulpal anesthesia, there has been little compelling reason for use of the PDL in the upper jaw (although there is absolutely no other reason not to recommend it in this area). Possibly the greatest potential benefit of the PDL injection lies in the fact that it provides pulpal and soft tissue anesthesia in a localized area (one tooth) of the mandible without producing extensive soft tissue (e.g., tongue and lower lip) anesthesia as well. Virtually all dental patients prefer this technique to any of the "mandibular nerve blocks." In a clinical trial, Malamed reported that 74% of patients preferred the PDL injection primarily because of its lack of lingual and labial soft tissue anesthesia.[12] It is interesting that those who preferred the inferior alveolar nerve block did so for an important reason: With the IANB, once the lip and tongue became numb, patients were able to relax, knowing that the remainder of their dental treatment would not hurt. Without lingual and labial soft tissue anesthesia in the PDL technique, patients were unable to fully relax because they were never certain that they had been adequately anesthetized.

Primary indications for the PDL injection include (1) the need for anesthesia of but one or two mandibular teeth in a quadrant, (2) treatment of isolated teeth in both mandibular quadrants (to avoid bilateral inferior alveolar nerve block), (3) treatment of children (because residual soft tissue anesthesia increases the risk of self-inflicted soft tissue injury), (4) treatment in which nerve block anesthesia is contraindicated (e.g., in hemophiliacs), and (5) its use as a possible aid in the diagnosis (e.g., localization) of mandibular pain.

Contraindications to the PDL injection include infection or severe inflammation at the injection site and the presence of primary teeth. Brannstrom and associates reported the development of enamel hypoplasia or hypomineralization or both in 15 permanent teeth after administration of the periodontal ligament injection.[13] Fortunately, there is rarely a need for the PDL injection in the primary dentition; other techniques, such as infiltration and nerve blocks, are effective and easy to administer.

Several concerns have been expressed about this technique, most of which were addressed in a status report on the PDL injection in the *Journal of the American Dental Association* in 1983.[14] Two of these concerns involve (1) the effect of injection and deposition of the local anesthetic under pressure into the confined space of the PDL, and (2) the effect of the drug or vasoconstrictor on pulpal tissues. Walton and Garnick concluded that the PDL injection (administered with a conventional syringe) causes slight damage to tissues in the region of needle penetration only.[15] Apical areas appeared normal; the epithelial and connective tissue attachment to enamel and cementum was not disturbed by the needle puncture; slight resorption of nonvital bone occurred in the crestal regions, forming a wedge-shaped defect; soft tissue damage was minimal; the disruption of tissue that did occur showed repair in 25 days, with absence of inflammation and with the formation of new bone in the regions of resorption; and injection of the solution was not in itself damaging. Damage produced by needle penetration alone (no drug administered) appeared similar to that seen when a drug had been deposited with the injection. The authors concluded that the PDL injection is safe to the periodontium.[15] In addition, no evidence to date suggests that inclusion of a vasoconstrictor in the local anesthetic solution has any detrimental effect on pulpal microcirculation after the PDL injection.

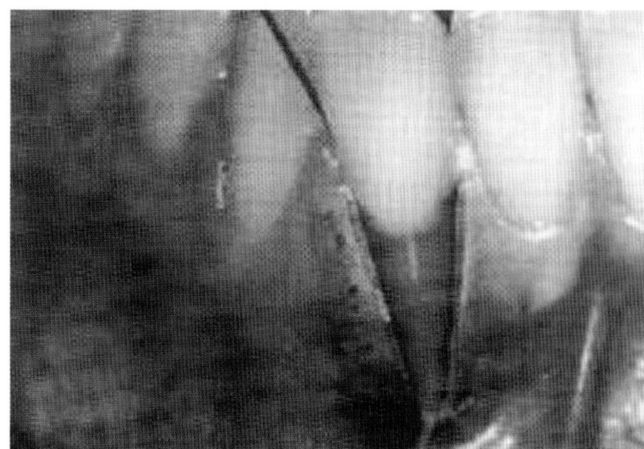

Figure 15-3. Periodontal ligament injection is intraosseous. Note the dispersion of ink into surrounding bone.

It appears that the mechanism whereby local anesthetic solution reaches the periapical tissues with the PDL injection consists of diffusion apically and into the marrow spaces surrounding the teeth. The solution is not forced apically through the periodontal tissues, a procedure that might lead (as Nelson reported) to avulsion of a tooth (premolar) because of the increased hydrostatic pressure exerted in a confined space.[16] Therefore the PDL injection appears to produce anesthesia in much the same way as IO and intraseptal injections—by diffusion of anesthetic solution apically through marrow spaces in the intraseptal bone (Fig. 15-3).[17,18]

Postinjection complications are also of concern with the PDL injection. Reported complications have included mild to severe postoperative discomfort, swelling and discoloration of soft tissues at the injection site, and prolonged ischemia of the interdental papilla, followed by sloughing and exposure of crestal bone.[19,20] Some of these complications result directly from poor operator technique, lack of familiarity with the pressure syringe, and injection of excessive volumes of local anesthetic into the PDL. The most frequently voiced postinjection complications are mild discomfort and sensitivity to biting and percussion for 2 or 3 days. The most common causes of postinjection discomfort are (1) too rapid injection (producing edema and slight extrusion of the tooth, thus sensitivity on biting), and (2) injection of excessive volumes of local anesthetic into the site.

Before the PDL technique is described, it must be mentioned that although "special" PDL syringes can be used effectively and safely, usually there is no need for them. A conventional local anesthetic syringe is equally effective in providing PDL anesthesia. Use of a conventional syringe requires that the administrator apply significant force to deposit the local anesthetic into the periodontal tissues. Virtually all doctors and most hygienists are able to produce PDL anesthesia successfully without a special PDL syringe. Only when a doctor or a hygienist is unable to achieve adequate PDL anesthesia with a conventional syringe is use of a PDL syringe recommended.

Arguments against using the conventional syringe for PDL injections (and my rebuttals) include the following:

1. It is too difficult to administer the solution with a conventional syringe.
   Comment: Slow administration of the local anesthetic makes the PDL injection atraumatic. Improper use (fast injection) of the PDL syringe produces both immediate and postinjection pain.
2. The extreme pressure applied to the glass may shatter the cartridge. PDL syringes provide a metal or plastic covering for the glass cartridge, thereby protecting the patient from shards of glass should the cartridge shatter during injection.
   Comment: Although I have read and heard of cartridges shattering during PDL injection, I have yet to experience this personally. However, the risk can be minimized in several ways: Because only small volumes of solution are injected (0.2 mL per root), a full, 1.8 mL cartridge is not necessary. Eliminate all but about 0.6 mL of solution before starting the PDL injection. This minimizes the area of glass being subjected to increased pressures, decreasing the risk of breakage. In addition, glass cartridges have a thin Mylar plastic label that covers most or all of the glass. If a cartridge breaks, the glass will not shatter but will be contained by the plastic covering.
3. Many manufacturers of PDL syringes recommend use of 30-gauge short or ultrashort needles in this technique.
   Comment: In my early experience with the PDL technique, I used the 30-gauge needle only to find that whenever pressure was applied to it (as when pushing it apically into the PDL), the 30-gauge needle bent easily. It was too fragile to withstand pressure without bending. PDL injection failure rates were excessive.
   A 30-gauge ultrashort needle was manufactured specifically for use with this injection technique (10 mm length). Although somewhat more effective than the 30-gauge short, there was no need to use a "special" needle for this injection. I have had great clinical success, with no increase in patient discomfort, using the more readily available 27-gauge short needle.
   In summary, the PDL injection is an important component of the armamentarium of local anesthetic techniques for providing mandibular and, to a lesser degree, maxillary pain control.
4. The PDL injection administered with a conventional or PDL syringe is painful.
   Comment: Use of a computer-controlled local anesthetic delivery (C-CLAD) device for administration of painless PDL injections has been strongly advocated.[21] Many dentists have related to me that their PDL injections, although effective in providing anesthesia, are painful to the patient during administration. Although this has not been my experience, there are

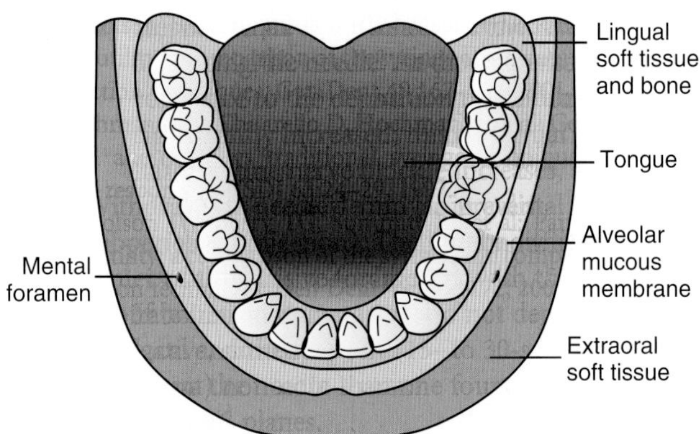

Figure 15-4. Area anesthetized by a periodontal ligament injection.

enough reports to convince me that many doctors believe this to be so. Use of C-CLAD systems (e.g., STA-Single Tooth Anesthesia System, Milestone Scientific, Inc., Livingston, NJ) does enable the PDL injection to be delivered painlessly (e.g., 0 to 1 on a visual analog scale [VAS]). The PDL technique utilizing a C-CLAD device is described in detail in the section immediately following this.

Other Common Names. Peridental (original name) injection, intraligamentary injection (ILI).

Nerves Anesthetized. Terminal nerve endings at the site of injection and at the apex of the tooth.

Areas Anesthetized. Bone, soft tissue, and apical and pulpal tissues in the area of injection (Fig. 15-4).

Indications

1. Pulpal anesthesia of one or two teeth in a quadrant
2. Treatment of isolated teeth in two mandibular quadrants (to avoid bilateral IANB)
3. Patients for whom residual soft tissue anesthesia is undesirable
4. Situations in which regional block anesthesia is contraindicated
5. As a possible aid in the diagnosis of pulpal discomfort
6. As an adjunctive technique after nerve block anesthesia if partial anesthesia is present

Contraindications

1. Infection or inflammation at the site of injection
2. Primary teeth when the permanent tooth bud is present[13]
   a. Enamel hypoplasia has been reported to occur in a developing permanent tooth when a PDL injection was administered to the primary tooth above it.
   b. There appears to be little reason for use of the PDL technique in primary teeth because infiltration anesthesia and the incisive nerve block are effective in primary dentition.
3. Patient who requires a "numb" sensation for psychological comfort

Advantages

1. There is no anesthesia of the lip, tongue, and other soft tissues, thus facilitating treatment in multiple quadrants during a single appointment.
2. Minimum dose of local anesthetic necessary to achieve anesthesia (0.2 mL per root)
3. An alternative to partially successful regional nerve block anesthesia
4. Rapid onset of profound pulpal and soft tissue anesthesia (30 seconds)
5. Less traumatic than conventional block injections
6. Well suited for procedures in children, extractions, and periodontal and endodontic single-tooth and multiple-quadrant procedures

Disadvantages

1. Proper needle placement is difficult to achieve in some areas (e.g., distal of the second or third molar).
2. Leakage of local anesthetic solution into the patient's mouth produces an unpleasant taste.
3. Excessive pressure or overly rapid injection may break the glass cartridge.
4. A special syringe may be necessary.
5. Excessive pressure can produce focal tissue damage.
6. Postinjection discomfort may persist for several days.
7. The potential for extrusion of a tooth exists if excessive pressure or volumes are used.

Positive Aspiration. 0%.

Alternative. Supraperiosteal injection (entire maxilla and the mandibular incisor region).

Technique

1. A 27-gauge short needle is recommended.
2. *Area of insertion:* Long axis of the tooth to be treated on its mesial or distal root (one-rooted tooth) or on the mesial and distal roots (of multirooted tooth) interproximally (Fig. 15-5)
3. *Target area:* depth of the gingival sulcus
4. Landmarks:
   a. Root(s) of the tooth
   b. Periodontal tissues
5. *Orientation of the bevel:* Although not significant to the success of the technique, it is recommended that the bevel of the needle face toward the root to permit easy advancement of the needle in an apical direction.
6. Procedure:
   a. Assume the correct position. (This varies significantly with PDL injections on different teeth.) Sit comfortably, have adequate visibility of the injection site, and maintain control over the needle. It may be necessary to bend the needle to achieve the

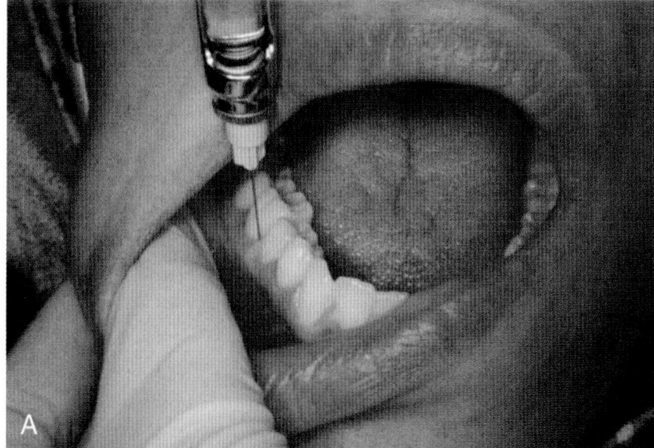

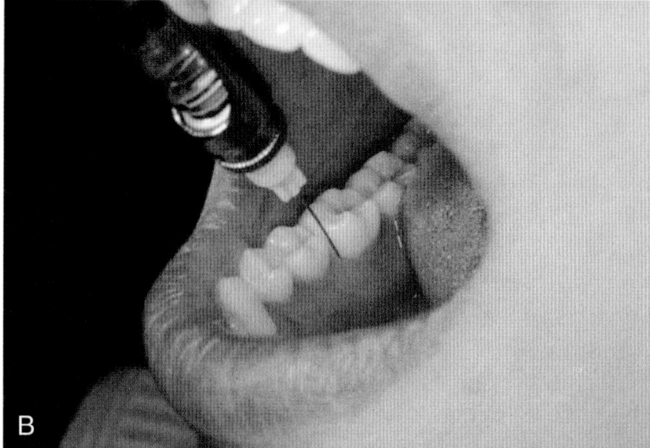

Figure 15-5. Area of insertion for a periodontal ligament injection. **A,** Buccal. **B,** Lingual.

proper angle, especially on the distal aspects of second and third molars.*

b. Position the patient supine or semisupine, with the head turned to maximize access and visibility.
c. Stabilize the syringe and direct it along the long axis of the root to be anesthetized.
   (1) The bevel faces the root of the tooth.
   (2) If interproximal contacts are tight, the syringe should be directed from the lingual or buccal surface of the tooth but maintained as close to the long axis as possible.
   (3) Stabilize the syringe and your hand against the patient's teeth, lips, or face.
d. With the bevel of the needle on the root, advance the needle apically until resistance is met.
e. Deposit 0.2 mL of local anesthetic solution in a minimum of 20 seconds.
   (1) When using a conventional syringe, note that the thickness of the rubber stopper in the local anesthetic cartridge is equal to 0.2 mL of solution. This may be used as a gauge for the volume of local anesthetic to be administered.
   (2) With a PDL syringe, each squeeze of the "trigger" provides a volume of 0.2 mL.
f. There are two important indicators of success of the injection:
   (1) Significant resistance to the deposition of local anesthetic solution
      (a) This is especially noticeable when the conventional syringe is used; resistance is similar to that felt with the nasopalatine injection and is thought to be the reason for reports of PDL injections being painful.
      (b) The local anesthetic should not flow back into the patient's mouth. If this happens, repeat the injection at the same site but from a different angle. Two tenths of a milliliter of solution must be deposited and must remain within the tissues for the PDL to be effective.
   (2) Ischemia of the soft tissues adjacent to the injection site. (This is noted with all local anesthetic solutions but is more prominent with vasoconstrictor-containing local anesthetics.)
g. If the tooth has only one root, remove the syringe from the tissue and cap the needle. Dental treatment usually may start within 30 seconds.
h. If the tooth is multirooted, remove the needle and repeat the procedure on the other root(s).

*Although the author dislikes bending needles for most injections, it may become necessary for the success of the PDL and intrapulpal injections to bend the needle to gain access to certain areas of the oral cavity. Because the needle does not enter into tissues more than a few millimeters, bending it is not as risk-prone as when the needle enters more completely into soft tissue.

Signs and Symptoms

1. *Subjective:* There are no signs that absolutely assure adequate anesthesia; the anesthetized area is quite circumscribed. When the following two signs are present, there is an excellent chance that profound anesthesia is present:
   a. Ischemia of soft tissues at the injection site
   b. Significant resistance to injection of solution (with a traditional syringe)
2. *Objective:* Use of electrical pulp testing (EPT) with no response from the tooth with maximal EPT output (80/80)

Safety Feature. Intravascular injection is extremely unlikely to occur.

Precautions

1. Keep the needle against the tooth to prevent overinsertion into soft tissues on the lingual aspect.
2. Do not inject too rapidly (minimum 20 seconds for 0.2 mL).
3. Do not inject too much solution (0.2 mL per root retained within tissues).
4. Do not inject directly into infected or highly inflamed tissues.

Failures of Anesthesia

1. Infected or inflamed tissues. The pH and vascularity changes at the apex and periodontal tissues minimize the effectiveness of the local anesthetic.
2. Solution not retained. In this case, remove the needle and reenter at a different site(s) until 0.2 mL of local anesthetic is deposited and retained in the tissues.
3. Each root must be anesthetized with 0.2 mL of solution.

Complications

1. Pain during insertion of the needle
   Cause #1: The needle tip is in soft tissues. To correct: Keep the needle against tooth structure.
   Cause #2: The tissues are inflamed.
   To correct: Avoid use of the PDL technique, or apply a small amount of topical anesthetic for a minimum of 1 minute before injection.
2. Pain during injection of solution
   Cause: Too rapid injection of local anesthetic solution
   To correct: Slow down the rate of injection to a minimum 20 seconds for a 0.2 mL solution, regardless of the syringe being used.
3. Postinjection pain
   Cause: Too rapid injection, excessive volume of solution, too many tissue penetrations. (The patient usually complains of soreness and premature contact when occluding.)
   To correct: Manage symptomatically with warm saline rinses and mild analgesics, if necessary (usually resolves within 2 to 3 days).

Duration of Expected Anesthesia. The duration of pulpal anesthesia obtained with a successful PDL injection is quite variable and is not related to the drug administered. Administration of lidocaine with 1:100,000 epinephrine, for example, provides pulpal anesthesia ranging in duration from 5 to 55 minutes. The PDL injection may be repeated if necessary to permit completion of the dental procedure. It appears that the volume of anesthetic solution used with the PDL is too small to provide the usually expected duration of anesthesia of the drug. The question of anesthetic volume is discussed further in the following description of PDL injections given using a C-CLAD device.

STA-Intraligamentary (PDL) Injection

The technique used to perform the PDL injection, as described previously, has remained relatively unchanged since it was first introduced in the early 1900s.[22] A variety of mechanical syringes have been developed throughout the years to enable high pressures to be generated during the administration of anesthetic solution into these tissues.[23] These mechanical syringes produce considerably high pressures, thereby creating a pressure gradient to promote diffusion of anesthetic solution from the coronal region of the crestal bone to the apex of the tooth. The anesthetic solution diffuses through the cortical and medullary bone to eventually surround or envelope the neurovascular bundle at the apex of a tooth.[24,25] This localized "bathing" of the nerve entering into the apex of a tooth provides anesthesia of a single tooth without the often undesirable collateral anesthesia of the lip and tongue. Additionally, this localized administration has a rapid onset because of the localized nature of the injection technique. With the production of high pressures, only a small volume (typically 0.2 to 0.4 mL) can be injected and absorbed.[18] Last, patients routinely report moderate to severe discomfort when injections are performed using high-pressure syringe techniques.[26,27]

With the introduction of the STA-Single Tooth Anesthesia System C-CLAD device, a change in the basic concepts related to performing the PDL injection occurred as a result of the mechanical and technological differences between a hand-driven mechanical syringe versus a computer-regulated electromechanical instrument.[28] The difference between the STA System versus a hand-driven syringe is that in the former, a precisely regulated flow rate and controlled low-pressure injection are used to perform the intraligamentary injection.[29] These fundamental changes in fluid dynamics have led to the following clinically relevant changes: a consistent and measurable reduction in patient pain perception,[30,31] a histologically demonstrated reduction in tissue damage, and the ability to administer larger volumes of anesthetic safely and effectively when the PDL injection is performed.[32] The ability to administer a larger volume of anesthetic solution results in an increased duration of effective dental local anesthesia.[33] In addition, the STA System incorporates a new technology that allows the PDL injection to be performed as a "guided" injection by providing real-time feedback during positioning of the needle in the intended target area, thereby improving the efficacy and predictability of PDL injection.[34,35]

The STA System precisely regulates and measures fluid pressure at the needle tip while a subcutaneous injection is performed, providing the clinician with continuous real-time audible and visual feedback during the injection.[32]

Clinical studies in medicine and dentistry have demonstrated that using real-time exit-pressure sensing allows identification of a specific tissue type related to objective measurement of tissue density (i.e., tissue compliance) while a subcutaneous injection is performed.[30,36-38] One study led researchers to the use of this technology to more accurately identify tissue type and to perform the epidural nerve block technique commonly used for obstetric and surgical procedures of the lower extremities.[38] Hochman and coworkers published the results of a clinical study in which more than 200 dental injections were given using dynamic pressure-sensing technology to differentiate specific tissues of the oral cavity: periodontal ligament, attached gingiva, and unattached gingival mucosal tissues.[30] Investigators concluded that specific tissue types require a specific pressure range with a given flow rate to be used to perform a safe and effective dental injection.

The STA instrument provides continuous audible and visual feedback to the clinician as the dental needle is introduced into the tissues during the injection. This system has

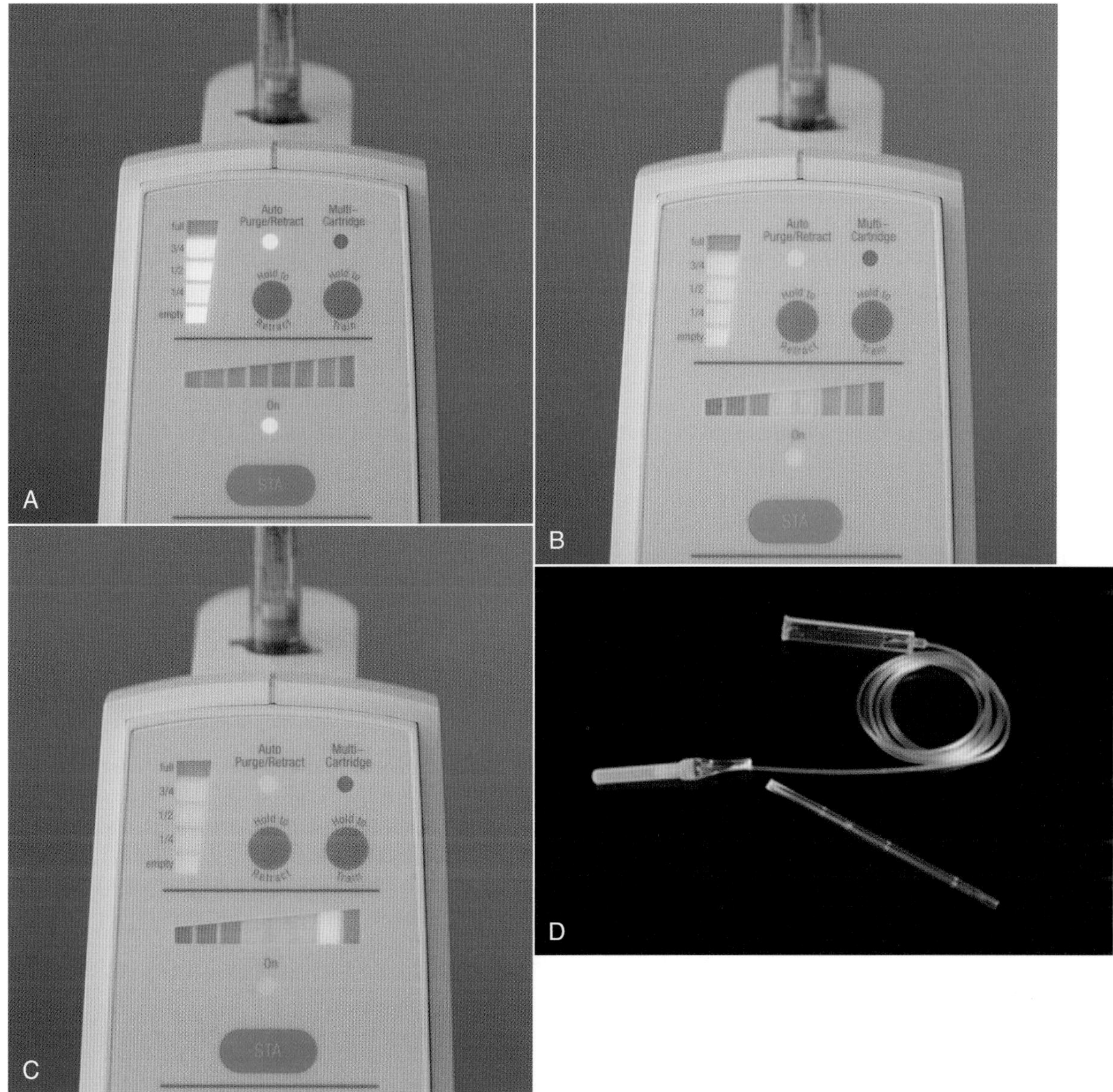

Figure 15-6. Dynamic Pressure Sensing (DPS) on the STA Single Tooth Anesthesia C-CLAD device provides both visual and audible feedback regarding placement of the needle tip during the periodontal ligament (PDL) injection. Horizontal color bars indicate pressure at the tip of the needle. **A,** Red—pressure is too low. **B,** Orange and dark yellow—increasing pressure but not yet adequate. **C,** Light yellow—correct pressure for PDL injection. At this point **(C)** the STA unit will also provide an audible clue "PDL. PDL, PDL" that the needle tip is properly situated. STA Wand handpiece is lightweight (less than 10 grams) and can easily be shortened to aid in administration of some injections **(D)**, such as the AMSA or other palatal techniques.

a visual pressure-sensing scale on the front of the unit that is composed of a series of light-emitting diode (LED) lights (orange, yellow, and green) (Fig. 15-6, *A-C*). Orange lights indicate minimal pressure at the needle tip, yellow indicates mild to moderate pressure, and green indicates moderate tissue pressure indicative of the PDL space. PDL tissue may be identified at pressures of the yellow LED at high range as well.[39]

Through auditory feedback, the clinician becomes aware of how to maintain correct needle-to-intraligamentary position throughout the injection. Auditory feedback consists of a series of sounds with a pressure-sensing scale composed of ascending tones to guide the clinician. When the clinician hears the ascending sequence, this indicates that the pressure is rising. When the periodontal ligament is identified, the letters "P-D-L" are spoken, indicating that correct needle position has been achieved. Maintaining a consistent level of moderate pressure throughout the injection process is necessary for success. Audible and visual feedback provides this important information. When the STA-PDL injection is performed, it is not uncommon for the clinician to reposition the needle to find the optimal position within periodontal ligament tissues, allowing a high degree of predictability and accuracy when this injection is performed. This transforms the "blind" syringe approach, described above, into an objective method of locating and maintaining correct needle position when performing the PDL injection.

Ferrari and coworkers published data on 60 patients in whom they compared the STA System versus two standard PDL hand-driven manual syringes: a high-pressure mechanical syringe (Ligmaject) and a conventional dental syringe.[32] Electrical pulp testing was performed on all tested teeth at regular intervals to determine success or failure of these different instruments and the techniques used. In addition to EPT results, subjective pain responses of the patient were recorded after treatment. Ferrari reported a success rate of 100% for the STA System. In addition, a rapid onset of anesthesia was observed. In this study, the PDL injection was performed as the primary injection for restorative dental care in mandibular teeth. Investigators reported subjective pain responses of "minimal or no pain" in all patients receiving the PDL injection performed with the STA device. In contrast, injections performed with the other two systems (high-pressure mechanical syringe and conventional syringe) were found to result in higher pain scores throughout testing and required repeated attempts to achieve a successful outcome. Researchers concluded the STA System device resulted in a more predictable, more reliable, and more comfortable anesthesia technique than the high-pressure mechanical syringe and/or the conventional dental syringe.

Pediatric Use. Brannstrom and associates reported on the use of a high-pressure PDL injection to anesthetize 16 monkey primary teeth.[13] Hypoplasia or hypomineralization defects developed on 15 of the permanent teeth, but none in controls. The PDL injection, when delivered by a hand-driven mechanical syringe, produces uncontrolled high pressures and is associated with damage to the periodontal tissues.[40] Other reports have also recommended avoidance of the PDL injection on primary teeth when a traditional syringe or PDL syringe is used.[13]

In 2010, Ashekenzi and coworkers published the first long-term, clinical controlled study using a low-pressure PDL injection with the STA System with dynamic pressure-sensing (DPS) technology.[31] The study population consisted of 78 children (ages, 4.1 to 12.8 years) who received STA intraligamentary injections in 166 primary molar teeth. Teeth receiving conventional dental anesthesia or that were not anesthetized by local anesthesia served as controls. After reviewing data collected between 1999 and 2007, Ashekenzi concluded that performing the PDL injection using a low-pressure C-CLAD injection instrument, specifically the STA System with DPS, did not produce damage to the underlying developing permanent tooth bud and was deemed safe and effective. The same authors, in another study, demonstrated that children exhibited minimal disruptive pain-related behavior and minimal levels of dental-related stress during and immediately after STA intraligamentary anesthesia.[41] These findings represent a new perspective on dental local anesthesia and the treatment of primary teeth of the pediatric patient.

The PDL injection performed with the STA System device represents a single-tooth injection technique that provides a level of safety, comfort, and predictability previously unattainable. The system provides the clinician with multiple benefits that cannot be achieved with use of the manually driven conventional syringe, the pistol-grip high-pressure syringe, or previous C-CLAD instruments.

Other Common Names. Peridental (original name) injection, intraligamentary injection (ILI).

Nerves Anesthetized. Terminal nerve endings at the site of injection and at the apex of the tooth.

Areas Anesthetized. Bone, soft tissue, and apical and pulpal tissues in the area of the injection.

Indications

1. Pulpal anesthesia of one or two teeth in a quadrant
2. Treatment of isolated teeth in two mandibular quadrants (to avoid bilateral IANB)
3. Patients for whom residual soft tissue anesthesia is undesirable
4. Pediatric dental patient in treatment of the primary dentition
   a. A recent study conclusively reported that using the STA System does not present the previous risk of enamel hypoplasia that was reported with a manually driven syringe, and that using the STA System instrument does not adversely affect the developing permanent tooth when PDL injection is performed.
5. Situations in which regional block anesthesia is contraindicated
6. As a possible aid in diagnosis of pulpal discomfort
7. As an adjunctive technique after nerve block anesthesia if partial anesthesia is present

Contraindications

1. Infection or inflammation at the site of injection
2. Patients who require a "numb" sensation for psychological comfort

Advantages

1. The STA System device with dynamic pressure-sensing technology provides an objective means by which to identify the correct target location to perform a PDL injection, improving the predictability of this injection when compared with previous techniques and instruments.
2. The STA System device uses a controlled **low-pressure** fluid dynamic that has been shown to reduce the risk of tissue injury and to minimize subjective pain responses.
3. The STA System device, through use of a controlled low-pressure fluid dynamic, allows a greater volume of anesthetic solution (0.45 mL to 0.90 mL) to be safely administered, thereby increasing the effective working time of this PDL injection (30 to 45 minutes).
4. The STA System device with dynamic pressure-sensing technology can detect local anesthetic solution leakage into the patient's mouth, avoiding an unpleasant taste.
5. The STA System device with dynamic pressure-sensing technology can detect excessive pressure and can

safeguard patient and operator from glass cartridge breakage.

Disadvantages

1. Requires the use of a specialized C-CLAD instrument and associated costs of purchase and use
2. Requires additional training

Positive Aspiration. 0%.

Technique

1. A STA-Wand bonded handpiece with a 30-gauge ½ inch needle
2. Set the STA instrument to the STA mode.
3. Area of insertion:
   a. The needle should be placed at a 45-degree angle to the long axis of the tooth.
   b. When a PDL injection is performed on a single-rooted tooth, only a single site is necessary.
   c. When a PDL injection is performed on a multirooted tooth, it is recommended that two sites be used: one on the distal root and a second on the mesial root.
   d. Start with the distal aspect of the tooth.
   e. The injection can be performed anywhere from the lingual line angle to the interproximal contact for each root.
4. To improve accessibility in difficult areas, shorten the STA handpiece by breaking off a section of the handle. This will allow easier access (Fig. 15-6, *D*).
5. Place the needle very slowly into the gingival sulcus as if it was a periodontal probe, while simultaneously initiating the ControlFlo (0.005 mL/sec) flow rate. Advance the needle slowly into the sulcus, moving it gently down into the sulcus until you encounter resistance.
6. The ControlFlo rate can be initiated by pressing on the foot control; after three audible beeps, you will hear the unit announce "Cruise." Once you hear the word "Cruise," you may remove your foot. The STA system will continue the flow of anesthetic solution.
7. Once you feel you are at the base of the sulcus, you need to minimize movement for 10 to 15 seconds as the dynamic pressure-sensing technology analyzes the location of the needle tip.
8. As the STA system DPS senses pressure building, you will see a sequential illumination of LED lights on the front of the unit. The visual pressure sensing scale consists of a series of orange, yellow, and green LED lights. If after 20 to 30 seconds, pressure does not build, you will need to relocate the needle. The STA System also provides audible pressure feedback, with a series of three ascending tones indicating that the system is detecting pressure at the needle tip.
9. After 20 to 30 seconds with the needle tip in the correct location, the STA System will announce "P-D-L, P- D-L." This will be followed by a series of two longer "beeps," indicating that proper pressure is being maintained, and that you have identified the correct needle tip position for the PDL injection.
10. It is important to note that a successful PDL may occur when the LED lights are in green or high yellow zones. It is necessary to maintain the LED light indicators throughout the injection process to achieve success. Note that you will not hear the audible spoken word "PDL" in the yellow zone.
11. Deposit 0.45 mL to 0.90 mL of local anesthetic per root.

Signs and Symptoms

1. Indicators of success:
   Subjective: There are no signs that absolutely assure adequate anesthesia; the anesthetized area is quite circumscribed. When the following sign is present, there is an excellent chance that profound anesthesia is present:
   Subjective: Ischemia of soft tissues at the injection site
   Subjective: Maintenance of high yellow and green LED zones on the front of the STA drive unit throughout the injection process
2. *Objective:* Use of electrical pulp testing (EPT) with no response from the tooth with maximal EPT output (80/80)

Safety Feature. The STA System instrument DPS technology precisely regulates and monitors fluid exit-pressures within the tissues, thereby preventing buildup of excessive pressure and ensuring a safe and effective controlled flow rate of local anesthetic solution.

Precautions

1. Maintain direct vision of the needle as it enters the sulcus of the tooth.
2. Keep the needle at a 45-degree angle to the long axis of the tooth to ensure that the needle is inserted into the entrance to the PDL space at the level of the crest of bone.
3. Do not inject directly into infected or highly inflamed tissues.

Failures of Anesthesia

1. Infected or inflamed tissues. The pH and vascularity changes at the apex of, and periodontal tissues surrounding, infected teeth minimize the effectiveness of the local anesthetic.
2. Inability to generate STA System in the high yellow or green LED zone. In this case, remove and reenter at a different site(s) until the STA System can generate and maintain the proper DPS outcome.

Complications

1. Pain during insertion of the needle
   Cause: The needle is inserted into the sulcus too rapidly.
   To correct: Enter and move the needle very slowly

into the sulcus while simultaneously initiating the ControlFlo of local anesthetic solution.

2. Inability to maintain high yellow or green LED zone on the STA System
   Cause #1: Have not located the entrance to the intraligamentary tissue (PDL space). To correct: Relocate the needle.
   Cause #2: Have not allowed adequate time (10 to 15 seconds) for back-pressure and analysis of DPS technology to occur. To correct: Position needle and allow 10 to 15 seconds for the ascending tones and sequential illumination of the LED lights.
3. Over-pressure announcement by the STA System:
   Cause #1: Excessive hand pressure on the STA-Wand handpiece can jam the needle into the bone, resulting in obstruction of flow of the anesthetic solution at the needle tip. To correct: Restart the STA System and use gentler forward hand pressure when placing the needle into the sulcus.
   Cause #2: Clogged needle tip from plaque or dental calculus. To correct: Stop, remove needle, and restart, verifying that local anesthetic solution is flowing from the tip of the needle before reentry into PDL tissues.
4. Postinjection pain or tissue necrosis
   Cause #1: Excessive volume of anesthetic solution was used. To correct: Limit the volume of anesthetic solution.
   Cause #2: Too many tissue penetrations with needle and/or excessive forward hand force placed on the needle, causing mechanical trauma to the tissues. To correct: Limit the number of needle entries to a given site, and use a moderate amount of forward hand pressure on the STA-Wand handpiece.

Suggested Drug/Volume

1. 2% Lidocaine HCl 1:100,000 epinephrine
   Adult:
   a. Drug volume no greater than 0.9 mL (½ cartridge) is suggested for a single-rooted tooth.
   b. Drug volume no greater than 1.8 mL (full cartridge) is suggested for a multirooted tooth.
   Child:
   a. Drug volume no greater than 0.45 mL (¼ cartridge) is suggested for a single-rooted tooth.
   b. Drug volume no greater than 0.9 mL (½ cartridge) is suggested for a multirooted tooth.
2. 4% Articaine HCl 1:200,000 epinephrine
   Adult:
   a. Drug volume no greater than 0.45 mL (¼ cartridge) is suggested for a single-rooted tooth.
   b. Drug volume no greater than 0.9 mL (½ cartridge) is suggested for a multirooted tooth.
   Child:
   a. Drug volume no greater than 0.4 mL is suggested for a single-rooted tooth.
   b. Drug volume no greater than 0.8 mL is suggested for a multirooted tooth.

BOX 15-1 Advantages and Disadvantages of the Wand/STA System

Advantages

- Dynamic pressure-sensing (DPS) technology provides continuous real-time feedback when an injection is performed, resulting in a more predictable injection.
- Allows the PDL injection to be used as a predictable primary injection
- Allows all traditional injections techniques to be performed
- Allows newer injection techniques—AMSA, P-ASA, and STA-intraligamentary injections—to be performed
- Reduces pain-disruptive behavior in children and adults
- Reduces stress for patient
- Reduces stress for operator

Disadvantages

- Requires additional armamentarium
- Cost

AMSA, Anterior middle superior alveolar; *P-ASA,* posterior anterior superior alveolar; *PDL,* periodontal ligament.

Duration of Expected Anesthesia. The expected pulpal anesthesia duration is directly correlated with the volume of local anesthetic solution administered. The recommended dosages provide pulpal anesthesia ranging from 30 to 45 minutes. The PDL injection may be repeated if necessary to permit completion of the dental procedure.

Advantages and disadvantages of the Wand/STA System are presented in Box 15-1.

Intraseptal Injection

The intraseptal injection is similar in technique and design to the PDL injection. It is included for discussion because it is useful in providing osseous and soft tissue anesthesia and hemostasis for periodontal curettage and surgical flap procedures. In addition, it may be effective when the condition of periodontal tissues in the gingival sulcus precludes use of the PDL injection (e.g., infection, acute inflammation). Saadoun and Malamed have shown that the path of diffusion of the anesthetic solution is through medullary bone, as in the PDL injection.[42]

Other Common Names. None.

Nerves Anesthetized. Terminal nerve endings at the site of injection and in adjacent soft and hard tissues.

Areas Anesthetized. Bone, soft tissue, root structure in the area of injection (Fig. 15-7).

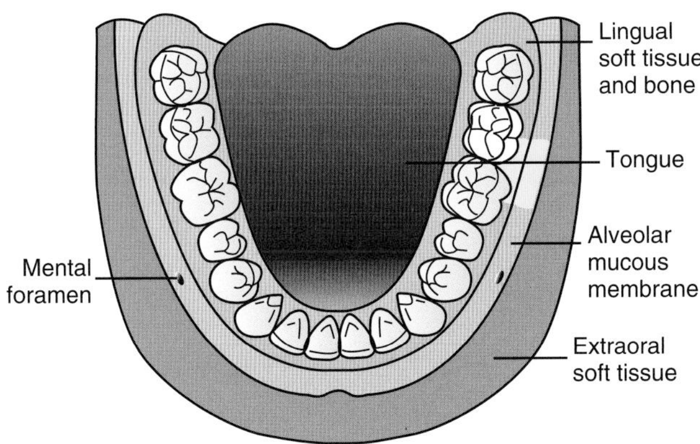

Figure 15-7. Area anesthetized by an intraseptal injection.

Indication. When both pain control and hemostasis are desired for soft tissue and osseous periodontal treatment.

Contraindication. Infection or severe inflammation at the injection site.

Advantages
1. Lack of lip and tongue anesthesia (appreciated by most patients)
2. Minimum volumes of local anesthetic necessary
3. Minimized bleeding during the surgical procedure
4. Atraumatic
5. Immediate (<30 second) onset of action
6. Few postoperative complications
7. Useful on periodontally involved teeth (avoids infected pockets)

Disadvantages
1. Multiple tissue punctures may be necessary.
2. Bitter taste of the anesthetic drug (if leakage occurs)
3. Short duration of pulpal anesthesia; limited area of soft tissue anesthesia (may necessitate reinjection)
4. Clinical experience necessary for success

Positive Aspiration. 0%.

Alternatives
1. PDL injection in the absence of infection or severe periodontal involvement
2. IO anesthesia
3. Regional nerve block with local infiltration for hemostasis

Technique
1. A 27-gauge short needle is recommended.
2. *Area of insertion:* Center of the interdental papilla adjacent to the tooth to be treated (Fig. 15-8)
3. *Target area:* Same
4. *Landmarks:* Papillary triangle, about 2 mm below the tip, equidistant from adjacent teeth
5. *Orientation of the bevel:* Not significant, although Saadoun and Malamed recommend toward the apex[42]

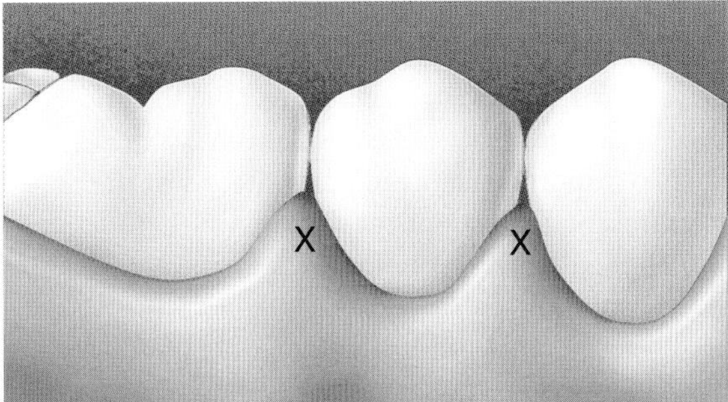

Figure 15-8. Area of insertion for an intraseptal injection.

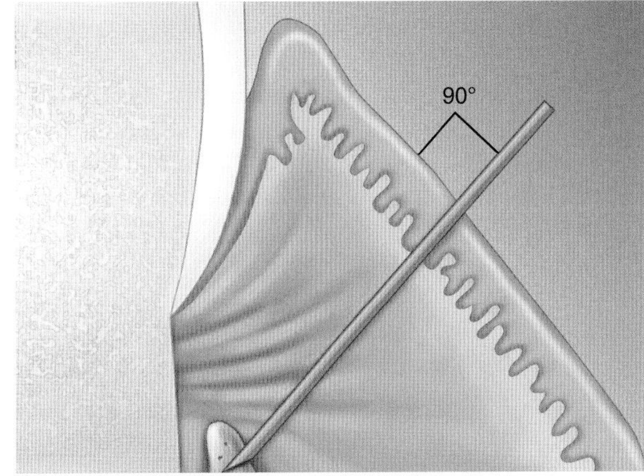

Figure 15-9. Orientation of the needle for an intraseptal injection.

6. Procedure:
   a. Assume the correct position, which varies significantly from tooth to tooth. The administrator should be comfortable, have adequate visibility of the injection site, and maintain control over the needle.
   b. Position the patient supine or semisupine with the head turned to maximize access and visibility.
   c. Prepare tissue at the site of penetration.
      (1) Dry with sterile gauze.
      (2) Apply topical antiseptic (optional).
      (3) Apply topical anesthetic for minimum of 1 minute.
   d. Stabilize the syringe and orient the needle correctly (Fig. 15-9).
      (1) Frontal plane: 45 degrees to the long axis of the tooth
      (2) Sagittal plane: At right angle to the soft tissue
      (3) Bevel facing the apex of the tooth
   e. Slowly inject a few drops of local anesthetic as the needle enters soft tissue, and advance the needle until contact with bone is made.
   f. While applying pressure to the syringe, push the needle slightly deeper (1 to 2 mm) into the interdental septum.

g. Deposit 0.2 to 0.4 mL of local anesthetic in not less than 20 seconds.
   (1) With a conventional syringe, the thickness of the rubber plunger is equivalent to 0.2 mL.
h. Two important items indicate success of the intraseptal injection:
   (1) Significant resistance to the deposition of solution
      (a) This is especially noticeable when a conventional syringe is used. Resistance is similar to that felt with nasopalatine and PDL injections.
      (b) Anesthetic solution should not come back into the patient's mouth. If this occurs, repeat the injection with the needle slightly deeper.
   (2) Ischemia of soft tissues adjacent to the injection site (although noted with all local anesthetic solutions, this is more prominent with local anesthetics containing a vasoconstrictor)
i. Repeat the injection as needed during the surgical procedure.

Signs and Symptoms

1. As with the PDL injection, no objective symptoms ensure adequate anesthesia. The anesthetized area is too circumscribed.
2. Subjective: Ischemia of soft tissues is noted at the injection site.
3. Subjective: Resistance to the injection of solution is felt.

Safety Feature. Intravascular injection is extremely unlikely to occur.

Precautions

1. Do not inject into infected tissue.
2. Do not inject rapidly (not faster than 20 seconds).
3. Do not inject too much solution (0.2 to 0.4 mL per site).

Failures of Anesthesia

1. Infected or inflamed tissues. Changes in tissue pH minimize the effectiveness of the local anesthetic.
2. Solution not retained in tissue. To correct: Advance the needle further into the septal bone and readminister 0.2 to 0.4 mL.

Complication. Postinjection pain is unlikely to develop because the injection site is within the area of surgical treatment. Saadoun and Malamed demonstrated that postsurgical periodontal discomfort after the use of intraseptal anesthesia is no greater than after a regional nerve block.[42]

Duration of Expected Anesthesia. The duration of osseous and soft tissue anesthesia is variable after an intraseptal injection. Using an epinephrine concentration of 1:50,000, Saadoun and Malamed found pain control and hemostasis adequate for completion of the planned procedure without reinjection in most patients.[42] However, some patients require a second intraseptal injection.

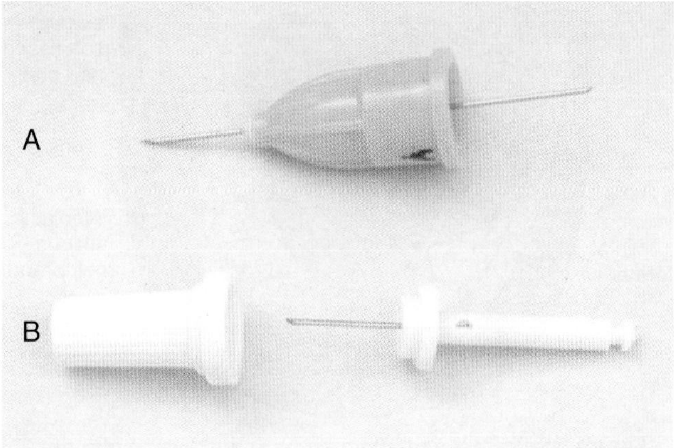

Figure 15-10. Intraosseous anesthesia—Stabident. Components: **A,** Needle. **B,** Perforator.

Intraosseous Injection

Deposition of local anesthetic solution into the interproximal bone between two teeth has been practiced in dentistry since the start of the twentieth century.[23] Originally, IO anesthesia necessitated the use of a half-round bur to provide entry into interseptal bone that had been surgically exposed. Once the hole had been made, a needle would be inserted into this hole and local anesthetic deposited.

The PDL and intraseptal injections previously described are variations of IO anesthesia. With the PDL injection, local anesthetic enters interproximal bone through the periodontal tissues surrounding a tooth, whereas in intraseptal anesthesia, the needle is embedded into the interproximal bone without the use of a burr.

In recent years, the IO technique has been modified with the introduction of several devices* that simplify the procedure. The Stabident System was introduced, followed later by the X-Tip, and most recently by the IntraFlow. The Stabident System consists of two parts: a perforator—a burr that perforates the cortical plate of bone with a conventional slow-speed contra-angle handpiece—and an 8-mm long, 27-gauge needle that is inserted into this predrilled hole for anesthetic administration (Fig. 15-10).

Experience with the IO technique has shown that perforation of the interproximal bone is almost always entirely atraumatic. However, some persons initially had difficulty placing the needle of the local anesthetic syringe back into the previously drilled hole in the interproximal bone. Introduction of the X-Tip eliminated this problem. The X-Tip is composed of a drill and a guide sleeve (Fig. 15-11). The drill leads the guide sleeve through the cortical plate of bone, after which it is separated and withdrawn. The guide sleeve remains in the bone and easily accepts a 27-gauge short

*Stabident Local Anesthesia System, Fairfax Dental, Inc., Miami, Fla; www.stabident.com.
X-Tip: (1) CE-Magic, (2) Dentsply, Victoria, Australia; www.dentsply.com.
IntraFlow, IntraVantage, Inc., Plymouth, Minn; www.intravantageinc.com.

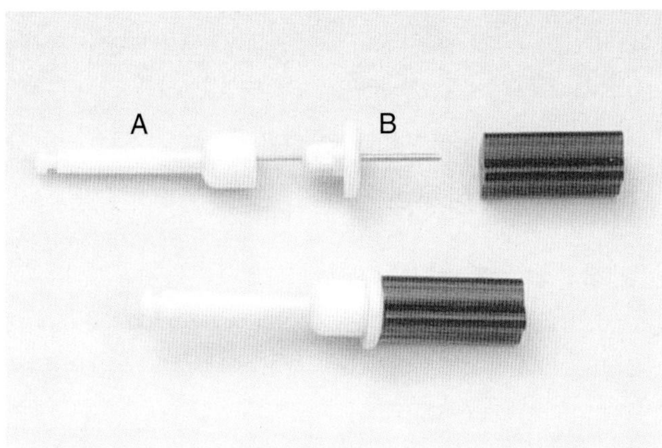

Figure 15-11. Intraosseous anesthesia—X-Tip. Components: *A*, Drill. *B*, Guide sleeve.

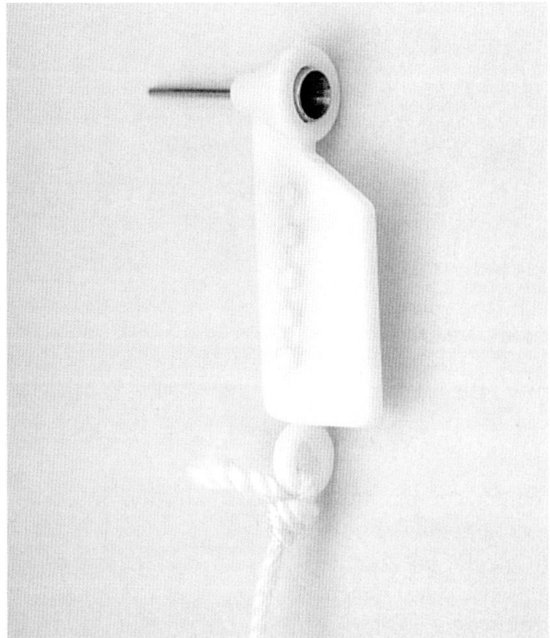

Figure 15-12. Alternative Stabident System. Guide sleeve remains in hole in bone, permitting easy access for needle.

needle, which is recommended by the manufacturer for injection of local anesthetic into the cancellous bone. The Alternative Stabident System introduced shortly thereafter eliminated the problem of locating the "hole" by inserting a conical-shaped "guide sleeve" into the hole. The 27-gauge short needle could then be easily placed into the hole (Fig. 15-12).

The IntraFlow HTP Anesthesia Delivery System, which was recently introduced, combines the two steps previously described into one (Fig. 15-13).[3] The IntraFlow handpiece is attached to a standard four-hole air hose on a treatment room delivery unit and is controlled by a foot rheostat. The IntraFlow is a specially modified slow-speed handpiece that consists of four main parts:

1. A needle or drill that makes the perforation through the bone and delivers the local anesthetic
2. A transfuser that acts as a conduit from the local anesthetic cartridge to the needle or drill
3. A latch tip or clutch that drives and governs the rotation of the needle or drill
4. A motor or infusion drive that powers the rotation of the needle or drill and, while holding the local anesthetic cartridge in place, powers the infusion plunger. A 24-gauge dual-beveled needle is provided.

The IO injection technique can provide anesthesia of a single tooth or multiple teeth in a quadrant. To a significant degree, the area of anesthesia is dependent on both the site of injection and the volume of local anesthetic deposited. It is recommended that 0.45 to 0.6 mL of anesthetic be administered when treatment is to be confined to not more than one or two teeth. Greater volumes (up to 1.8 mL) may be administered when treatment of multiple teeth in one quadrant is contemplated. The IO injection may be used when six or eight mandibular anterior teeth (e.g., first premolar to first premolar bilaterally) are managed. Bilateral IO injections are necessary, the perforation being made between the canine and the first premolar on both sides. This provides pulpal anesthesia of eight teeth. It should be remembered, however, that the incisive nerve block provides pulpal anesthesia of these same teeth without the need for perforation of bone.

Because IO injections deposit local anesthetic into a vascular site, it is suggested that the volume of local anesthetic delivered be kept to the recommended minimum to avoid possible overdose.[43] In addition, because of the high incidence of palpitations noted when vasopressor-containing local anesthetics are used, a "plain" local anesthetic is recommended in the IO injection. However, discussion with endodontists who use IO frequently indicates that the quality and depth of anesthesia are not as great when plain local anesthetics are used.

Other Common Names. None.

Nerves Anesthetized. Terminal nerve endings at the site of injection and in adjacent soft and hard tissues.

Areas Anesthetized. Bone, soft tissue, and root structure in the area of injection (Fig. 15-14).

Indication. Pain control for dental treatment on single or multiple teeth in a quadrant.

Contraindication. Infection or severe inflammation at the injection site.

Advantages

1. Lack of lip and tongue anesthesia (appreciated by most patients)
2. Atraumatic
3. Immediate (<30 seconds) onset of action
4. Few postoperative complications

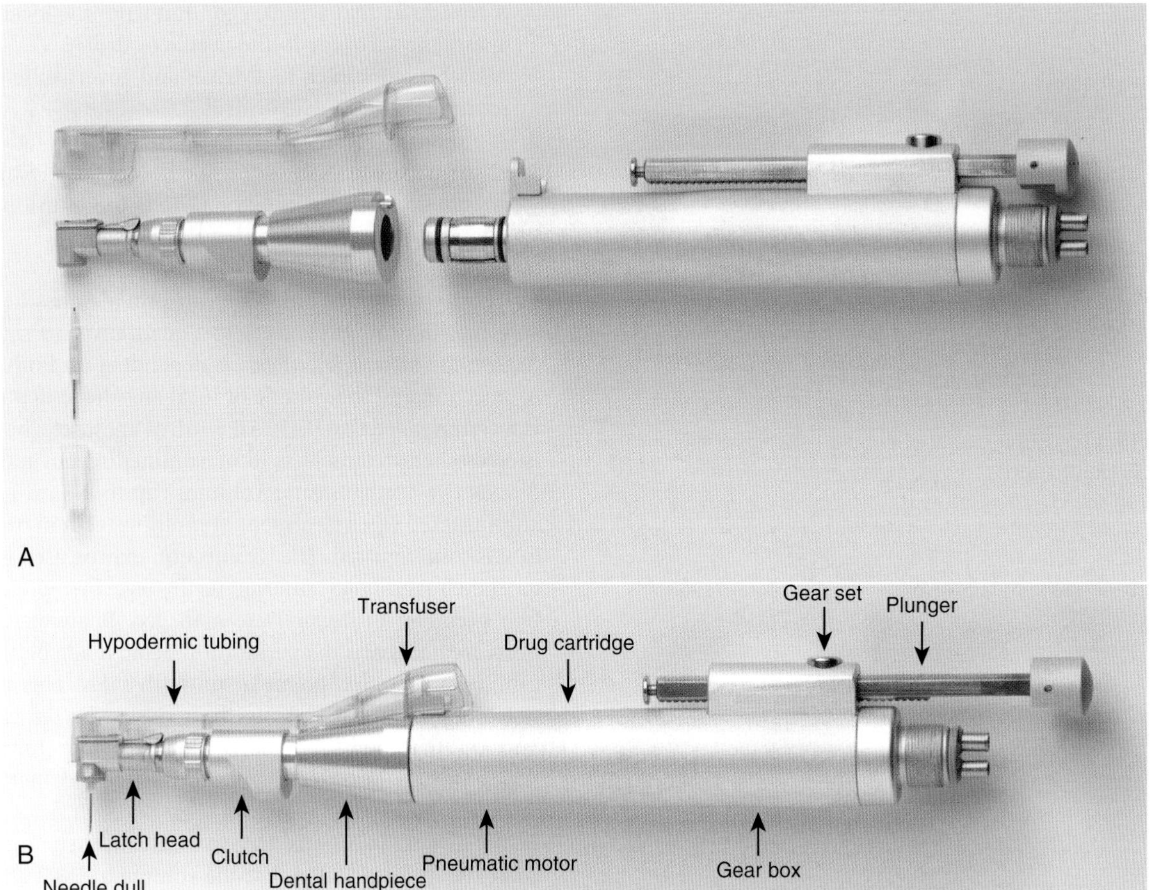

Figure 15-13. Intraosseous anesthesia—IntraFlow HTP Anesthesia Delivery System. Components: **A,** Disassembled. **B,** Assembled.

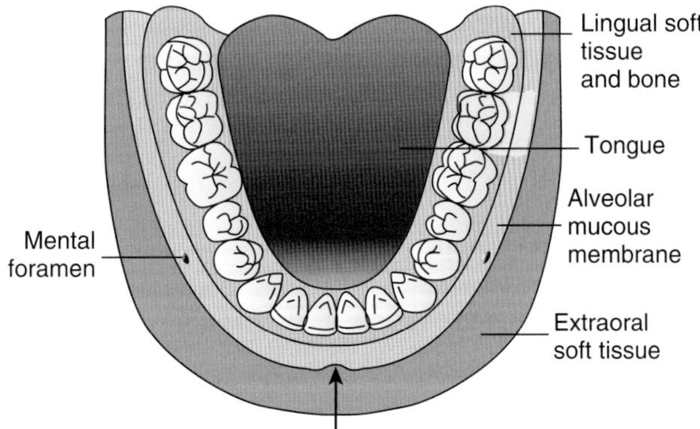

Figure 15-14. Area anesthetized by intraosseus injection.

Disadvantages

1. Requires a special syringe (e.g., Stabident System, X-Tip, IntraFlow)
2. Bitter taste of the anesthetic drug (if leakage occurs)
3. Occasional (rare) difficulty in placing anesthetic needle into predrilled hole (primarily in mandibular second and third molar regions)
4. High occurrence of palpitations when vasopressor-containing local anesthetic is used

Positive Aspiration. 0%.

Alternatives

1. PDL injection, in the absence of infection or severe periodontal involvement
2. Intraseptal injection
3. Supraperiosteal injection
4. Regional nerve block

Technique*

1. Selection of site for injection
   a. Lateral perforation
      (1) At a point 2 mm apical to the intersection of lines drawn horizontally along the gingival margins of the teeth and a vertical line through the interdental papilla
      (2) The site should be located distal to the tooth to be treated, if possible, although this technique provides anesthesia in most cases when injected anterior to the tooth being treated.
      (3) Avoid injecting in the mental foramen area (increased risk of nerve damage).
   b. Vertical perforation (for edentulous areas)
      (1) Perforate at a point on the alveolar crest mesial or distal to the treatment area (also called the *crestal anesthesia technique*).

*From the instruction manual, CE-Magic, 1-877-478-9748; www.CE-Magic.com.

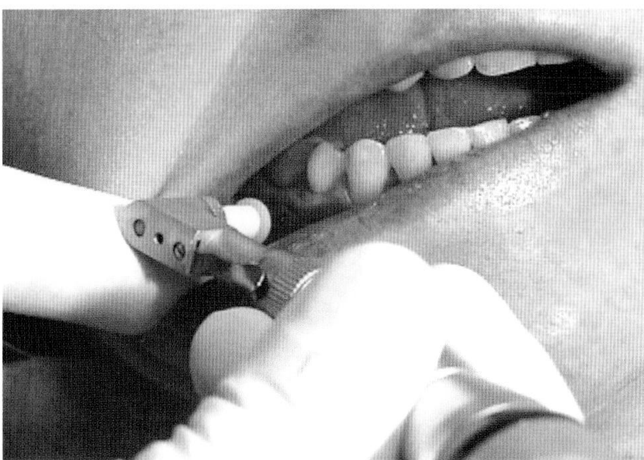

Figure 15-15. Drill hole using a gentle "pecking" motion.

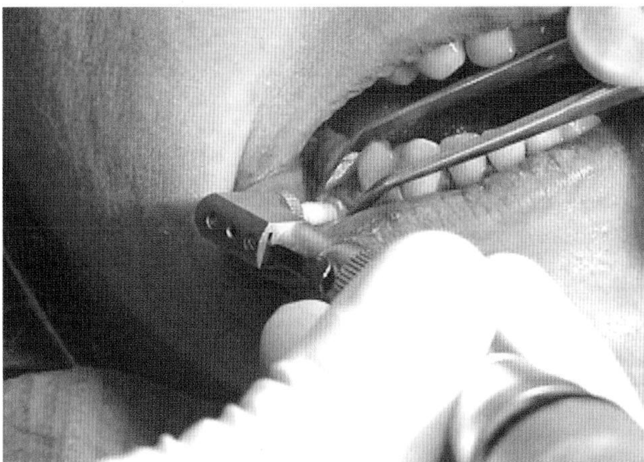

Figure 15-16. Hold the guide sleeve in place as the drill is withdrawn.

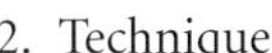

2. Technique
   a. Remove the X-Tip from its sterile vial.
      (1) Hold the protective cover as you insert the X-Tip onto the slow speed handpiece (20,000 rpm).
   b. Prepare soft tissues at perforation site:
      (1) Prepare tissue at the injection site with 2 × 2 inch sterile gauze.
      (2) Apply topical anesthetic to the injection site for minimum of 1 minute.
      (3) Place bevel of needle against gingiva, injecting a small volume of local anesthetic until blanching occurs.
      (4) Check soft tissue anesthesia using a cotton pliers.
         (a) Cotton pliers leave a slight dimple marking of the perforation site.
      (5) Inject a few drops of local anesthetic into the dimple.
   c. Perforation of the cortical plate
      (1) While holding the perforator perpendicular to the cortical plate, gently push the perforator through the attached gingiva until its tip rests against bone (without activating the handpiece).
      (2) Activate the handpiece, using a gentle "pecking" motion on the perforator until a sudden loss of resistance is felt. Cortical bone will be perforated within 2 seconds (Fig. 15-15).
      (3) Hold the guide sleeve in place as the drill is withdrawn (Fig. 15-16). Withdraw the perforator and dispose of it safely (sharps container).
         (a) The guide sleeve remains in place until you are certain you have adequate anesthesia.
   d. Injection into cancellous bone:
      (1) It is easy to insert the needle into the hole when a short needle is used (Fig. 15-17).
      (2) Press the tapered needle gently against the guide sleeve to minimize local anesthetic leakage.
         (a) Compress a cotton roll or 2 × 2 sterile gauze against the mucosa to absorb any excess local anesthetic.
      (3) Slowly and gently inject the local anesthetic solution.

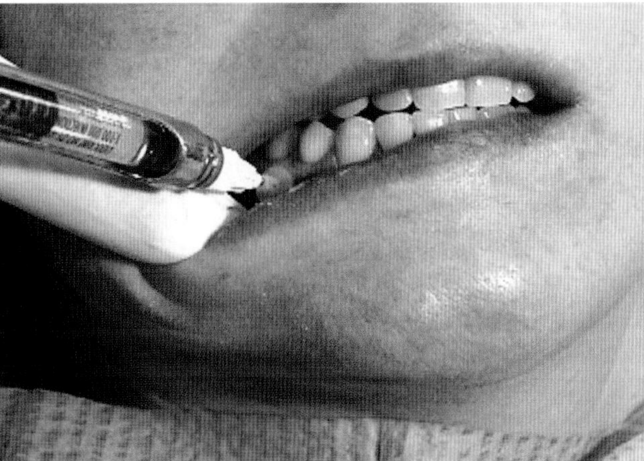

Figure 15-17. Insert needle into guide sleeve and inject local anesthetic solution.

   e. X-Tip doses: Recommended dosages for the X-Tip are the same for each local anesthetic solution as is recommended for other injections.
   f. Stabident doses (Table 15-1)
   g. Recommended technique for the IntraFlow IO syringe system is presented in Box 15-2.

Signs and Symptoms

1. Subjective: Ischemia of soft tissues at the injection site
2. Objective: Use of electrical pulp testing with no response from tooth with maximal EPT output (80/80)

Safety Feature. Intravascular injection is extremely unlikely, although the area injected into is quite vascular. Slow injection of the recommended volume of solution is important to keeping IO anesthesia safe.

Precautions

1. Do not inject into infected tissue.
2. Do not inject rapidly.
3. Do not inject too much solution. (See recommended dosages in Table 15-1.)

TABLE 15-1
Stabident Dosages*

To Anesthetize	Injection Site	Dose (number of 1.8 mL cartridges)
STABIDENT MANDIBULAR DOSAGES		
One tooth	Immediately distal OR immediately mesial	¼ to ⅓
Two adjacent teeth	Between the two teeth OR immediately distal to the more distal tooth	⅓ to ½
Three adjacent teeth	Immediately distal to the middle tooth	½
Six front teeth plus the first premolars (i.e., total of eight teeth)	Give two injections, one on each side, between the canine and the first premolar	½ on each side (total of 1)
STABIDENT MAXILLARY DOSAGES		
One tooth	Immediately distal OR immediately mesial	¼
Two adjacent teeth	Between the two teeth	¼
Four adjacent teeth (e.g., 1, 2, 3, and 4)	Midway (e.g., two teeth distal and two teeth mesial to the injection site)	½
Up to eight teeth on one side	Midway (e.g., four teeth distal and four teeth mesial to the injection site)	1

*From www.stabident.com/manualall.htm.

BOX 15-2 Recommended Technique for the IntraFlow Intraosseous Syringe System

1. Select injection site, and then prepare tissue with topical anesthetic and soft tissue anesthesia.
2. Depress foot pedal to perforate tissue and bone, and begin injection.
3. Engage clutch when full depth of perforation is reached to stop rotation of the perforator (see Fig. 15-12).
4. Continue injecting the anesthetic.
5. Disengage the clutch to start rotation and remove drill.
6. Wait 1 minute, then begin the procedure.

4. Do not use a vasopressor-containing local anesthetic unless necessary, and then only 1:200,000 or 1:100,000. Try to avoid use of 1:50,000 epinephrine.

Failures of Anesthesia

1. Infected or inflamed tissues. Changes in tissue pH minimize the effectiveness of the anesthetic.
2. Inability to perforate cortical bone. If cortical bone is not perforated within 2 seconds, it is recommended that drilling be stopped and an alternative site be used.

Complications

1. Palpitation: This reaction frequently occurs when a vasopressor-containing local anesthetic is used. To minimize its occurrence, use a "plain" local anesthetic, if possible, or the most dilute epinephrine concentration available (e.g., 1:200,000).
2. Postinjection pain is unlikely after IO anesthesia. The use of mild analgesics (nonsteroidal anti-inflammatory drugs) is recommended if discomfort occurs in the postinjection period.

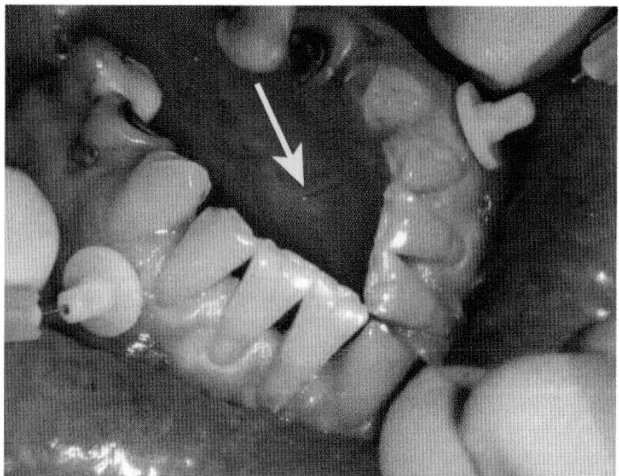

Figure 15-18. Accidental perforation of lingual plate *(arrow)*.

3. Fistula formation at the site of perforation has been reported on occasions. In most instances, this can be prevented by employing a gentle "pecking" motion with the handpiece as the perforator goes through the cortical plate of bone. Application of constant pressure against the bone presumably leads to the buildup of heat with possible bony necrosis and fistula formation.
4. Separation of the perforator or cannula: Rare, but reported. The metal shaft of the burr or cannula separates and remains in bone. Usually easy to remove with a hemostat
5. Perforation of lingual plate of bone (Fig. 15-18). Prevented by proper technique

Duration of Expected Anesthesia. Pulpal anesthesia of between 15 and 30 minutes can be expected. If a vasopressor-containing solution is used, the duration approaches 30 minutes. If a plain solution is used, a 15-minute duration is usual. The depth of anesthesia is greater with a vasopressor-containing local anesthetic.

INTRAPULPAL INJECTION

Obtaining profound anesthesia in the pulpally involved tooth was a significant problem before the rediscovery of IO anesthesia. Specifically the problem occurred with mandibular molars, because few alternative anesthetic techniques were available with which the doctor could obtain profound anesthesia. Maxillary teeth usually are anesthetized with a supraperiosteal injection or a nerve block such as the posterior superior alveolar (PSA), anterior superior alveolar (ASA), anterior middle superior alveolar (AMSA), or (rarely) maxillary (second division; V_2) nerve block. Mandibular teeth anterior to the molars are anesthetized with the incisive nerve block. Anesthesia of mandibular molars, however, commonly is limited to nerve block anesthesia, which may prove to be ineffective in the presence of infection and inflammation. Methods of obtaining anesthesia for endodontics are described in Chapter 16.

Deposition of local anesthetic directly into the coronal portion of the pulp chamber of a pulpally involved tooth provides effective anesthesia for pulpal extirpation and instrumentation where other techniques have failed. The intrapulpal injection may be used on any tooth when difficulty in providing profound pain control exists, but from a practical view, it is necessary most commonly on mandibular molars.

The intrapulpal injection provides pain control through both the pharmacologic action of the local anesthetic and applied pressure. This technique may be used once the pulp chamber is exposed surgically or pathologically.

Other Common Names. None.

Nerves Anesthetized. Terminal nerve endings at the site of injection in the pulp chamber and canals of the involved tooth.

Areas Anesthetized. Tissues within the injected tooth.

Indication. When pain control is necessary for pulpal extirpation or other endodontic treatment in the absence of adequate anesthesia from other techniques.

Contraindication. None. The intrapulpal injection may be the only local anesthetic technique available in some clinical situations.

Advantages

1. Lack of lip and tongue anesthesia (appreciated by most patients)
2. Minimum volumes of anesthetic solution necessary
3. Immediate onset of action
4. Very few postoperative complications

Disadvantages

1. Traumatic
   a. The intrapulpal injection is associated with a brief period of pain as anesthetic is deposited.
2. Bitter taste of the anesthetic drug (if leakage occurs)
3. May be difficult to enter certain root canals
   a. Bending of the needle may be necessary
4. A small opening into the pulp chamber is needed for optimum effectiveness.
   a. Large areas of decay make it more difficult to achieve profound anesthesia with the intrapulpal injection.

Positive Aspiration. 0%.

Alternatives. IO. However, when IO fails, intrapulpal injection may be the only viable alternative to provide clinically adequate pain control.

Technique

1. Insert a 25- or 27-gauge short or long needle into the pulp chamber or the root canal as needed (Fig. 15-19).
2. Ideally, wedge the needle firmly into the pulp chamber or root canal.

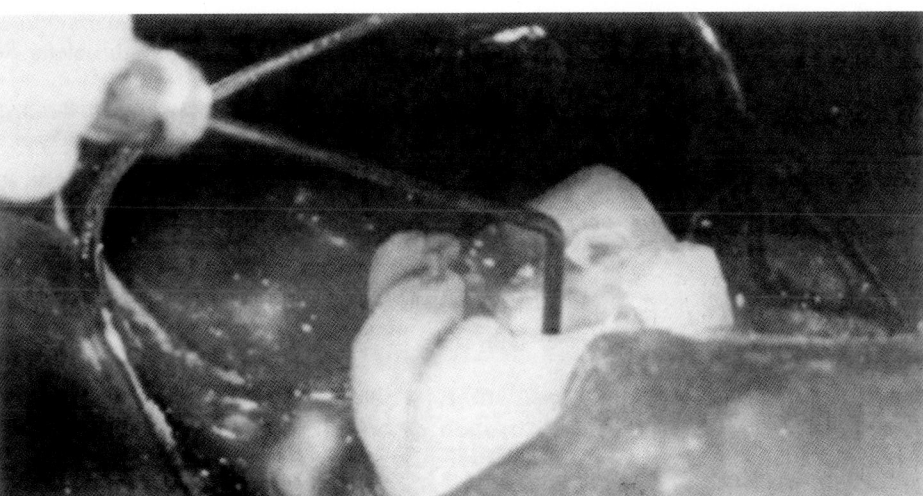

Figure 15-19. For the intrapulpal injection, a 25-gauge 1 or 1⅝ inch needle is inserted into the pulp chamber or a specific root canal. Bending the needle may be necessary to gain access. (From Cohen S, Burns RC: Pathways of the pulp, ed 8, St Louis, 2001, Mosby.)

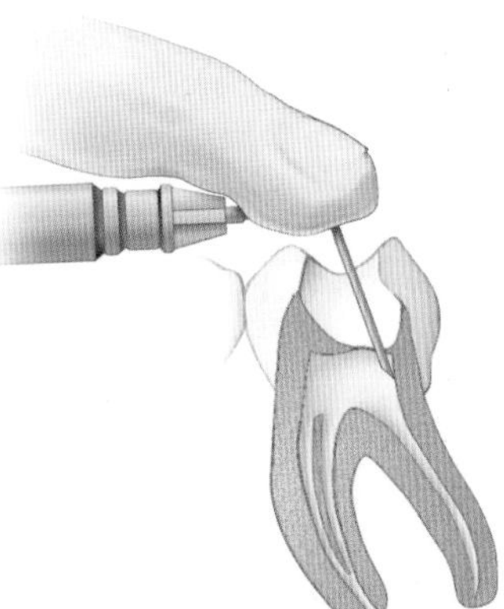

Figure 15-20. The needle may have to be bent to gain access to a canal. (Modified from Cohen S, Burns RC: Pathways of the pulp, ed 8, St Louis, 2001, Mosby.)

   a. Occasionally, the needle does not fit snugly into the canal. In this situation, the anesthetic can be deposited in the chamber or canal. Anesthesia in this case is produced only by the pharmacologic action of the local; there is no pressure anesthesia.
3. Deposit anesthetic solution under pressure.
   a. A small volume of anesthetic (0.2 to 0.3 mL) is necessary for successful intrapulpal anesthesia, if the anesthetic stays within the tooth. In many situations, the anesthetic simply flows back out of the tooth into the aspirator (vacuum) tip.
4. Resistance to injection of the drug should be felt.
5. Bend the needle, if necessary, to gain access to the pulp chamber (Fig. 15-20).
   a. Although there is a greater risk of breakage with a bent needle, this is not a problem during intrapulpal anesthesia, because the needle is inserted into the tooth itself, not into soft tissues. Retrieval is relatively simple if the needle breaks.
6. When the intrapulpal injection is performed properly, a brief period of sensitivity (ranging from mild to very painful) usually accompanies the injection. Pain relief usually occurs immediately thereafter, permitting instrumentation to proceed atraumatically.
7. Instrumentation may begin approximately 30 seconds after the injection is given.

Signs and Symptoms
1. As with PDL, intraseptal, and IO injections, no subjective symptoms ensure adequate anesthesia. The area is too circumscribed.
2. Objective: The endodontically involved tooth may be treated painlessly.

Safety Features
1. Intravascular injection is extremely unlikely to occur.
2. Small volumes of anesthetic are administered.

Precautions
1. Do not inject into infected tissue.
2. Do not inject rapidly (not less than 20 seconds).
3. Do not inject too much solution (0.2 to 0.3 mL).

Failures of Anesthesia
1. Infected or inflamed tissues. Changes in tissue pH minimize the effectiveness of the anesthetic. However, intrapulpal anesthesia invariably works to provide effective pain control.
2. Solution not retained in tissue. To correct: Try to advance the needle farther into the pulp chamber or root canal, and readminister 0.2 to 0.3 mL of anesthetic drug.

Complication. Discomfort during the injection of anesthetic. The patient may experience a brief period of intense discomfort as the injection of the anesthetic drug is started. Within a second (literally), the tissue is anesthetized and the discomfort ceases. The use of inhalation sedation (nitrous oxide or oxygen) can help to minimize or alter the feeling experienced.

Duration of Expected Anesthesia. The duration of anesthesia is variable after intrapulpal injection. In most instances, the duration is adequate to permit atraumatic extirpation of the pulpal tissues.

MANDIBULAR INFILTRATION IN ADULTS

Providing effective pain control is one of the most important aspects of dental care. Indeed, patients rate a dentist "who does not hurt" and one who can "give painless injections" as meeting the second and first most important criteria used in evaluating dentists.[44] Unfortunately, the ability to attain consistently profound anesthesia for dental procedures in the mandible of adult patients has proved extremely elusive. This is even more of a problem when infected teeth are involved, primarily mandibular molars. Anesthesia of maxillary teeth on the other hand, although on occasion difficult to achieve, is rarely an insurmountable problem. Reasons for this, as discussed in Chapter 12, include the fact that the cortical plate of bone overlying the maxillary teeth is normally thin, thus allowing the local anesthetic drug to diffuse when administered by supraperiosteal injection (infiltration). Additionally, relatively simple nerve blocks, such as the PSA, MSA, ASA (infraorbital), and AMSA, are available as alternatives to infiltration. Maxillary anesthesia technique was discussed in Chapter 13.

It is commonly stated that the significantly higher failure rate for mandibular anesthesia is related to the thickness of the cortical plate of bone in the adult mandible. Indeed it is generally acknowledged that mandibular infiltration is successful where the patient has a full primary dentition (see discussion of pediatric local anesthesia in Chapter 16).[45,46] Once a mixed dentition develops, it is a general rule of teaching that the mandibular cortical plate of bone has thickened to the degree that infiltration might not be effective, leading to the recommendation that "mandibular block" techniques should now be employed.[47]

A second difficulty with the traditional Halsted approach to the inferior alveolar nerve (e.g., IANB, "mandibular block") is the absence of consistent landmarks. Multiple authors have described numerous approaches to this oftentimes elusive nerve.[48-50] Reported failure rates for the IANB are commonly high, ranging from 31% and 41% in mandibular second and first molars to 42%, 38%, and 46% in second and first premolars and canines, respectively,[51] and 81% in lateral incisors.[52]

Not only is the inferior alveolar nerve elusive, studies using ultrasound[53] and radiography[54,55] to accurately locate the inferior alveolar neurovascular bundle or the mandibular foramen revealed that accurate needle location did not guarantee successful pain control.[56] The central core theory best explains this problem.[57,58] Nerves on the outside of the nerve bundle supply the molar teeth, while nerves on the inside (core fibers) supply the incisor teeth. Therefore the local anesthetic solution deposited near the IAN may diffuse and block the outermost fibers but not those located more centrally, leading to incomplete mandibular anesthesia.

This difficulty in achieving mandibular anesthesia has led to the development of alternative techniques to the traditional (Halsted approach) inferior alveolar nerve block. These have included the Gow-Gates mandibular nerve block, the Akinosi-Vazirani closed-mouth nerve block, the periodontal ligament (PDL, intraligamentary) injection, intraosseous anesthesia, and, most recently, buffered local anesthetics.[59] Although all maintain some advantages over the traditional Halsted approach, none is without its own faults and contraindications.

The ability to provide localized areas of anesthesia by infiltration injection without the need for nerve block injections has a number of benefits. Meechan[60] has enumerated them as follows: (1) technically simple, (2) more comfortable for patients, (3) can provide hemostasis when needed, (4) in many cases obviate the presence of collateral innervation, (5) avoid the risk of potential damage to nerve trunks, (6) lesser risk of intravascular injection, (7) safer in patients with clotting disorders, (8) reduce risk of needle-stick injury, and (9) preinjection application of topical anesthetic masks needle penetration discomfort.

Attempts at mandibular infiltration in adult patients have been made in the past. In a 1976 study of 331 subjects receiving IANB with lidocaine HCl 2% with epinephrine 1:80,000, 23.7% had unsuccessful anesthesia.[61] Supplemental infiltration of 1.0 mL of the same drug on the buccal aspect of the mandible proved successful in 70 of the 79 failures. Of the remaining 9, 7 were successfully anesthetized following additional infiltration of 1.0 mL on the lingual aspect of the mandible.

Yonchak and colleagues investigated infiltration on incisors, reporting 45% success following labial infiltration (lidocaine 2% with 1:100,000 epinephrine) and 50% success with lingual infiltrations of the same solution for lateral incisors, and 63% and 47% for central incisors on labial and lingual infiltration.[62]

Meechan and Ledvinka found similar success rates (50%) on central incisor teeth following labial or lingual infiltration of 1.0 mL of lidocaine 2% with 1:80,000 epinephrine.[63]

In 1990, Haas and coworkers compared mandibular buccal infiltrations for canines with prilocaine HCl versus articaine HCl and found no significant differences.[64] Success rates were 50% for prilocaine and 65% for articaine (both 4% with epinephrine 1:200,000). A second study noted a 63% success rate on mandibular second molars with articaine and 53% with prilocaine (both 4% with epinephrine 1:200,000).[65]

Since the introduction of articaine HCl 4% with epinephrine 1:100,000 into the U.S. dental market in June 2000, numerous anecdotal reports have been received from doctors who claimed that they no longer needed to administer the IANB to work painlessly in the adult mandible. They claimed that mandibular infiltration with articaine HCl was uniformly successful. These claims were initially met with skepticism. In the past 5 years, four well-designed clinical trials have been reported comparing infiltration in the adult mandible of articaine HCl 4% with epinephrine 1:100,000 versus lidocaine 2% with epinephrine 1:100,000 or 1:80,000.[7,8,52,66]

Following is a summary of these papers.

Kanaa MD, Whitworth JM, Corbett IP, Meechan JG: Articaine and lidocaine mandibular buccal infiltration anesthesia: a prospective randomized double-blind cross-over study, J Endod 32:296–298, 2006[8]

Design. Infiltrations were administered to 31 subjects in the buccal fold adjacent to the mandibular first molar. A dose of 1.8 mL was administered at a rate of 0.9 mL per 15 seconds. The order of drug administration was randomized, with the second injection administered at least 1 week after the first. The same investigator administered all injections. Electrical pulp testing (EPT) was used to determine pulpal sensitivity. Baseline readings were obtained, and EPT was repeated once every 2 minutes after injection for 30 minutes. If no response (to maximal EPT stimulation of 80 μA) occurred, the number of episodes of no response at maximal stimulation was recorded. The criterion for successful anesthesia was no volunteer response to maximal stimulation on two or more consecutive episodes of testing. (This had been established as the criterion for success in many previous clinical trials.)

Results. The total number of episodes of no sensation on maximal stimulation in first molars over the period of the trial (32 minutes) was greater for articaine (236 episodes) than for lidocaine (129) ($P < .001$). Twenty (64.5%) subjects experienced anesthetic success following articaine, whereas 12 (38.7%) did so with lidocaine ($P < .08$). The design of the trial allowed for a maximal possible duration of anesthesia of 28 minutes. Six subjects receiving articaine achieved 28 minutes of anesthesia compared with two for lidocaine.

Discussion. The difference between articaine and lidocaine was most obvious toward the end of the study period. The percentage of patients showing no response at maximal stimulation was reduced at all reference points after 22 minutes with lidocaine. With articaine, however, the greatest percentage of nonresponders was noted at the end of the trial (32 minutes).

Conclusion. It was noted that 4% articaine with epinephrine was more effective than 2% lidocaine with epinephrine in producing pulpal anesthesia in lower molars following buccal infiltration.

Robertson D, Nusstein J, Reader A, Beck M, McCartney M: The anesthetic efficacy of articaine in buccal infiltration of mandibular posterior teeth, J Am Dent Assoc 138:1104–1112, 2007.[7]

Design. Sixty blinded subjects randomly received buccal infiltration injections of 1.8 mL of 2% lidocaine with epinephrine 1:100,000 and 4% articaine with epinephrine 1:100,000 at two separate appointments at least 1 week apart. Each subject served as his or her own control. Sixty infiltrations were administered on the right side and 60 on the left side. For the second infiltration in each subject, the investigator used the same side randomly chosen for the first infiltration. The teeth chosen for evaluation were the first and second molars and the first and second premolars. The same investigator administered all injections. Before injections were administered, baseline values were determined on the experimental teeth with EPT. A single infiltration was administered buccal to the first mandibular molar, bisecting the approximate location of the mesial and distal roots. The 1.8 mL was deposited over a period of 1 minute. One minute after injection, the first and second molars were pulp tested. At 2 minutes, the premolars were tested. At 3 minutes, the control canine (contralateral side) was tested. This testing cycle was repeated every 3 minutes for 60 minutes. Complete absence of sensation to maximal EPT stimulation on two or more consecutive readings was the criterion for successful anesthesia. Onset of anesthesia was defined as the time at which the first of two consecutive no responses to EPT of 80 occurred.

Results. Articaine was significantly better than lidocaine in achieving pulpal anesthesia in each of the four teeth ($P < .0001$ for all four teeth). Table 15-2 summarizes these findings.

The onset of successful anesthesia was significantly faster for articaine than for lidocaine for all four teeth tested (Table 15-3).

Discussion. The exact mechanism of the increased efficacy of articaine is not known. One theory relates to the 4% concentration of articaine versus the 2% lidocaine solution. However, Potocnik and associates found that 4% and 2% articaine were superior to 2% lidocaine in blocking nerve conduction.[67] A second theory is that the thiophene ring of articaine enables it to diffuse more effectively than the benzene ring found in other local anesthetics.

Regarding onset of anesthesia, previous studies with onset of lidocaine following IANB found onset times ranging from 8 to 11 minutes for the first molar and from 8 to 12 minutes for the first premolar.[68-73] Articaine provided a more rapid onset of pulpal anesthesia for all tested teeth than was provided by IANB. However, pulpal anesthesia declined steadily over the 60 minute test period. Therefore, if profound pulpal anesthesia is required for 60 minutes, buccal infiltration of 4% articaine with epinephrine 1:100,000 will not provide the duration needed because of declining pulpal anesthesia.

Conclusion. Buccal infiltration of the first mandibular molar with 1.8 mL of 4% articaine with epinephrine 1:100,000 is significantly better than similar infiltration of 2% lidocaine with epinephrine 1:100,000 in achieving pulpal anesthesia in mandibular posterior teeth. Clinicians should keep in mind that pulpal anesthesia will likely decline slowly over 60 minutes.

TABLE 15-2
Summary of Articaine vs. Lidocaine Success

Tooth	Articaine % Success	Lidocaine % Success
Second molar	75	45
First molar	87	57
Second premolar	92	67
First premolar	86	61

[1]P < .0001 for all teeth tested.

TABLE 15-3
Results of the Onset of Successful Anesthesia, Articaine vs. Lidocaine

Tooth	Articaine Onset (min) ± Standard Deviation	Lidocaine Onset (min) ± Standard Deviation	*P* Value
Second molar	4.6 ± 4.0	11.1 ± 9.5	.0001
First molar	4.2 ± 3.1	7.7 ± 4.3	.0002
Second premolar	4.3 ± 2.3	6.9 ± 6.6	.0014
First premolar	4.7 ± 2.4	6.3 ± 3.1	.0137

Haase A, Reader A, Nusstein J, Beck M, Drum M: Comparing anesthetic efficacy of articaine versus lidocaine as a supplemental buccal infiltration of the mandibular first molar after an inferior alveolar nerve block, J Am Dent Assoc 139:1228–1235, 2008.[66]

Design. Seventy-three subjects participated in a prospective, randomized, double-blinded, crossover study comparing the degree of pulpal anesthesia achieved by means of a mandibular buccal infiltration of two anesthetic solutions: 4% articaine with epinephrine 1:100,000, and 2% lidocaine with epinephrine 1:100,000, following an IANB with 4% articaine with epinephrine 1:100,000. The subject served as his/her own control. The side chosen for the first infiltration was used again for the second infiltration. Injections were administered at least 1 week apart. The same investigator administered all injections. An EPT was used to test the first molar for anesthesia in 3 minute cycles for 60 minutes. The IANB was administered over 60 seconds. Fifteen minutes after completion of the IANB, the infiltration was administered buccal to the first mandibular molar, bisecting the approximate location of the mesial and distal roots. The 1.8 mL was deposited over a period of 1 minute. Sixteen minutes after completion of the IANB (1 minute following the infiltration), EPT testing of the first molar was performed. At 3 minutes, the contralateral canine was tested. This cycle was repeated every 3 minutes for 60 minutes. Anesthesia was considered successful when two consecutive EPT readings of 80 were obtained within 10 minutes of the IANB and infiltration injection, and the 80 reading was maintained continuously through the 60th minute.

Results. The articaine formulation was significantly better than the lidocaine formulation with regard to anesthetic success: 88% versus 71% for lidocaine ($P < .01$), with anesthesia developing within 10 minutes after IANB and buccal infiltration, sustaining the 80 reading on the EPT continuously for the 60 minute testing period.

Discussion. Anesthetic success was significantly better with the 4% articaine formulation than the 2% lidocaine formulation. Both anesthetic formulations demonstrated a gradual increase in pulpal anesthesia. This is likely a result of the effect of the infiltrations' overcoming failure or the slow onset of anesthesia following IANB. Therefore, for a maximum effect with 4% articaine infiltration, a waiting time is required before onset of pulpal anesthesia is achieved. It may be prudent to wait for signs of lip numbness before administering the infiltration. Without an effective IANB, buccal infiltration of articaine alone has a relatively short duration (see previous two citations). A fairly high percentage of patients receiving the articaine infiltration maintained pulpal anesthesia through the 50th minute. Articaine infiltration demonstrated a decline in the incidence of pulpal anesthesia after the 52nd minute. Because most dental procedures require less than 50 minutes for completion, this injection protocol should prove successful for most dental treatments. The 2% lidocaine demonstrated a decline after the 60th minute.

Conclusion. Buccal infiltration of the first molar with a cartridge of 4% articaine with epinephrine 1:100,000 resulted in a significantly higher success rate (88%) than was attained with buccal infiltration of a cartridge of 2% lidocaine with epinephrine 1:100,000 (71%) after an IANB with 4% articaine with epinephrine 1:100,000.

Kanaa MD, Whitworth JM, Corbett IP, Meechan JG: Articaine buccal infiltration enhances the effectiveness of lidocaine inferior alveolar nerve block, Int Endod J 42:238–246, 2009.[52]

Design. The goal of this study was to compare mandibular tooth anesthesia following lidocaine IANB with and without supplementary articaine buccal infiltration. In this prospective randomized, double-blind, crossover study, 36 subjects received two IANB injections with 2.2 mL lidocaine 2% with epinephrine 1:80,000 over two visits. At one visit, an infiltration of 2.2 mL of articaine 4% with epinephrine 1:100,000 was administered in the mucobuccal fold opposite the mandibular first molar. At the other visit, a dummy injection was performed. At least 1 week separated the two visits. Pulpal anesthesia of first molar, first premolar, and lateral incisor teeth was assessed with an EPT every 2 minutes for the first 10 minutes, and then at 5 minute intervals for 45 minutes post injection. Successful anesthesia was defined as the absence of sensation on two or more consecutive maximal EPT stimulations. The number of episodes of no response to maximal EPT stimulation was also recorded. Onset of pulpal anesthesia was considered the first episode of no response to maximal stimulation (two consecutive readings), whereas duration of anesthesia was taken as the time from the first of at least two consecutive maximal readings with no response until the onset of more than two responses at less than maximal stimulation or the end of the 45 minute test period, whichever was sooner.

Results. IANB with supplemental articaine infiltration produced greater success than IANB alone in first molars (33 vs. 20 subjects, respectively; $P < .001$), premolars (32 vs. 24; $P = .021$), and lateral incisors (28 vs. 7; $P < .001$). Additionally, IANB with articaine supplemental infiltration produced significantly more episodes of no response than IANB alone for first molars (339 vs. 162 cases, respectively; $P < .001$), premolars (333 vs. 197; $P < .001$), and lateral incisors (227 vs. 63; $P < .001$) (Table 15-4).

Discussion. Onset of pulpal anesthesia: In this study, the anesthetic effect for mandibular first molars peaked 25 minutes post injection with the dummy injection versus 6 minutes following articaine infiltration. For first premolars, peak anesthetic effect occurred at 30 minutes post injection versus 8 minutes following articaine infiltration, and for lateral incisors, peak anesthetic effect occurred at 40 minutes

TABLE 15-4
Success of IANB with Supplemental Articaine Infiltration vs. IANB Alone

	First Molar	First Premolar	Lateral Incisor
Success IANB + dummy	55.6%	66.7%	19.4%
Success IANB + infiltration	91.7%	88.9%	77.8%
	(*P* < .001)	(*P* = .021)	(*P* < .001)
Onset (mean) IANB + dummy (minutes)	6.8	8.9	10.9
Onset (mean) IANB + infiltration(minutes)	4.5	4.2	6.9
	(*P* < .06)	(*P* < .002)	(*P* = .40)
Duration of pulpal anesthesia (mean) IANB + dummy (minutes)	29.0	31.3	29.1
Duration of pulpal anesthesia (mean) IANB + infiltration (minutes)	38.8	37.8	30.0
	(*P* < .001)	(*P* = .013)	(*P* = .90)

IANB, Inferior alveolar nerve block.

post injection versus 20 minutes following articaine infiltration in the first molar region.

Duration of Pulpal Anesthesia. The maximum duration of anesthesia possible in this trial was 43 minutes. The duration of pulpal anesthesia was significantly longer for first molars and first premolars but not for lateral incisors (see previous chart).

Conclusions. IANB injection supplemented with articaine by buccal infiltration was more successful than IANB alone for pulpal anesthesia in mandibular teeth. Articaine infiltration increased the duration of pulpal anesthesia in premolar and molar teeth when given in combination with a lidocaine IANB and produced a more rapid onset for premolars.

These four clinical trials clearly demonstrate that articaine given by mandibular buccal infiltration in the mucobuccal fold by the first mandibular molar can provide more successful anesthesia of longer duration to mandibular teeth when administered alone or as a supplement to IANB.

One thing to consider is that in each of these trials, buccal infiltration of articaine was administered adjacent to the first mandibular molar. These trials demonstrated the effectiveness of articaine in improving pulpal anesthesia success rates in molars and premolars. However, success rates and duration of anesthesia were not improved as significantly in lateral incisors—teeth at a distance from the site of local anesthetic deposition.

Meechan JG, Ledvinka JI: Pulpal anaesthesia for mandibular central incisor teeth: a comparison of infiltration and intraligamentary injections, Int Endod J 35:629–634, 2002.[63]

In 2002, Meechan and Ledvinka studied the effect of infiltrating 1.0 mL of 2% lidocaine with 1:80,000 epinephrine buccally or lingually to the mandibular central incisor.[63]

A success rate of 50% was achieved with the buccal or lingual injection site. However, when the injection dose was split (0.5 mL per site) between buccal AND lingual, the success rate increased to a statistically significant 92%.

Jaber A, Al-Baqshi B, Whitworth B, et al: The efficacy of infiltration anesthesia for adult mandibular incisors, J Dent Res 88:Special Issue A (Abstract 702), 2009.[74]

Jaber and colleagues used a split dose (0.9 mL per site) of 2% lidocaine with 1:100,000 epinephrine to confirm this finding.[74]

For buccal infiltration of 1.8 mL alone, successful anesthesia of the central incisor was 77% vs. 97% for the split buccal/lingual dose. Investigators also compared articaine 4% with epinephrine 1:100,000 versus lidocaine 2% with epinephrine 1:100,000 as an anesthetic for infiltration in the anterior mandible and found that articaine was superior to lidocaine in obtaining pulpal anesthesia of the central incisor when infiltrated adjacent to the tooth buccally alone (94%) or with split buccal/lingual injections (97%).

The increased success rate for infiltration in the adult mandibular incisor region is thought to be due to the fact that the cortical plate of bone, both buccal and lingual, is thin and might provide little resistance to infiltration.

SUMMARY AND CONCLUSIONS

Failure rates for profound pulpal anesthesia following the traditional inferior alveolar nerve block (IANB) on non–pulpally involved teeth are quite high. This has led to the development of several alternative techniques, including the Gow-Gates mandibular nerve block, the Akinosi-Vazirani closed-mouth mandibular nerve block, periodontal ligament injection, and intraosseous anesthesia. The introduction of articaine HCl spurred interest in its use by infiltration in the adult mandible.

Initial studies infiltrating articaine in the buccal fold adjacent to the first mandibular molar showed significantly greater success rates compared with lidocaine 2% infiltration (all with epinephrine). Additional studies using articaine mandibular infiltration (by the first molar) as a supplement to IANB (with lidocaine or articaine) demonstrated the same significant increases. In each of these studies, a full cartridge of local anesthetic was administered (1.8 mL [USA] or 2.2 mL [UK]). Further research is needed to determine the minimal volume of LA solution needed to produce the best clinical result. At this time, the recommendation is to administer a full cartridge of articaine 4% with epinephrine 1:100,000 (or 1:200,000) in the mucobuccal fold adjacent to the mandibular first molar when treating molars or premolars in the adult mandible.

When treating mandibular incisors, the recommendation is to administer a split dose of articaine 0.9 mL in the buccal fold adjacent to the tooth being treated and 0.9 mL on the lingual aspect of the same tooth. Splitting of the LA dose is *not* effective in the mandibular molar region.

The articaine mandibular infiltration injection can be repeated later in the dental procedure if pulpal anesthesia begins to resolve and the patient starts to become sensitive.

An electrical pulp tester (EPT) can be used effectively do assess pulpal anesthesia before invasive dental treatment is begun.[7] Studies have demonstrated that the absence of patient response to an 80 reading was an assurance of pulpal anesthesia in vital asymptomatic teeth.[6,75] Two consecutive EPT readings at maximal output (80 μA) 2 or 3 minutes apart is almost always indicative of profound anesthesia. Certosimo and Archer demonstrated that patients who had EPT readings of less than 80 experienced pain during operative procedures in asymptomatic teeth.[6]

References

1. Masselink BH: The advent of painless dentistry, Dent Cosmos 52:868–872, 1910.
2. Magnes GD: Intraosseous anesthesia, Anesth Prog 15:264–267, 1968.
3. Klebber CH: Intraosseous anesthesia: implications, instrumentation and techniques, J Am Dent Assoc 134:487–491, 2003.
4. Brown R: Intraosseous anesthesia: a review, J Calif Dent Assoc 27:785–792, 1999.
5. Weathers A, Jr: Taking the mystery out of endodontics, Part 6. Painless anesthesia for the "hot" tooth, Dent Today 18:90–93, 1999.
6. Certosimo AJ, Archer RD: A clinical evaluation of the electric pulp tester as an indicator of local anesthesia, Oper Dent 21:25–30, 1996
7. Robertson D, Nusstein J, Reader A, et al: The anesthetic efficacy of articaine in buccal infiltration of mandibular posterior teeth, J Am Dent Assoc 138:1104–1112, 2007.
8. Kanaa MD, Whitworth JM, Corbett IP, et al: Articaine and lidocaine mandibular buccal infiltration anesthesia: a prospective randomized double-blind cross-over study, J Endod 32:296–298, 2006.
9. Bethel LP, editor: Dental summary, vol 32, Toledo, Ohio, 1912, Ranson & Randolph, p 167.
10. Fischer G: Local anesthesia in dentistry, ed 3, Philadelphia, 1923, Lea & Febiger, p 197.
11. Illustrated catalogue of dental furniture, instruments, and materials, ed 4, Pittsburgh, 1905, Lee S Smith & Son.
12. Malamed SF: The periodontal ligament (PDL) injection: an alternative to inferior alveolar nerve block, Oral Surg 53:117–121, 1982.
13. Brannstrom M, Lindskog S, Nordenvall KJ: Enamel hypoplasia in permanent teeth induced by periodontal ligament anesthesia of primary teeth, J Am Dent Assoc 109:735–736, 1984.
14. Council on Dental Materials, Instruments, and Equipment: Status report: the periodontal ligament injection, J Am Dent Assoc 106:222–224, 1983.
15. Walton RE, Garnick JJ: The periodontal ligament injection: histologic effects on the periodontium in monkeys, J Endodod 8:22–26, 1982.
16. Nelson PW: Injection system, J Am Dent Assoc 103:692, 1981 (letter).
17. Shepherd PA, Eleazer PD, Clark SJ, et al: Measurement of intraosseous pressures generated by the Wand, high-pressure periodontal ligament syringe, and the Stabident system, J Endodont 27:381–384, 2001.
18. Meechan JG: Supplementary routes to local anaesthesia, Intern Endod J 35:885–896, 2002.
19. Wong JK: Adjuncts to local anesthesia: separating fact from fiction, Can Dent Assoc 67:391–397, 2001.
20. Quinn CL: Injection techniques to anesthetize the difficult tooth, J Calif Dent Assoc 26:665–667, 1998.
21. Hochman M, Chiarello D, Hochman C, et al: Computerized local anesthesia vs. traditional syringe technique: subjective pain response, NY State Dent J 63:24–29, 1997.
22. Cassamani C: Une Nouvelle Technique d'Anesthesia Intraligamentarire [PhD thesis], Paris, 1924.
23. Fischer G: Local anesthesia in dentistry, ed 4, Philadelphia, 1933, Lea & Febiger.
24. Hoffmann-Axtheim W: History of dentistry, Chicago, 1981, Quintessence.
25. Dreyer WP, van Heerden JD, de V Joubert JJ: The route of periodontal ligament injection of local anesthetic solution, J Endod 9:471–474, 1983.
26. Walton RE, Abbott BJ: Periodontal ligament injection: a clinical evaluation, J Am Dent Assoc 103:571–575, 1981.
27. Meechan JG: Intraligamentary anaesthesia, J Dent 20:325–332, 1992.
28. Smith GN, Walton RE, Abbott BJ: Clinical evaluation of periodontal ligament anesthesia using a pressure syringe, J Am Dent Assoc 107:953–956, 1983.
29. Hochman MN: Single-tooth anesthesia: pressure sensing technology provides innovative advancement in the field of dental local anesthesia, Compendium 28:186–193, 2007.
30. Hochman MN, Friedman MF, Williams WP, et al: Interstitial pressure associated with dental injections: a clinical study, Quintessence Int 37:469–476, 2006.
31. Ashkenazi M, Blumer S, Eli I: Effect of computerized delivery intraligamental injection in primary molars on their corresponding permanent tooth buds, Int J Paediatr Dent 20:270–275, 2010.
32. Ferrari M, Cagidiaco MC, Vichi A, et al: Efficacy of the computer-controlled injection system STA, the Ligamaject, and the dental syringe for intraligamentary anesthesia in restorative patients, Int Dent SA 11:4–12, 2010.
33. Froum SJ, Tarnow D, Caiazzo A, et al: Histologic response to intraligament injections using a computerized local anesthetic delivery system: a pilot study in mini-swine, J Periodontol 71:1453–1459, 2000.
34. Berlin J, Nusstein J, Reader A, et al: Efficacy of articaine and lidocaine in a primary intraligamentary injection administered with a computer controlled local anesthetic delivery system, Oral Surg Oral Med Oral Path Oral Radiol Endod 99:361–366, 2005.
35. Hochman MN: Single-tooth anesthesia: pressure sensing technology provides innovative advancement in the field of dental local anesthesia, Compendium 28:186–193, 2007.

36. Hochman MN, inventor: Computer controlled drug delivery system with dynamic pressure sensing. U.S. Patent # 7 618:409, 2006.
37. Ghelber O, Gebhard R, Szmuk P, et al: Identification of the epidural space: a pilot study of a new technique, Anesth Analg 22:S255, 2005.
38. Ghelber O, Gebhard RE, Vora S, et al: Identification of the epidural space using pressure measurement with the CompuFlo injection pump: a pilot study, Reg Anesth Pain Med 33:346–352, 2008.
39. Hochman MN: Single-tooth anesthesia: pressure sensing technology provides innovative advancement in the field of dental local anesthesia, Compendium 28:186–193, 2007.
40. Pertot WJ, Dejou J: Bone and root resorption: effects of the force developed during periodontal ligament injections in dogs, Oral Surg Oral Med Oral Pathol 74:357–365, 1992.
41. Ashkenazi M, Blumer S, Eli I: Effective computerized delivery of intrasulcular anesthetic in primary molars, J Am Dent Assoc 136:1418–1425, 2005.
42. Saadoun A, Malamed SF: Intraseptal anesthesia in periodontal surgery, J Am Dent Assoc 111:249–256, 1985.
43. Leonard M: The efficacy of an intraosseous injection system of delivering local anesthetic, J Am Dent Assoc 126:81–86, 1995.
44. De St Georges J: How dentists are judged by patients, Dent Today 23:96, 98–99, 2004.
45. Oulis CJ, Vadiakis GP, Vasilopoulou A: The effectiveness of mandibular infiltration compared to mandibular block anesthesia in treating primary molars in children, Pediatr Dent 18:301–305, 1996.
46. Sharaf AA: Evaluation of mandibular infiltration versus block anesthesia in pediatric dentistry, J Dent Child 64:276–281, 1997.
47. Malamed SF: Local anesthetic considerations in dental specialties. In Malamed SF, editor: Handbook of local anesthesia, ed 5, St Louis, 2004, CV Mosby.
48. Bennett CR: Techniques of regional anesthesia and analgesia. In Bennett CR, editor: Monheim's local anesthesia and pain control in dental practice, ed 7, St Louis, 1984, CV Mosby.
49. Evers H, Haegerstam G: Anaesthesia of the lower jaw. In Evers H, Haegerstam G, editors: Introduction to dental local anaesthesia, Fribourg, Switzerland, 1990, Mediglobe SA.
50. Trieger N: New approaches to local anesthesia. In Pain control, ed 2, St Louis, 1994, CV Mosby.
51. OnPharma Inc.: Results of 38 studies on LA success rates, unpublished. Available at: www.onpharma.com. Accessed September 22, 2011.
52. Kanaa MD, Whitworth JM, Corbett IP, et al: Articaine buccal infiltration enhances the effectiveness of lidocaine inferior alveolar nerve block, Int Endod J 42:238–246, 2009.
53. Hannan L, Reader A, Nist R, et al: The use of ultrasound for guiding needle placement for inferior alveolar nerve blocks, Oral Surg Oral Med Oral Pathol Oral Radiol Endod 87:658–665, 1999.
54. Berns JM, Sadove MS: Mandibular block injection: a method of study using an injected radiopaque material, J Am Dent Assoc 65:736–745, 1962.
55. Galbreath JC: Tracing the course of the mandibular block injection, Oral Surg Oral Med Oral Pathol 30:571–582, 1970.
56. Reader A, American Association of Endodontists: Taking the pain out of restorative dentistry and endodontics: current thoughts and treatment options to help patients achieve profound anesthesia. Endodontics: Colleagues for Excellence Winter 2009.
57. DeJong RH: Local anesthetics, St Louis, 1994, CV Mosby, pp 110–111.
58. Strichartz G: Molecular mechanisms of nerve block by local anesthetics, Anesthesiology 45:421–444, 1976.
59. Whitcomb M, Drum M, Reader A, et al: A prospective, randomized, double-blind study of the anesthetic efficacy of sodium bicarbonate buffered 2% lidocaine with 1:100,000 epinephrine in inferior alveolar nerve blocks, Anesth Prog 57:59–66, 2010.
60. Meechan JG: Infiltration anesthesia in the mandible, Dent Clin N Am 54:621–629, 2010.
61. Rood JP: The analgesia and innervation of mandibular teeth, Br Dent J 140:237–239, 1976
62. Yonchak T, Reader A, Beck M, et al: Anesthetic efficacy of infiltrations in mandibular anterior teeth, Anesth Prog 48:55–60, 2001.
63. Meechan JG, Ledvinka JI: Pulpal anaesthesia for mandibular central incisor teeth: a comparison of infiltration and intraligamentary injections, Int Endod J 35:629–634, 2002.
64. Haas DA, Harper DG, Saso MA, et al: Comparison of articaine and prilocaine anesthesia by infiltration in maxillary and mandibular arches, Anesth Prog 37:230–237, 1990.
65. Haas DA, Harper DG, Saso MA, et al: Lack of differential effect by Ultracaine (articaine) and Citanest (prilocaine) in infiltration anaesthesia, J Can Dent Assoc 57:217–223, 1991.
66. Haase A, Reader A, Nusstein J, et al: Comparing anesthetic efficacy of articaine versus lidocaine as a supplemental buccal infiltration of the mandibular first molar after an inferior alveolar nerve block, J Am Dent Assoc 139:1228–1235, 2008.
67. Potocnik I, Tomsic M, Sketelj J, et al: Articaine is more effective than lidocaine or mepivacaine in rat sensory nerve conduction block in vitro, J Dent Res 85:162–166, 2006.
68. Vreeland DL, Reader A, Beck M, et al: An evaluation of volumes and concentrations of lidocaine in human inferior alveolar nerve block, J Endod 15:6–12, 1989.
69. Hinkley SA, Reader A, Beck M, et al: An evaluation of 4 percent prilocaine with 1:200,000 epinephrine and 2% mepivacaine with 1:20,000 levonordefrin compared with 2% lidocaine with 1:100,000 epinephrine for inferior alveolar nerve block, Anesth Prog 38:84–89, 1991.
70. Chaney MA, Kerby R, Reader A, et al: An evaluation of lidocaine hydrocarbonate compared with lidocaine hydrochloride for inferior alveolar nerve block, Anesth Prog 38:212–216, 1991.
71. McClean C, Reader A, Beck M, et al: An evaluation of 4% prilocaine and 3% mepivacaine compared with 2% lidocaine (1:100,000 epinephrine) for inferior alveolar nerve block, J Endod 19:146–150, 1993.
72. Ridenour S, Reader A, Beck M, et al: Anesthetic efficacy of a combination of hyaluronidase and lidocaine with epinephrine in inferior alveolar nerve blocks, Anesth Prog 48:9–15, 2001.
73. Steinkruger G, Nusstein J, Reader A, et al: The significance of needle bevel orientation in achieving a successful inferior alveolar nerve block, J Am Dent Assoc 137:1685–1691, 2006.
74. Jaber A, Al-Baqshi B, Whitworth C, et al: The efficacy of infiltration anesthesia for adult mandibular incisors, J Dent Res 88(Special Issue A):Abstract 702, 2009.
75. Dreven LJ, Reader A, Beck M, et al: An evaluation of the electric pulp tester as a measure of analgesia in human vital teeth, J Endod 13:233–238, 1987.

CHAPTER 16

Anesthetic Considerations in Dental Specialties

The techniques of local anesthesia described previously in this section are valuable to doctors in virtually all areas of dental practice. However, specific needs and problems are associated with pain control in particular areas of dentistry. This chapter discusses the dental specialties listed below and their peculiar needs in the area of pain control:

- Endodontics
- Pediatric dentistry
- Periodontics
- Oral and maxillofacial surgery
- Fixed prosthodontics
- Long-duration anesthesia (postsurgical pain control)
- Dental hygiene

ENDODONTICS

Effects of Inflammation on Local Anesthesia

Inflammation and infection lower tissue pH, altering the ability of a local anesthetic to provide clinically adequate pain control. As a review, local anesthetics are weak bases (pKa, 7.5 to 9.5) and are not water-soluble compounds. Combined with hydrochloric acid (HCl), local anesthetics are injected in their acid–salt form (e.g., lidocaine HCl), improving their water solubility and stability. The pH of a "plain" local anesthetic is approximately 6.5, and the pH of one containing a vasoconstrictor is approximately 3.5. In an acidic solution, hydrogen ions (H^+) are "floating around." If we abbreviate the anesthetic drug as RN (the un-ionized form of the local anesthetic), then some of these RNs will attach to an H^+, forming the cationic form of the local anesthetic (RNH^+). The more acidic the anesthetic solution, the greater the number of H^+ ions available, and the greater the percentage of RNH^+ found in the solution. Because only the RN ionic form is lipid soluble and is able to cross the lipid-rich nerve membrane, the lower the pH of the anesthetic solution and the tissue into which it is injected, the lower is the percentage of RN ions, the slower is the onset, and the less profound is the resultant anesthesia.

Once injected, the pH of the anesthetic solution is slowly increased toward the body's normal pH of approximately 7.4 by tissue fluid buffers. As this conversion occurs, RNH^+ ions lose H^+, becoming un-ionized RN ions (according to the Henderson-Hasselbalch equation; see Chapter 1), which now are able to diffuse across the nerve membrane to the interior of the nerve.

Pulpal and periapical inflammation or infection can cause significant alterations in tissue pH in the affected region, including decreased pH (e.g., pus has a pH of 5.5 to 5.6) and increased vascularity. Increased acidity has several negative aspects.[1] It severely limits the formation of RN, increasing the formation of RNH^+. RNs that do diffuse into the nerve find a normal tissue pH of 7.4 within the nerve and re-equilibrate into both RN and RNH^+ forms. These RNH^+ forms are then able to enter into and block sodium channels, blocking nerve conduction. But with fewer total anesthetic molecules (RN's and RNH^+'s) diffusing into the nerve, there is a greater likelihood that incomplete anesthesia will develop. The overall effect of ion entrapment is to delay the onset of anesthesia and possibly interfere with nerve blockade.[2] Ion entrapment changes the products of inflammation, so they inhibit anesthesia by directly affecting the nerve. Brown demonstrated that inflammatory exudates enhance nerve conduction by lowering the response threshold of the nerve,[1] which may inhibit local anesthesia. This causes blood vessels in the region of inflammation to become unusually dilated, allowing more rapid removal of the anesthetic from the site of injection. This leads to an increased possibility that resultant local anesthetic blood levels will be elevated (from those seen in normal tissue).[2]

Although there are no magic bullets for attaining profound pain control in teeth requiring pulpal extirpation, several methods may increase the likelihood of success. First, administer the local anesthetic at a site distant from the area of inflammation. It is undesirable to inject anesthetic solutions into infected tissue because this may cause the infection to spread to uninvolved regions.[3,4] Administration of local anesthetic solution into a site distant from the involved tooth is more likely to provide adequate pain control because of the existence of normal tissue conditions. Therefore, regional nerve block anesthesia is a major factor in pain control for the pulpally involved tooth. Second, use a buffered local anesthetic solution. Administration of a solution of local anesthetic with a pH in the range of 7.35 to 7.5 increases the percentage of RN ionic form approximately 6000-fold (lidocaine HCl with epinephrine [pH 3.5] = 0.004% of ionic forms RN; pH 7.4 = 24.03% RN). In studies with "normal" teeth, 71% of patients receiving a buffered local anesthetic achieved successful pulpal anesthesia within 2 minutes versus 5 minutes 17 seconds for unbuffered local anesthetic.[5] Although at the time of this writing (January 2012), no clinical trials of buffered local anesthetics have been published, anecdotal reports from endodontists indicate that they have seen a considerably greater incidence of successful anesthesia on teeth requiring pulpal extirpation.[6]

Methods of Achieving Anesthesia

The following techniques are recommended for providing pain control in pulpally involved teeth: local infiltration, regional nerve block, intraosseous injection, intraseptal injection, periodontal ligament injection, and intrapulpal injection. The order in which these techniques are discussed is the typical sequence in which they are normally used to achieve pain control when one seeks to extirpate pulpal tissues.

Local Infiltration (Supraperiosteal Injection). Local infiltration is commonly used to provide pulpal anesthesia in maxillary teeth. It is usually effective in endodontic procedures when severe inflammation or infection is not present. Local infiltration should not be attempted in a region where infection is obviously (clinically or radiographically) present because of the possible spread of infection to other regions and a greatly decreased rate of success. When infection is present, other techniques of pain control should be relied on. Infiltration anesthesia is often effective at subsequent endodontic visits, if adequate débridement and shaping of the canals have been previously accomplished.

Regional Nerve Block. Regional nerve block anesthesia is recommended in cases where infiltration anesthesia may be ineffective or contraindicated. These techniques are discussed in detail in Chapters 13 and 14. Regional nerve block is likely to be effective because the anesthetic solution is deposited at a distance from the inflammation, where tissue pH and other factors are more normal.

Intraosseous Injection. The intraosseous (IO) injection has experienced a resurgence of enthusiasm in recent years.[7-15] IO injections can provide anesthesia profound enough to allow painless access into the pulp chamber for removal of pulpal tissue. IO technique is described in Chapter 15 and is reviewed here (Figs. 16-1 and 16-2):

1. Apply topical anesthetic at the site of the injection to anesthetize the soft tissue.

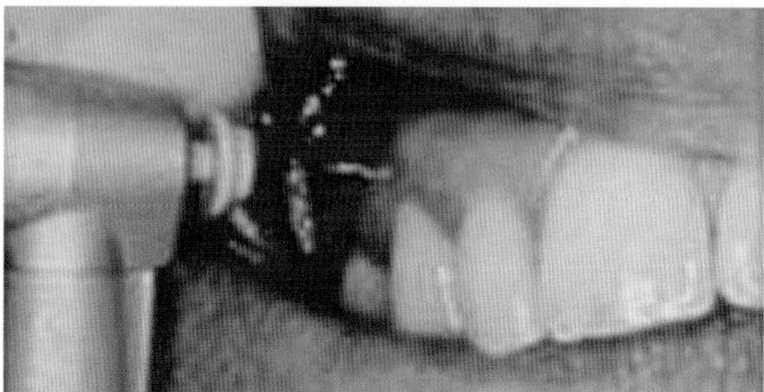

Figure 16-1. Stabident intraosseous injection technique.

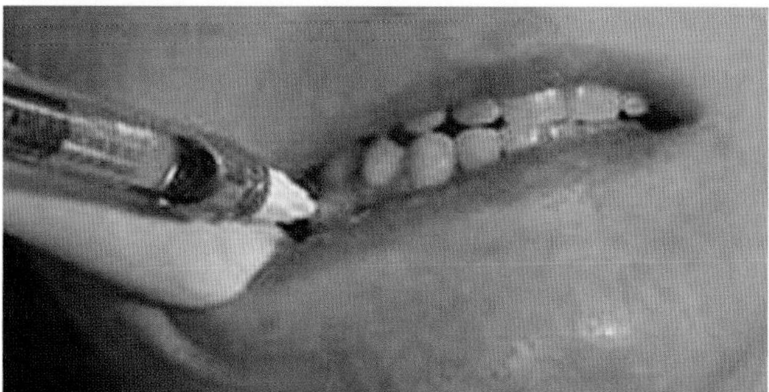

Figure 16-2. X-Tip intraosseous injection technique.

2. While holding the perforator perpendicular to the cortical plate, gently push it through the attached gingiva until its tip rests against bone.
3. Activate the handpiece and apply pressure on the perforator in a "pecking" motion until a sudden loss of resistance is felt.
4. Withdraw the perforator and dispose of it safely.
5. Insert the local anesthetic needle into the hole and deposit the volume of local anesthetic appropriate for the procedure (see charts in Chapter 15).

Cardiovascular absorption of the local anesthetic after IO injection is more rapid than after the other techniques described.[16,17] Transient elevations in heart rate were noted in 67% (28/42) of healthy patients receiving 2% lidocaine with 1:100,000 epinephrine via IO injection. The heart rate returned to within 5 beats of normal within 4 minutes in 79% of patients. No significant increase was noted when 3% mepivacaine was injected IO in the same patients.[17]

The use of epinephrine-containing local anesthetics in the IO technique is not contraindicated in healthy, non–cardiovascular risk patients. However, where significant cardiovascular risk or other relative contraindications to administration of epinephrine exist, a "plain" local anesthetic is a good alternative for IO anesthesia, keeping in mind that neither the depth nor duration of anesthesia will be as good as expected in a non-pulpally involved tooth.

Intraseptal Injection. This is a variation of IO and periodontal ligament (PDL) injections and may be used as an alternative to these techniques. It is more successful in

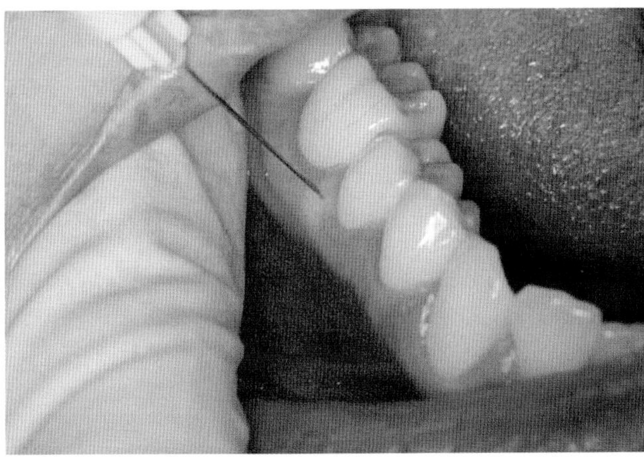

Figure 16-3. For the intraseptal injection, a 27-gauge short needle is inserted into the intraseptal bone distal to the tooth to be anesthetized.

younger patients because of decreased bone density. Intraseptal anesthesia is described in Chapter 15 and proceeds as follows[18]:

1. Anesthetize the soft tissues at the injection site via local infiltration.
2. Insert a 27-gauge short needle into the intraseptal bone distal to the tooth to be anesthetized (Fig. 16-3).
3. Advance the needle firmly into the cortical plate of bone.
4. Inject about 0.2 mL of anesthetic.

Considerable resistance must be encountered as the anesthetic is being deposited. If administration of the anesthetic is easy, the needle tip is most likely in soft tissue, not in bone.

Periodontal Ligament Injection. The PDL injection may be an effective method of providing anesthesia in pulpally involved teeth if infection and severe inflammation are not present. This technique is discussed in Chapter 15. By way of review, a 27-gauge short needle is firmly placed between the interproximal bone and the tooth to be anesthetized. The bevel of the needle should face the tooth (although bevel orientation is not critical for success). It is appropriate to bend the needle if necessary to gain access. A small volume (0.2 mL) of local anesthetic is deposited under pressure for each root of the tooth. It may be necessary to repeat the PDL injection on all four sides of the tooth. Computer-controlled local anesthetic delivery (C-CLAD) devices enable the PDL injection to be administered more successfully and more comfortably than an injection given with a traditional dental local anesthetic syringe.

Intrapulpal Injection. The intrapulpal injection provides pain control both by the pharmacologic action of the local anesthetic and by applied pressure. This technique may be used once the pulp chamber is exposed surgically or pathologically. The technique is described in Chapter 15.

When intrapulpal injections are administered properly, a brief period of sensitivity, ranging from mild to severe, may accompany the injection. Clinical pain relief follows almost immediately, permitting instrumentation to proceed atraumatically.

Occasionally, the anesthetic needle does not fit snugly into the canal, preventing the increased pressure normally encountered in the intrapulpal injection. In this situation, the anesthetic can be deposited in the chamber or canal. Anesthesia is produced only by the pharmacologic action of the drug; there is no pressure anesthesia. Instrumentation may begin approximately 30 seconds after the drug is deposited.

With the growing popularity of IO anesthesia, the need for intrapulpal injection to provide profound pain control in cases of irreversible pulpitis has decreased.

Today there are but few occasions when all of the techniques discussed fail to provide clinically acceptable pain control, and intrapulpal anesthesia cannot be attempted until the pulp is exposed. The following sequence of treatment may be of value on these rare occasions:

1. Use slow-speed high-torque instrumentation (which usually is less traumatic than the high-speed low-torque option).
2. Use (minimal or moderate) sedation (which helps to decrease the patient's response to painful stimuli). Nitrous oxide–oxygen inhalation sedation is a readily available, safe, and highly effective method of relaxing a patient and elevating his or her pain reaction threshold.
3. If, after steps 1 and 2, the pulp chamber is opened, administer direct intrapulpal anesthesia. This is usually effective despite the brief period of pain associated with intrapulpal administration.
4. If a high level of pain persists and it still is not possible to enter the pulp chamber, then the following sequence should be considered:
   a. Place a cotton pellet saturated with local anesthetic loosely on the pulpal floor of the tooth.
   b. Wait 30 seconds; then press the pellet more firmly into the dentinal tubules or the area of pulpal exposure. This area may be sensitive initially but should become insensitive within 2 to 3 minutes.
   c. Remove the pellet and continue use of the slow-speed drill until pulpal access is gained; then perform direct injection into the pulp.

With most endodontic procedures, difficulty in providing adequate anesthesia occurs only at the first appointment. Once the pulp tissue has been extirpated, the need for pulpal anesthesia disappears. Soft tissue anesthesia may be necessary at ensuing appointments for comfortable placement of the rubber dam clamp, but if adequate tooth structure remains, this may not be necessary. Some patients respond unfavorably to instrumentation of their root canals, even when the canals have been thoroughly débrided. If this occurs, infiltration (in the maxillary or mandibular incisor region [with articaine HCl]), intrapulpal anesthesia, or topical anesthetic may be used. Apply a small amount of topical anesthetic ointment onto the file or reamer before inserting it into the canal. This helps to desensitize the periapical tissues during instrumentation of the canals. Patients may react to filling of the canals. Local anesthesia should be considered before this stage of treatment is started.

PEDIATRIC DENTISTRY

Pain control is one of the most important aspects of behavioral management in children undergoing dental treatment. Unpleasant childhood experiences have made many adults acutely phobic with regard to dental treatment. Today, however, many local anesthetic drugs are available to make pain management relatively easy. Special concerns in pediatric dentistry relevant to local anesthetic include anesthetic overdose (toxic reaction), self-inflicted soft tissue injury related to the prolonged duration of soft tissue anesthesia, and technique variations related to the smaller skulls and differing anatomy of younger patients.

Local Anesthetic Overdose

Overdose from a drug occurs when its blood level in a target organ (e.g., brain and myocardium for local anesthetics) becomes excessive (see Chapter 18). Undesirable (toxic) effects may be caused by intravascular injection or administration of large volumes of the drug. Local anesthetic toxicity develops when the blood level of the drug in the brain or myocardium becomes too high. Therefore local anesthetic toxicity relates to the volume of drug reaching the cerebrovascular and cardiovascular systems and to the blood volume of the patient. Once the blood level of a drug reaches toxic levels, the drug exerts unwanted and possibly deleterious systemic actions that are consistent with its pharmacological properties. Local anesthetic toxicity produces central nervous system (CNS) and cardiovascular system (CVS) depression, with reactions ranging from mild tremor to tonic–clonic convulsions (CNS), or from a slight decrease in blood pressure and cardiac output to cardiac arrest (CVS).

Disproportionately high numbers of deaths and serious morbidities caused by local anesthetic overdose have occurred in children, leading to the assumption that local anesthetics are more toxic in children than in adults.[19,20] This is untrue; it is the safety margin of local anesthetics in small children that is low. Given an equal dose (mg) of local anesthetic, a healthy adult patient with a larger body weight and greater blood volume will have a lower blood level of anesthetic than the child patient of lesser weight and smaller blood volume. Blood volume, to a large degree, relates to body weight: the greater the body weight, the greater the blood volume (except in cases of marked obesity).

Maximum recommended doses (MRDs) of all drugs administered by injection should be calculated by body weight and should not be exceeded, unless it is absolutely essential to do so.[20] For example, two cartridges of 3% mepivacaine (54 mg per cartridge) exceed the MRD for a 15-kg (33-lb) child of 66 mg. Unfortunately, lack of awareness of maximum doses has led to fatalities in children.[21–25] The ease with which a lighter-weight child may be overdosed with local anesthetics is compounded by the practice of multiple-quadrant dentistry and the concomitant use of sedative drugs (especially opioids).[19] When treating a smaller child, the dentist should maintain strict adherence to MRDs (Table 16-1) and should anesthetize only that quadrant that is currently being treated.

TABLE 16-1
Maximum Recommended Doses (MRDs) of Local Anesthetics

Drug	Formulation	Manufacturer's MRD	mg/kg (mg/lb)
Articaine	4% with epinephrine	N/A	7.0 (3.2)
Lidocaine	Plain	300	4.4 (2.0)
Lidocaine	Epinephrine 1:100,000	500	7.0 (3.2)
Lidocaine	Epinephrine 1:50,000	500	7.0 (3.2)
Mepivacaine	Plain	400	6.6 (3.0)
Mepivacaine	With levonordefrin	400	6.6 (3.0)
Prilocaine	Plain	600	8.0 (3.6)
Prilocaine	With epinephrine	600	8.0 (3.6)
Bupivacaine	With epinephrine	90	—

Cheatham and associates surveyed 117 dentists who regularly treated children about their local anesthetic usage.[26] They found that the lighter the weight of the patient, the more likely the doctor was to administer an overly large dose of the local anesthetic, based on milligrams per kilogram of body weight. For example, a 13-kg patient should receive no more than 91 mg of lidocaine (based on an MRD of 7.0 mg/kg). The range of doses administered by dentists treating children was 0.9 to 19.3 mg/kg. As the patient's weight increased, the number of milligrams per pound or kilogram reached lower and safer levels, the maximum mg/kg range falling to 12.6 mg/kg in the 20-kg patient and to 7.2 mg/kg in the 35-kg patient. The mean dose of local anesthetic also fell when the patient's weight increased, from 5.4 mg/kg in the 13-kg patient to 4.8 mg/kg in the 20-kg patient to 3.8 mg/kg in the 35-kg patient (Table 16-2).

Administration of large volumes of local anesthetic is not necessary when one is seeking to achieve pain control in younger patients. Because of differences in anatomy (see the following discussion of "Techniques of Local Anesthesia in Pediatric Dentistry"), smaller volumes of local anesthetics provide the depth and duration of pain control usually necessary to successfully complete planned dental treatment in younger patients.

Because all injectable local anesthetics possess vasodilating properties, leading to more rapid vascular uptake and a shorter duration of adequate anesthesia, it is strongly recommended that a vasopressor be included in the local anesthetic solution unless there is a compelling reason for it to be excluded.[27] Many treatment appointments in pediatric dentistry do not exceed 30 minutes in duration; therefore

TABLE 16-2
Local Anesthetic Administration by Dentists Who Treat Children (n = 117)

Patient Age	Patient Weight, kg	Mean Dose, mg/kg	Mean, mg/kg	Range, mg	Range, mg/kg	Recommended (MRD), mg/kg
2	13	69.9	5.4	12-252	0.9-19.3	Lidocaine 4.4-7.0 Mepivacaine 4.4-6.0
5	20	96.5	4.8	18-252	0.9-12.6	
10	35	135	3.8	36-252	1.0-7.2	

Modified from Cheatham BD, Primosch RE, Courts FJ: A survey of local anesthetic usage in pediatric patients by Florida dentists, J Dent Child 59:401–407, 1992.

TABLE 16-3
Local Anesthetic Choice by Dentists Who Treat Children (n = 117)

Anesthetic Formulation	Percent Employing
2% lidocaine + 1:100,000 epinephrine	69
3% mepivacaine	11
2% lidocaine	8
2% mepivacaine + 1:20,000 levonordefrin	8
Other anesthetics	4

Adapted from Cheatham BD, Primosch RE, Courts FJ: A survey of local anesthetic usage in pediatric patients by Florida dentists, J Dent Child 59:401–407, 1992.

BOX 16-1 Factors Adding to Increased Risk of Local Anesthetic Overdose in Younger Patients

1. Treatment plan: all four quadrants treated using local anesthetic in one visit.
2. Local anesthetic administered is a plain (no vasopressor) solution.
3. Full cartridges (1.8 mL) administered with each injection.
4. Local anesthetic administered to all four quadrants at one time.
5. Exceeding the maximum dosage based on patient's body weight.

Adapted from Cheatham BD, Primosch RE, Courts FJ: A survey of local anesthetic usage in pediatric patients by Florida dentists, J Dent Child 59:401–407, 1992.

use of a local anesthetic containing a vasopressor is considered to be unnecessary and unwarranted. It is thought that increased duration of soft tissue anesthesia, especially after inferior alveolar nerve block, increases the risk of self-inflicted soft tissue injury. A non–vasopressor-containing local anesthetic is frequently used (most often, mepivacaine 3%). Providing 20 to 40 minutes of pulpal anesthesia, mepivacaine 3% is considered the appropriate drug for this group of patients; this is true, provided that treatment is limited to one quadrant per visit. However, when multiple quadrants are to be treated (and anesthetized) on a smaller, lighter-weight patient in a single visit, administration of a "plain" drug into multiple injection sites increases the potential risk of overdose. Use of a local anesthetic containing a vasopressor is strongly recommended whenever multiple quadrants are anesthetized in the smaller pediatric patient. Sixty-nine percent of doctors treating children administered lidocaine with epinephrine as their primary anesthetic (Table 16-3).[26]

Factors increasing the risk of local anesthetic overdosage in younger patients are presented in Box 16-1.[28]

Complications of Local Anesthesia

Self-inflicted soft tissue injury—accidental biting or chewing of the lip, tongue, or cheek—is a complication associated with residual soft tissue anesthesia (Fig. 16-4). Soft tissue anesthesia lasts considerably longer than pulpal anesthesia and may persist for 4 or more hours after local anesthetic administration. Fortunately, most patients do not encounter problems related to prolonged soft tissue anesthesia, but most of those who do are younger, oldest old (>85 years), or mentally or physically disabled. Problems related to soft tissue anesthesia most often involve the lower lip. Much less frequently, the tongue is injured, and rarely, the upper lip is involved.

College and associates reported an 18% incidence of self-inflicted soft tissue injury in patients younger than 4 years of age receiving inferior alveolar nerve block.[29] From 4 to 7 years, the rate was 16%, from 8 to 11 years, 13%, and from 12 years on, 7%.

Several preventive measures can be implemented:

1. Select a local anesthetic with a duration of action that is appropriate for the length of the planned procedure. Some local anesthetics provide pulpal anesthesia of adequate duration (20 to 40 minutes) for restorative procedures in children, with a relatively short duration of soft tissue anesthesia (1 to 3 hours, instead of 4 or 5) (Table 16-4). It should be kept in mind, however, that investigators have not demonstrated a relationship between the use of plain local anesthetics and a reduction in soft tissue trauma. The clinician must consider the advisability of using a local anesthetic containing a vasopressor when treating multiple

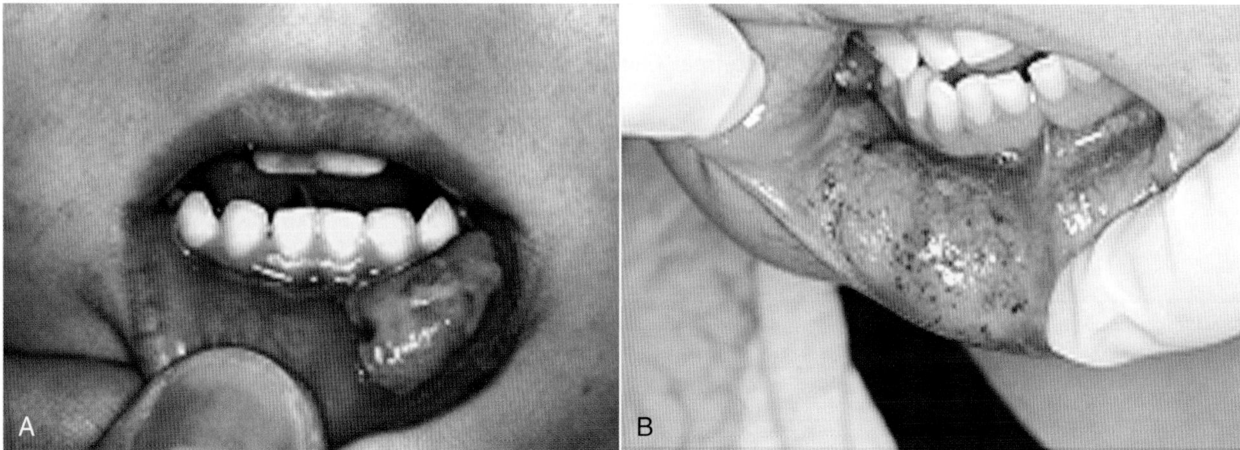

Figure 16-4. Lip trauma caused by biting while the area was anesthetized.

TABLE 16-4
Relative Durations of Pulpal and Soft Tissue Anesthesia

Drug	Approximate Pulpal Anesthesia, min	Approximate Soft Tissue Anesthesia, hr
Mepivacaine plain	20-40	3-4
Prilocaine plain	(infiltration) 10	1½-2
Lidocaine plain	5-10	1-1½

quadrants in view of the decreased margin of safety of local anesthetics in smaller children.

2. Administer phentolamine mesylate (Oraverse) at the conclusion of the traumatic portion of the dental procedure. Discussed more completely in Chapter 20, phentolamine mesylate is an alpha-adrenergic antagonist that, when injected into the site where local anesthetic with vasopressor was previously deposited, produces vasodilation, increasing blood flow through the area, thereby increasing the speed with which the local anesthetic drug diffuses out of the nerve. The duration of residual soft tissue anesthesia is significantly reduced. Phentolamine mesylate has been approved by the Food and Drug Administration (FDA) for use in patients 6 years of age and older and weighing more than 15 kg (33 lb).[30,31]
3. Advise both the patient and the accompanying adult about the possibility of injury if the patient bites, sucks, or chews on the lips, tongue, or cheeks, or ingests hot substances while anesthesia persists.
4. Some doctors reinforce the verbal warning to the patient and the adult by placing a cotton roll in the mucobuccal fold (held in position by dental floss through the teeth) if soft tissue anesthesia is still present at the time of the patient's discharge. Warning stickers are available to help prevent soft tissue trauma.

Management of self-inflicted soft tissue trauma consists of reassuring the patient, allowing time for anesthetic effects

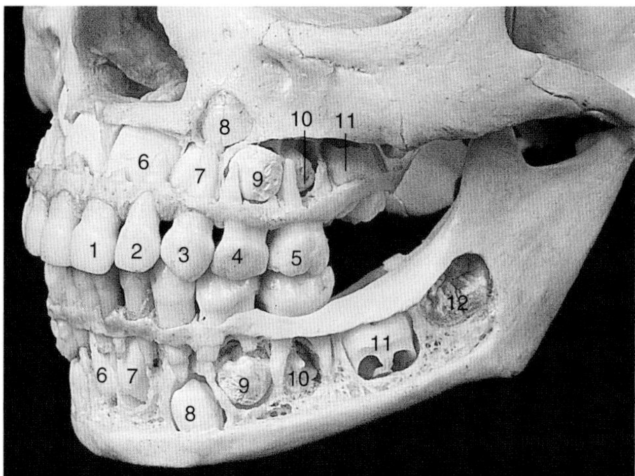

Figure 16-5. Upper and lower jaws in a 4-year-old child with erupted primary teeth and unerupted permanent teeth. 1, First (central) incisor of primary dentition; 2, second (lateral) incisor of primary dentition; 3, canine of primary dentition; 4, first molar of primary dentition; 5, second molar of primary dentition; 6, first (central) incisor of permanent dentition; 7, second (lateral) incisor of permanent dentition; 8, canine of permanent dentition; 9, first premolar of permanent dentition; 10, second premolar of permanent dentition; 11, first molar of permanent dentition; 12, second molar of permanent dentition. (From Abrahams PH, Marks SC Jr, Hutchings RT: McMinn's color atlas of human anatomy, ed 5, St Louis, 2003, Mosby.)

to diminish, and coating the involved area with a lubricant (petroleum jelly) to help prevent drying, cracking, and pain.

Techniques of Local Anesthesia in Pediatric Dentistry

Local anesthetic techniques in children do not differ greatly from those used in adults. However, the skulls of children do have some anatomic differences from those of adults. For instance, maxillary and mandibular bone in children generally is less dense, which works to the dentist's advantage (Fig. 16-5). Decreased bone density allows more rapid and complete diffusion of the anesthetic solution. Also, children are smaller; thus standard injection techniques usually can be completed with decreased depth of needle penetration.

Maxillary Anesthesia. All primary teeth and permanent molars can be anesthetized by supraperiosteal infiltration in the mucobuccal fold. The posterior superior alveolar (PSA) nerve block is rarely necessary because of the effectiveness of infiltration in children. However, in some individuals, the morphology of the bone surrounding the apex of the permanent first molar does not permit effective infiltration of local anesthetic, because the zygomatic process lies closer to the alveolar bone in children. A PSA nerve block may be warranted in this clinical situation. A 27-gauge short dental needle should be used and the depth of needle penetration modified to meet the smaller dimensions of the pediatric patient, to minimize the risk of overinsertion leading to hematoma. As an alternative to the PSA, Rood[32] has suggested using buccal infiltrations on both the mesial and the distal of the maxillary first molar to avoid a prominent zygomatic process. The anterior superior alveolar (ASA) nerve block also can be used in children, as long as it is realized that the depth of penetration is probably just slightly greater than with a supraperiosteal injection (because of the lower height of the maxillae in children). Generally, there are few indications for the PSA or ASA nerve block in children.

Occasionally, a maxillary tooth remains sensitive after a supraperiosteal injection because of accessory innervation from the palatal nerves[33] or widely flared palatal roots. Palatal anesthesia can be attained in children through the nasopalatine and greater (anterior) palatine nerve blocks. The technique for a nasopalatine nerve block proceeds exactly as described in Chapter 13. That for a greater palatine nerve block is as follows: The administrator visualizes a line from the gingival border of the most posterior molar that has erupted to the midline. The needle is inserted from the opposite side of the mouth, distal to the last molar, bisecting this line. If the child has only primary dentition, the needle is inserted approximately 10 mm posterior to the distal surface of the second primary molar, bisecting the line drawn toward the midline.

An intrapapillary injection also can be used to achieve palatal anesthesia in young children. Once buccal anesthesia is effective, the needle (27-gauge short) is inserted horizontally into the buccal papilla just above the interdental septum. Local anesthetic is injected as the needle is advanced toward the palatal side. This should cause ischemia of the soft tissue.[34]

Mandibular Anesthesia. Supraperiosteal infiltration usually is effective in providing pain control in mandibular primary teeth.[35,36] Sharaf reported that buccal infiltration in the mandible in 80 children (ages 3 to 9 years) was as effective as inferior alveolar nerve block (IANB) anesthesia in all situations, except when pulpotomy was performed on the primary second molar.[35] This was the result of decreased density of bone in the mandible in younger children. The rate of success of mandibular infiltration anesthesia decreases somewhat for primary mandibular molars as the child increases in age. The technique of supraperiosteal infiltration in the mandible is the same as in the maxilla. The tip of the needle is directed toward the apex of the tooth, in the mucobuccal fold, and approximately one fourth to one third (0.45 to 0.6 mL) cartridge is slowly deposited.

The IANB has a greater success rate in children than in adults because of the location of the mandibular foramen. The mandibular foramen in children lies distal and more inferior to the occlusal plane. Benham[37] demonstrated that the mandibular foramen lies at the height of the occlusal plane in children and extends an average of 7.4 mm above the occlusal plane in adults. He also found that there is no age-related difference as to the anteroposterior position of the foramen on the ramus.

The technique for an IANB is essentially identical for adults and children. The syringe barrel is placed in the corner of the mouth on the opposite side. The average depth of penetration to bone is approximately 15 mm, although this may vary significantly with the size of the mandible and the age of the patient. As with the adult, bone should be contacted before any solution is deposited. In general, the more inferior location of the mandibular foramen in children provides a greater opportunity for successful anesthesia. "Too low" injections are more likely to be successful. In clinical situations, the success rate for well-behaved children usually exceeds 90% to 95%.

Because of the decreased thickness of soft tissue overlying the inferior alveolar nerve (about 15 mm), a 25- or 27-gauge short needle may be recommended for the IANB in younger, smaller patients. This should be changed to a long needle once the patient is of sufficient size that a short needle does not reach the injection site without entering tissue almost to its hub.

The buccal nerve may be anesthetized if anesthesia of the buccal tissues in the permanent molar region is necessary. The needle tip is placed distal and buccal to the most posterior tooth in the arch. Approximately 0.3 mL of solution is deposited.

The Vazirani-Akinosi and Gow-Gates mandibular nerve blocks also can be used in children. Akinosi[38] advocates the use of short needles with this technique in children. He states that the technique appears less reliable in children, which he relates to the difficulty of judging the depth of penetration necessary in a growing child. The Gow-Gates mandibular block can be used successfully in children.[39] However, these injections are rarely necessary in pediatric dentistry because of the effectiveness of mandibular infiltration (when the dentition is composed entirely of primary teeth) and the relative ease with which one can achieve inferior alveolar and incisive nerve block anesthesia.

The incisive nerve block provides pulpal anesthesia to the five primary mandibular teeth in a quadrant. Deposition of anesthetic solution outside the mental foramen with application of finger pressure for 2 minutes provides a very high degree of success. The mental foramen usually is located between the two primary mandibular molars. A volume of 0.45 mL (¼ of a cartridge) is suggested.

The PDL injection has been well accepted in pediatric dentistry and can be used as an alternative to supraperiosteal injection. It provides the doctor with the means to achieve anesthesia of proper depth and duration on one tooth, without unwanted residual soft tissue anesthesia. The PDL is also useful when a child has discrete carious lesions in multiple quadrants. See Chapter 15 for a complete discussion of technique for the PDL injection. It is recommended that the described technique be scrupulously adhered to, to avoid physiologic (pain) and psychological (fear) trauma to the patient. The PDL injection is not recommended for use on primary teeth because of the possibility of enamel hypoplasia occurring in the developing permanent tooth.[40]

PERIODONTICS

Special requirements for local anesthesia in periodontal procedures center on the use of vasopressors to provide hemostasis and the use of long-duration local anesthetics for postoperative pain control. Postsurgical pain management, including the use of long-duration anesthesia, is discussed as a separate subject later in this chapter.

Soft tissue manipulation and surgical procedures are associated with hemorrhage, especially when the tissues involved are not healthy. Administration of local anesthetics without vasopressors proves to be counterproductive because the vasodilating property of the local anesthetic increases bleeding in the region of the injection.[41] Vasopressors are added to counteract this undesirable property of local anesthetics.

The pharmacology of vasopressors is more completely discussed in Chapter 3. As a review, vasopressors produce arterial smooth muscle contraction through direct stimulation of α receptors located in the wall of the blood vessel. Consequently, it follows that local anesthetics with vasopressors used for hemostasis must be injected directly into the region where the bleeding is to occur.

Pain control for periodontal procedures should be achieved through nerve block techniques, including posterior superior alveolar, inferior alveolar, and infraorbital nerve blocks. Saadoun[18] has shown that the intraseptal technique is very effective for periodontal flap surgical procedures. It decreases the total volume of administered anesthetic and the volume of blood lost during the procedure. Local anesthetic solutions used for nerve blocks should include a vasopressor in a concentration not greater than 1:100,000 epinephrine or 1:20,000 levonordefrin. An epinephrine concentration of 1:50,000 is not recommended for pain control because depth, duration, and success rates are no greater than those seen with anesthetics containing 1:100,000 or 1:200,000 epinephrine.

Epinephrine is the drug of choice for local hemostasis. Norepinephrine (which is not available in North America in dental local anesthetics) can produce marked tissue ischemia, which can lead to necrosis and sloughing and is not recommended for use in hemostasis.[42,43] Epinephrine is most commonly used for hemostasis in a concentration of 1:50,000 (0.2 mg/mL). Generally, small volumes (not exceeding 0.1 mL) are deposited when used for hemostasis. Epinephrine also provides excellent hemostasis in a concentration of 1:100,000, although surgical bleeding is inversely proportional to the concentration of vasopressor administered. When plain local anesthetic is infiltrated (e.g., 3% mepivacaine) during periodontal surgery, blood loss is two to three times that noted when 2% lidocaine with 1:100,000 epinephrine is administered.[44] Buckley and associates demonstrated that use of a 1:50,000 epinephrine concentration produced a 50% decrease in bleeding during periodontal surgery from that seen with a 1:100,000 concentration (with 2% lidocaine).[45] However, epinephrine is not a drug without systemic effects and some undesirable local effects. Studies have shown that even the small volumes of epinephrine used in dentistry can significantly increase the concentrations of plasma catecholamine and can alter cardiac function.[46] Therefore, it is prudent to administer the smallest volume of the least concentrated form of epinephrine that provides clinically effective hemostasis.

As tissue levels of epinephrine decrease after its injection for hemostasis, a rebound vasodilation develops. Sveen demonstrated that postsurgical bleeding (at 6 hours) occurred in 13 of 16 (81.25%) patients receiving 2% lidocaine with epinephrine for surgical removal of a third molar, whereas 0 of 16 patients who underwent surgery with 3% mepivacaine bled at 6 hours post surgery.[44] Bleeding interfered with postoperative healing in 9 of 16 (56.25%) patients receiving lidocaine with epinephrine, compared with 25% of patients receiving no epinephrine. Evidence also suggests that the use of epinephrine in local anesthetics during surgery may produce an increase in postoperative pain.[47]

Many doctors use a 30-gauge short needle to deposit anesthetics for hemostasis. Their rationale is that the thinner needle produces a smaller defect (puncture) in the tissue. If a small puncture is important, then the 30-gauge needle should be used, but only for this purpose (hemostasis). The 30-gauge short needle should not be used if there is the possibility of positive aspiration of blood, or if any depth of soft tissue must be penetrated. Aspiration of blood through a 30-gauge needle is difficult (although possible). A 27-gauge needle can be used for local infiltration to achieve hemostasis when vascularity is a problem, or in any other area of the oral cavity without an increase in patient discomfort.

ORAL AND MAXILLOFACIAL SURGERY

Pain control during surgical procedures is achieved through administration of local anesthetics, given alone or in combination with inhalation sedation, intravenous sedation, or general anesthesia. As is the case with periodontal surgery, long-duration local anesthetics play an important role in postoperative pain control and are discussed separately.

Local anesthetic techniques used in oral surgery do not differ from those employed in nonsurgical procedures.

Therefore it should be expected that instances of partial or incomplete anesthesia will occur. Oral and maxillofacial surgeons frequently treat patients who have received intravenous sedation or general anesthesia before the start of surgery. These techniques act to modify the patient's reaction to pain, leading to a decrease in the number of reported instances of inadequate local anesthesia.

Local anesthesia is administered almost routinely to patients for third molar extractions under general anesthesia. The reasons for this are as follows:

1. General anesthesia does not prevent pain. General anesthesia prevents the patient from responding outwardly to painful stimulation. Blood pressure (BP), heart rate (HR), and respiratory rate (RR) do respond to surgical stimulation (increases in BP, HR, and RR).
2. Pain control through local anesthetic administration during surgery permits lessened exposure to general anesthetic agents, allowing for a faster postanesthetic recovery period and minimizing drug-related complications.
3. Hemostasis is possible if a vasopressor is included.
4. Residual local anesthesia in the postoperative period aids in postsurgical pain control.

The volume of drug and the rate at which it is administered are important in all areas of dental practice, but probably are most important during extraction of teeth from multiple quadrants. When four third molars are extracted, effective pain control must be obtained in all four quadrants. This requires multiple injections of local anesthetics, which usually occur within a relatively short time. Four cartridges or more of local anesthetic are frequently used.* The rate at which these local anesthetics are administered must be closely monitored to lessen the occurrence of complications. Complications arising from rapid administration of local anesthetic include any of the following:

1. Pain during injection
2. Greater possibility of a serious overdose reaction, if the local anesthetic is administered intravascularly (the speed of IV drug administration significantly affects the clinical manifestations of toxicity)
3. Postanesthetic pain caused by tissue trauma during the injection

These complications and their prevention, recognition, and management are discussed in greater detail in Chapters 17 and 18.

It should be noted that in some persons, the inferoposterior border of the mandible is not innervated by the trigeminal nerve. Any of the mandibular nerve blocks described in Chapter 14 provide only partial anesthesia in this situation. The PDL injection usually corrects the lack of pain control in this circumstance.

*Typical local anesthetic injections for extraction of four third molars include the following:

1. Right and left inferior alveolar nerve blocks, 1.8 mL each (3.6 mL)
2. Right and left posterior superior alveolar nerve blocks or supraperiosteal infiltration over each third molar, 1.3 to 1.8 mL each (2.6 to 3.6 mL)
3. Right and left palatal infiltration over the maxillary third molars, 0.45 mL each, or right and left greater palatine nerve block, 0.45 mL each (0.09 mL)

Total volume of local anesthetic: 8.1 mL or 162 mg or a 2% solution, 243 mg of a 3%, or 324 mg of a 4%.

FIXED PROSTHODONTICS

When preparing a tooth for full coverage (crown or bridge), it is necessary to place a provisional restoration over the prepared tooth. Although achieving pain control might not be difficult at the initial visit, it may be difficult at subsequent visits to adequately anesthetize the prepared tooth. The reason for this is probably the provisional restoration. Overly high restorations produce traumatic occlusion, which can lead to considerable sensitivity after about a day. Poorly adapted gingival margins develop microleakage, also causing sensitivity. Preparation of the tooth itself can cause sensitivity, through desiccation of tooth structure, possible pulpal involvement, and periodontal irritation. The longer these sources of irritation are present, the greater the trauma to the tooth is likely to be, and the more difficult it is to achieve adequate anesthesia. Usually a regional nerve block is effective. Supraperiosteal injections generally do not provide adequate pain control in these situations (depth may be adequate, but duration is considerably shorter than that usually expected from the drug).

LONG-DURATION LOCAL ANESTHESIA

Prolonged Dental or Surgical Procedures

Several specialty areas of dental practice require longer than usual pulpal or soft tissue anesthesia. They include fixed prosthodontics, oral surgery, and periodontics. During longer procedures (2 or more hours), an adequate duration of pulpal anesthesia may be difficult to achieve with more commonly used anesthetics such as articaine, lidocaine, mepivacaine, and prilocaine. Bupivacaine is a long-acting local anesthetic that can then be used. It is discussed more completely in Chapter 4.

Bupivacaine, a homolog of mepivacaine, has a long duration of clinical effectiveness when used for regional nerve block. Its duration of action when administered by supraperiosteal injection, although still long, is somewhat shorter (shorter even than that of lidocaine with epinephrine).[48] Its postoperative analgesic period lasts an average of 8 hours in the mandible and 5 hours in the maxilla.

Bupivacaine is available with a vasopressor (1:200,000 epinephrine). It is interesting to note that the addition of vasopressor to bupivacaine does not prolong its duration of action.[49]

Postsurgical Management of Pain

Frequently, after extensive surgical procedures, patients experience intense pain when the local anesthetic effect dissipates. It was, and still is in many cases, common practice to treat postoperative pain through the use of opioid analgesics. However, opioids have a high incidence of undesirable side effects such as nausea, vomiting, constipation, respiratory depression, and postural hypotension, especially in ambulatory patients.[50] Additionally, opioid analgesics are not very effective in the management of pain following dental surgery.[51]

Long-acting local anesthetics administered to surgical patients offer a means of providing successful postoperative pain control with minimal risk of developing adverse reactions. An advantage of using long-duration local anesthetics is their longer postoperative analgesia, which leads to a reduced need for the administration of postoperative opioid analgesic drugs.[52] Dentists often use an intermediate-acting local anesthetic such as articaine, lidocaine, mepivacaine, or prilocaine with a vasopressor for the surgical procedure, administering a long-acting local anesthetic just before the termination of surgery. Danielsson and associates compared bupivacaine, etidocaine, and lidocaine with regard to their effects on postoperative pain, and found that both bupivacaine and etidocaine were more effective in controlling postoperative pain when compared with lidocaine.[48] They also reported that bupivacaine was more effective than etidocaine in providing postoperative analgesia, and that patients receiving bupivacaine used significantly fewer analgesics.

It is pertinent to note that there appears to be a difference between etidocaine and bupivacaine with respect to their ability to provide adequate hemostasis, even though they contain the same concentration of vasopressor (1:200,000). Danielsson and associates noted that bupivacaine and lidocaine provided adequate hemostasis in 90% and etidocaine in only 75% of procedures.[49] It is possible that a higher concentration of local anesthetic may necessitate a higher concentration of vasopressor to provide comparable hemostasis. Also keep in mind the different vasodilating properties of the solutions.[53] Etidocaine HCl is no longer available in dental cartridges in North America.

TABLE 16-5
Oxford League of Analgesic Efficacy (Drugs Available in the United States and Canada)*†

Analgesic & Dose (mg)	NNT	Patients with at least 50% pain relief
Ibuprofen 600/800	1.7	86
Ketorolac 20	1.8	57
Ketorolac 60 (IM)	1.8	56
Diclofenac 100	1.8	69
Piroxicam 40	1.9	80
Celecoxib 400	2.1	52
Paracetamol 1000 + Codeine 60	2.2	57
Oxycodone IR 5 + Paracetamol 500	2.2	60
Oxycodone IR 15	2.3	73
Aspirin 1200	2.4	61
Ibuprofen 400	2.4	55
Oxycodone IR 10 + Paracetamol 1000	2.7	67
Naproxen 400/440	2.7	51
Pirocicam 20	2.7	63
Meperidine 100 (IM)	2.9	54
Tramadol 150	2.9	48
Morphine 10 (IM)	2.9	50
Ketorolac 30 (IM)	3.4	53
Placebo	n/a	18

Modified from the Oxford League Table of Analgesics in Acute Pain, Bandolier Website, 2007. Available at: http://www.medicine.ox.ac.uk/bandolier/booth/painpag/acutrev/analgesics/leagtab.html. Accessed 6 October 2011.
*Paracetamol is known as acetaminophen in the United States and Canada.
†Intramuscular drugs (IM) are highlighted in red.

Protocol for Perioperative and Postoperative Pain Control in Surgical Patients. Postoperative pain associated with most uncomplicated dental surgical procedures is mild and is well managed by oral administration of nonsteroidal anti-inflammatory drugs (NSAIDs) such as aspirin and ibuprofen.[51] Preoperative administration of NSAIDs appears to delay the onset of postoperative pain and to lessen its severity.[52,54] When a patient is unable to tolerate aspirin or other NSAIDs, acetaminophen can provide acceptable analgesia.

Other dental surgical procedures, such as removal of bony impactions and osseous periodontal or endodontic surgery, are more traumatic and typically are associated with more intense and prolonged postoperative pain. The onset of such pain can be delayed by presurgical administration of an NSAID followed by administration of a long-acting local anesthetic (bupivacaine) at the completion of surgery.[54]

The Oxford League Table of Analgesic Efficacy presents a meta-analysis of randomized, double-blind, single-dose, placebo-controlled studies in patients with moderate to severe postoperative dental, orthopedic, gynecologic, and general surgical pain.[51] Analgesic efficacy is expressed as number needed to treat (NNT), the number of patients who need to receive the active drug for one to achieve at least 50% relief of pain compared with placebo over a 4- to 6-hour treatment period.[55] The most effective analgesics have an NNT of just over 2 (Table 16-5). Effective pain relief for dental surgery normally can be achieved with oral nonopioid, nonsteroidal anti-inflammatory drugs, coxibs, and combinations of acetaminophen (paracetamol) and codeine.[51]

As noted in Table 16-5, few, if any, analgesics are better than NSAIDs for acute pain. All NSAIDs on the League table have NNTs of 1.6 to 3.0. Alternative analgesics, such as codeine 60 mg and tramadol 50 mg, have NNTs of 16 and 8, respectively. Parenteral morphine 10 mg and meperidine 100 mg have NNTs of 2.9.[51,56] Acetaminophen (paracetamol), administered orally at a dose of 1000 mg, has an NNT of almost 4. When combined with codeine 60 mg, its NNT improves to 2.2. Ibuprofen 400 mg at 2.4 and diclofenac 50 mg and rofecoxib 50 mg at about 2.3 are better. NSAIDs generally do well with lower (better) NNTs.[51]

For effective postsurgical pain management (i.e., no breakthrough pain), it is important to maintain a therapeutic

TABLE 16-6
Nonsteroidal Anti-Inflammatory Drugs

Generic	Proprietary	Availabiity, mg	Dosage Regimen
Ibuprofen	Advil, Caldolor, Motrin, and others	100, 200, 400, 600, 800	Adults: 400 mg PO every 4-6 hours as needed
Ketorolac	Toradol	10	10 mg PO q4-6h; max 40 mg/day Start 20 mg PO if <65 yo and >50 kg *Note:* PO only for patients who have received parenteral treatment; duration of combined PO/IM/IV treatment not to exceed 5 days
Diclofenac potassium	Cambia, Zipsor	50	50 mg PO tid Start 100 mg PO; 200 mg/day first 24 hours only, 150 mg/day thereafter
Piroxicam	Feldene	10, 20	Adults: 20 mg PO once daily. Adjust dose, as needed. Daily dose may be divided into two doses, if desired.
Celecoxib	Celebrex	50, 100, 200, 400	Start 400 mg PO, then 200 mg PO bid
Naproxen	Naprosyn	250, 375, 500	250-500 mg PO q12h. Max: 1250 mg/day
Tramadol	Ultram, Ryzolt	50, 100, 200 ER	50-100 mg PO q4-6h; Max: 400 mg/day

Data from Mosby's dental drug reference, St Louis, 2012, Mosby.

BOX 16-2 Pain Control Regimen for Surgical Procedures

Preoperative: Administer one oral dose of nonsteroidal anti-inflammatory drug (NSAID), minimally 1 hour before the scheduled surgical procedure.

Perioperative: Administer local anesthetic of adequate duration for procedure (articaine, lidocaine, mepivacaine, prilocaine with vasopressor).

If surgery of approximately 30 minutes' duration is planned, immediately follow initial local anesthetic injection with long-acting local anesthetic (bupivacaine).

If surgery of 1 hour or longer duration is planned, at the conclusion of the surgical procedure reinject the patient with long-acting local anesthetic (bupivacaine).

Postoperative: Have patient continue to take oral NSAID on a timed basis (e.g., bid, tid, qid) for the number of days considered necessary by the surgeon.

Contact patient via telephone the evening of the surgery to determine level of comfort. If considerable pain is present, add opioid to NSAID: codeine.

Modified from Malamed SF: Local anesthetics: dentistry's most important drugs, J Am Dent Assoc 125:1571–1576, 1994.

blood level of the analgesic via time-based dosage administration of the appropriate oral analgesic. A therapeutic dose of the drug (e.g., ibuprofen 600 mg) should be administered every 4 to 6 hours. The drug package insert for ibuprofen states the following regarding its administration for mild to moderate dental pain[57]:

> *Oral dosage:* ***Adults:*** *400 mg PO every 4–6 hours as needed. Doses greater than 400 mg have not provided greater relief of pain.* ***Elderly:*** *See adult dosage; as elderly patients may be at a higher risk of adverse events, treat with the lowest effective dose and shortest possible duration.* ***Adolescents:*** *400 mg PO every 4–6 hours as needed. Doses greater than 400 mg have not provided greater relief of pain.*

Despite the statement above regarding larger doses than 400 mg ibuprofen, the Oxford League clearly shows that ibuprofen 600 mg (NNT of 1.7) is more efficacious than ibuprofen 400 mg (NNT of 2.4).

Box 16-2 outlines a recommended protocol for the management of intraoperative and postoperative pain associated with dental surgical procedures.[58] Common NSAIDs and their recommended doses are listed in Table 16-6.

DENTAL HYGIENE

In 1997 when the fourth edition of this textbook was published, registered dental hygienists in 20 states in the United States and several provinces in Canada were permitted to administer local anesthesia to dental patients. This number increased to 32 in 2003 and today (2011) stands at 44 states (Fig. 16-6).[59] Inclusion of this expanded function in the Dental Practice Act in these areas has proved of great benefit to the hygienist, doctor, and dental patient.[60,61]

Though not all patients need local anesthesia for scaling, root planing, and subgingival curettage, many do. The periodontal tissues being treated normally are sensitive to stimuli and are even more so when inflammation is present. Such is frequently the case when a patient is treated by the dental hygienist.

The hygienist who is permitted to administer local anesthetics to dental patients requires the same technique armamentarium as the doctor. Regional block anesthesia, especially in the maxilla (posterior superior or anterior superior alveolar nerve block), is an integral part of the hygienist's anesthetic armamentarium because hygienists usually treat whole quadrants during a single appointment. The hygiene patient requires the same depth of anesthesia as is attained by the doctor doing restorative dentistry or surgery. Root

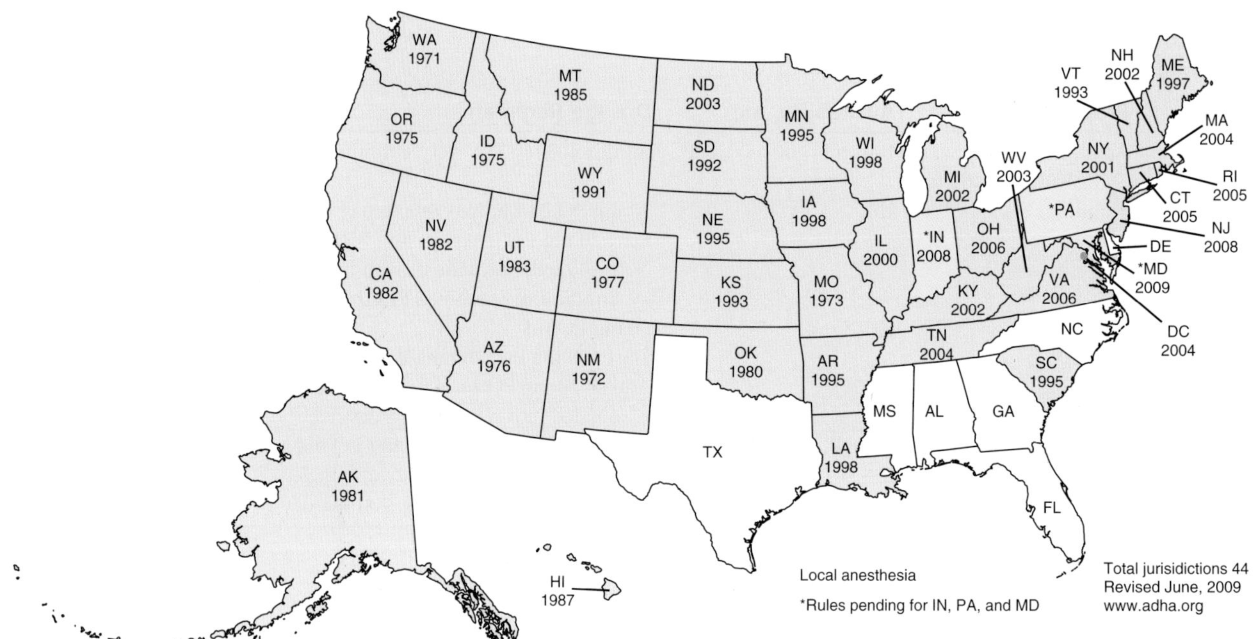

Figure 16-6. Dental Hygiene local anesthesia map.

planing without discomfort requires pulpal anesthesia, along with soft tissue and osseous anesthesia.[60] More than 70% of respondents to a survey on dental hygiene patients' need for pain control reported that their patients needed anesthesia but did not receive it.[61]

Feedback from dentists whose hygienists administer local anesthesia has been uniformly positive; negative comments have been extremely rare.[62] Dental patients themselves are aware of the difference between local anesthesia administered by the dental hygienist and that administered by the dentist. They frequently comment on the lack of discomfort when the hygienist injects the local anesthetic. Be it a slower rate of administration, greater attention to the details of atraumatic injection technique, or greater empathy, it works.

References

1. Brown RD: The failure of local anaesthesia in acute inflammation, Br Dent J 151:47–51, 1981.
2. Vandermeulen E: Pain perception, mechanisms of action of local anesthetics and possible causes of failure, Rev Belge Medecine Dent 55:19–40, 2000.
3. Kitay D, Ferraro N, Sonis ST: Lateral pharyngeal space abscess as a consequence of regional anesthesia, J Am Dent Assoc 122:56–59, 1991.
4. Connor JP, Edelson JG: Needle tract infection: a case report, Oral Surg 65:401–403, 1988.
5. Malamed SF: Buffering local aesthetics in dentistry, ADSA Pulse. In press.
6. Personal communication, Onpharma Inc., February 2011.
7. Coggins R, Reader A, Nist R, et al: Anesthetic efficacy of the intraosseous injection in maxillary and mandibular teeth, Oral Surg Oral Med Oral Pathol Oral Radiol Endodont 81:634–641, 1996.
8. Reisman D, Reader A, Nist R, et al: Anesthetic efficacy of the supplemental intraosseous injection of 3% mepivacaine in irreversible pulpitis, Oral Surg Oral Med Oral Pathol Oral Radiol Endodont 84:676–682, 1997.
9. Leonard M: The efficacy of an intraosseous injection system of delivering local anesthetic, J Am Dent Assoc 126:11–86, 1995.
10. Coury KA: Achieving profound anesthesia using the intraosseous technique, Tex Dent J 114:34–39, 1997.
11. Nusstein J, Reader A, Nist R, et al: Anesthetic efficacy of the supplemental intraosseous injection of 2% lidocaine with 1:100,000 epinephrine in irreversible pulpitis, J Endodont 24:478–491, 1998.
12. Quinn CL: Injection techniques to anesthetize the difficult tooth, J Calif Dent Assoc 26:665–667, 1998.
13. Parente SA, Anderson RW, Herman WW, et al: Anesthetic efficacy of the supplemental intraosseous injection for teeth with irreversible pulpitis, J Endodont 24:826–828, 1998.
14. Brown R: Intraosseous anesthesia: a review, J Calif Dent Assoc 27:785–792, 1999.
15. Weathers A Jr: Taking the mystery out of endodontics. Part 6. Painless anesthesia for the "hot" tooth, Dent Today 18:90–93, 1999.
16. Stabile P, Reader A, Gallatin E, et al: Anesthetic efficacy and heart rate effects of the intraosseous injection of 1.5% etidocaine (1:200,000 epinephrine) after an inferior alveolar nerve block, Oral Surg Oral Med Oral Pathol Oral Radiol Endodont 89:407–411, 2000.
17. Replogle K, Reader A, Nist R, et al: Cardiovascular effects of intraosseous injections of 2% lidocaine with 1:100,000 epinephrine and 3% mepivacaine, J Am Dent Assoc 130:549–657, 1999.
18. Saadoun AP, Malamed SF: Intraseptal anesthesia in periodontal surgery, J Am Dent Assoc 111:249-256, 1985.
19. Goodsen JM, Moore PA: Life-threatening reactions after pedodontic sedation: an assessment of narcotic, local anesthetic, and antiemetic drug interaction, J Am Dent Assoc 107:239–245, 1983.
20. Moore PA: Preventing local anesthesia toxicity, J Am Dent Assoc 123:60–64, 1992.

21. Berquist HC: The danger of mepivacaine 3% toxicity in children, Can Dent Assoc J 3:13, 1975.
22. Malamed SF: Morbidity, mortality and local anesthesia, Prim Dent Care 6:11–15, 1999.
23. American Academy on Pediatric Dentistry Council on Clinical Affairs: Guideline on appropriate use of local anesthesia for pediatric dental patients, Pediatr Dent 30(Suppl 7):134–139, 2008-2009.
24. Meechan JG, Rood JP: Adverse effects of dental local anaesthesia, Dent Update 24:315–318, 1997.
25. Davis MJ, Vogel LD: Local anesthetic safety in pediatric patients, N Y State Dent J 62:22–35, 1996.
26. Cheatham BD, Primosch RE, Courts FJ: A survey of local anesthetic usage in pediatric patients by Florida dentists, J Dent Child 59:401–407, 1992.
27. Yagiela JA: Regional anesthesia for dental procedures, Int Anesthesiol Clin 27:28–82, 1989.
28. Malamed SF: Allergic and toxic reactions to local anesthetics, Dent Today 22:114–121, April 2003.
29. College C, Feigal R, Wandera A, et al: Bilateral versus unilateral mandibular block anesthesia in a pediatric population, Pediatr Dent 22:453–457, 2000.
30. FDA approves OraVerse. Available at: www.drugs.com. Accessed February 7, 2011.
31. Tavares M, Goodson JM, Studen-Pavlovich D, et al, and The Local Anesthetic Reversal Group: Reversal of soft tissue anesthesia with phentolamine mesylate in pediatric patients, J Am Dent Assoc 139:1095–1104, 2008.
32. Rood JP: Notes on local analgesia for the child patient, Dent Update 8:377–381, 1981.
33. Kaufman L, Sowray JH, Rood JP: General anaesthesia, local analgesia, and sedation in dentistry, Oxford, UK, 1982, Blackwell Scientific.
34. O'Sullivan VR, Holland T, O'Mullane DM, et al: A review of current local anaesthetic techniques in dentistry for children, J Irish Dent Assoc 32:17–27, 1986.
35. Sharaf AA: Evaluation of mandibular infiltration versus block anesthesia in pediatric dentistry, ASDC J Dent Child 64:276–281, 1997.
36. Oulis CJ, Vadiakis GP, Vasilopoulou A: The effectiveness of mandibular infiltration compared to mandibular block anesthesia in treating primary molars in children, Pediatr Dent 18:301–305, 1996.
37. Benham NR: The cephalometric position of the mandibular foramen with age, J Dent Child 43:233–237, 1976.
38. Akinosi JO: A new approach to the mandibular nerve block, Br J Oral Surg 15:83–87, 1977.
39. Yamada A, Jastak JT: Clinical evaluation of the Gow-Gates block in children, Anesth Prog 28:106–109, 1981.
40. Brannstrom M, Lindskog S, Nordenvall KJ: Enamel hypoplasia in permanent teeth induced by periodontal ligament anesthesia of primary teeth, J Am Dent Assoc 109: 535–736, 1984.
41. Davenport RE, Porcelli RJ, Iacono VJ, et al: Effects of anesthetics containing epinephrine on catecholamine levels during periodontal surgery, J Periodontol 61:553–558, 1990.
42. van der Bijl P, Victor AM: Adverse reactions associated with norepinephrine in dental local anesthesia, Anesth Prog 39:37–89, 1992.
43. Jakob W: Local anaesthesia and vasoconstrictive additional components, Newslett Int Fed Dent Anesthesiol Soc 2:1, 1989.
44. Sveen K: Effect of the addition of a vasoconstrictor to local anesthetic solution on operative and postoperative bleeding, analgesia and wound healing, Int J Oral Surg 8:301–306, 1979.
45. Buckley JA, Ciancio SG, McMullen JA: Efficacy of epinephrine concentration in local anesthesia during periodontal surgery, J Periodontol 55:653–657, 1984.
46. Jastak JT, Yagiela JA: Vasoconstrictors and local anesthesia; a review and rationale for use, J Am Dent Assoc 107:623–630, 1983.
47. Skoglund LA, Jorkjend L: Postoperative pain experience after gingivectomies using different combinations of local anaesthetic agents and periodontal dressings, J Clin Periodontol 18:204–209, 1991.
48. Danielsson K, Evers H, Nordenram A: Long-acting local anesthetics in oral surgery: an experimental evaluation of bupivacaine and etidocaine for oral infiltration anesthesia, Anesth Prog 32:65–68, 1985.
49. Danielsson K, Evers H, Holmlund A, et al: Long-acting local anaesthetics in oral surgery, Int J Oral Maxillofac Surg 15:119–126, 1986.
50. Hardman JG, Limbird LE, editors: Goodman & Gilman's the pharmacological basis of therapeutics, ed 10, New York, 2001, McGraw-Hill.
51. The Oxford League Table of Analgesics in Acute Pain, Bandolier Website, 2007. Available at: http://www.medicine.ox.ac.uk/bandolier/booth/painpag/Acutrev/Analgesics/Leagtab.html. Accessed October 6, 2011.
52. Jackson DL, Moore PA, Hargreaves KM: Pre-operative nonsteroidal anti-inflammatory medication for the prevention of postoperative dental pain, J Am Dent Assoc 119:641–647, 1989.
53. Linden ET, Abrams H, Matheny J, et al: A comparison of postoperative pain experience following periodontal surgery using two local anesthetic agents, J Periodontol 57:637–642, 1986.
54. Acute Pain Management Guideline Panel: Acute pain management: operative or medical procedures and trauma. Clinical practice guideline, AHCPR Pub. No. 92-0032, Rockville, Md, 1992, Agency for Health Care Policy and Research, Public Health Service, U.S. Department of Health and Human Services.
55. Cook RJ, Sackett DL: The number needed to treat: a clinically useful measure of treatment effect, BMJ 310:452–454, 1995.
56. Ong CKS, Lirk P, Tan CH, et al: An evidence-based update on nonsteroidal anti-inflammatory drugs, Clin Med Res 5:19–34, 2007.
57. Ibuprofen monograph. Indications—Dosage. Available at: www.mdconsult.com. Updated August 16, 2010. Accessed October 6, 2011.
58. Malamed SF: Local anesthetics: dentistry's most important drugs, J Am Dent Assoc 125:1571–1576, 1994.
59. American Dental Hygienists Association: Available at: www.adha.org, January 2011. Accessed October 6, 2011.
60. Sisty-LePeau N, Boyer EM, Lutjen D: Dental hygiene licensure specifications on pain control procedures, J Dent Hyg 64:179–185, 1990.
61. Sisty-LePeau N, Nielson-Thompson N, Lutjen D: Use, need and desire for pain control procedures by Iowa hygienists, J Dent Hyg 66:137–146, 1992.
62. DeAngelis S, Goral V: Utilization of local anesthesia by Arkansas dental hygienists, and dentists' delegation/satisfaction relative to this function, J Dent Hyg 74:196–204, 2000.

IN THIS PART

PART IV

Complications, Legal Considerations, Questions, and Future

In spite of careful patient evaluation, proper tissue preparation, and meticulous technique of administration, local and systemic complications associated with dental anesthesia occasionally develop. These problems are addressed in Chapters 17 and 18. Emphasis is placed on prevention, recognition, and management of the complications.

Dr. Daniel Orr II discusses legal considerations associated with the administration of local anesthetics in Chapter 19.

Chapter 20, "Future Trends in Pain Control," first appeared in the third edition and is updated here. Starting in the late 1990s, there has been a renewal of interest in the field of local anesthesia…a renaissance of sorts…beginning with the introduction of computer-controlled local anesthetic delivery (C-CLAD), and in 2000, the introduction of articaine HCl in the United States. Most recently, the local anesthesia reversal agent phentolamine mesylate (2008) and buffered local anesthetics (2011) have been introduced. As for the future, research is now being conducted into providing maxillary pulpal anesthesia without the need for injection of local anesthetics.

Chapter 21 presents a series of questions related to local anesthesia and pain control in dentistry. These frequently asked questions (FAQs) come from doctors who have had peculiar situations arise in connection with local anesthetic administration. The more common questions are presented here as a matter of interest and in the hope that the answers to specific questions or problems might be included.

CHAPTER 17

Local Complications

A number of potential complications are associated with the administration of local anesthetics. For purposes of convenience, these complications may be separated into those that occur locally in the region of the injection and those that are systemic. Systemic complications associated with the administration of local anesthesia are discussed in Chapter 18, and include overdosage (toxic reaction), allergy, and psychogenic reactions. The following localized complications are described in this chapter:

- Needle breakage
- Prolonged anesthesia or paresthesia
- Facial nerve paralysis
- Trismus
- Soft tissue injury
- Hematoma
- Pain on injection
- Burning on injection
- Infection
- Edema
- Sloughing of tissues
- Postanesthetic intraoral lesions

It must be emphasized that with any complication associated with the administration of a local anesthetic, a written note should be entered onto the patient's dental chart. For complications that become chronic, a note should appear whenever the patient is re-evaluated.

NEEDLE BREAKAGE

Since the introduction of non-reusable, stainless steel dental local anesthetic needles, needle breakage has become an extremely rare complication of dental local anesthetic injections (Fig. 17-1). Pogrel has (roughly) estimated the risk of needle breakage among Northern California dentists at 1 in 14 million inferior alveolar nerve blocks.[1] In the United States, 1.43 million boxes of dental needles (100 needles per box; 143,000,000 needles) were sold by one needle manufacturer in 2004, 1.56 million boxes in 2005, and 1.43 million boxes in 2006.[2] Reports of broken dental needles in the published literature appear only infrequently, but they do appear. A MedLine search for broken dental needles from 1951 through February 2010 uncovered 26 published reports of broken dental needles, including their cause and management.[1,3-27] Review of 20 of these reports, for which information regarding needle gauge and length and technique of anesthesia employed is available, reveals that 15 were inferior alveolar nerve block (IANB) and 5 were posterior superior alveolar (PSA) nerve block. All 5 PSA reports described adult patients, whereas 9 of the 15 broken needle reports following IANB occurred in children. Needle gauge and/or length was presented in 11 papers. Ten of the 11 needles were 30-gauge short; only one case reported long needle breakage (27-gauge) with the needle remaining in the tissues.[12]

Pogrel reported on 16 patients whom he evaluated over a 25-year period (1983-2008) following needle breakage.[1] Fifteen patients had received IANB, one a PSA. Thirteen of the 16 needles were 30-gauge short, 3 were 27-gauge short.

Independent of the cited literature, this author is aware of 51 cases that progressed to litigation in which broken dental needle fragments remained within the soft tissues of the patient receiving the injection.[28] Fifty of these events involved 30-gauge short needles; a 27-gauge short was involved in the other case. All but 1 involved administration of an IANB. A posterior superior alveolar nerve block was used in the other case.

A manufacturer of dental local anesthetic needles reported that over a 6-year period (1997-2002), 27 doctors contacted the company reporting instances of broken dental needles. All incidents involved 30-gauge short needles.[29]

Long dental needles most likely have broken during injection. However, because the long needle is unlikely to have been inserted to its full length (approximately 32 mm) into soft tissue, some portion of the needle would remain visible in the patient's mouth. Retrieval of the fragment with a hemostat is easily accomplished. Litigation does not occur in such incidents.

Table 17-1 summarizes the accumulated findings presented to this point. Although some reports may have been

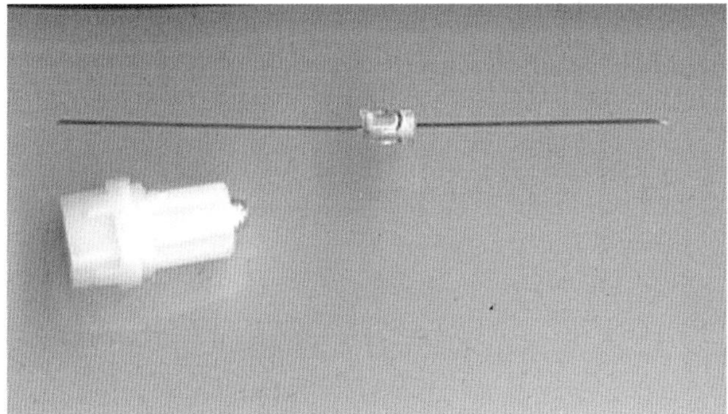

Figure 17-1. Metal disposable needle, disassembled.

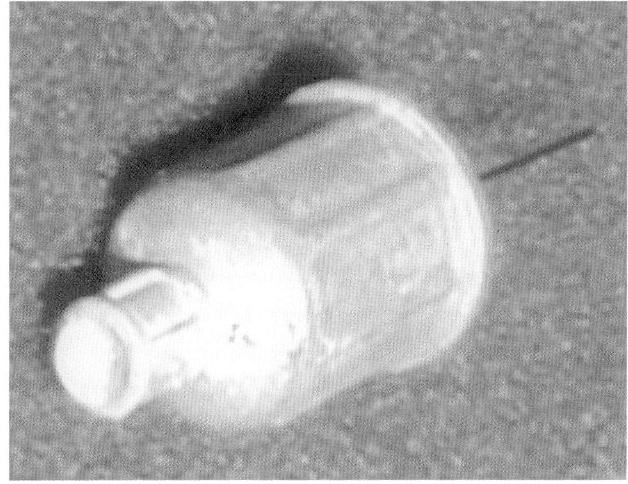

Figure 17-2. Hub of broken needle from Figure 17-3, B.

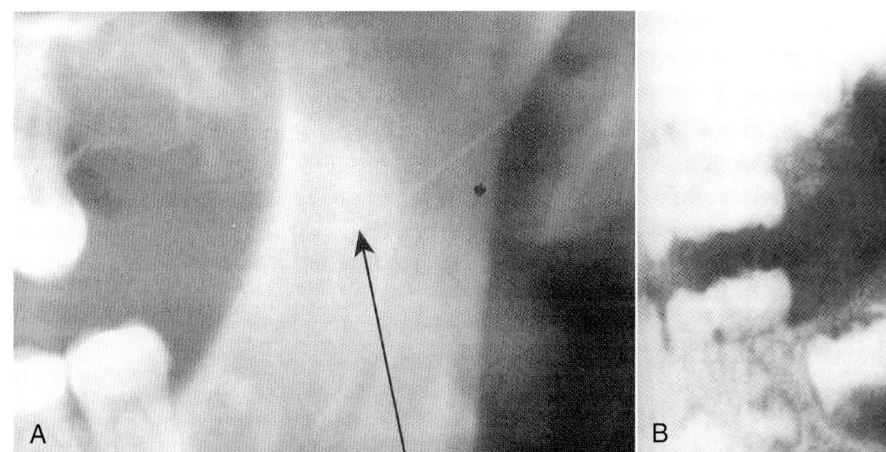

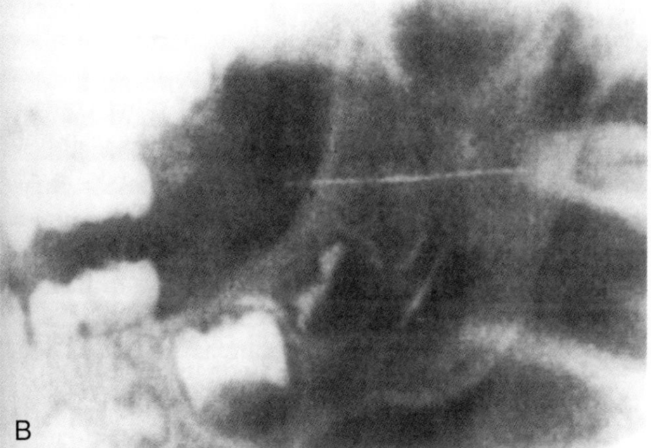

Figure 17-3. **A,** Radiograph of a broken dental needle (note bend in needle: arrow). **B,** Radiograph of a broken dental needle in the pterygomandibular space. (**B,** From Marks RB, Carlton DM, McDonald S: Management of a broken needle in the pterygomandibular space: report of a case, J Am Dent Assoc 109:263–264, 1984. Reprinted by permission.)

TABLE 17-1
Summary of Reports of Broken Dental Needles

	IANB	PSA	30-Gauge	27-Gauge
Individual citations	15	5	10	1
Pogrel[21]	15	1	13	3
Malamed	32	1	33	1
Reed	17	0	17	0
Manufacturer	N/A	N/A	27	0
Total	79	7	100	5

From Malamed SF, Reed K, Poorsattar S: Needle breakage: incidence and prevention, Dent Clin N Am 54:745–756, 2010.
N/A, Not applicable.

duplicated, the factual information clearly identifies commonalities in most cases: use of 30-gauge short or ultrashort needles in injection techniques in which the needle is inserted to its hub ("hubbing the needle"). All reported cases involved the inferior alveolar or posterior superior alveolar nerve block. In all situations in which it is mentioned, needle fracture occurred at the hub—never along the shaft of the needle (Fig. 17-2). Additional factors include (1) intentional bending of the needle by the doctor before injection (Fig. 17-3, *A*) (2) sudden unexpected movement by the patient while the needle is still embedded in tissue; and (3) forceful contact with bone.

The exact cause of needle breakage is rarely discernible. In cases in which the needle has been surgically retrieved and/or forensic metallurgists have examined the hub of the needle, no evidence has revealed manufacturing defects in the needle (Fig. 17-4).

Problem

Needle breakage per se is not a significant problem if the needle can be removed without surgical intervention. Ready access to a hemostat enables the doctor or the assistant to grasp the visible proximal end of the needle fragment and remove it from the soft tissue.

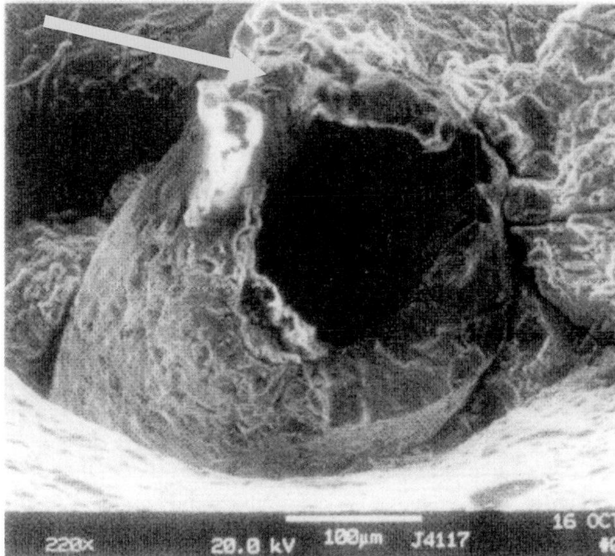

Figure 17-4. Scanning electron microscopy of a broken dental needle. Arrow at 11 o'clock position indicates area where needle was bent superiorly before injection, per court testimony of forensic metallurgist.

Where the needle has been inserted to its hub and the soft tissue has dimpled under pressure from the syringe, the broken fragment will not be visible when the syringe is withdrawn from the patient's mouth.The needle fragment remaining in the tissue poses a risk of serious damage being inflicted on the soft tissues for as long as the fragment remains. Although it does not often occur, needle fragments can migrate, as is illustrated by the series of panoramic films taken at 3-month intervals (Fig. 17-5).

Management

Management of the broken dental needle involves immediate referral of the patient to an appropriate specialist (e.g., an oral and maxillofacial surgeon) for evaluation and possible attempted retrieval. Conventional management involves locating the retained fragment through panoramic and computed tomographic (CT) scanning.[25]

More recently, three-dimensional CT scanning has been recommended to identify the location of the retained needle fragment.[1,30] A surgeon in the operating theater then removes the retained needle fragment while the patient is under general anesthesia (Fig. 17-6).

Prevention

Although rare, dental needle breakage can, and does, occur. Review of the literature and personal experience of the authors bring into focus several commonalities, which, when avoided, can minimize the risk of needle breakage with the fragment being retained. These include the following:

- Do not use short needles for inferior alveolar nerve block in adults or larger children.
- Do not use 30-gauge needles for inferior alveolar nerve block in adults or children.
- Do not bend needles when inserting them into soft tissue.
- Do not insert a needle into soft tissue to its hub, unless it is absolutely essential for the success of the injection.
- Observe extra caution when inserting needles in younger children or in extremely phobic adult or child patients.

PROLONGED ANESTHESIA OR PARESTHESIA

On occasion, a patient reports feeling numb ("frozen") many hours or days after a local anesthetic injection. Normal distribution of patient response to drugs allows for the rare individual (e.g., hyperreactor) who may experience prolonged soft tissue anesthesia after local anesthetic administration that persists for many hours longer than expected. This is not a problem.

When anesthesia persists for days, weeks, or months, the potential for the development of problems is increased. Paresthesia or persistent anesthesia is a disturbing yet often-times unpreventable complication of local anesthetic administration. Paresthesia is one of the most frequent causes of dental malpractice litigation.

A patient's clinical response to this can be profuse and varied, including sensations of numbness, swelling, tingling, and itching. Associated oral dysfunction, including tongue biting, drooling, loss of taste, and speech impediment, may be noted.[31-34]

Paresthesia is defined as persistent anesthesia (anesthesia well beyond the expected duration), or altered sensation well beyond the expected duration of anesthesia. In addition, the definition of paresthesia should include hyperesthesia and dysesthesia, in which the patient experiences both pain and numbness.[35]

Causes

Trauma to any nerve may lead to paresthesia. Paresthesia is a not uncommon complication of oral surgical procedures and mandibular dental implants.[32,36-38] In an audit of 741 mandibular third molar extractions, Bataineh found postoperative lingual nerve anesthesia in 2.6%; inferior alveolar nerve paresthesia was 3.9%, developing in 9.8% of patients younger than 20 years of age. Also, a significant correlation was noted between the incidence of paresthesia and the experience of the operator.[38]

Injection of a local anesthetic solution contaminated by alcohol or sterilizing solution near a nerve produces irritation, resulting in edema and increased pressure in the region of the nerve, leading to paresthesia. These contaminants, especially alcohol, are neurolytic and can produce long-term trauma to the nerve (paresthesia lasting for months to years).

Trauma to the nerve sheath can be produced by the needle during injection. Many patients report the sensation of an "electric shock" throughout the distribution of the involved nerve. Although it is exceedingly difficult (and is highly unlikely) to actually sever a nerve trunk or even its fibers

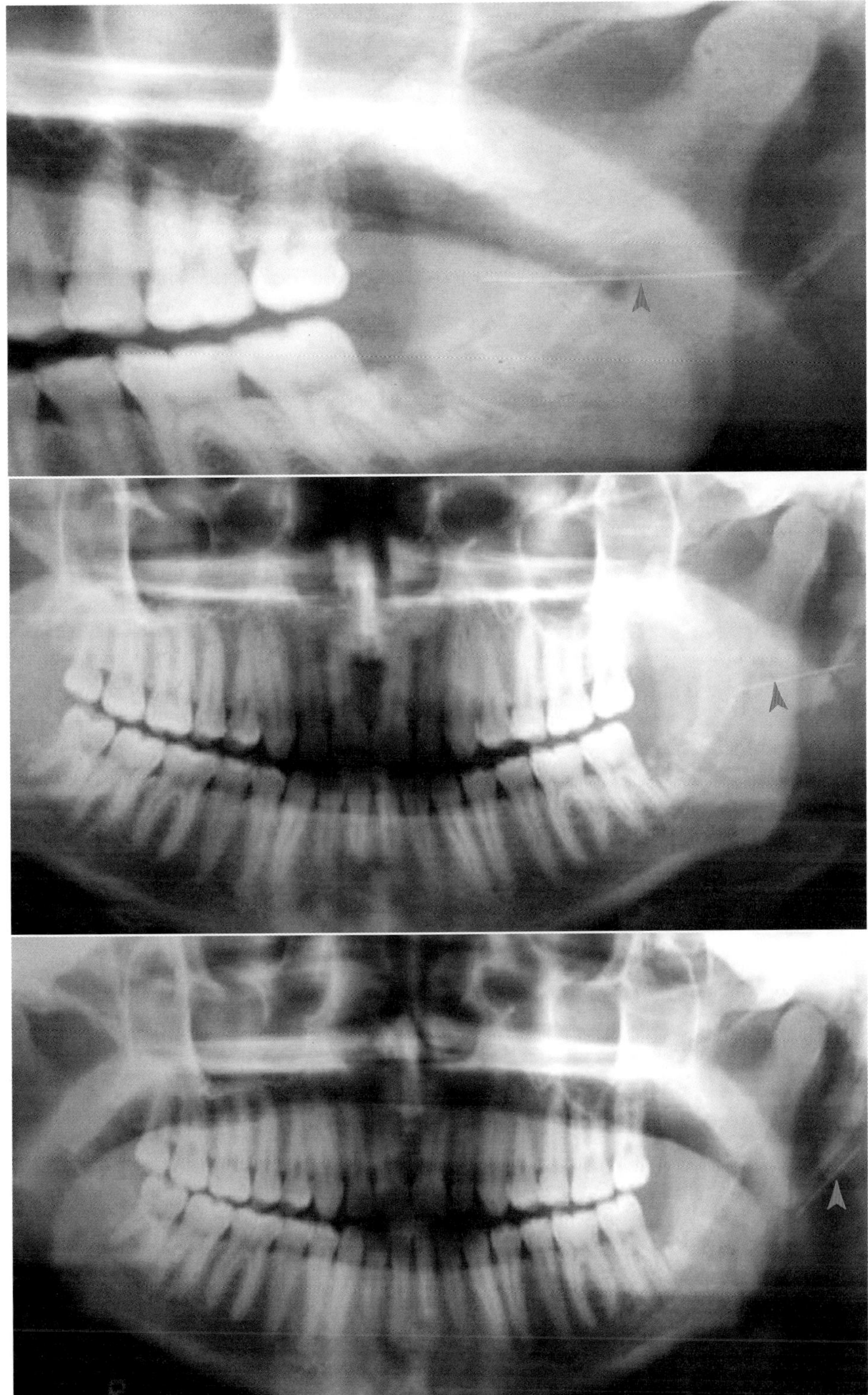

Figure 17-5. Needle fragments can migrate as is shown in the series of panoramic films taken at 3-month intervals. (Courtesy Dr. Carlos Elias De Freitas. From Malamed SF, Reed KR, Poorsattar S: Needle breakage: incidence and prevention, Dent Clin N Amer 54:745–756, 2010.)

with the small needles used in dentistry, trauma to a nerve produced by contact with the needle is all that may be needed to produce paresthesia.[32,33] Insertion of a needle into a foramen, as in the second division (maxillary) nerve block via the greater palatine foramen, also increases the likelihood of nerve injury.

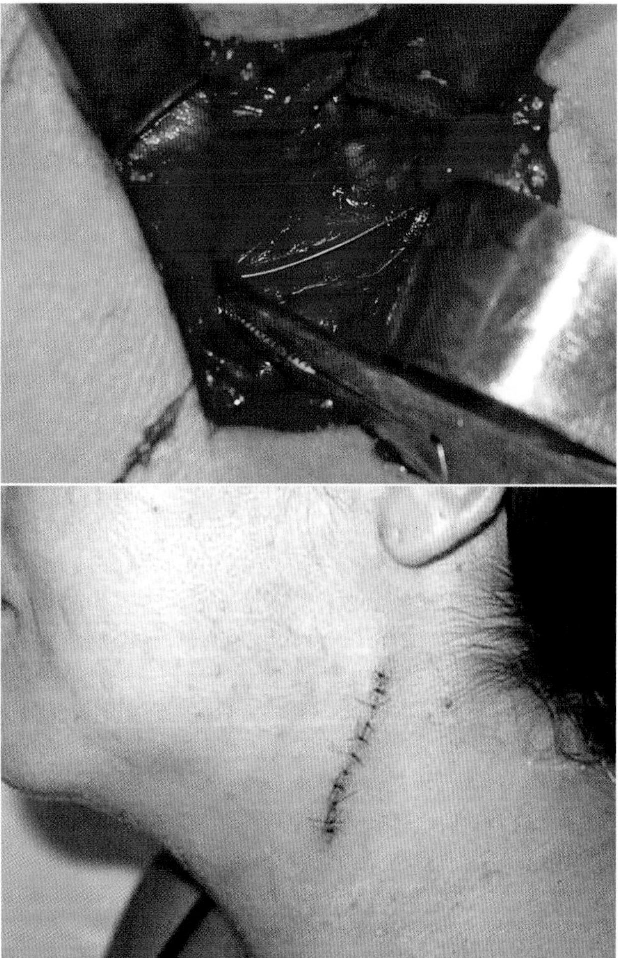

Figure 17-6. Surgical excision of needle fragment (see patient from Fig. 17-5). Courtesy Dr. Carlos Elias De Freitas CVM. From Malamed SF, Reed KR, Poorsattar S: Needle breakage: incidence and prevention, Dent Clin N Amer 54:745–756, 2010.)

Hemorrhage into or around the neural sheath is another cause. Bleeding increases pressure on the nerve, leading to paresthesia.[31-33,35]

The local anesthetic solution itself may contribute to the development of paresthesia after local anesthetic injection.[39] Haas and Lennon took a retrospective look at paresthesia after injection of local anesthetic in dentistry in the province of Ontario, Canada, over a 20-year period (1973-1993).[31] This report included voluntary submissions by dentists to their insurance carriers for claims of paresthesia. Only cases where no surgery was performed were considered. One hundred forty-three cases of paresthesia unrelated to surgery were reported in this period. All reported cases involved the inferior alveolar or the lingual nerve or both, with anesthesia of the tongue reported most often, followed by anesthesia of the lip. Pain (hyperesthesia) was reported by 22% of patients. Paresthesia was reported more often after administration of a 4% local anesthetic—prilocaine HCl and articaine HCl. Observed frequencies of paresthesia after administration of articaine HCl and prilocaine HCl were greater than expected, based on the distribution of local anesthetic use in Ontario in 1993.[31] According to Haas, the incidence of paresthesia resulting from all local anesthetics is approximately 1:785,000; for 0.5%, 2%, and 3% local anesthetics, it is approximately 1:1,250,000, and for 4% local anesthetics, it is approximately 1:485,000.[31]

In 2006 Hillerup and Jensen in Denmark, reviewing insurance claims, suggested that articaine should not be used by inferior alveolar nerve block because it had, in their opinion, a greater propensity for paresthesia.[40] Yet, of the 54 case reports of paresthesia reviewed, 42 (77%) involved not the inferior alveolar nerve but the lingual nerve (see later discussion) (Table 17-2).

In response to Hillerup and Jensen's article, the Pharmacovigilance Working Committee of the European Union reviewed reports of paresthesia associated with articaine and other local anesthetics in 57 countries, estimating that the number of patients treated with articaine is approximately 100 million annually.[41] Their published report (October 30, 2006) states the following: "This investigation is a follow-up to an inquiry initiated in 2005. This enquiry resulted from suspicions that were raised in Denmark, that a local anesthetic, articaine, was responsible for an increased risk of nerve injuries compared with the risk associated with other

TABLE 17-2
Distribution of Analgesic Solution and Nerve Affected, Including 54 Nerve Injuries in 52 Patients

	Inferior Alveolar Nerve	Lingual Nerve	Sum, N (%)
Articaine 4%	5	24	29 (54)
Prilocaine 3%	4	6	10 (19)
Lidocaine 2%	3	7	10 (19)
Mepivacaine 3%	0	4	4 (7)
Mepivacaine 3% + Articaine 4%	0	1	1 (2)
Number of nerve injuries	12	42	54 (100)

From Hillerup S, Jensen R: Nerve injury caused by mandibular block analgesia, Int J Oral Maxillofac Surg 35:437–443, 2006.

TABLE 17-3
Number of cases of nerve damage with percentage of U.S. National Sales Figures

Anesthetic	# of Cases (%)	Approximate Share of LA Market in United States, %	Ratio (1.0 Expected)
Lidocaine HCl	20 (35)	54	0.64
Prilocaine HCl	17 (29.8)	6	4.96
Articaine HCl	17 (29.8)	25	1.19
Articaine HCl + Lidocaine HCl	1 (1.75)		
Lidocaine HCl + Prilocaine HCl	1 (1.75)		
Bupivacaine HCl	1 (1.75)		
Mepivacaine HCl	0 (0)	15	

From Pogrel MA: Permanent nerve damage from inferior alveolar nerve blocks—an update to include articaine, J Calif Dent Assoc 35:271–273, 2007 (modified to include ratio).

local anesthetics (mepivacaine, prilocaine, lidocaine)." The report concluded: "Regarding articaine, the conclusion is that [the] safety profile of the drug has not significantly evolved since its initial launch (1999). Thus, no medical evidence exists to prohibit the use of articaine according to the current guidelines listed in the summary of product characteristics.[41] All local anesthetics may cause nerve injury (they are neurotoxic in nature). The occurrence of sensory impairment is apparently slightly more frequent following use of articaine and prilocaine. However, considering the number of patients treated, sensory impairments rarely occur. For example, the incidence of sensory impairment following the use of articaine is estimated to be 1 case in 4.6 million treated patients." Further they report, "Nerve injuries may result from several incidents: mechanical injury due to needle insertion; direct toxicity from the drug; and neural ischaemia."

In 2007 Pogrel reported the first, and still the only, clinical evaluation of cases of paresthesia.[42] Evaluation of 57 cases of paresthesia following local anesthetic administration (over a 3-year period) revealed that lidocaine was responsible for 35% of cases, articaine 29.8%, and prilocaine 29.8%. He presented the following as the reason for his research and writing of the paper: "We were aware of the discussion in dental circles as to the use of articaine for inferior alveolar nerve blocks, and are aware of recommendations suggesting that it not be used for IANBs. This was the predominant reason for submitting this paper at this time."

Table 17-3 presents the incidence of paresthesia as reported by Pogrel along with the market share of each drug at that time.[12] If all local anesthetics were equally neurotoxic, then the percentage of reported cases of paresthesia for any given drug would be equal to its percentage of market share. For example, if a drug had a 30% market share, it should then account for 30% of the reported cases of paresthesia—a 1:1 ratio (reported as 1.0).

From Pogrel's statistics, lidocaine, with 54% of the market share and 35% of the reported cases of paresthesia, had a 0.64% ratio—better than expected. Prilocaine, on the other hand, with a 6% market share, had 29.8% of the reported cases—a 4.96% ratio. Articaine, with 25% market share at the time, had 29.8% of the reported cases—a 1.19% ratio.

TABLE 17-4
Reported incidences of paresthesia to AERS from 1997 to 2008

Mepivacaine	1:623,112,900
Lidocaine	1:181,076,673
Bupivacaine	1:124,286,050
Overall	1:13,800,970
Articaine	1:4,159,848
Prilocaine	1:2,070,678
Being struck by lightning (annual risk)	1:750,000

Data derived and modified from Garisto GA, Gaffen AS, Lawrence HP, et al: Occurrence of paresthesia after dental local anesthetic administration in the United States, J Am Dent Assoc 141:836–844, 2010.
AERS, Adverse event reporting system.

Pogrel concluded, "using our previous assumption that approximately half of local anesthetic used is for inferior alveolar nerve blocks, then on the figures we have generated from our clinic, we do not see disproportionate nerve involvement for articaine."

A meta-analysis of the efficacy and safety of articaine versus lidocaine, published in 2010, concluded, "This systematic review supports the argument that articaine as compared with lignocaine provides a higher rate of anaesthetic success, with comparable safety to lignocaine when used as infiltration or blocks for routine dental treatments."[43]

In July of 2010, Garisto and associates reported on the occurrence of paresthesia after dental local anesthetic administration in the United States.[44] Data were gathered from the U.S. Food and Drug Administration Adverse Event Reporting System (AERS). Over a 10-year reporting period (November 1997–August 2008), 248 cases of paresthesia following dental local anesthesia were reported, of which 94.5% involved inferior alveolar nerve block. Of the reported cases, 89.0% involved only the lingual nerve. Table 17-4 reports the incidence of paresthesia calculated for each dental local anesthetic. As a comparison, the reported risk of being struck by lightning in a given year in the United States is 1:750,000.[45]

Of the 248 cases, 108 reported on resolution of the paresthesia, which ranged from 1 day to 736 days. Confirmed resolution occurred in 34 of the 108 cases (31.4%). Of these, 25 resolved within 2 months, and the remaining 9 resolved within 240 days.[44]

However, the report by Garisto and colleagues relied on data from the AERS. The FDA Website for AERS displays the following warning: "AERS data do have limitations. First, there is no certainty that the reported event was actually due to the product. FDA does not require that a causal relationship between a product and event be proven, and reports do not always contain enough detail to properly evaluate an event. Further, FDA does not receive all adverse event reports that occur with a product. Many factors can influence whether or not an event will be reported, such as the time a product has been marketed and publicity about an event. Therefore, AERS cannot be used to calculate the incidence of an adverse event in the U.S. population."[46]

So, as of January 2012, "the jury is still out," as the saying goes. Proponents of one side of the argument adamantly believe that 4% local anesthetics do carry a greater risk of paresthesia, be it transient or permanent, but the others believe that other factors are usually involved, primarily mechanical trauma, especially when the paresthesia involves only the lingual nerve, as is the case in 89% of the cases cited by Garisto and colleages.[44]

So what should the doctor do? As with all procedures under consideration for use by a doctor, as well as with any drugs being considered for administration, the doctor must weigh the benefit to be gained from use of the drug or therapeutic procedure against the risks involved in its use. Only when, in the mind of the treating doctor, the benefit to be gained clearly outweighs the risk should the drug or the procedure be used.

Problem

Persistent anesthesia, rarely total, in most cases partial, can lead to self-inflicted soft tissue injury. Biting or thermal or chemical insult can occur without a patient's awareness until the process has progressed to a serious degree. When the lingual nerve is involved, the sense of taste (via the chorda tympani nerve) also may be impaired.

In some instances, loss of sensation (paresthesia) is not the clinical manifestation of nerve injury. Hyperesthesia (an increased sensitivity to noxious stimuli) and dysesthesia (a painful sensation occurring to usually nonnoxious stimuli) also may be noted. Haas and Lennon reported that pain was present in 22% of the 143 cases of paresthesia that they reviewed.[31]

Prevention

Strict adherence to injection protocol and proper care and handling of dental cartridges help minimize the risk of paresthesia. Nevertheless, cases of paresthesia will still occur in spite of care taken during the injection. Whenever a needle is inserted into soft tissues, anywhere in the body, in an attempt to deposit a drug (e.g., local anesthetic) as close to a nerve as possible without actually contacting it, it is simply a matter of time before such contact does occur. As Pogrel opined: "It is reasonable to suggest that during a career, each dentist may encounter at least one patient with an inferior alveolar nerve block resulting in permanent nerve involvement. The mechanisms are unknown and there is no known prevention or treatment."[32]

Management

Nichol reported that most paresthesias resolve within approximately 8 weeks without treatment.[47] Only when damage to the nerve is severe will the paresthesia be permanent, and this occurs only rarely.

In most situations, paresthesia is minimal, with the patient retaining most of the sensory function to the affected area. Therefore, the risk of self-inflicted tissue injury is minimal.

Garisto and coworkers, in reviewing 248 reports of paresthesia, had data on resolution in 108 cases. The period of resolution ranged from as little as 1 day to as many as 736 days. Confirmed resolution of paresthesia was reported in 34 of the 108 cases (31.4%). Of the 34 cases that did resolve, 25 did so within 2 months; the remaining 9 cases resolved within 240 days.[44]

McCarthy[48] and Orr[49] have recommended the following sequence in managing the patient with a persistent sensory deficit after local anesthesia:

1. Be reassuring. The patient usually telephones the office the day after the dental procedure complaining of still being a little numb.
   a. Speak with the patient personally. Do not relegate the duty to an auxiliary. Remember that if patients cannot get through to speak to their doctor, they can always get the doctor's attention through litigation.
   b. Explain that paresthesia is not uncommon after local anesthetic administration. Sisk and associates have reported that paresthesia may develop in up to 22% of patients in very select circumstances.[50]
   c. Arrange an appointment to examine the patient.
   d. Record the incident on the dental chart.
2. Examine the patient in person.
   a. Determine the degree and extent of paresthesia.
   b. Explain to the patient that paresthesia normally persists for at least 2 months before resolution begins, and that it may last up to a year or longer.
   c. "Tincture of time" (e.g., observation) is the recommended treatment, although surgery might be considered as an option.
   d. Record all findings on the patient's chart using the patient's own descriptors, such as "hot," "cold," "painful," "tingling," "increasing," "decreasing," and "staying the same."
   e. Suggest that simple observation for 1 to 2 months is recommended, but on that same day, offer to send the patient for a second opinion to an oral and maxillofacial surgeon (OMS), who will be able to map out the affected area and would be able to

perform the surgical repair, if that is deemed necessary.

f. If surgical repair is suggested by this first consultant, a second opinion should be sought from another OMS. It generally is deemed appropriate to observe the situation for minimally 1 to 2 months before considering the surgical option.

3. Reschedule the patient for examination every 2 months for as long as the sensory deficit persists.
4. Dental treatment may continue, but avoid readministering local anesthetic into the region of the previously traumatized nerve. Use alternate local anesthetic techniques if possible.
5. It would be prudent to contact your liability insurance carrier should the paresthesia persist without evident improvement beyond 1 to 2 months.

FACIAL NERVE PARALYSIS

The seventh cranial nerve carries motor impulses to the muscles of facial expression, of the scalp and external ear, and of other structures. Paralysis of some of its terminal branches occurs whenever an infraorbital nerve block is administered, or when maxillary canines are infiltrated. Muscle droop is also observed when, occasionally, motor fibers are anesthetized by inadvertent deposition of local anesthetic into their vicinity. This may occur when anesthetic is introduced into the deep lobe of the parotid gland, through which terminal portions of the facial nerve extend (Fig. 17-7).

The facial nerve branches and the muscles they innervate are listed below:

1. Temporal branches
   a. Frontalis
   b. Orbicularis oculi
   c. Corrugator supercilii
2. Zygomatic branches
   a. Orbicularis oculi
3. Buccal branches: supplying the region inferior to the eye and around the mouth
   a. Procerus
   b. Zygomaticus
   c. Levator labii superioris
   d. Buccinator
   e. Orbicularis oris
4. Mandibular branch: supplying muscles of the lower lip and chin
   a. Depressor anguli oris
   b. Depressor labii inferioris
   c. Mentalis

Cause

Transient facial nerve paralysis is commonly caused by the introduction of local anesthetic into the capsule of the parotid gland, which is located at the posterior border of the mandibular ramus, clothed by the medial pterygoid and

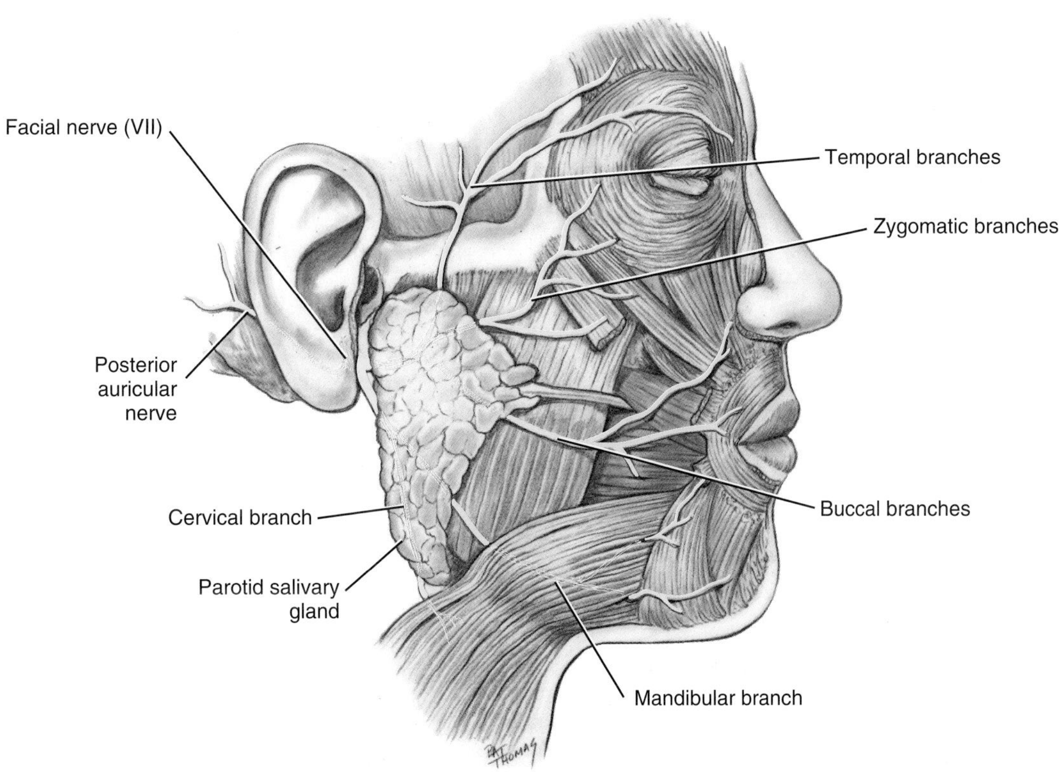

Figure 17-7. Facial nerve distribution.

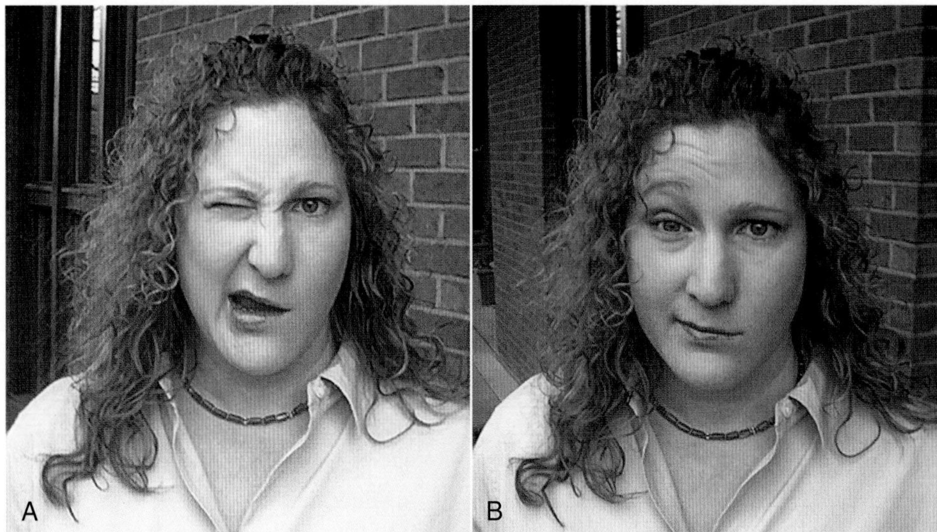

Figure 17-8. Facial nerve paralysis. Inability to close eyelid (**A**) and drooping of lip on affected side (patient's left) (**B**).

masseter muscles.[35,50-53] Directing the needle posteriorly or inadvertently deflecting it in a posterior direction during an IANB, or overinserting during a Vazirani-Akinosi nerve block, may place the tip of the needle within the body of the parotid gland. If local anesthetic is deposited, transient paralysis can result. The duration of the paralysis is equal to that of the soft tissue anesthesia usually noted for that drug.

Problem

Loss of motor function to the muscles of facial expression produced by local anesthetic deposition is normally transitory. It lasts no longer than several hours, depending on the local anesthetic formulation used, the volume injected, and proximity to the facial nerve. Usually, minimal or no sensory loss occurs.

During this time, the patient has unilateral paralysis and is unable to use these muscles (see Fig. 17-8). The primary problem associated with transient facial nerve paralysis is cosmetic: the person's face appears lopsided. No treatment is known, other than waiting until the action of the drug resolves.

A secondary problem is that the patient is unable to voluntarily close one eye. The protective lid reflex of the eye is abolished. Winking and blinking become impossible. The cornea, however, does retain its innervation; thus if it is irritated, the corneal reflex is intact, and tears lubricate the eye.

Prevention

Transient facial nerve paralysis is almost always preventable by adhering to protocol with the inferior alveolar and Vazirani-Akinosi nerve blocks (as described in Chapter 14), although in some situations, branches of the facial nerve may lie close to the site of local anesthetic deposition in the IANB and Vazirani-Akinosi nerve blocks.

A needle tip that comes in contact with bone (medial aspect of the ramus) before depositing local anesthetic solution essentially precludes the possibility that anesthetic will be deposited into the parotid gland during an IANB. If the needle deflects posteriorly during this block and bone is not contacted, the needle should be withdrawn almost entirely from the soft tissues, the barrel of the syringe brought posteriorly (thereby directing the needle tip more anteriorly), and the needle readvanced until it contacts bone.

Because no contact is made with bone during the Vazirani-Akinosi nerve block, overinsertion of the needle, either absolute (>25 mm) or relative (25 mm in a smaller patient), should be avoided, if possible.

Management

Within seconds to minutes after deposition of local anesthetic into the parotid gland, the patient senses weakening of the muscles on the affected side of the face. Sensory anesthesia is not present in this situation. Management includes the following:

1. Reassure the patient. Explain that the situation is transient, will last for a few hours, and will resolve without residual effect. Mention that it is produced by the normal action of local anesthetic drugs on the facial nerve, which is a motor nerve to the muscles of facial expression.
2. Contact lenses should be removed until muscular movement returns.
3. An eye patch should be applied to the affected eye until muscle tone returns. If resistance is offered by the patient, advise the patient to manually close the affected eyelid periodically to keep the cornea lubricated.
4. Record the incident on the patient's chart.
5. Although no contraindication is known to reanesthetizing the patient to achieve mandibular anesthesia, it may be prudent to forego further dental care at this appointment.

TRISMUS

Trismus, from the Greek *trismos,* is defined as a prolonged, tetanic spasm of the jaw muscles by which the normal opening of the mouth is restricted (locked jaw). This designation was originally used only in tetanus, but because an inability to open the mouth may be seen in a variety of other conditions, the term is currently used in restricted jaw movement, regardless of the cause.[54] Although postinjection pain is the most common local complication of local anesthesia, trismus can become one of the more chronic and complicated problems to manage.[55-57]

Causes

Trauma to muscles or blood vessels in the infratemporal fossa is the most common causative factor in trismus associated with dental injection of local anesthetics.

Local anesthetic solutions into which alcohol or cold sterilizing solutions have diffused produce irritation of tissues (e.g., muscle), leading potentially to trismus. Local anesthetics have been demonstrated to be slightly myotoxic to skeletal muscles. The injection of local anesthetic solution intramuscularly or supramuscularly leads to a rapidly progressive necrosis of exposed muscle fibers.[58-60]

Hemorrhage is another cause of trismus. Large volumes of extravascular blood can produce tissue irritation, leading to muscle dysfunction as the blood is slowly resorbed (over approximately 2 weeks). Low-grade infection after injection can also cause trismus.[61]

Every needle insertion produces some damage to the tissue through which it passes. It stands to reason, then, that multiple needle penetrations correlate with a greater incidence of postinjection trismus. In addition, Stacy and Hajjar found that of 100 needles used for the administration of IANB, 60% were barbed on removal from the tissues. The barb occurred when the needle came into contact with the medial aspect of the mandibular ramus. Withdrawal of the needle from tissue increased the likelihood of involvement of the lingual or inferior alveolar nerve (e.g. paresthesia) and the development of trismus.[62]

Excessive volumes of local anesthetic solution deposited into a restricted area produce distention of tissues, which may lead to postinjection trismus. This is more common after multiple missed IANBs.

Problem

Although the limitation of movement associated with postinjection trismus is usually minor, it is possible for much more severe limitation to develop. The average interincisal opening in cases of trismus is 13.7 mm (range, 5 to 23 mm).[59] Average interincisal opening for males is 44.8 (±9.4) mm and for females is 39.2 (±10.8) mm.[83] Stone and Kaban reported four cases of severe trismus after multiple inferior alveolar (IA) or PSA nerve blocks, three of which required surgical intervention.[63] Before surgery, patients had limited mandibular openings of approximately 2 mm, despite usual treatment regimens.

In the acute phase of trismus, pain produced by hemorrhage leads to muscle spasm and limitation of movement.[64,65] The second, or chronic, phase usually develops if treatment is not begun. Chronic hypomobility occurs secondary to organization of the hematoma, with subsequent fibrosis and scar contracture.[66] Infection may produce hypomobility through increased pain, increased tissue reaction (irritation), and scarring.[61]

Prevention

1. Use a sharp, sterile, disposable needle.
2. Properly care for and handle dental local anesthetic cartridges.
3. Use aseptic technique. Contaminated needles should be changed immediately.
4. Practice atraumatic insertion and injection technique.
5. Avoid repeat injections and multiple insertions into the same area by gaining knowledge of anatomy and proper technique. Use regional nerve blocks instead of local infiltration (supraperiosteal injection) wherever possible and rational.
6. Use minimum effective volumes of local anesthetic. Refer to specific protocols for recommendations. **Trismus is not always preventable.**

Management

In most instances of trismus, the patient reports pain and some difficulty opening his or her mouth on the day after dental treatment in which a posterior superior alveolar or, more commonly, an inferior alveolar nerve block was administered. Hinton and associates reported that the onset of trismus occurred 1 to 6 days post treatment (average, 2.9 days).[59] The degree of discomfort and dysfunction varies but is usually mild.

With mild pain and dysfunction, the patient reports minimum difficulty opening his or her mouth. Arrange an appointment for examination. In the interim, prescribe heat therapy, warm saline rinses, analgesics, and, if necessary, muscle relaxants to manage the initial phase of muscle spasm.[67,68] Heat therapy consists of applying hot, moist towels to the affected area for approximately 20 minutes every hour. For a warm saline rinse, a teaspoon of salt is added to a 12-ounce glass of warm water; the rinse is held in the mouth on the involved side (and spit out) to help relieve the discomfort of trismus. Aspirin (325 mg) is usually adequate as an analgesic in managing pain associated with trismus. Its anti-inflammatory properties are also beneficial. Diazepam (approximately 10 mg bid) or another benzodiazepine is used for muscle relaxation if deemed necessary.

The patient should be advised to initiate physiotherapy consisting of opening and closing the mouth, as well as lateral excursions of the mandible, for 5 minutes every 3 to 4 hours. Chewing gum (sugarless, of course!) is yet another means of providing lateral movement of the temporomandibular joint.

Record the incident, findings, and treatment on the patient's dental chart. Avoid further dental treatment in the involved region until symptoms resolve and the patient is more comfortable.

If continued dental care in the area is urgent, as with an infected painful tooth, it may prove difficult to achieve effective pain control when trismus is present. The Vazirani-Akinosi mandibular nerve block usually provides relief of the motor dysfunction, permitting the patient to open his or her mouth, allowing administration of the appropriate injection for clinical pain control, if needed.

In virtually all cases of trismus related to intraoral injections that are managed as described, patients report improvement within 48 to 72 hours. Therapy should be continued until the patient is free of symptoms. If pain and dysfunction continue unabated beyond 48 hours, consider the possibility of infection. Antibiotics should be added to the treatment regimen described and continued for 7 full days. Complete recovery from injection-related trismus takes about 6 weeks (range, 4 to 20 weeks).[59]

For severe pain or dysfunction, if no improvement is noted within 2 or 3 days without antibiotics or within 5 to 7 days with antibiotics, or if the ability to open the mouth has become limited, the patient should be referred to an oral and maxillofacial surgeon for evaluation. Other therapies, including the use of ultrasound or appliances, are available for use in these situations.[69,70]

Temporomandibular joint involvement is rare in the first 4 to 6 weeks after injection. Surgical intervention to correct chronic dysfunction may be indicated in some instances.[59,63]

SOFT TISSUE INJURY

Self-inflicted trauma to the lips and tongue is frequently caused by the patient inadvertently biting or chewing these tissues while still anesthetized (see Fig. 17-9).

Cause

Trauma occurs most frequently in younger children, in mentally or physically disabled children or adults, and in older-old patients; however, it can and does occur in patients of all ages. The primary reason is the fact that soft tissue anesthesia lasts significantly longer than does pulpal anesthesia. Dental patients receiving local anesthetic during their treatment usually are dismissed from the dental office with residual soft tissue numbness. (See the discussion in Chapter 20 of the local anesthesia reversal agent, phentolamine mesylate.)

Problem

Trauma to anesthetized tissues can lead to swelling and significant pain when the anesthetic effects resolve. A young child or a handicapped individual may have difficulty coping with the situation, and this may lead to behavioral problems. The possibility that infection will develop is remote in most instances.

Prevention

A local anesthetic of appropriate duration should be selected if dental appointments are brief. (Refer to the discussion of lip chewing and duration of anesthesia for specific drugs, p. 281.)

A cotton roll can be placed between the lips and the teeth if they are still anesthetized at the time of discharge. The cotton roll is secured with dental floss wrapped around the teeth (to prevent inadvertent aspiration of the roll) (Fig. 17-10).

Warn the patient and the guardian against eating, drinking hot fluids, and biting on the lips or tongue to test for anesthesia. A self-adherent warning sticker may be used on children (Fig. 17-11).

Management

Management of the patient with self-inflicted soft tissue injury secondary to lip or tongue biting or chewing is symptomatic:

1. Analgesics for pain, as necessary.
2. Antibiotics, as necessary, in the unlikely situation that infection results.
3. Lukewarm saline rinses to aid in decreasing any swelling that may be present.
4. Petroleum jelly or other lubricant to cover a lip lesion and minimize irritation.

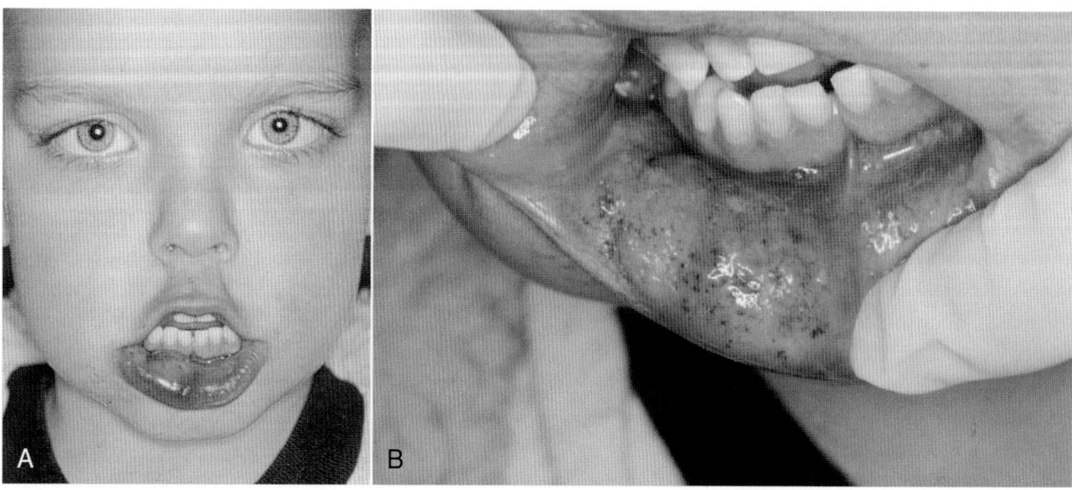

Figure 17-9. A and B, Traumatized lip caused by inadvertent biting while it was still anesthetized.

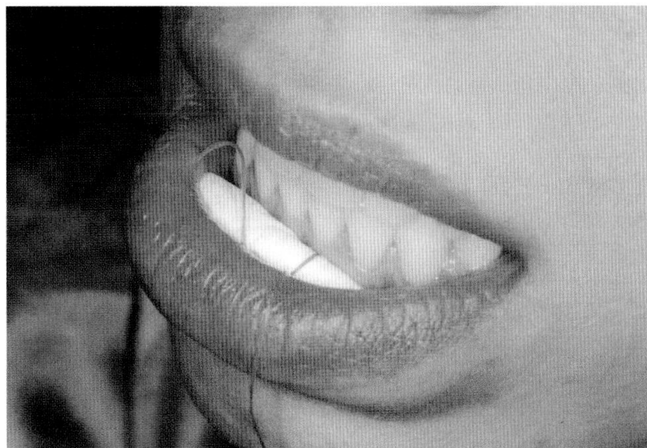

Figure 17-10. Cotton roll placed between lips and teeth, secured with dental floss, minimizes risk of accidental mechanical trauma to anesthetized tissues.

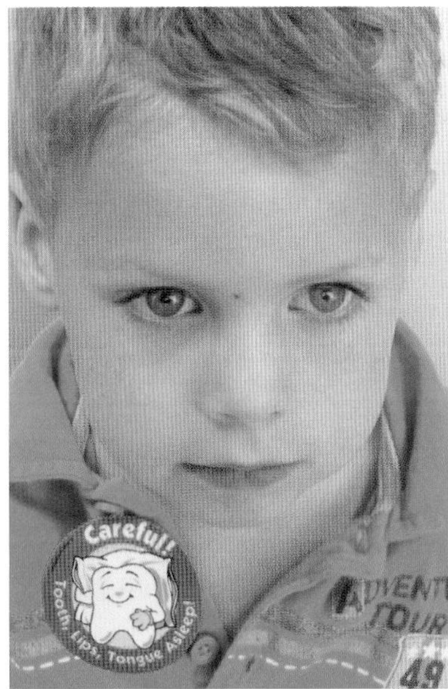

Figure 17-11. Self-adherent warning sticker to help prevent accidental trauma to anesthetized tissues in children.

HEMATOMA

The effusion of blood into extravascular spaces can be caused by inadvertent nicking of a blood vessel (artery or vein) during administration of a local anesthetic. A hematoma that develops subsequent to the nicking of an artery usually increases rapidly in size until treatment is instituted because of the significantly greater pressure of blood within an artery. Nicking of a vein may or may not result in the formation of a hematoma. Tissue density surrounding the injured vessel is a determining factor. The denser the surrounding tissues (e.g., palate), the less likely a hematoma is to develop, but in looser tissue (e.g., infratemporal fossa), large volumes of blood may amass before a swelling is ever noted and therapy instituted.

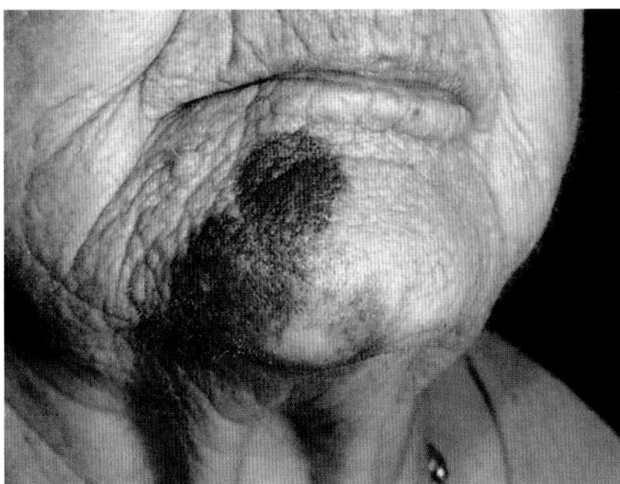

Figure 17-12. Hematoma that developed after bilateral mental nerve blocks.

Cause

Because of the density of tissue in the hard palate and its firm adherence to bone, hematoma rarely develops after a palatal injection. A rather large hematoma may result from arterial or venous puncture after a posterior superior alveolar or inferior alveolar nerve block. The tissues surrounding these vessels more readily accommodate significant volumes of blood. The blood effuses from vessels until extravascular exceeds intravascular pressure, or until clotting occurs. Hematomas that occur after the inferior alveolar nerve block usually are only visible intraorally, whereas PSA hematomas are visible extraorally.

Problem

A hematoma rarely produces significant problems, aside from the resulting "bruise," which may or may not be visible extraorally. Possible complications of hematoma include trismus and pain. Swelling and discoloration of the region usually subside gradually over 7 to 14 days.

A hematoma constitutes an inconvenience to the patient and an embarrassment to the person administering the drug (Fig. 17-12).

Prevention

1. Knowledge of the normal anatomy involved in the proposed injection is important. Certain techniques are associated with a greater risk of visible hematoma. The PSA nerve block is the most common, followed by the IANB (a distant second) and the mental/incisive nerve block (a close third when the foramen is entered, a distant third if the technique described in Chapter 14 is adhered to).
2. Modify the injection technique as dictated by the patient's anatomy. For example, the depth of penetration for a PSA nerve block may be decreased in a patient with smaller facial characteristics.[71,72]

3. Use a short needle for the PSA nerve block to decrease the risk of hematoma.
4. Minimize the number of needle penetrations into tissue.
5. Never use a needle as a probe in tissues.

Hematoma is not always preventable. Whenever a needle is inserted into tissue, the risk of inadvertent puncturing of a blood vessel is present.

Management

Immediate. When swelling becomes evident during or immediately after a local anesthetic injection, direct pressure should be applied to the site of bleeding. For most injections, the blood vessel is located between the surface of the mucous membrane and the bone; localized pressure should be applied for not less than 2 minutes. This effectively stops the bleeding.

Inferior Alveolar Nerve Block. Pressure is applied to the medial aspect of the mandibular ramus. Clinical manifestations of the hematoma, which are visible intraorally, include possible tissue discoloration and probable tissue swelling on the medial (lingual) aspect of the mandibular ramus.

Anterior Superior Alveolar (Infraorbital) Nerve Block. Pressure is applied to the skin directly over the infraorbital foramen. The clinical manifestation is discoloration of the skin below the lower eyelid. Hematoma is unlikely to occur with anterior superior alveolar (ASA) nerve block because the technique described requires application of pressure to the injection site throughout drug administration and for a period of at least 1 to 2 minutes thereafter.

Incisive (Mental) Nerve Block. Pressure is placed directly over the mental foramen, externally on the skin or intraorally on the mucous membrane. Clinical manifestations include discoloration of the skin of the chin in the area of the mental foramen and/or swelling in the mucobuccal fold in the region of the mental foramen (see Fig. 17-12). As with the ASA nerve block, pressure applied during administration of the drug effectively minimizes the risk of hematoma formation during incisive (but not mental) nerve block.

Buccal Nerve Block or Any Palatal Injection. Place pressure at the site of bleeding. In these injections, the clinical manifestations of hematoma usually are visible only within the mouth.

Posterior Superior Alveolar Nerve Block. The PSA nerve block usually produces the largest and most esthetically unappealing hematoma. The infratemporal fossa, into which bleeding occurs, can accommodate a large volume of blood. The hematoma usually is not recognized until a colorless swelling appears on the side of the face around the temporomandibular joint area (usually a few minutes after the injection is completed). It progresses over a period of days, extending inferiorly and anteriorly toward the lower anterior region of the cheek. It is difficult to apply pressure to the site of bleeding in this situation because of the location of the involved blood vessels. It is also relatively difficult to apply pressure directly to the posterior superior alveolar artery (the primary source of bleeding), the facial artery, and the pterygoid plexus of veins. They are located posterior, superior, and medial to the maxillary tuberosity. Bleeding normally ceases when external pressure on the vessels exceeds internal pressure, or when clotting occurs. Digital pressure can be applied to the soft tissues in the mucobuccal fold as far distally as can be tolerated by the patient (without eliciting a gag reflex). Apply pressure in a medial and superior direction. If available, ice should be applied (extraorally) to increase pressure on the site and help constrict the punctured vessel.

Subsequent. The patient may be discharged once bleeding stops. Note the hematoma on the patient's dental chart. Advise the patient about possible soreness and limitation of movement (trismus). If either of these develops, begin treatment as described for trismus. Discoloration will likely occur as a result of extravascular blood elements; it is gradually resorbed over 7 to 14 days.

If soreness develops, advise the patient to take an analgesic such as aspirin or NSAID. Do not apply heat to the area for at least 4 to 6 hours after the incident. Heat produces vasodilation, which may further increase the size of the hematoma if applied too soon. Heat may be applied to the region beginning the next day. It serves as an analgesic, and its vasodilating properties may increase the rate at which blood elements are resorbed, although the latter benefit is debatable. The patient should apply warm moist heat to the affected area for 20 minutes every hour.

Ice may be applied to the region immediately on recognition of a developing hematoma. It acts as both an analgesic and a vasoconstrictor, and it may aid in minimizing the size of the hematoma. Time (tincture of time) is the most important element in managing a hematoma. With or without treatment, a hematoma will be present for 7 to 14 days. Avoid additional dental therapy in the region until symptoms and signs resolve.

PAIN ON INJECTION

Pain on injection of a local anesthetic can best be prevented through careful adherence to the basic protocol of atraumatic injection. (See Chapter 11.)

Causes

1. Careless injection technique and a callous attitude ("Palatal injections always hurt" or "This will hurt a little") all too often become self-fulfilling prophecies.
2. A needle can become dull from multiple injections.
3. Rapid deposition of the local anesthetic solution may cause tissue damage.
4. Needles with barbs (from impaling bone) may produce pain as they are withdrawn from tissue.[62]

Problem

Pain on injection increases patient anxiety and may lead to sudden unexpected movement, increasing the risk of needle breakage, traumatic soft tissue injury to the patient, or needle-stick injury to the administrator.

Prevention

1. Adhere to proper techniques of injection, both anatomic and psychological.
2. Use sharp needles.
3. Use topical anesthetic properly before injection.
4. Use sterile local anesthetic solutions.
5. Inject local anesthetics slowly.
6. Make certain that the temperature of the solution is correct. A solution that is too hot or too cold may be more uncomfortable than one at room temperature.
7. Buffered local anesthetics, at a pH of approximately 7.4, have been demonstrated to be more comfortable on administration.[73,74] Buffered local anesthetics are discussed further in Chapter 20.

Management

No management is necessary. However, steps should be taken to prevent the recurrence of pain associated with the injection of local anesthetics.

BURNING ON INJECTION

Causes

A burning sensation that occurs during injection of a local anesthetic is not uncommon. Several potential causes are known.

The primary cause of a mild burning sensation is the pH of the solution being deposited into the soft tissues. The pH of "plain" local anesthetics (i.e., no vasopressor included) is approximately 6.5, whereas solutions that contain a vasopressor are considerably more acidic (around 3.5). Wahl and associates compared the pain on injection of prilocaine plain versus lidocaine with epinephrine (1 : 100,000) and found no statistical difference in patient perception[75]; however, when bupivacaine with epinephrine (1 : 200,000) was compared with prilocaine plain, significantly more pain was reported by patients receiving bupivacaine.[76]

Rapid injection of local anesthetic, especially in the denser, more adherent tissues of the palate, produces a burning sensation.

Contamination of local anesthetic cartridges can result when they are stored in alcohol or other sterilizing solutions, leading to diffusion of these solutions into the cartridge. Solutions warmed to normal body temperature usually are considered "too hot" by the patient.

Problem

Although usually transient, the sensation of burning on injection of a local anesthetic indicates that tissue irritation is occurring. If this is caused by the pH of the solution, it rapidly disappears as the anesthetic action develops. Usually no residual sensitivity is noted when the anesthetic action terminates.

When a burning sensation occurs as a result of rapid injection, a contaminated solution, or an overly warm solution, the likelihood that tissue may be damaged is greater, and subsequent complications such as postanesthetic trismus, edema, or possible paresthesia are reported.

Prevention

By buffering the local anesthetic solution to a pH of approximately 7.4 immediately before injection, it is possible to eliminate the burning sensation that some patients experience during injection of a local anesthetic solution containing a vasopressor.[73,74]

Slowing the speed of injection also helps. The ideal rate of injectable drug administration is 1 mL/min. Do not exceed the recommended rate of 1.8 mL/min.

The cartridge of anesthetic should be stored at room temperature in the container (blister-pack or tin) in which it was shipped, or in a suitable container without alcohol or other sterilizing agents. (See Chapter 7 for proper care and handling of dental cartridges.)

Management

Because most instances of burning on injection are transient and do not lead to prolonged tissue involvement, formal treatment usually is not indicated. In those few situations in which postinjection discomfort, edema, or paresthesia becomes evident, management of the specific problem is indicated.

INFECTION

Infection subsequent to local anesthetic administration in dentistry is an extremely rare occurrence since sterile disposable needles and glass cartridges have been introduced.

Causes

The major cause of postinjection infection is contamination of the needle before administration of the anesthetic. Contamination of a needle always occurs when the needle touches mucous membrane in the oral cavity. This cannot be prevented, nor is it a significant problem because the normal flora of the oral cavity does not lead to tissue infection.

Improper technique in the handling of local anesthetic equipment and improper tissue preparation for injection are other possible causes of infection.

Injecting Local Anesthetic Solution Into an Area of Infection. As discussed in the section on local anesthetic requirements in endodontics (see Chapter 16), local anesthetics are less effective when injected into infected tissues. However, if deposited under pressure, as in the periodontal ligament injection, the force of their administration might transport bacteria into adjacent, healthy tissues, thereby spreading infection.

Problem

Contamination of needles or solutions may cause a low-grade infection when the needle or solution is placed in deeper tissue. This may lead to trismus if it is not recognized and if proper treatment is not initiated.[61]

Prevention

1. Use sterile disposable needles.
2. Properly care for and handle needles. Take precautions to avoid contamination of the needle through contact with nonsterile surfaces; avoid multiple injections with the same needle, if possible.
3. Properly care for and handle dental cartridges of local anesthetic.
   a. Use a cartridge only once (one patient).
   b. Store cartridges aseptically in their original container, covered at all times.
   c. Cleanse the diaphragm with a sterile disposable alcohol wipe immediately before use.
4. Properly prepare the tissues before penetration. Dry them and apply topical antiseptic (optional).

Management

Low-grade infection, which is rare, is seldom recognized immediately. The patient usually reports postinjection pain and dysfunction 1 or more days after dental care. Overt signs and symptoms of infection occur rarely. Immediate treatment consists of those procedures used to manage trismus: heat and analgesic if needed, muscle relaxant if needed, and physiotherapy. Trismus produced by factors other than infection normally responds with resolution or improvement within several days. If signs and symptoms of trismus do not begin to respond to conservative therapy within 3 days, the possibility of a low-grade infection should be entertained and the patient started on a 7- to 10-day course of antibiotics. Prescribe 29 (or 41, if 10 days) tablets of penicillin V (250-mg tablets). The patient takes 500 mg immediately and then 250 mg four times a day until all tablets have been taken. Erythromycin may be substituted if the patient is allergic to penicillin.

Record the progress and management of the patient on the dental chart.

EDEMA

Swelling of tissues is not a syndrome, but it is a clinical sign of the presence of some disorder.

Causes

1. Trauma during injection
2. Infection
3. Allergy: Angioedema is a possible response to ester-type topical anesthetics in an allergic patient (localized tissue swelling occurs as a result of vasodilation secondary to histamine release).
4. Hemorrhage (effusion of blood into soft tissues produces swelling)
5. Injection of irritating solutions (alcohol- or cold sterilizing solution–containing cartridges)
6. Hereditary angioedema is a condition characterized by the sudden onset of brawny nonpitting edema affecting the face, extremities, and mucosal surfaces of the intestine and respiratory tract, often without obvious precipitating factors. Manipulation within the oral cavity, including local anesthetic administration, may precipitate an attack. Lips, eyelids, and the tongue are often involved.[77] Karlis and associates noted that 15% to 33% of untreated angioedema patients died from acute airway obstruction as a result of laryngeal edema.[78]

Problem

Edema related to local anesthetic administration is seldom intense enough to produce significant problems such as airway obstruction. Most instances of local anesthetic–related edema result in pain and dysfunction of the region and embarrassment for the patient.

Angioneurotic edema produced by topical anesthetic in an allergic individual, although exceedingly rare, can compromise the airway. Edema of the tongue, pharynx, or larynx may develop and represents a potentially life-threatening situation that requires vigorous management.[79]

Prevention

1. Properly care for and handle the local anesthetic armamentarium.
2. Use atraumatic injection technique.
3. Complete an adequate medical evaluation of the patient before drug administration.

Management

The management of edema is predicated on reduction of the swelling as quickly as possible and on the cause of the edema. When produced by traumatic injection or by introduction of irritating solutions, edema is usually of minimal degree and resolves in several days without formal therapy. In this and all situations in which edema is present, it may be necessary to prescribe analgesics for pain.

After hemorrhage, edema resolves more slowly (over 7 to 14 days) as extravasated blood elements are resorbed into the vascular system. If signs of hemorrhage (e.g., bluish discoloration progressing to green, yellow, and other colors) are evident, management follows that discussed for hematoma.

Edema produced by infection does not resolve spontaneously but may, in fact, become progressively more intense if untreated. If signs and symptoms of infection (pain, mandibular dysfunction, edema, warmth) do not appear to resolve within 3 days, antibiotic therapy should be instituted as outlined previously.

Allergy-induced edema is potentially life threatening. Its degree and location are highly significant. If swelling develops in buccal soft tissues and there is absolutely no airway involvement, treatment consists of intramuscular and oral histamine blocker administration and consultation with an allergist to determine the precise cause of the edema.

If edema occurs in any area where it compromises breathing, treatment consists of the following:

1. P (position): if unconscious, the patient is placed supine.

2. A-B-C (airway, breathing, circulation): basic life support is administered, as needed.
3. D (definitive treatment): emergency medical services (e.g., 9-1-1) is summoned.
4. Epinephrine is administered: 0.3 mg (0.3 mL of a 1:1000 epinephrine solution) (adult), 0.15 mg (0.15 mL of a 1:1000 epinephrine solution) (child [15 to 30 kg]), intramuscularly (IM) or 3 mL of a 1:10,000 epinephrine solution intravenously (IV-adult), every 5 minutes until respiratory distress resolves.
5. Histamine blocker is administered IM or IV.
6. Corticosteroid is administered IM or IV.
7. Preparation is made for cricothyrotomy if total airway obstruction appears to be developing. This is extremely rare but is the reason for summoning emergency medical services early.
8. The patient's condition is thoroughly evaluated before his or her next appointment to determine the cause of the reaction.

SLOUGHING OF TISSUES

Prolonged irritation or ischemia of gingival soft tissues may lead to a number of unpleasant complications, including epithelial desquamation and sterile abscess.

Causes

Epithelial Desquamation

1. Application of a topical anesthetic to the gingival tissues for a prolonged period
2. Heightened sensitivity of the tissues to either topical or injectable local anesthetic
3. Reaction in an area where a topical has been applied

Sterile Abscess

1. Secondary to prolonged ischemia resulting from the use of a local anesthetic with vasoconstrictor (usually norepinephrine)
2. Usually develops on the hard palate

Problem

Pain, at times severe, may be a consequence of epithelial desquamation or a sterile abscess. It is remotely possible that infection may develop in these areas.

Prevention

Use topical anesthetics as recommended. Allow the solution to contact the mucous membranes for 1 to 2 minutes to maximize its effectiveness and minimize toxicity.

When using vasoconstrictors for hemostasis, do not use overly concentrated solutions. Norepinephrine (Levophed) 1:30,000 is the agent most likely to produce ischemia of sufficient duration to cause tissue damage and a sterile abscess (Fig. 17-13). Norepinephrine is not available in any dental local anesthetic solution in North America. Epinephrine (1:50,000) also may produce this problem, if reinjection of the solution occurs whenever ischemia resolves, over a long period of time (e.g., several hours). The palatal tissues are likely the only place in the oral cavity where this phenomenon may arise.

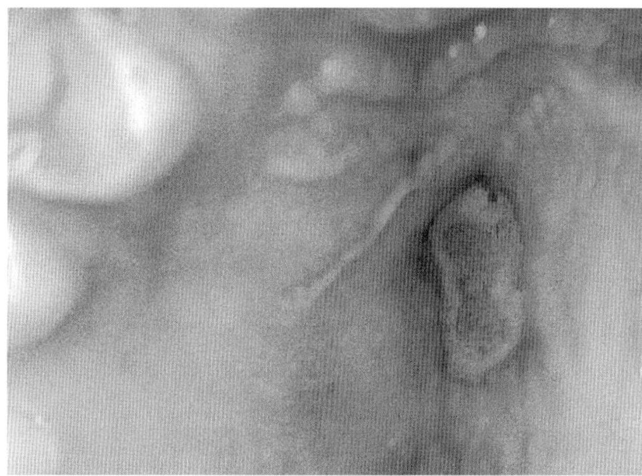

Figure 17-13. Sloughing of tissue on the palate caused by prolonged ischemia secondary to the use of local anesthetic with high concentration (1:50,000) of epinephrine.

Management

Usually, no formal management is necessary for epithelial desquamation or sterile abscess. Be certain to reassure the patient of this fact.

Management may be symptomatic. For pain, analgesics such as aspirin or other NSAIDs and a topically applied ointment (Orabase) are recommended to minimize irritation to the area. Epithelial desquamation resolves within a few days; the course of a sterile abscess may run 7 to 10 days. Record data on the patient's chart.

POSTANESTHETIC INTRAORAL LESIONS

Patients occasionally report that approximately 2 days after an intraoral injection of local anesthetic, ulcerations developed in their mouth, primarily around the site(s) of the injection(s). The primary initial symptom is pain, usually of a relatively intense nature.

Cause

Recurrent aphthous stomatitis or herpes simplex can occur intraorally after a local anesthetic injection or after any trauma to the intraoral tissues.

Recurrent aphthous stomatitis (recurrent aphthous ulceration) is the most common oral mucosal disease known to human beings.[80] Recurrent aphthous stomatitis is more frequently observed than herpes simplex, typically developing on gingival tissues that are not attached to underlying bone (e.g., movable tissue), such as the buccal vestibule (Fig. 17-14). In spite of much continuing research, the causes remain poorly understood, the ulcers are not preventable, and treatment remains symptomatic.

Herpes simplex can develop intraorally, although more commonly it is observed extraorally. It is viral and becomes

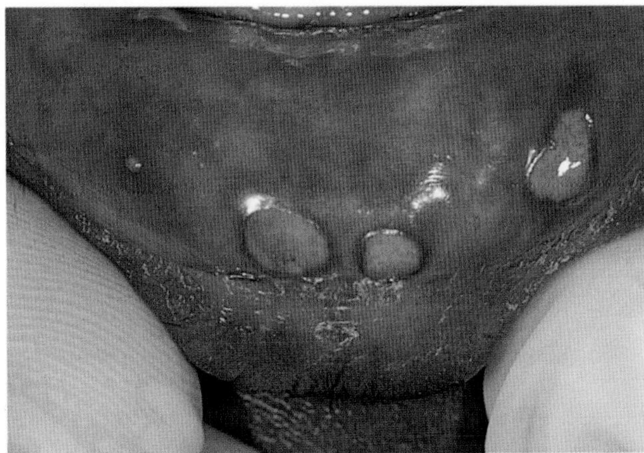

Figure 17-14. Aphthous stomatitis. (From Eisen D, Lynch D: The mouth: diagnosis and treatment, St Louis, 1998, Mosby.)

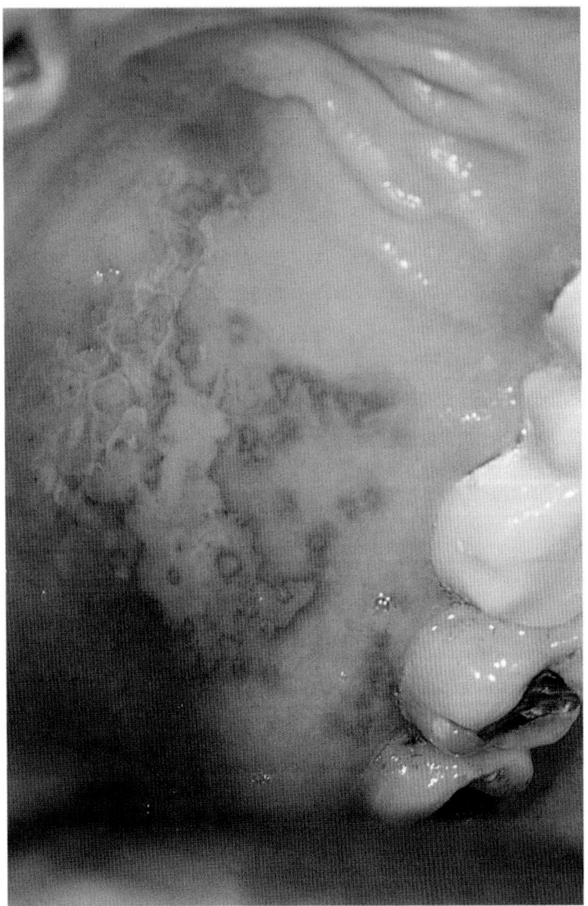

Figure 17-15. Intraoral lesion (herpes simplex) on the palate. (From Eisen D, Lynch D: The mouth: diagnosis and treatment, St Louis, 1998, Mosby.)

manifest as small bumps on tissues that are attached to underlying bone (e.g., fixed) such as the soft tissue of the hard palate (Fig. 17-15).

Trauma to tissues by a needle, a local anesthetic solution, a cotton swab, or any other instrument (e.g., rubber dam clamp, handpiece) may activate the latent form of the disease process that was present in the tissues before injection.

Problem

The patient describes acute sensitivity in the ulcerated area. Many consider that the tissue has become infected as a result of the local anesthetic injection they received; however, the risk of a secondary infection developing in this situation is minimal.

Prevention

Unfortunately, there is no means of preventing these intraoral lesions from developing in susceptible patients. Extraoral herpes simplex, on occasion, may be prevented or its clinical manifestations minimized if treated in its prodromal phase. The prodrome consists of a mild burning or itching sensation at the site where the virus is present (e.g., lip). Antiviral agents, such as acyclovir, applied qid to the affected area effectively minimize the acute phase of this process.

Management

Primary management is symptomatic. Pain is the major initial symptom, developing approximately 2 days after injection. Reassure the patient that the situation is not caused by a bacterial infection secondary to the local anesthetic injection, but in fact is an exacerbation of a process that was present, in latent form, in the tissues before injection. Indeed, most of these patients have experienced this response before and are resigned to it happening again.

No management is necessary if the pain is not severe. However, if pain causes the patient to complain, treatment can be instituted, usually with varying degrees of success. The objective is to keep the ulcerated areas covered or anesthetized.

Topical anesthetic solutions (e.g., viscous lidocaine) may be applied as needed to the painful areas. A mixture of equal amounts of diphenhydramine (Benadryl) and milk of magnesia rinsed in the mouth effectively coats the ulcerations and provides relief from pain. Orabase, a protective paste, without Kenalog can provide a degree of pain relief. Kenalog, a corticosteroid, is not recommended because its anti-inflammatory actions increase the risk of viral or bacterial involvement. A tannic acid preparation (Zilactin) can be applied topically to the lesions extraorally or intraorally (dry the tissues first). Studies from the University of Alabama have demonstrated that most patients achieve substantial pain relief for up to 6 hours.[81,82]

The ulcerations usually last 7 to 10 days with or without treatment. Maintain records on the patient's chart.

References

1. Pogrel MA: Broken local anesthetic needles: a case series of 16 patients, with recommendations, J Am Dent Assoc 140:1517–1522, 2009.
2. 2006 Septodont reported wholesale sales, Newark, Del, 2006, Septodont NA.
3. Amies AB: Broken needles, Aust Dent J 55:403–406, 1951.

4. Muller EE, Lernoud R: Surgical extraction of needles broken during local anesthesia of the mandibular nerve, Acta Odontol Venez 5:229–237, 1967.
5. Dudani IC: Broken needles following mandibular injections, J Indian Dent Assoc 43:14–17, 1971.
6. Kennett S, Curran JB, Jenkins GR: Management of a broken hypodermic needle: report of a case, J Can Dent Assoc 38:414–416, 1972.
7. Kennett S, Curran JB, Jenkins GR: Management of a broken hypodermic needle: report of a case, Anesth Prog 20:48–50, 1973.
8. Bump RL, Roche WC: A broken needle in the pterygomandibular space: report of a case, Oral Surg Oral Med Oral Pathol 36:750–752, 1973.
9. Hai HK: Retrieval of a broken hypodermic needle: a new technique of localising, Singapore Dent J 8:27–29, 1983.
10. Orr DL 2nd: The broken needle: report of case, J Am Dent Assoc 107:603–604, 1983.
11. Marks RB, Carlton DM, McDonald S: Management of a broken needle in the pterygomandibular space: report of case, J Am Dent Assoc 109:263–264, 1984.
12. Burke RH: Management of a broken anesthetic needle, J Am Dent Assoc 112:209–210, 1986.
13. Fox IJ, Belfiglio EJ: Report of a broken needle, Gen Dent 34:102–106, 1986.
14. Pietruszka JF, Hoffman D, McGivern BE Jr: A broken dental needle and its surgical removal: a case report, N Y State Dent J 52:28–31, 1986.
15. Chaikin L: Broken needles, N Y State Dent J 53:8, 1987.
16. Burgess JO: The broken dental needle—a hazard, Spec Care Dentist 8:71–73, 1986.
17. Ho KH: A simple technique for localizing a broken dental needle in the pterygomandibular region, Aust Dent J 33:308–309, 1988.
18. Mima T, Shirasuna K, Morioka S, et al: A broken needle in the pterygomandibular space, Osaka Daigaku Shigaku Zasshi 34:418–422, 1989.
19. McDonogh T: An unusual case of trismus and dysphagia, Br Dent J 180:465–466, 1996.
20. Bhatia S, Bounds G: A broken needle in the pterygomandibular space: report of a case and review of the literature, Dent Update 25:35–37, 1998.
21. Bedrock RD, Skigen A, Dolwick MF: Retrieval of a broken needle in the pterygomandibular space, J Am Dent Assoc 130:685–687, 1999.
22. Faura-Sole M, Sanchez-Garces MA, Berini-Aytes L, et al: Broken anesthetic injection needles: report of 5 cases, Quintessence Int 30:461–465, 1999.
23. Dhanrayani PJ, Jonaidel O: A forgotten entity: "broken needle while inferior dental block," Dent Update 27:101, 2000.
24. Murray M: A forgotten entity: "broken needle while administering inferior dental block," Dent Update 27:306, 2000.
25. Zeltser R, Cohen C, Casap N: The implications of a broken needle in the pterygomandibular space: clinical guidelines for prevention and retrieval, Pediatr Dent 24:153–156, 2002.
26. Thompson M, Wright S, Cheng LH, et al: Locating broken dental needles, Int J Oral Maxillofac Surg 32:642–644, 2003.
27. Baart JA, van Amerongen WE, de Jong KJ, et al: Needle breakage during mandibular block anaesthesia: prevention and retrieval, Ned Tijdschr Tandheelkd 113:520–523, 2006.
28. Malamed SF, Reed K, Poorsattar S: Needle breakage: incidence and prevention, Dent Clin N Am 54:745–756, 2010.
29. Personal communication, Dentsply-MPL Technologies. Franklin Park, Ill, 2003.
30. Ethunandan M, Tran AL, Anand R, et al: Needle-breakage following inferior alveolar nerve block: implications and management, Br Dent J 202:395–397, 2007.
31. Haas DA, Lennon D: A 21 year retrospective study of reports of paresthesia following local anesthetic administration, J Can Dent Assoc 61:319–320, 323–326, 329–330, 1995.
32. Pogrel MA, Thamby S: Permanent nerve involvement resulting from inferior alveolar nerve blocks, J Am Dent Assoc 131:901–907, 2000.
33. Pogrel MA, Thamby S: The etiology of altered sensation in the inferior alveolar, lingual, and mental nerves as a result of dental treatment, J Calif Dent Assoc 27:531–538, 1999.
34. Dower JS Jr: A review of paresthesia in association with administration of local anesthesia, Dent Today 22:64–69, 2003.
35. Haas DA: Localized complications from local anesthesia, J Calif Dent Assoc 26:677–682, 1998.
36. Malden NJ, Maidment YG: Lingual nerve injury subsequent to wisdom teeth removal: a 5-year retrospective audit from a High Street dental practice, Br Dent J 193:203–205, 2002.
37. Heller AA, Shankland WE II: Alternative to the inferior alveolar nerve block anesthesia when placing mandibular dental implants posterior to the mental foramen, J Oral Implantol 27:127–133, 2001.
38. Bataineh AB: Sensory nerve impairment following mandibular third molar surgery, J Oral Maxillofac Surg 59:1012–1017, 2001.
39. Kasaba T, Onizuka S, Takasaki M: Procaine and mepivacaine have less toxicity in vitro than other clinically used local anesthetics, Anesth Analg 97:85–90, 2003.
40. Hillerup S, Jensen R. Nerve injury caused by mandibular block analgesia, Int J Oral Maxillofac Surg 35:437–443, 2006.
41. Stenver DI: Pharmacovigilance Working Party of the European Union—Laegemiddelstyrelsen Danish Medicines Agency. Adverse effects from anaesthetics used in relation with dental care with a special focus on anesthetics containing articaine, October 20, 2006.
42. Pogrel MA: Permanent nerve damage from inferior alveolar nerve blocks—an update to include articaine, J Calif Dent Assoc 35:271–273, 2007.
43. Katyal V: The efficacy and safety of articaine versus lignocaine in dental treatments: a meta-analysis, J Dent 38:307–317, 2010.
44. Garisto GA, Gaffen AS, Lawrence HP, et al: Occurrence of paresthesia after dental local anesthetic administration in the United States, J Am Dent Assoc 141:836–844, 2010.
45. National Weather Service, Lightning Safety: Odds of becoming a lightning victim. Available at: www.lightningsafety.noaa.gov/medical. Accessed February 15, 2011.
46. U.S. Food and Drug Administration Center for Drug Evaluation and Research Office of Post-Marketing Drug Risk Assessment: Available at: www.fda.gov/Drugs/GuidanceCompliance RegulatoryInformation/Surveillance/AdverseDrugEffects. Accessed October 14, 2011.
47. Nickel AA Jr: A retrospective study of paresthesia of the dental alveolar nerves, Anesth Prog 37:42–45, 1990.
48. Personal communication. F. M. McCarthy, 1979.
49. Personal communication. D. Orr, 2011.
50. Sisk AL, Hammer WB, Shelton DW, et al: Complications following removal of impacted third molars, J Oral Maxillofac Surg 44:855–859, 1986.

51. Cooley RL, Coon DE: Transient Bell's palsy following mandibular block: a case report, Quintessence Int 9:9, 1978.
52. Crean SJ, Powis A: Neurological complications of local anaesthetics in dentistry, Dent Update 26:344–349, 1999.
53. Malamed SF: The possible secondary effects in cases of local anesthesia, Rev Belge Medec Dent 55:19–28, 2000.
54. Tveter-as K, Kristensen S: The aetiology and pathogenesis of trismus, Clin Otolaryngol 11:383–387, 1986.
55. Dhanrajani PJ, Jonaidel O: Trismus: etiology, differential diagnosis and treatment, Dent Update 29:88–92, 94, 2002.
56. Leonard M: Trismus: what is it, what causes it, and how to treat it, Dent Today 18:74–77, 1999.
57. Marien M Jr: Trismus: causes, differential diagnosis, and treatment, Gen Dent 45:350–355, 1997.
58. Benoit PW, Yagiela JA, Fort NF: Pharmacologic correlation between local anesthetic-induced myotoxicity and disturbances of intracellular calcium distribution, Toxic Appl Pharmacol 52:187–198, 1980.
59. Hinton RJ, Dechow PC, Carlson DS: Recovery of jaw muscle function following injection of a myotonic agent (lidocaine-epinephrine), Oral Surg Oral Med Oral Pathol 59:247–251, 1986.
60. Jastak JT, Yagiela JA, Donaldson D: Complications and side effects. In Jastak JT, Yagiela JA, Donaldson D, editors: Local anesthesia of the oral cavity, Philadelphia, 1995, WB Saunders.
61. Kitay D, Ferraro N, Sonis ST: Lateral pharyngeal space abscess as a consequence of regional anesthesia, J Am Dent Assoc 122:56–59, 1991.
62. Stacy GC, Hajjar G: Barbed needle and inexplicable paresthesias and trismus after dental regional anesthesia, Oral Surg Oral Med Oral Pathol 77:585–588, 1994.
63. Stone J, Kaban LB: Trismus after injection of local anesthetic, Oral Surg 48:29–32, 1979.
64. Eanes WC: A review of the considerations in the diagnosis of limited mandibular opening, Cranio 9:137–144, 1991.
65. Luyk NH, Steinberg B: Aetiology and diagnosis of clinically evident jaw trismus, Aust Dent J 35:523–529, 1990.
66. Brooke RI: Postinjection trismus due to formation of fibrous band, Oral Surg Oral Med Oral Pathol 47:424–426, 1979.
67. Himel VT, Mohamed S, Luebke RG: Case report: relief of limited jaw opening due to muscle spasm, LDA J 47:6–7, 1988.
68. Kouyoumdjian JH, Chalian VA, Nimmo A: Limited mandibular movement: causes and treatment, J Prosthet Dent 59:330–333, 1988.
69. Carter EF: Therapeutic ultrasound for the relief of restricted mandibular movement, Dent Update 13:503, 504, 506, 508–509, 1986.
70. Lund TW, Cohen JI: Trismus appliances and indications for use, Quintessence Int 24:275–279, 1993.
71. Harn SD, Durham TM, Callahan BP, Kent DK: The triangle of safety: a modified posterior superior alveolar injection technique based on the anatomy of the PSA artery, Gen Dent 50:554–557, 2002.
72. Harn SD, Durham TM, Callahan BP, et al: The posterior superior alveolar injection technique: a report on technique variations and complications, Gen Dent 50:544–550, 2002.
73. Malamed SF, Hersh E, Poorsattar S, Falkel M. Reduction of local anesthetic injection pain using an automated dental anesthetic cartridge buffering system: A randomized, double-blind, crossover study, J Amer Dent Assoc October 2011.
74. Malamed SF: Buffering local anesthetics in dentistry, ADSA Pulse 44(1):3, 8–9, 2011.
75. Wahl MJ, Overton D, Howell J, et al: Pain on injection of prilocaine plain vs. lidocaine with epinephrine: a prospective double-blind study, J Am Dent Assoc 132:1398–1401, 2001.
76. Wahl MJ, Schmitt MM, Overton DA, et al: Injection pain of bupivacaine with epinephrine vs. prilocaine plain, J Am Dent Assoc 133:1652–1656, 2002.
77. Nzeako U, Frigas E, Tremaine W: Hereditary angioedema: a broad review for clinicians, Arch Intern Med 161:2417–2429, 2001.
78. Karlis V, Glickman RS, Stern R, et al: Hereditary angioedema: case report and review of management, Oral Surg Oral Med Oral Pathol Oral Radiol Endodont 83:462–464, 1997.
79. Hayes SM: Allergic reaction to local anesthetic: report of a case, Gen Dent 28:30–31, 1980.
80. Ship JA: Recurrent aphthous stomatitis: an update, Oral Surg Oral Med Oral Pathol Oral Radiol Endodont 82:118, 1996.
81. Raborn GW, McGaw WT, Grace M, et al: Herpes labialis treatment with acyclovir 5% modified aqueous cream: a double-blind randomized trial, Oral Surg Oral Med Oral Pathol 67:676–679, 1989.
82. Raborn GW, McGaw WT, Grace M, et al: Treatment of herpes labialis with acyclovir: review of three clinical trials, Am J Med 85:39–42, 1988.
83. Mezitis M, Rallis G, Zachariades N: The normal range of mouth opening, J Oral Maxillofac Surg 47:1028–1029, 2009.

CHAPTER 18

Systemic Complications

The therapeutic use of drugs is commonplace in dentistry, with the administration of local anesthetics considered essential whenever potentially painful procedures are contemplated. It is estimated (conservatively) that dental professionals in the United States administer in excess of 6 million dental cartridges per week, or more than 300 million per year.

Local anesthetics are extremely safe drugs when used as recommended. However, whenever any drug, including local anesthetics, is used, the potential for unwanted and undesirable responses exists. In this chapter, systemic adverse reactions to drugs in general, and local anesthetics in particular, are reviewed.

Several general principles of toxicology (the study of the harmful effects of chemicals or drugs on biological systems) are presented to further an understanding of the material in this chapter.

Harmful effects of drugs range from those that are inconsequential to the patient and entirely reversible once the drug is withdrawn, to those that are uncomfortable but not seriously harmful, to those that can seriously incapacitate or prove fatal to the patient.

Whenever any drug is administered, two types of actions may be observed: (1) desirable actions, which are clinically sought and usually beneficial; and (2) undesirable actions, which are additional and are not sought.

- **Principle 1: No drug ever exerts a single action.** All drugs exert many actions, desirable and undesirable. In ideal circumstances, the right drug in the right dose is administered via the right route to the right patient at the right time for the right reason and does not produce any undesirable effects.[1] This ideal clinical situation is rarely, if ever, attained, because no drug is so specific that it produces only the desired actions in all patients.
- **Principle 2: No clinically useful drug is entirely devoid of toxicity.** The aim of rational drug treatment is to maximize the therapeutic and to minimize the toxic effects of any given drug. No drug is completely safe or completely harmful. All drugs are capable of producing harm if handled improperly; conversely, any drug may be handled safely if proper precautions are observed.
- **Principle 3: The potential toxicity of a drug rests in the hands of the user.** A second factor in the safe use of drugs (after the drug itself) is the person to whom the drug is being administered. Individuals react differently to the same stimulus. Therefore, patients vary in their reactions to a drug. Before administering any drug, the doctor must ask the patient specific questions about his or her medical and drug history. Physical evaluation and the ensuing dialogue history related to local anesthetic administration are presented in Chapters 4 and 10.

CLASSIFICATION OF ADVERSE DRUG REACTIONS

Classifying adverse drug reactions, in the past, has been the object of much confusion; reactions were labeled as side effects, adverse experiences, drug-induced disease, diseases of medical progress, secondary effects, and intolerance. The term *adverse drug reaction (ADR)* is preferred at this time.

Box 18-1 outlines the three major methods by which drugs produce adverse reactions.

Overdose reactions, allergy, and idiosyncrasy are important topics in relation to local anesthetics and pain control in dentistry. A brief overview of each is presented, followed by an in-depth look at overdose and allergy.

Overdose reactions are those clinical signs and symptoms that manifest as a result of an absolute or relative overadministration of a drug, which leads to elevated blood levels of the drug in its target organs (places in the body where the drug exerts a clinical action). Signs and symptoms of overdose are related to direct extension of the normal pharmacologic actions of the drug in its target organs. Local anesthetics are drugs that act to depress excitable membranes (e.g., the central nervous system [CNS] and myocardium are the target organs for local anesthetics). When administered properly and in therapeutic dosages, they cause little or no clinical evidence of CNS or cardiovascular system

BOX 18-1 Causes of Adverse Drug Reactions

Toxicity Caused by *Direct Extension of the Usual Pharmacologic Effects* of the Drug:
1. Side effects
2. Overdose reactions
3. Local toxic effects

Toxicity Caused by *Alteration in the Recipient* of the Drug:
1. A disease process (hepatic dysfunction, heart failure, renal dysfunction)
2. Emotional disturbances
3. Genetic aberrations (atypical plasma cholinesterase, malignant hyperthermia)
4. Idiosyncrasy

Toxicity Caused by *Allergic Responses* to the Drug

TABLE 18-1 Comparison of Allergy and Overdose

	Allergy	Overdose
Clinical Response		
Dose	Non–dose related	Dose related
S&S	Similar, regardless of allergen	Relate to pharmacology of drug administered
Management	Similar (epinephrine, histamine blockers)	Different: specific for drug administered

S&S, Signs and symptoms.

(CVS) depression. However, signs and symptoms of selective CNS and CVS depression develop with increased blood levels in the cerebral circulation or myocardium. *Toxic reaction* is a synonym for *overdose.* Toxins are poisons. All drugs are poisons when administered to excess, thus the term *toxic reaction.*

Allergy is a hypersensitive state acquired through exposure to a particular allergen (a substance capable of inducing altered bodily reactivity), re-exposure to which brings about a heightened capacity to react. Clinical manifestations of allergy vary and include the following:
- Fever
- Angioedema
- Urticaria
- Dermatitis
- Depression of blood-forming organs
- Photosensitivity
- Anaphylaxis

In stark contrast to the overdose reaction, in which clinical manifestations are related directly to the normal pharmacology of the causative agent, the clinically observed reaction in allergy is always produced by an exaggerated response of the patient's immune system. Allergic responses to a local anesthetic, an antibiotic, latex, shellfish, bee sting, peanuts, or strawberries are produced by the same mechanism and may present clinically similar signs and symptoms. All allergies require the same basic management. Overdose reactions to these substances appear clinically dissimilar, necessitating entirely different modes of emergency management.

Another point of contrast between overdose and allergy relates to the amount of "drug" necessary to produce or provoke the reaction. For an overdose reaction to develop, a large enough amount of the drug must be administered to result in excessive blood levels in the drugs target organ(s). *Overdose reactions are dose related.* In addition, the degree of intensity (severity) of the clinical signs and symptoms relates directly to the blood level of the drug. The greater the dose administered, the higher the blood level, and the more severe the reaction. By contrast, *allergic reactions are not dose related.* A large dose of a drug administered to a nonallergic patient does not provoke an allergic response, whereas a minuscule amount (e.g., 0.1 mL or less) of a drug to which the patient is allergic can provoke life-threatening anaphylaxis.

Idiosyncrasy, the third category of true adverse drug reactions, is a term used to describe a qualitatively abnormal, unexpected response to a drug, differing from its usual pharmacologic actions and thus resembling hypersensitivity. However, idiosyncrasy does not involve a proven, or even suspected, allergic mechanism. A second definition considers an idiosyncratic reaction to be any adverse response that is neither overdose nor an allergic reaction. An example is stimulation or excitation that develops in some patients after administration of a CNS-depressant drug (e.g., a histamine blocker). Unfortunately, it is virtually impossible to predict which persons will have idiosyncratic reactions or the nature of the resulting idiosyncrasy.

It is thought that virtually all instances of idiosyncratic reaction have an underlying genetic mechanism. These aberrations remain undetected until the individual receives a specific drug, which then produces its bizarre (nonpharmacologic) clinical expression.

Specific management of idiosyncratic reactions is difficult to discuss because of the unpredictable nature of the response. Treatment is necessarily symptomatic and includes positioning, airway, breathing, circulation, and definitive care.

Table 18-1 compares allergy versus overdose.

OVERDOSE

A *drug overdose reaction* is defined as those clinical signs and symptoms that result from an overly high blood level of a drug in various target organs and tissues. Overdose reactions are the most common of all true ADRs, accounting for up to 99% in some estimates.[2]

For an overdose reaction to occur, the drug first must gain access to the circulatory system in quantities sufficient to produce adverse effects on various tissues of the body. Normally, both constant absorption of the drug from its site

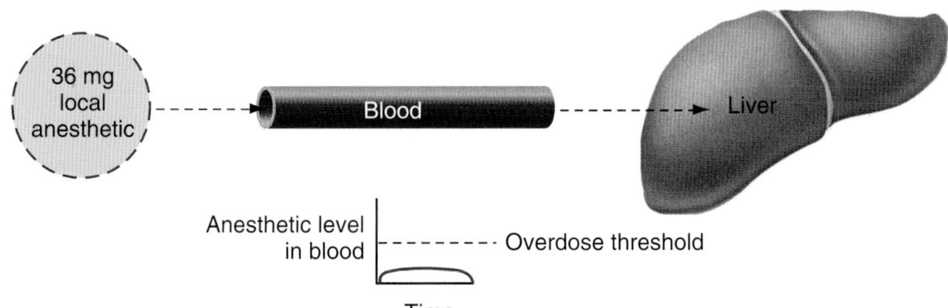

Figure 18-1. Under normal conditions, both constant absorption of local anesthetic from the site of deposition into the cardiovascular system and constant removal of the drug from the blood by the liver occur. Local anesthetic levels in the blood remain low and below the threshold for overdose.

of administration into the circulatory system and steady removal of the drug from the blood as it undergoes redistribution (e.g., to skeletal muscle and fat) and biotransformation in other parts of the body (e.g., liver) are noted. Overly high drug levels in the blood and target organs rarely occur (Fig. 18-1) in this situation.

However, this "steady state" can be altered in various ways, leading to rapid or more gradual elevation of the drug's blood level. In either case, a drug overdose reaction is caused by a level of a drug in the blood that is sufficiently high to produce adverse effects in various organs and tissues of the body in which the drug exerts a clinical action (these are termed the *target organs* of the drug). The reaction continues for only as long as the blood level of the drug in the target organs remains above its threshold for overdose.

Predisposing Factors

Overdose to local anesthetics is related to the blood level of the local anesthetic that occurs in certain tissues after the drug is administered. Many factors influence the rate at which this level is elevated and the length of time it remains elevated. The presence of one or more of these factors predisposes the patient to the development of overdose. The first group of factors relates to the patient, the second group to the drug and the area into which the drug is administered (Box 18-2).

BOX 18-2 Local Anesthetic Overdose: Predisposing Factors

Patient Factors
Age
Weight
Other drugs
Sex
Presence of disease
Genetics
Mental attitude and environment

Drug Factors
Vasoactivity
Concentration
Dose
Route of administration
Rate of injection
Vascularity of the injection site
Presence of vasoconstrictors

Patient Factors

Age. Although ADRs, including overdose, can occur in persons of any age, individuals at both ends of the age spectrum experience a higher incidence of such reactions.[3-8] The functions of absorption, metabolism, and excretion may be imperfectly developed in very young persons and may be diminished in older-old persons, thereby increasing the half-life of the drug, elevating circulating blood levels, and increasing the risk of overdose.[9]

Weight. The greater the (lean) body weight of a patient (within certain limits), the larger the dose of a drug that can be tolerated before overdose reactions occur (providing the patient responds "normally" to the drug). Most drugs are distributed evenly throughout the body. Larger individuals have a greater blood volume and consequently a lower level of the drug per milliliter (mL) of blood. Maximum recommended doses (MRDs) of local anesthetics normally are calculated on the basis of milligram of drug per kilogram or pound of body weight. One of the major factors involved in producing local anesthetic overdose in the past was lack of consideration of this extremely important factor. Determination of maximum doses according to milligram per kilogram or milligram per pound of body weight is based on the responses of the "normal-responding" patient, which are calculated from the responses of many thousands of patients. An individual patient's response to drug administration, however, may demonstrate significant variation. The normal distribution curve (Fig. 18-2) illustrates this fact. The usual

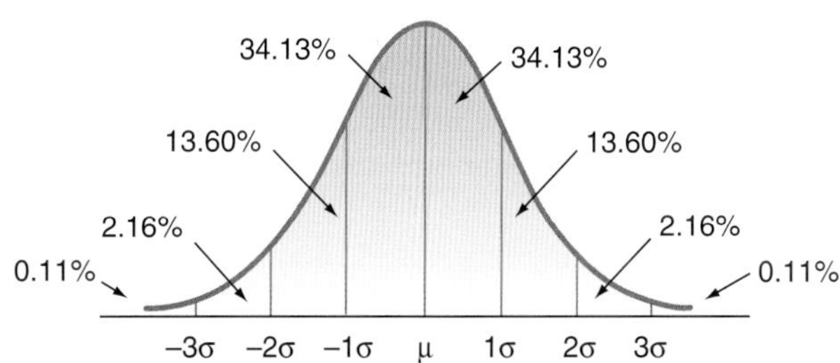

Figure 18-2. Normal distribution curve (bell curve).

cerebral blood level of lidocaine necessary to induce seizure activity is approximately 7.5 μg/mL. However, patients on the hyporesponding side of this curve may not convulse until a significantly higher brain–blood level is reached, whereas others (hyperresponders) may convulse at a brain–blood level considerably lower than 7.5 μg/mL.

Other Medications. Administration of concomitant medications may influence local anesthetic drug levels. Patients taking meperidine (Demerol), phenytoin (Dilantin), quinidine (an antidysrhythmic), or desipramine (a tricyclic antidepressant) have increased local anesthetic blood levels and thus may experience toxic actions of the local anesthetic at lower administered doses because of protein binding competition. The H_2-histamine blocker cimetidine slows the biotransformation of lidocaine by competing with the local anesthetic for hepatic oxidative enzymes, leading to somewhat elevated lidocaine blood levels.[10-12]

Sex. Studies in animals have shown that sex is a factor in drug distribution, response, and metabolism, although it is not of major significance in humans. In humans, the only instance of sexual difference affecting a drug response is pregnancy. During pregnancy, renal function may be disturbed, leading to impaired excretion of certain drugs, their accumulation in the blood, and increased risk of overdose. However, local anesthetic seizure thresholds for the fetus, newborn, and mother are significantly different.[11-15] In the adult woman, the seizure threshold is reported to be 5.8 mg/kg, in the newborn 18.4 mg/kg, and in the fetus 41.9 mg/kg. This is thought to be a result of the efficient placental clearance of lidocaine into the mother's plasma.

Presence of Disease. Disease may affect the ability of the body to transform a drug into an inactive by-product. Hepatic and renal dysfunction impairs the body's ability to break down and excrete the local anesthetic, leading to an increased anesthetic blood level, whereas heart failure decreases liver perfusion (the volume of blood flowing through the liver during a specific period), thereby increasing the half-lives of amide local anesthetics and increasing the risk of overdose.[16,17]

Genetics. Genetic deficiencies may alter a patient's response to certain drugs. A genetic deficiency in the enzyme serum pseudocholinesterase (serum cholinesterase, plasma pseudocholinesterase, plasma cholinesterase) is an important example. This enzyme, produced in the liver, circulates in the blood and is responsible for biotransformation of the ester local anesthetics. A deficiency in this enzyme quantitatively or qualitatively can prolong the half-life of an ester local anesthetic, thereby increasing its blood level. Approximately 1 in 2820 individuals, or 6% to 7% of patients in most surgical populations, possesses atypical serum pseudocholinesterase.[18]

Mental Attitude and Environment. A patient's psychological attitude influences the ultimate effect of a drug. Although of greater importance with regard to antianxiety or analgesic drugs, it is also important with regard to local anesthetics. Psychological attitude affects the patient's response to various stimuli. The apprehensive patient who overreacts to stimulation (experiencing pain when gentle pressure is applied) is more likely to receive a larger dose of local anesthetic, which would seemingly increase his or her risk of local anesthetic overdose. However, a recent study in rats demonstrated that stress-induced changes in arterial carbon dioxide tension (decreased $paCO_2$) and in partial pressure of oxygen in arterial blood (increased paO_2) significantly *raised* the seizure threshold for both lidocaine and articaine.[19] Stress significantly increased the latency period for the first tonic–clonic seizure induced by toxic doses of both lidocaine and articaine.[19]

Drug Factors

Vasoactivity. All local anesthetics currently used by injection in dentistry are vasodilators. Injection into soft tissues increases perfusion in the area, leading to an increased rate of drug absorption from the site of injection into the cardiovascular system. This causes two undesirable effects: a shorter duration of clinical anesthesia and an increased blood level of the local anesthetic.

Concentration. The greater the concentration (percent solution injected) of the local anesthetic administered, the greater the number of milligrams per milliliter of solution and the greater the circulating blood volume of the drug in the patient. For example, 1.8 mL of a 4% solution is 72 mg of the drug, but 1.8 mL of a 2% solution represents only 36 mg. If the drug is clinically effective as a 2% concentration, higher concentrations should not be used. The lowest concentration of a given drug that is clinically effective should be selected for use. For commonly used local anesthetics in dentistry, these "ideal" concentrations have been determined and are represented in the commercially available forms of these drugs.

Dose. The larger the volume of a local anesthetic administered, the greater the number of milligrams injected and the higher the resulting circulating blood level. The smallest dose of a given drug that is clinically effective should be administered. For each of the injection techniques discussed in this book, a recommended dose has been presented. Where possible, this dose should not be exceeded. Although "dental" doses of local anesthetics are relatively small compared with those used in many nondental nerve blocks, significantly high blood levels of the local anesthetic can be achieved in dental situations because of the greater vascularity of the intraoral injection site or inadvertent intravascular injection.

Route of Administration. Local anesthetics, when used for pain control, exert their clinical effects in the area of deposition. Ideally then, a local anesthetic drug should *not* enter into the cardiovascular system. Almost all other therapeutic agents *must* enter the CVS and achieve a minimum therapeutic blood level before their clinical action(s) occur. Local anesthetics administered for antidysrhythmic purposes must reach such a therapeutic blood level to be effective. Indeed, one factor involved in terminating pain control by a local anesthetic consists of its diffusion out of the nerve tissue and its subsequent entry into the CVS and removal from the site of deposition.

A factor in local anesthetic overdose in dentistry is "inadvertent" intravascular injection. Extremely high drug levels can be obtained in a short time, leading to serious overdose reactions.

Absorption of local anesthetics through oral mucous membranes is also potentially dangerous because of the rate at which some topically applied anesthetics enter the circulatory system. Lidocaine HCl and tetracaine HCl are absorbed well after topical application to mucous membranes. Benzocaine, which is not water soluble, is poorly absorbed.

Rate of Injection. The rate at which a drug is injected is a very important factor in the causation or prevention of overdose reactions. (According to the author, rate of injection is the single most important factor.) Whereas intravascular injection may or may not produce signs and symptoms of overdose (indeed, lidocaine is frequently administered intravenously in doses of 1.0 to 1.5 mg/kg to treat ventricular ectopy), the rate at which the drug is injected is a major factor in determining whether drug administration will prove clinically safe or hazardous. Malagodi and associates demonstrated that the incidence of seizures with etidocaine went up when the rate of intravenous (IV) infusion was increased.[20]

Rapid IV administration (15 seconds or less) of 36 mg of lidocaine produces greatly elevated levels and virtually ensures an overdose reaction. Slow (60-second or more) IV administration produces significantly lower levels in the blood, with a lesser risk that a severe overdose reaction will develop.

Vascularity of the Injection Site. The greater the vascularity of the injection site, the more rapid the absorption of the drug from that area into the circulation. Unfortunately (as regards local anesthetic overdose) for dentistry, the oral cavity is one of the most highly vascular areas of the entire body. However, some areas within the oral cavity are less well perfused (e.g., the site for the Gow-Gates nerve block), and these usually are more highly recommended than other, better-perfused, sites (e.g., those for the inferior alveolar or posterior superior alveolar nerve block).

Presence of Vasoconstrictors. The addition of vasoconstrictor to a local anesthetic produces a decrease in the perfusion of an area and a decreased rate of systemic absorption of the drug. This, in turn, decreases the clinical toxicity of the local anesthetic (see Table 3-1).

Causes

Elevated blood levels of local anesthetics may result from one or more of the following:

1. Biotransformation of the drug is unusually slow.
2. The unbiotransformed drug is too slowly eliminated from the body through the kidneys.
3. Too large a total dose is administered.
4. Absorption from the injection site is unusually rapid.
5. Intravascular administration.

Biotransformation and Elimination. Ester local anesthetics, as a group, undergo more rapid biotransformation in the liver and blood than the amides. Plasma pseudocholinesterase is primarily responsible for their hydrolysis to para-aminobenzoic acid.

Atypical pseudocholinesterase occurs in approximately 1 out of every 2820 individuals, or 6% to 7% of patients in a surgical population.[18] Patients with a familial history of this disorder may be unable to biotransform ester agents at the usual rate, and subsequently, higher levels of ester anesthetics may develop in their blood.

Atypical pseudocholinesterase represents a relative contraindication to the administration of ester local anesthetics. Amide local anesthetics may be used without increased risk of overdose in patients with pseudocholinesterase deficiency.

Amide local anesthetics are biotransformed in the liver by hepatic microsomal enzymes. A history of liver disease, however, does not absolutely contraindicate their use. In an ambulatory patient with a history of liver disease (American Society of Anesthesiologists [ASA] Physical Status classification system 2 or 3), amide local anesthetics may be used judiciously (relative contraindication) (Fig. 18-3).

Minimum effective volumes of anesthetic should be used. Average, even low-average, doses may be capable of producing an overdose if liver function is compromised to a great enough degree (ASA 4 or 5); however, this situation is unlikely to occur in an ambulatory patient.[17]

Renal dysfunction also can delay elimination of the active local anesthetic from the blood. A percentage of all anesthetics is eliminated unchanged through the kidneys: 2% procaine, 10% lidocaine, 5% to 10% articaine, and 1% to 15% mepivacaine and prilocaine. Renal dysfunction may lead to a gradual increase in the level of active local anesthetic in the blood.[16]

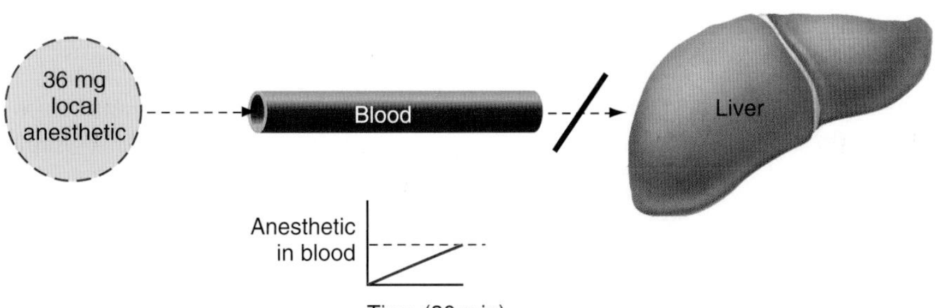

Figure 18-3. In patients with significant liver dysfunction, removal of a local anesthetic from the blood may be slower than its absorption into the blood, leading to a slow but steady rise in the blood anesthetic level.

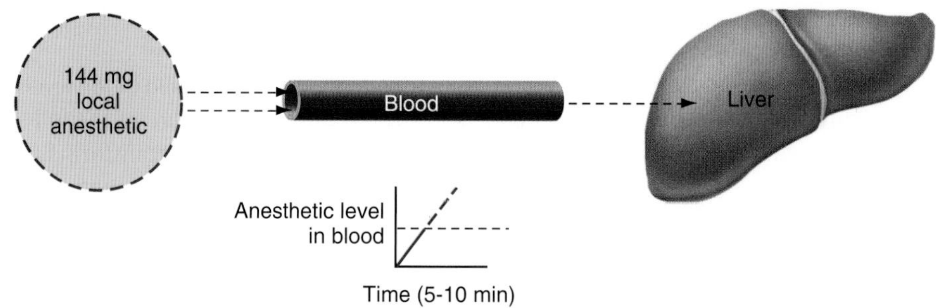

Figure 18-4. Even in a patient with normal liver function, a large dose of local anesthetic may be absorbed into the cardiovascular system more rapidly than the liver can remove it. This produces a relatively rapid elevation of the anesthetic blood level.

TABLE 18-2
Maximum Recommended Doses of Local Anesthetics

Drug	Formulation	MRD	mg/lb	(mg/kg)
Articaine	With epinephrine	None listed*	3.2	(7.0)
Lidocaine	Plain	300†	2.0	(4.4)†
	With epinephrine	500†	3.3	(7.0)†
Mepivacaine	Plain	400†	2.6	(5.7)†
	With levonordefrin	400†	2.6	(5.7)†
Prilocaine	Plain	600†	4.0	(8.8)†
	With epinephrine	600†	4.0	(8.8)†

*Manufacturer's recommendation: Prescribing information, New Castle, Del, 2000.
†Manufacturer's recommendation: Prescribing information, dental, Westborough, Mass, 1990, Astra Pharmaceutical Products.

Excessive Total Dose. Given in excess, all drugs are capable of producing signs and symptoms of overdose (Fig. 18-4). Precise milligram dosages or the blood levels at which clinical effects are noted are impossible to predict. Biological variability has a great influence on the manner in which persons respond to drugs.

The MRD of parenterally administered (injected) drugs is commonly calculated after consideration of a number of factors, including the following:

1. **Patient's age.** Individuals at either end of the age spectrum may be unable to tolerate normal doses, which should be decreased accordingly.
2. **Patient's physical status.** For medically compromised individuals (ASA 3, 4, and 5) the calculated MRD should be decreased.
3. **Patient's weight.** The larger the person (within limits), the greater is the volume of distribution of the drug. With a usual dose, the blood level of the drug is lower in the larger patient, and a larger milligram dose can be administered safely. Although this rule is generally valid, there are always exceptions; care must be exercised whenever any drug is administered.

MRDs of local anesthetics should be determined after consideration of the patient's age, physical status, and body weight. Table 18-2 provides maximum recommended doses based on body weight for lidocaine, mepivacaine, prilocaine, and articaine.

It is highly unlikely that the maximum figures indicated in Table 18-2 will be reached in the typical dental practice. There is rarely an occasion to administer more than three or four cartridges during a dental appointment. Regional block anesthesia is capable of obtunding the full mouth in an adult with six cartridges, and with two cartridges in the primary dentition. Yet despite this ability to achieve widespread anesthesia with minimum volumes of anesthetic, the administration of excessive volumes is the most frequently seen cause of local anesthetic overdose.[21,22]

Rapid Absorption Into the Circulation. Vasoconstrictors are considered an integral component of all local anesthetics whenever depth and duration of anesthesia are important. There are but few indications for the use of local anesthetics without a vasoconstrictor in dentistry. Vasoconstrictors increase both the depth and the duration of anesthesia and reduce the systemic toxicity of most local anesthetics by delaying their absorption into the CVS. Vasoconstrictors should be included in local anesthetic solutions unless specifically contraindicated by the medical status of the patient or the duration of the planned treatment.[23] The American Dental Association and the American Heart Association have summarized this as follows: "Vasoconstrictor agents should be used in local anesthetic solutions during dental practice only when it is clear that the procedure will be shortened or the analgesia rendered more profound. When a vasoconstrictor is indicated, extreme care should be taken to avoid intravascular injection. The minimum possible amount of vasoconstrictor should be used."[24] Rapid absorption of local anesthetics also may occur after their application to oral mucous membranes. Absorption of some topically applied local anesthetics into the circulation is rapid, exceeded in rate only by direct intravascular injection.[25] Local anesthetics designed for topical application are used in a higher concentration than formulations suitable for parenteral administration.

From the perspective of overdose, amide topical anesthetics, when applied to wide areas of mucous membrane, increase the risk of serious reactions. Benzocaine, an ester anesthetic, which is poorly, if at all, absorbed into the cardiovascular system, is less likely to produce an overdose reaction than amides, although cases of methemoglobinemia from excessive benzocaine administration have been reported.[26-28] The risk of allergy (more likely with esters than amides) must be addressed before any drug is used. Serious overdose reactions have been reported after topical application of amide local anesthetics.[29-32]

The area of application of a topical anesthetic should be limited. There are few indications for applying a topical to more than a full quadrant (buccal and lingual/palatal) at one time. Application of an amide topical to a wide area requires a large quantity of the agent and increases the likelihood of overdose.

When a spray topical anesthetic is needed, the use of metered dosage forms is strongly recommended. Disposable nozzles for metered sprays make maintenance of sterility simpler (Fig. 18-5). Ointments or gels, if used in small amounts (as on the tip of a cotton applicator stick), may be applied with minimal risk of overdose.

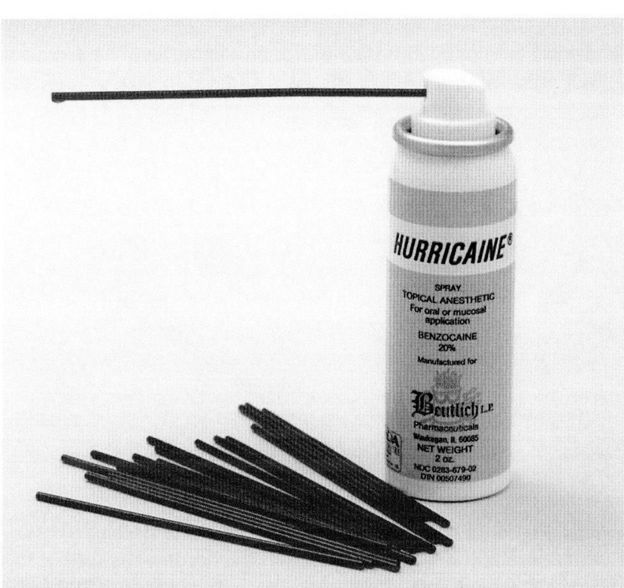

Figure 18-5. Metered spray with disposable nozzle.

Intravascular Injection. Intravascular injection may occur with any type of intraoral injection but is more likely when a nerve block is administered[33]:

Nerve Block	Positive Aspiration Rate, %
Inferior alveolar	11.7
Mental or incisive	5.7
Posterior superior alveolar	3.1
Anterior superior alveolar	0.7
(Long) buccal	0.5

Both IV and intra-arterial (IA) injections are capable of producing overdose (Fig. 18-6). Aldrete demonstrated that a rapidly administered IA injection may cause retrograde blood flow in the artery as the anesthetic drug is deposited (Fig. 18-7).[34] Intravascular injections of local anesthetic within the usual practice of dentistry should not occur. With knowledge of the anatomy of the site to be anesthetized and proper technique of aspiration before the anesthetic solution is deposited, overdose as a result of intravascular injection is minimized.

Prevention. To prevent intravascular injection, use an aspirating syringe. In an unpublished survey conducted by the author, 23% of dentists questioned stated that they routinely use nonaspirating syringes to administer local anesthetics. There is no justification for the use of a nonaspirating syringe for any intraoral injection technique, because it is impossible to determine the precise location of the needle tip without aspirating.

Use a needle no smaller than 25 gauge when the risk of aspiration is high. Although aspiration of blood is possible through smaller-gauge needles, resistance to the return of blood into the lumen of smaller-gauge needles is increased, leading to an increased likelihood of an unreliable aspiration test. Therefore, injection techniques with a greater likelihood of positive aspiration dictate the use of a 25-gauge needle. A 27-gauge needle can be utilized in lieu of 25-gauge as it provides relatively reliable aspiration; however, 30-gauge needles should be avoided, if at all possible, when injections are administered into more vascular areas of the oral cavity.

Aspirate in at least two planes before injection. Figure 18-8 illustrates how an aspiration test may be negative even though the needle tip lies within the lumen of a blood vessel. The use of multiple aspiration tests before injection of solution, with the needle bevel in different planes, overcomes this potential problem. After the initial aspiration, rotate the

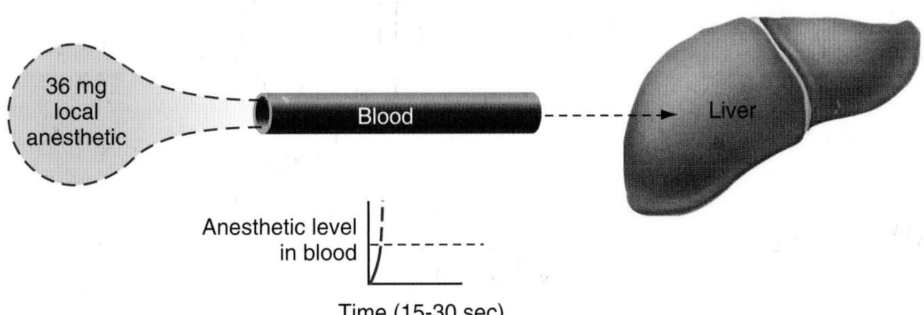

Figure 18-6. Direct rapid intravascular administration of one cartridge of local anesthesia produces marked elevation of the anesthetic blood level in a very short time.

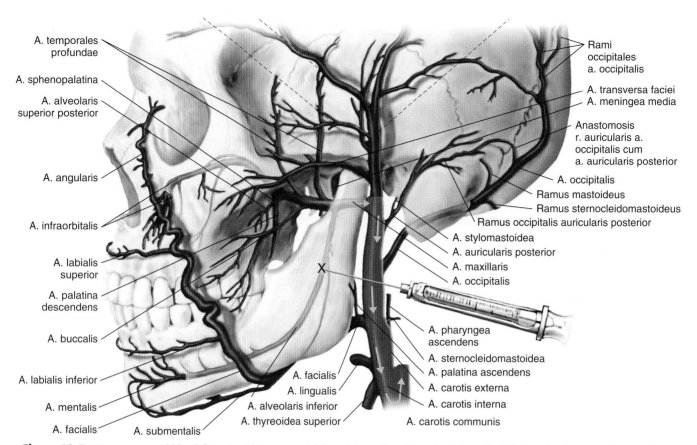

Figure 18-7. Reverse carotid blood flow. Rapid intra-arterial deposition of local anesthetic into the inferior alveolar artery (X) produces an overdose reaction. Blood flow in the arteries is reversed because of the high pressure produced by the rate of injection. Arrows indicate the path of the solution into the internal carotid artery and cerebral circulation.

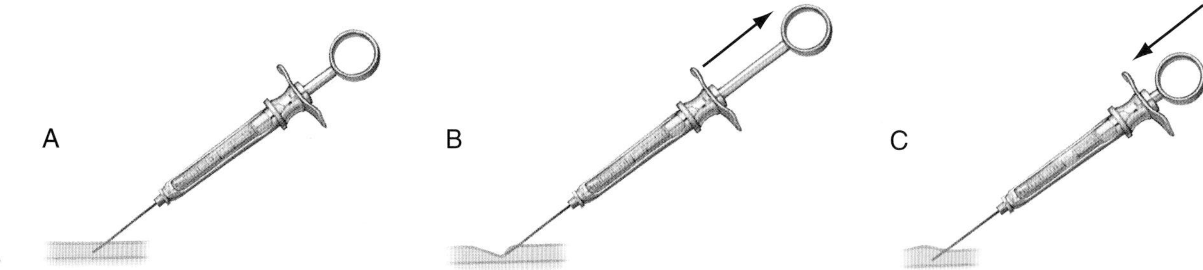

Figure 18-8. Intravascular injection of local anesthetic. **A,** Needle is inserted into the lumen of the blood vessel. **B,** Aspiration test is performed. Negative pressure pulls the vessel wall against the bevel of the needle; therefore no blood enters the syringe (negative aspiration). **C,** Drug is injected. Positive pressure on the plunger of the syringe forces local anesthetic solution out through the needle. The wall of the vessel is forced away from the bevel, and anesthetic solution is deposited directly into the lumen of the blood vessel.

syringe about 45 degrees to reorient the needle bevel relative to the wall of the blood vessel, and reaspirate.

Slowly inject the anesthetic. Rapid intravascular injection of 1.8 mL of a 2% local anesthetic solution produces a blood level in excess of that necessary for overdose. Rapid injection is defined (by the author) as administration of the entire volume of a dental cartridge in 30 seconds or less. The same volume of anesthetic deposited intravascularly slowly (minimum, 60 seconds) produces slightly elevated blood levels that are still below the minimum for serious overdose (seizure). In the event that the level does exceed this minimum, onset of the reaction will be slower and signs and symptoms will be less severe than those observed after more rapid injection. *Slow injection is the most important factor in preventing adverse drug reactions—it is even more important than aspiration.* The ideal rate of local anesthetic administration is 1.0 mL/min. Given that many dentists administer LA more rapidly than this ideal, the recommended rate of LA administration is deposition of a 1.8-mL cartridge in not less than 60 seconds. Because the recommended volumes of local anesthetic for most intraoral injection techniques are considerably less than 1.8 mL, most injections can be administered safely (and comfortably) in less than 1 minute.

• • •

The truth about local anesthetic overdosage in dentistry[35]: Administration of too large an LA dose relative to the weight (and age) of the patient is the most common cause of serious local anesthetic overdose reactions in dentistry. Although some serious cases of local anesthetic overdose have occurred in adult patients,[5] an overwhelming majority of problems commonly develop in the child who is young (2 to 6 years), lightweight (<30 kg [66 lb]), and well behaved; requires multiple procedures in four quadrants; and is managed in the office of an inexperienced general dentist.[3]

Review of many of the cases that resulted in serious morbidity or death reveals a number of shared factors, none of which in itself might pose a serious problem; however, when added together, they act to produce clinical signs and symptoms of local anesthetic overdose. These factors are presented in Box 18-3.

1. *Treatment plan:* In interviews with trained pediatric dentists, it has been the author's experience that when presented with the patient described in the preceding section (young, lightweight, well behaved), the pediatric dentist (with few exceptions) will not treat all four quadrants at one visit using local anesthetic alone. Limiting treatment to one or two quadrants per visit represents a more rational approach to this patient's needs, and enhances safety.
   A dentist confronted with a (well-meaning) parent or grandparent who complains of the difficulties of getting to the dental office and the inconvenience of having to miss a half-day of work, and wanting to have the child's dental care accomplished in one visit (not two or more), might feel pressured into agreeing to this request, thus increasing the risk for local anesthetic overdose. This is more likely to occur in offices of younger (by which I mean "inexperienced") dentists who are developing their practice and wish to keep their patients "happy."
2. *Choice of local anesthetic:* In most instances where serious LA overdose has occurred in children, the local anesthetic administered has been a "plain" drug, either mepivacaine HCl 3% (usually) or prilocaine HCl 4%. Both of these are excellent local anesthetics—when used properly. The rationale behind the clinician's selection of a short-acting drug for children includes that (1) most pediatric appointments are of short duration, and (2) "plain" local anesthetics possess a shorter duration of residual soft tissue anesthesia, minimizing the likelihood of inadvertent soft tissue injury as the child bites or chews his or her numb lip or tongue.
   As a rule, the pediatric dentist administers a "plain" local anesthetic only when treatment is limited to one quadrant. If treatment extends to two or more quadrants in one visit, a vasopressor-containing LA is selected. Prolonged posttreatment soft tissue anesthesia leads to the increased possibility of soft tissue damage; however, this risk is outweighed by benefits accrued through delayed absorption of the local anesthetic into the CVS (the risk of overdose is diminished).
   Postoperative soft tissue injury can be prevented in many ways, such as securing a cotton roll in the buccal fold and advising the parent to watch the child. (See Chapters 16 and 17.) Availability of the local anesthesia reversal agent—phentolamine mesylate—decreases residual soft tissue anesthesia duration significantly.[36,37] Reversal of local anesthesia is discussed fully in Chapter 20.
   Table 18-3 presents the local anesthetic of choice for 117 dentists who treat children.[38]
3. *Volume of local anesthetic administered:* Pain control for the entire primary dentition can be achieved with approximately two cartridges of local anesthetic. In the smaller child patient, there is rarely a compelling need to administer a 1.8-mL volume of local anesthetic in any one injection. Yet full cartridges are commonly administered when children receive local anesthetic administered by nonpediatric dentists. In many of the instances where a death resulted, a total of five, six, or seven cartridges were administered.[3]

BOX 18-3 Factors Adding to Increased Risk of Local Anesthetic Overdose in Younger Patients

1. Treatment plan where all four quadrants are treated with local anesthetic in one visit.
2. Local anesthetic administered is a plain (no vasopressor) solution.
3. Full cartridges (1.8 mL) administered with each injection.
4. Local anesthetic administered to all four quadrants at one time.
5. Exceeding the maximum dosage based on patient's body weight.

TABLE 18-3
Local Anesthetic of Choice for 117 Dentists Who Treat Children

Local Anesthetic Formulation	Percent Preferentially Employing Drug
2% lidocaine + epinephrine	69
3% mepivacaine	11
2% lidocaine	8
2% mepivacaine + levonordefrin	8
Other	4

Data from Cheatham BD, Primosch RE, Courts FJ: A survey of local anesthetic usage in pediatric patients by Florida dentists, J Dent Child 59:401–407, 1992.

In those situations where LA must be administered to all four quadrants of a smaller child, pain control can be achieved with not more than two cartridges, as follows: one fourth of a cartridge each for the right and left incisive nerve blocks (anesthetizing all mandibular primary teeth); or one half of a cartridge each for right and left inferior alveolar nerve blocks; one quarter of a cartridge each for the right and left anterior superior alveolar nerve blocks. In lieu of the anterior superior alveolar nerve block, maxillary infiltrations may be administered with one sixth of a cartridge per injection (Table 18-4).

4. *Local anesthetic administered to all four quadrants at one time*: Administration, over 1 or 2 minutes, of four or more cartridges of a local anesthetic without a vasopressor to all four quadrants makes little therapeutic sense and considerably increases the risk of an overdose. Administration of local anesthetic to one quadrant, treating that area, then anesthetizing the next quadrant, and so on, makes considerably more sense from both a therapeutic and a safety perspective. For equal volumes of local anesthetic, administration over a longer time frame (e.g., 1 to 2 hours) results in a lower blood level when compared with administration of the entire dose at one time.

TABLE 18-4
Recommended Volumes of Local Anesthetic for Intraoral Injections

Technique	Adult Volume, mL	Pediatric Volume, mL
Infiltration (supraperiosteal)	0.6	0.3
Inferior alveolar	1.5	0.9
Gow-Gates mandibular	1.8	0.9
Mental or incisive	0.6	0.45
Posterior superior alveolar	0.9	0.45
Anterior superior alveolar (infraorbital)	0.9	0.45
Greater (anterior) palatine	0.45	0.2
Nasopalatine	0.2	0.2
Maxillary (second division)	1.8	0.9

5. *Exceeding the maximum dosage based on patient's body weight:* An important factor, especially when younger, lighter-weight patients are managed, is maximum recommended dose (MRD). Determine the weight of the patient (in kilograms [kg] or pounds [lb]) *before* the start of treatment. It is preferable to weigh the child on a scale, because parents frequently can offer only a rough estimate of their child's weight (usually underestimating it). One must always remember that these figures are not absolutes. Exceeding the MRD of a drug does not guarantee that an overdose will happen (see Table 18-5 and discussion). On the other hand, administering dosages below the maximum calculated by body weight is no guarantee that adverse reactions will not be seen. The likelihood of ADRs developing is dose related. Smaller dosages minimize (but do not eliminate) this risk; larger doses increase (but do not guarantee) it.
Maximum recommended dosages of commonly administered local anesthetics are summarized in Table 18-5.

The intrinsic safety of local anesthetics is illustrated in Table 18-6, which presents the volume of local anesthetic administered on 65 occasions by a general dentist who removed third molars from college-aged individuals.

None of these patients experienced an adverse response to the local anesthetic, although many received dosages many times the MRD.[39] This is one indication that local anesthetics are extremely safe drugs when administered to healthy, younger (teenage to mid-20s) adult patients. Unfortunately, when they are administered in overly large doses to younger, lightweight patients, overdose *is* a significant risk.

Virtually all local anesthetic overdose reactions are preventable if the clinician adheres to the very basic, simple recommendations presented in the preceding section. In the unlikely situation that an overdose reaction develops, adherence to the basic steps of emergency management will lead to a successful outcome in essentially all cases.

Clinical Manifestations

Clinical signs and symptoms of overdose appear whenever the blood level in that drug's target organ(s) becomes overly high for that individual (Box 18-4). Target organs for local

TABLE 18-5
Maximum Recommended Dosages of Local Anesthetics

Drug	Clinical Percent mg	/ mL	mg/Cartridge (1.8 mL)	Recommended* mg/kg	mg/lb	Absolute Maximum,* mg
Articaine	4	40	72	7.0	3.2	None listed
Lidocaine	2	20	36	4.4	2.0	300
Mepivacaine	2	20	36	4.4	2.0	300
Mepivacaine	3	30	54	4.4	2.0	300
Prilocaine	4	40	72	6.0	2.7	400
Bupivacaine	0.5	5	9	1.3	0.6	90

*Maximum recommended doses of local anesthetics are for local anesthetic solutions containing vasoconstrictors or without vasoconstrictors.

TABLE 18-6
Local Anesthetic Administration for Removal of Third Molars

Procedure (Number of Third Molars Extracted at Visit)	Number of Patients in Category	Number of Cartridges (Range)	Number of Cartridges (Average)
1	5	4-10	6.2
2	13	4-23	12.18
3	8	10-20	15.33
4	39	6-26	19.24

From Malamed SF: Unpublished data, 2002.

BOX 18-4 Overdose Levels

Minimal to Moderate Overdose Levels

Signs	Symptoms (progressive with increasing blood levels)
Talkativeness	Lightheadedness and dizziness
Apprehension	Restlessness
Excitability	Nervousness
Slurred speech	Numbness
Generalized stutter, leading to muscular twitching and tremor distal extremities	Sensation of twitching before actual twitching is observed (see "Generalized Stutter" under "Signs")
Euphoria	Metallic taste
Dysarthria	Visual disturbances (inability to focus)
Nystagmus	Auditory disturbances (tinnitus)
Sweating	Drowsiness and disorientation
Vomiting	Loss of consciousness
Failure to follow commands or be reasoned with	
Disorientation	
Loss of response to painful stimuli	
Elevated blood pressure	
Elevated heart rate	
Elevated respiratory rate	

Moderate to High Overdose Levels

Signs

Tonic–clonic seizure activity followed by:

- Generalized central nervous system depression
- Depressed blood pressure, heart rate, and respiratory rate

anesthetics include CNS and the myocardium. The rate of onset of signs and symptoms and, to an extent, their severity correspond to this level. Table 18-7 compares the various modes of local anesthetic overdose.

> **NOTE:** It is possible that the "excitatory" phase of the overdose reaction may be extremely brief or may not occur at all, in which case the first clinical manifestation of overdose may be drowsiness progressing to unconsciousness and respiratory arrest. This appears to be more common with lidocaine than with other local anesthetics.[40]

The clinical manifestations of LA overdose will persist until the anesthetic blood level in the affected organs (brain, heart) falls below the minimum value (through redistribution), or until clinical signs and symptoms are terminated through administration of appropriate drug therapy.

Pathophysiology

The blood or plasma level of a drug is the amount absorbed into the circulatory system and transported in plasma throughout the body. Levels are measured in micrograms per milliliter (μg/mL) (1000 μg equals 1 mg). Figure 18-9 illustrates clinical manifestations observed with increasing blood levels of lidocaine in the CNS and heart. Blood levels are estimates because significant individual variation can occur.

Local anesthetics exert a depressant effect on all excitable membranes. In the clinical practice of anesthesia, a local anesthetic is applied to a specific region of the body, where it produces its primary effect: reversible depression of peripheral nerve conduction. Other actions are related to its absorption into the circulation and its subsequent actions on excitable membranes, including smooth muscle, the myocardium, and the CNS.

Following intraoral administration of 40 to 160 mg of lidocaine, the blood level rises to a maximum of approximately 1 μg/mL. (The usual range is between 0.5 and 2 μg/mL, but remember that response to drugs varies according to the individual.) Adverse reactions to the anesthetic are extremely uncommon in most individuals at these normal blood levels.

Central Nervous System Actions. The CNS is extremely sensitive to the actions of local anesthetics. As the cerebral blood level of LA increases, clinical signs and symptoms are observed.

Local anesthetics cross the blood–brain barrier, producing CNS depression. At nonoverdose levels of lidocaine (<5 μg/mL), no clinical signs or symptoms of adverse CNS effects are noted. Indeed, therapeutic advantage may be taken at blood levels between 0.5 and 4 μg/mL, because in this range, lidocaine demonstrates anticonvulsant

TABLE 18-7
Comparison of Forms of Local Anesthetic Overdose

	Rapid Intravascular	Too Large a Total Dose	Rapid Absorption	Slow Biotransformation	Slow Elimination
Likelihood of occurrence	Common	Most common	Likely with "high normal" doses if no vasoconstrictors are used	Uncommon	Least common
Onset of signs and symptoms	Most rapid (seconds); intra-arterial faster than intravenous	3-5 min	3-5 min	10-30 min	10 min–several hr
Intensity of signs and symptoms	Usually most intense	Gradual onset with increased intensity; may prove quite severe		Gradual onset with slow increase in intensity of symptoms	
Duration of signs and symptoms	1-2 min	Usually 5-30 min; depends on dose and ability to metabolize or excrete		Potentially longest duration because of inability to metabolize or excrete agents	
Primary prevention	Aspirate, slow injection	Administer minimal doses	Use vasoconstrictor; limit topical anesthetic use or use nonabsorped type (base)	Adequate pretreatment physical evaluation of patient	
Drug groups	Amides and esters	Amides; esters only rarely	Amides; esters only rarely	Amides and esters	Amides and esters

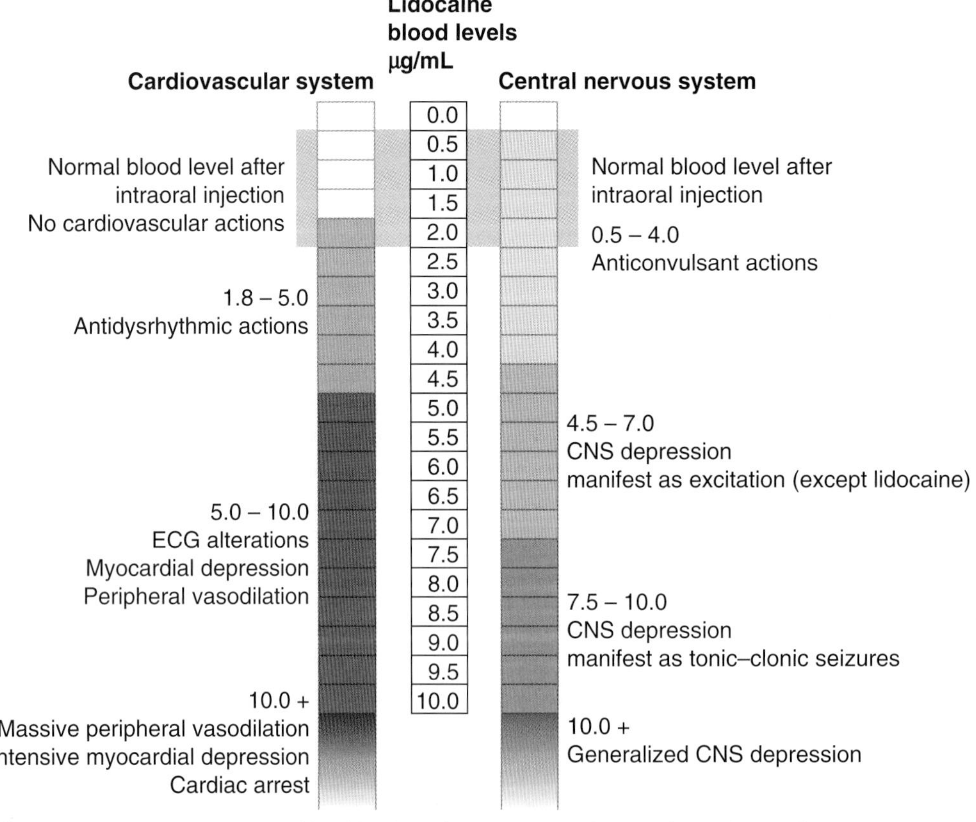

Figure 18-9. Local anesthetic blood levels and actions on cardiovascular and central nervous systems.

actions.[41-43] The mechanism of this action is depression of hyperexcitable neurons found in the amygdala of seizing patients.

Signs and symptoms of CNS toxicity appear at a cerebral blood level greater than 4.5 µg/mL. Generalized cortical sensitivity is noted: agitation, talkativeness, and irritability. Tonic–clonic seizures generally occur at levels greater than 7.5 µg/mL. With further increases in the lidocaine blood level, seizure activity ceases and a state of generalized CNS depression develops. Respiratory depression and arrest (apnea) are manifestations of this. Chapter 2 describes the method through which a CNS-depressant drug, such as a local anesthetic, can produce clinical signs and symptoms of apparent CNS stimulation.

Cardiovascular System Actions. The CVS is considerably less sensitive to the actions of local anesthetics. Adverse CVS responses do not usually develop until long after adverse CNS actions have appeared.

Local anesthetics, primarily lidocaine, have been used in the management of cardiac dysrhythmias, especially ventricular extrasystoles (premature ventricular contractions [PVCs]) and ventricular tachycardia. The minimum effective level of lidocaine for this action is 1.8 µg/mL, and the maximum is 5 µg/mL—the level at which undesirable actions become more likely.[44]

Increased blood levels (5 to 10 µg/mL) lead to minor alterations on the electrocardiogram, myocardial depression, decreased cardiac output, and peripheral vasodilation. At levels above 10 µg/mL, these effects are intensified: primarily massive peripheral vasodilation, marked reduction in myocardial contractility, severe bradycardia, and possible cardiac arrest.[45,46]

Management

Management of all medical emergencies is predicated on keeping the victim alive until he or she recovers, or until help arrives on scene to take over management. With prompt implementation of the basic emergency management protocol, a local anesthetic overdose reaction will resolve within minutes. Management of the LA overdose is based on the severity of the reaction. In most cases, the reaction is mild and transitory, requiring little or no specific treatment beyond basic treatment. In other instances, however, the reaction may be more severe and longer lasting, in which case more aggressive therapy is warranted.

Most local anesthetic overdose reactions are self-limiting because the blood level in the target organs (e.g., brain and heart) continues to decrease over time as the reaction progresses and the local anesthetic is redistributed (if the heart is still pumping effectively—as it usually is). Only rarely will drugs other than oxygen be necessary to terminate a local anesthetic overdose. Whenever signs and symptoms of overdose develop, do not simply label the patient "allergic" to local anesthetics, because this will further complicate future treatment (see p. 326).

Mild Overdose Reaction. Signs and symptoms of a mild overdose include retention of consciousness, talkativeness, and agitation, along with increased heart rate, blood pressure, and respiratory rate, which usually develop slowly—approximately 5 to 10 minutes after injection(s).

Slow Onset (≥5 minutes after administration). Possible causes of reactions with a slow onset include unusually rapid absorption, and too large a total dose. Management follows the usual P→A→B→C→D algorithm used in the management of all medical emergencies. Box 18-5 summarizes basic emergency management.

BOX 18-5 Basic Emergency Management

P...POSITION
- Unconscious...supine with feet elevated slightly
- Conscious...based on patient comfort

A...AIRWAY
- Unconscious...assess and maintain airway
- Conscious...assess airway

B...BREATHING
- Unconscious...assess and ventilate if necessary
- Conscious...assess breathing

C...CIRCULATION
- Unconscious...assess and provide external cardiac compression if necessary
- Conscious...assess circulation

D...DEFINITIVE CARE
- Diagnosis:
- Management: Emergency drugs and/or assistance (emergency medical services, dial 9-1-1)

Use the following protocol to deal with slow onset of symptoms.

P→A→B→C. Position the conscious patient comfortably. A, B, and C are assessed as adequate (patient is conscious and talking).

D (definitive care):

1. Reassure the patient that everything is all right and under control.
2. Administer oxygen via nasal cannula or nasal hood. This is indicated as a means of preventing acidosis, a situation during which the seizure threshold of the local anesthetic is decreased. The greater the arterial carbon dioxide tension, the lower the local anesthetic blood level necessary to induce or perpetuate tonic–clonic activity.[47]
3. Monitor and record vital signs. Postexcitation depression is usually mild, with little or no therapy necessary.
4. *(optional)* If trained and if equipment is available, establish an IV infusion. Use of anticonvulsants (e.g., midazolam) usually is not indicated at this time, although midazolam may be administered slowly intravenously and titrated at a rate of 1 mg/min if CNS stimulation appears to be intensifying toward a more severe reaction. If midazolam is administered, activate emergency medical services (dial 9-1-1).
5. Permit the patient to recover for as long as necessary. Dental care may or may not be continued after the patient's physical and emotional status have been evaluated. The patient may leave the dental office unescorted only if you are convinced that full recovery has occurred. Vital signs should be recorded and compared with baseline values, and the patient evaluated thoroughly before discharge. If an anticonvulsant drug was administered, or if doubt exists

as to the patient's degree of recovery, do not permit the patient to leave the office alone; consider emergency medical assistance (e.g., dial 9-1-1).

Slower Onset (≥15 minutes after administration). Possible causes of reactions of a slower onset include abnormal biotransformation and renal dysfunction. Follow this protocol for dealing with the slower onset of signs and symptoms in a conscious patient.

P→A→B→C. Position the conscious patient comfortably. A, B, and C are assessed as adequate (patient is conscious and talking).

D (definitive care):

1. Reassure the patient.
2. Administer oxygen.
3. Monitor vital signs.
4. Administer an anticonvulsant. Overdose reactions caused by abnormal biotransformation or renal dysfunction usually progress somewhat in intensity and last longer (because the drug cannot be eliminated rapidly). If venipuncture can be performed and if equipment is available, titrate 1 mg of midazolam/min until the clinical signs and symptoms of overdose subside.
5. Summon medical assistance. When venipuncture is not practical, or when an anticonvulsant drug has been administered, seek emergency medical assistance as soon as possible. Postexcitement depression usually is moderate after a mild excitement phase. Administration of midazolam or any other anticonvulsant will intensify this depression to varying degrees. Monitoring of the patient's status and adherence to the steps of basic life support are normally more than adequate for this situation.
6. After termination of the reaction, be sure that the patient is examined by a physician or a hospital staff member to determine possible causes. The examination could include blood tests and hepatic and renal function tests.
7. If the patient is not transported to a hospital by emergency medical services (EMS), do not let him or her leave the dental office alone. Arrangements should be made for an adult companion if hospitalization is deemed unnecessary.
8. Determine the cause of the reaction before proceeding with therapy requiring additional local anesthetics.

Severe Overdose Reaction

Rapid Onset (within 1 minute). Signs and symptoms include loss of consciousness with or without convulsions. The probable cause is intravascular injection.

P→A→B→C. Place the unconscious patient in the supine position. A, B, and C are assessed and maintained, as necessary. Remove the syringe from the mouth (if still present), and place the patient supine with feet elevated slightly. Subsequent management is based on the presence or absence of convulsions.

D (definitive care): In the presence of tonic–clonic convulsions:

1. Protect the patient's arms, legs, and head. Loosen tight clothing, such as ties, collars, and belts, and remove the pillow (or "doughnut") from the headrest.
2. Immediately summon emergency medical assistance (i.e., 9-1-1).
3. Continue basic life support. Maintenance of an adequate airway and adequate ventilation are of the utmost importance during management of local anesthetic–induced tonic–clonic seizures. Increased oxygen utilization and hypermetabolism, with increased production of CO_2 and lactic acid, occur during the seizure, leading to acidosis, which, in turn, lowers the seizure threshold (the blood level at which local anesthetic–induced seizures begin), prolonging the reaction.[48] Cerebral blood flow during such a seizure is also increased, elevating still further local anesthetic blood levels within the CNS.
4. Administer an anticonvulsant. The blood level of the local anesthetic declines as the drug undergoes redistribution; if acidosis is not present, seizures cease usually within about 1 to 3 minutes. Anticonvulsant therapy is not indicated for most seizures. If the seizure is prolonged (4 to 5 minutes with no indication of terminating), consider administering an anticonvulsant, but only if trained in parenteral drug administration (IV, intramuscular [IM], intranasal [IN]) and ventilation of a possibly apneic patient. IV midazolam, titrated at a rate of 1 mg/min until seizures cease, is the preferred treatment.[49,50] If venipuncture is not feasible, 5 mg/mL midazolam may be administered IM at a dose of 0.2 mg/kg for adult or pediatric patients.[51,52] The vastus lateralis is the preferred site for IM injection. Intranasal (IN) midazolam can be administered in patients weighing less than 50 kg at a dose of 0.2 mg/kg (up to 10 mg).[53] Seizures usually stop within 1 to 2 minutes after IN midazolam. Maintain basic life support, and obtain the assistance of emergency medical personnel.

Postseizure (Postictal) Phase. CNS depression is usually present at an intensity equal that of the excitation phase (Fig. 18-10). The patient may be drowsy or unconscious; breathing may be shallow or absent; the airway may be partially or totally obstructed; blood pressure and heart rate may be depressed or absent. A more intense postseizure state is noted when anticonvulsants have been administered to terminate the seizure.

P→A→B→C. Implementation of the steps of basic life support is crucial: airway, breathing, and circulation must be provided as needed. In all postictal situations, maintenance of an adequate airway is necessary; in some other cases, assisted or controlled ventilation may be indicated; for a small percentage of the most severe reactions, chest compression must be added to the first two steps of basic life support.

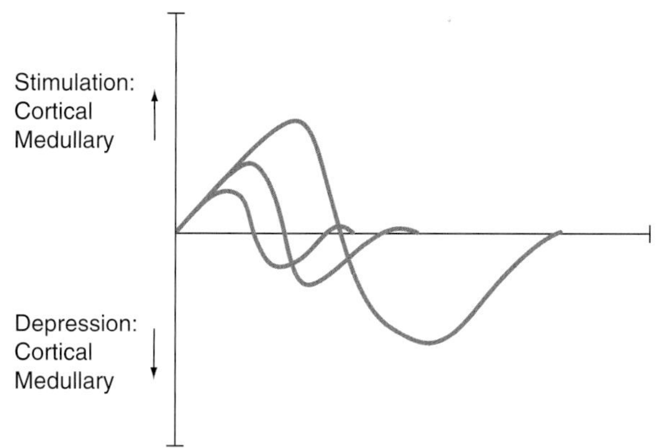

Figure 18-10. Effects of local anesthetics on the central nervous system. Notice that the intensity of depression is equal to the intensity of the preceding stimulation. (From Bennett CR: Monheim's local anesthesia and pain control in dental practice, ed 7, St Louis, 1984, Mosby.)

D (definitive care):

1. Additional management, such as use of a vasopressor (ephedrine) IM, is indicated if hypotension persists for extended periods (30 minutes). Preferred initial management for hypotension in this situation consists of positioning of the patient and administration of IV fluids.
2. Allow the patient to rest until recovery is sufficient to permit transfer to a hospital emergency department. This means a return of vital signs to baseline levels. In all situations in which local anesthetic–induced seizures occur and emergency medical services are necessary, evaluation of the patient in a hospital emergency department is necessary.

Slow Onset (5 to 15 minutes). Possible causes of severe reactions of slow onset include (1) too large a total dose, (2) rapid absorption, (3) abnormal biotransformation, and (4) renal dysfunction.

> **NOTE:** Overdose reactions that develop very slowly (15 to 30 min) are unlikely to progress to severe clinical manifestations if the patient is continually observed and management is started promptly.
>
> Terminate dental treatment as soon as the signs of toxicity first appear.

P→A→B→C. Provide basic life support (BLS) as necessary. As in the preceding protocol, prevention of acidosis and hypoxia through airway management and adequate pulmonary ventilation is of primary importance for a successful outcome.

D (definitive care):

1. Administer an anticonvulsant. If symptoms are mild at the onset but progress in severity, and if an IV line can be established, definitive treatment with IV anticonvulsants and continued oxygen administration are indicated. IM or IN midazolam may be considered when the IV route is not available.
2. Summon emergency medical assistance immediately if seizures develop.
3. Postseizure management includes BLS and IM or IV administration of a vasopressor for hypotension, as needed. Administration of IV fluids is recommended for management of hypotension.
4. Permit the patient to recover for as long as necessary before discharge to hospital. Completely evaluate the patient's condition at future appointments before readministering a local anesthetic.

• • •

Overdose reactions are the most common "true" ADRs associated with administration of amide local anesthetics. Most overdose reactions are preventable through adequate pretreatment evaluation of the patient and sensible administration of these drugs. In the few instances in which clinical manifestations of overly high local anesthetic blood levels become evident, a successful outcome usually results if the condition is promptly recognized and the patient treated efficiently and effectively. Primary among the steps of management are maintenance of a patent airway and adequate oxygenation. Data indicate that if local anesthetic–induced seizures are brief and well managed, no permanent neurologic or behavioral sequelae remain postictally.[54] In other words, ischemic CNS damage is not inevitable with well-managed, brief, local anesthetic–induced seizures.

Epinephrine Overdose

Precipitating Factors and Prevention. Epinephrine and levonordefrin are the vasoconstrictors presently included in dental local anesthetic cartridges in the United States and Canada. Table 18-8 outlines the milligram per milliliter concentrations of vasoconstrictors currently used in dentistry worldwide.

The optimum concentration of epinephrine for prolongation of pain control (with lidocaine) appears to be 1:400,000.[55] Use of a 1:50,000 epinephrine concentration for pain control cannot be recommended. Epinephrine 1:50,000 or 1:100,000 is useful via local infiltration in the control of bleeding when applied directly into the surgical site. Epinephrine or local anesthetic overdose reactions occurring under these conditions are rare.

Epinephrine overdose is more common when used in gingival retraction cord before impressions are taken for a crown and bridge procedure. Currently available cords contain approximately 225.5 μg of racemic epinephrine per inch of cord.[56] Epinephrine is readily absorbed through gingival epithelium that has been disturbed (abraded) by the dental procedure. About 64% to 94% of applied epinephrine is absorbed into the CVS.[56] Variability in absorption is extreme, according to the degree and duration of vascular exposure (bleeding). With regard to vasoconstrictors used for gingival retraction purposes, the American Dental Association states the following in *Accepted Dental*

TABLE 18-8
Dilutions of Vasoconstrictors Used in Dentistry

Dilution	Drug Available	mg/mL	mg per Cartridge (1.8 mL)	Maximum No. of Cartridges Used for Healthy Patient and Cardiac-Impaired Patient
1:1000	Epinephrine (emergency kit)	1.0	Not applicable	Not available in local anesthetic cartridge
1:10,000	Epinephrine (emergency kit)	0.1	Not applicable	Not available in local anesthetic cartridge
1:20,000	Levonordefrin	0.5	0.09	10 (H), 2 (C)
1:30,000	Levarterenol	0.034	0.06	5 (H), 2 (C)
1:50,000	Epinephrine	0.02	0.036	5 (H), 1 (C)
1:100,000	Epinephrine	0.01	0.018	10 (H), 2 (C)
1:200,000	Epinephrine	0.005	0.009	20 (H), 4 (C)

C, Cardiac-impaired patient; *H,* healthy patient.

BOX 18-6 Signs and Symptoms of Epinephrine or Other Vasopressor Overdose

Signs	Symptoms
Sharp elevation in blood pressure, primarily systolic	Fear, anxiety
Elevated heart rate	Tenseness
Possible cardiac dysrhythmias (premature ventricular contractions, ventricular tachycardia, ventricular fibrillation)	Restlessness
	Throbbing headache
	Tremor
	Perspiration
	Weakness
	Dizziness
	Pallor
	Respiratory difficulty
	Palpitations

Therapeutics: "Since effective agents which are devoid of systemic effects are available, it is not advisable to use epinephrine for gingival retraction, and its use is contraindicated in individuals with a history of cardiovascular disease."[57]

Clinical Manifestations. Clinical signs and symptoms of epinephrine overdose are listed in Box 18-6.

Management. Most instances of epinephrine overdose are of such short duration that little or no formal management is necessary. On occasion, however, the reaction may be prolonged and some management is desirable.

Terminate the Procedure. If possible, remove the source of epinephrine. Stopping the injection of local anesthetic does not remove epinephrine that has been deposited; however, release of endogenous epinephrine and norepinephrine from the adrenal medulla and nerve endings is lessened once the anxiety-inducing stimulus is eliminated. Epinephrine-impregnated gingival retraction cord, if present, should be removed.

Basic management follows the usual P→A→B→C→D algorithm used in management of all medical emergencies.

P→A→B→C. Position the conscious patient comfortably. The supine position often is not desired by the patient because it tends to accentuate the CVS effects. A semi-sitting or erect position minimizes any further elevation in cerebral blood pressure. A, B, and C are assessed as adequate (patient is conscious and talking).

D (definitive care):

1. Reassure the patient that the signs and symptoms are transient and will subside shortly. Anxiety and restlessness are common clinical manifestations of epinephrine overdose.
2. Monitor vital signs and administer oxygen. Blood pressure and heart rate should be checked every 5 minutes during the episode. Striking elevations in both parameters may be noted but gradually return toward baseline. Oxygen may be administered if necessary. The patient may complain of difficulty breathing. An apprehensive patient may hyperventilate (increased rate and depth of breathing). Oxygen is not indicated in the management of hyperventilation because it can exacerbate symptoms, possibly leading to carpopedal tetany.
3. Recovery. Permit the patient to remain in the dental chair as long as necessary to recover. The degree of postexcitation fatigue with depression noted varies but is usually prolonged. Do not discharge the patient if any doubt remains about his or her ability to provide self-care.

ALLERGY

Allergy is a hypersensitive state, acquired through exposure to a particular allergen, re-exposure to which produces a heightened capacity to react. Allergic reactions cover a broad spectrum of clinical manifestations ranging from mild and delayed responses occurring as long as 48 hours after exposure to the allergen, to immediate and life-threatening reactions developing within seconds of exposure (Table 18-9).

Predisposing Factors

The incidence of allergy in the population is not low: about 15% of patients with allergy have conditions severe enough to require medical management, and some 33% of all chronic disease in children is allergic in nature.[58]

TABLE 18-9
Classification of Allergic Diseases (After Gell and Coombs)

Type	Mechanism	Principal Antibody or Cell	Time of Reactions	Clinical Examples
I	Anaphylactic (immediate, homocytotropic, antigen induced, antibody mediated)	IgE	Seconds to minutes	Anaphylaxis (drugs, insect venom, antisera) Atopic bronchial asthma Allergic rhinitis Urticaria Angioedema Hay fever
II	Cytotoxic (antimembrane)	IgG IgM (activate complement)	—	Transfusion reactions Goodpasture's syndrome Autoimmune hemolysis Hemolytic anemia Certain drug reactions Membranous glomerulonephrosis
III	Immune complex (serum sickness–like)	IgG (form complexes with complement)	6-8 hr	Serum sickness Lupus nephritis Occupational allergic alveolitis Acute viral hepatitis
IV	Cell-mediated (delayed) or tuberculin-type response	—	48 hr	Allergic contact dermatitis Infectious granulomas (tuberculosis, mycoses) Tissue graft rejection Chronic hepatitis

Adapted from Krupp MA, Chatton MJ: Current medical diagnosis and treatment, Los Altos, Calif, 1994, Lange Medical.

Allergy to local anesthetics does occur, but its incidence has decreased dramatically since the introduction of amide anesthetics in the 1940s. Brown and associates stated, "The advent of the amino-amide local anesthetics which are not derivatives of para-aminobenzoic acid markedly changed the incidence of allergic type reactions to local anesthetic drugs. Toxic reactions of an allergic type to the amino amides are extremely rare, although several cases have been reported in the literature in recent years which suggest that this class of agents can on rare occasions produce an allergic type of phenomenon."[59]

Allergic responses to local anesthetics include dermatitis (common in dental office personnel), bronchospasm (asthmatic attack), and systemic anaphylaxis. The most frequently encountered are localized dermatologic reactions. Life-threatening allergic responses related to local anesthetics are indeed rare.[60,61]

Hypersensitivity to the ester-type local anesthetics—procaine, propoxycaine, benzocaine, tetracaine, and related compounds such as procaine penicillin G and procainamide—is much more frequent.

Amide-type local anesthetics are essentially free of this risk. However, reports from the literature and from medical history questionnaires indicate that alleged allergy to amide drugs appears to be increasing, despite the fact that subsequent evaluation of these reports usually finds them describing cases of overdose, idiosyncrasy, or psychogenic reactions.[62-65] Allergy to one amide local anesthetic does not preclude the use of other amides, because cross-allergenicity does not occur.[66] With ester anesthetic allergy, however, cross-allergenicity does occur; thus all ester-type local anesthetics are contraindicated with a documented history of ester allergy.[66]

TABLE 18-10
Contents of Local Anesthetic Cartridge

Ingredient	Function
Local anesthetic agent	Conduction blockade
Vasoconstrictor	Decreases absorption of local anesthetic into blood, thus increasing duration of anesthesia and decreasing toxicity of anesthetic
Sodium metabisulfite	Antioxidant for vasoconstrictor
Methylparaben*	Preservative to increase shelf life; bacteriostatic
Sodium chloride	Isotonicity of solution
Sterile water	Diluent

*Methylparaben has been excluded from all local anesthetic cartridges manufactured in the United States since January 1984, although it is still found in multidose vials of medication.

Allergic reactions have been documented for the various contents of the dental cartridge. Table 18-10 lists the functions of these components. Of special interest with regard to allergy is the bacteriostatic agent methylparaben. The parabens (methyl-, ethyl-, and propyl-) are included, as bacteriostatic agents, in all multiple-use formulations of drugs,

TABLE 18-11
Frequency of Dermal Reactions in Patients Exposed to Various Local Anesthetic Agents

Agent	Nonallergic Patients (n = 60)	Allergic Patients (n = 11)
NaCl	0	0
Procaine	20	8
Chloroprocaine	11	8
Tetracaine	25	8
Lidocaine	0	0
Mepivacaine	0	0
Prilocaine	0	0
Methylparaben	8	NA

Data from Aldrete JA, Johnson DA: Evaluation of intracutaneous testing for investigation of allergy to local anesthetic agents, Anesth Analg 49:173–183, 1970.
NA, Not available.

cosmetics, and some foods. Their increasing use has led to more frequent sensitization to them. In evaluating local anesthetic allergy, Aldrete and Johnson demonstrated positive reactions to methylparaben but negative reactions to the amide anesthetic without the bacteriostatic agent.[2] Table 18-11 presents Aldrete and Johnson's dermal reaction findings in patients exposed to various ester and amide local anesthetic solutions. The authors reported no signs of systemic anaphylaxis occurring in any of the subjects. Dental local anesthetic cartridges available in the United States and Canada are single-use items and as such no longer contain paraben preservatives.

Sodium Bisulfite Allergy. Allergy to sodium bisulfite or metabisulfite is being reported today with increasing frequency.[67-70] Bisulfites are antioxidants that are commonly sprayed onto prepared fruits and vegetables to keep them appearing "fresh" for long periods of time. For example, apple slices sprayed with bisulfite do not turn brown (become oxidized). People who are allergic to bisulfites (most often steroid-dependent asthmatic individuals) may develop a severe response (bronchospasm).[69,71] The U.S. Food and Drug Administration has enacted regulations that limit the use of bisulfites on foods. A history of allergy to bisulfites should alert the dentist to the possibility of this same type of response if sodium bisulfite or metabisulfite is included in the local anesthetic solution. Sodium bisulfite or metabisulfite is found in all dental local anesthetic cartridges that contain a vasoconstrictor, but is not found in "plain" local anesthetic solutions.

In the presence of a documented sulfite allergy, it is suggested that a local anesthetic solution without a vasopressor ("plain local anesthetic") should be used (e.g., mepivacaine HCl 3%, prilocaine HCl 4%) if possible. No cross-allergenicity is present between sulfites and the "sulfa-" type antibiotics (sulfonamides).

Epinephrine Allergy. Allergy to epinephrine cannot occur in a living person. Questioning of the "epinephrine-allergic" patient (see "Dialogue History," p. 329) immediately reveals signs and symptoms related to increased blood levels of circulating catecholamines (tachycardia, palpitation, sweating, nervousness), likely the result of fear of receiving injections (release of endogenous catecholamines [epinephrine and norepinephrine]). Management of the patient's fear and anxiety over receipt of the injection is in order in most of these situations.

Latex Allergy. The thick plunger (also known as the *stopper* or *bung*) at one end of the local anesthetic cartridge and the thin diaphragm at the other end of the cartridge (see Fig. 7-1), through which the needle penetrates, at one time contained latex. Because latex allergy is a matter of concern among all health care professionals, the risk of provoking an allergic reaction in a latex-sensitive patient must be considered. A review of the literature on latex allergy and local anesthetic cartridges by Shojaei and Haas reveals that latex allergen can be released into the local anesthetic solution as the needle penetrates the diaphragm, but no reports or case studies have described an allergic response to the latex component of the cartridge containing a dental local anesthetic.[70] Dental cartridges presently (January 2012) available in the United States and Canada are latex free.

Topical Anesthetic Allergy. Topical anesthetics possess the potential to induce allergy. The most commonly used topical anesthetics in dentistry are esters, such as benzocaine and tetracaine. The incidence of allergy to this classification of local anesthetics far exceeds that to amide local anesthetics. However, because benzocaine (an ester topical anesthetic) is poorly absorbed systemically, allergic responses that develop in response to its use normally are limited to the site of application.[72] When other topical formulations, ester or amide, that are absorbed systemically are applied to mucous membranes, allergic responses may be localized or systemic. Many contain preservatives such as methylparaben, ethylparaben, or propylparaben.

Prevention

Medical History Questionnaire. Most medical history questionnaires contain several questions related to allergy.

QUESTION: Are you allergic to (e.g., have itching, rash, swelling of hands, feet, or eyes) or made sick by penicillin, aspirin, codeine, or any other medications?

QUESTION: Have you ever had asthma, hay fever, sinus trouble, or allergies or hives?

These questions seek to determine whether the patient has experienced any adverse drug reactions. ADRs are not uncommon; those most frequently reported are labeled as allergy. If the patient mentions any unusual reaction to local anesthetics, the following protocol should be observed before use of the questionable drug is carried out. If the patient relates a history of alleged local anesthetic allergy, it is imperative that the dentist consider the following factors:

1. Assume that the patient *is* truly allergic to the drug in question and then take whatever steps are necessary to determine whether the alleged "allergy" is indeed an allergy. A recent paper on food allergy revealed that 30% of Americans have reported (alleged) one or more food allergies, but true food allergy in the U.S. population actually occurs at a rate of approximately 4% in adults and 5% in children.[73]
2. Any drug or closely related drug to which a patient claims to be allergic must not be used until the alleged allergy can be absolutely disproved.
3. For almost all drugs commonly implicated in allergic reactions, equally effective alternate drugs exist (e.g., antibiotics, analgesics).
4. The only drug group in which alternatives are not equally effective consists of local anesthetics.

• • •

Two major components are useful for determining the veracity of a claim of allergy: (1) dialogue history, whereby additional information is sought directly from the patient, and (2) consultation for a more thorough evaluation if doubt persists.

Dialogue History. The following questions are included in the dialogue history between the dentist and a patient with an alleged allergy to local anesthetics. The first two questions are the most critical, for they immediately establish in the evaluator's mind a sense of whether allergy does or does not exist.[74]

QUESTION: Describe exactly what happened. (Describe your "allergic" reaction.)

QUESTION: What treatment was given?

Following these two questions, the evaluator may consider others that will help elucidate the actual reaction.

QUESTION: What position were you in during injection of the local anesthetic?

QUESTION: What was the time sequence of events?

QUESTION: Were the services of emergency medical personnel necessary?

QUESTION: What drug was used?

QUESTION: What volume of the drug was administered?

QUESTION: Did the local anesthetic solution contain a vasoconstrictor?

QUESTION: Were you taking any other drugs or medications at the time of the incident?

QUESTION: Can you provide the name, address, and telephone number of the doctor (dentist or physician) who was treating you when the incident occurred?

Answers to these questions provide enough information to permit a doctor to make an informed determination as to whether a true allergic reaction to a drug occurred. This is the initial step in managing alleged local anesthetic allergy. The dialogue history follows.

QUESTION: Describe exactly what happened.

This is probably the most important question because it allows the patient to describe the actual sequence of events. The "allergy," in most instances, is explained by the answer to this question. The symptoms described by the patient should be recorded and evaluated to help in formulating a tentative diagnosis of the adverse reaction. Did the patient lose consciousness? Did convulsions occur? Was there skin involvement or respiratory distress? The manifestations of allergic reactions are discussed in the following paragraph. Knowing them can aid the evaluator in rapidly determining the nature of the reaction that occurred.

Allergic reactions involve one or more of the following: skin (itching, hives, rash, edema), gastrointestinal system (cramping, diarrhea, nausea, vomiting), exocrine glands (runny nose, watery eyes), respiratory system (wheezing, laryngeal edema), and cardiovascular system (angioedema, vasodilation, hypotension). Most patients describe their local anesthetic "allergy" as one in which they experienced palpitations, severe headache, sweating, and mild shaking (tremor). Such reactions are almost always of psychogenic origin or are related to the administration of overly large doses of vasoconstrictor (e.g., epinephrine). They are not allergic in nature. Hyperventilation, an anxiety-induced reaction in which patients lose control over their breathing (inhaling and exhaling rapidly and deeply), is accompanied by dizziness, lightheadedness, and peripheral paresthesias (fingers, toes, and lips). Complaints of itching, hives, rash, or edema lead to the presumptive conclusion that an allergic reaction actually may have occurred.

QUESTION: What treatment was given?

When the patient is able to describe his or her management, the evaluator usually can determine its cause. Were drugs injected? If so, what drugs? Epinephrine, histamine blockers, corticosteroids, or anticonvulsants? Was aromatic ammonia used? Oxygen? Knowledge of the specific management of these situations can lead to an accurate diagnosis.

Drugs used in the management of allergic reactions include three categories: vasopressors (epinephrine [Adrenalin]), histamine blockers (diphenhydramine [Benadryl] or chlorpheniramine [Chlor-Trimeton]), and corticosteroids (hydrocortisone sodium succinate [Solu-Cortef] or dexamethasone [Decadron]).

Mention of the use of one or more of these drugs increases the likelihood that an allergic response did occur. Anticonvulsants, such as diazepam or midazolam, are administered intravenously to terminate seizures induced by overdose of local anesthetic. Aromatic ammonia is frequently used in the treatment of syncopal episodes. Oxygen may be administered in any or all of these reactions but is not specific for allergy.

QUESTION: What position were you in when the reaction took place?

Injection of a local anesthetic into an upright patient is most likely to produce a psychogenic reaction (vasodepressor syncope). This does not exclude the possibility that another type of reaction may occur, but with the patient supine during the injection, vasodepressor syncope is a less likely cause, even though transient loss of consciousness may (on very rare occasions) occur in these circumstances.[75] In some of the evaluations of allergy to local anesthetics that the author has carried out, the patient had been given an intracapsular injection of corticosteroid in the knee. Seated upright on a table in the physician's treatment room, the patient was able to watch the entire procedure, which was profoundly disturbing. In an effort to make such injections more tolerable, lidocaine or another local anesthetic is added to the steroid mixture. In spite of this, however, the intracapsular injection of corticosteroid and lidocaine is extremely uncomfortable. Many patients experience their "allergic reaction" at this time. Therefore, the supine position is recommended as being physiologically best tolerated for the administration of all local anesthetic injections.

QUESTION: What was the time sequence of events?

When, in relation to administration of the local anesthetic, did the reaction occur? Most adverse drug reactions associated with local anesthetic administration occur during or immediately (within seconds) after the injection. Syncope, hyperventilation, overdose, and (sometimes) anaphylaxis are most likely to develop immediately during the injection or within minutes thereafter, although all may occur later, during dental therapy. Also, seek to determine the amount of time that elapsed during the entire episode. How long was it before the patient was discharged from the office? Did dental treatment continue after the episode? The fact that dental treatment continued after this episode indicates that the response was probably minor and of a nonallergic nature.

QUESTION: Were the services of a physician, emergency medical services, or a hospital necessary?

A positive response to this usually indicates the occurrence of a more serious reaction. Most psychogenic reactions are ruled out by a positive answer, although an overdose or allergic reaction indeed may have occurred.

QUESTION: What local anesthetic was administered?

A patient who is truly allergic to a drug should be told the exact (generic) name of the substance. Many persons with documented allergic histories wear a medical alert tag or bracelet (Fig. 18-11) that lists specific items to which they are sensitive. However, some patients respond to this question with, "I'm allergic to local anesthetics" or "I'm allergic to Novocain" or "I'm allergic to all 'caine' drugs." Of 59 patients reporting allergy to local anesthetics, 54 could name one or more local anesthetics they believed were responsible. Five referred to only caine drugs.[76] Novocain (procaine) and other esters rarely are used today as injectable local anesthetics in dentistry (although the esters (primarily tetracaine) maintain some popularity in medicine); the amides have replaced the esters in clinical practice. Yet patients throughout the world frequently call the local anesthetics they receive "shots of Novocain." Two reasons exist for this. First, many older patients at one time received Novocain as a dental local anesthetic, and its name has become synonymous with intraoral dental injections. Second, despite the fact that United States dentists do not inject procaine or procaine-propoxycaine, many still describe local anesthetics as Novocain when talking with their patients. Thus the usual response of a patient to this question

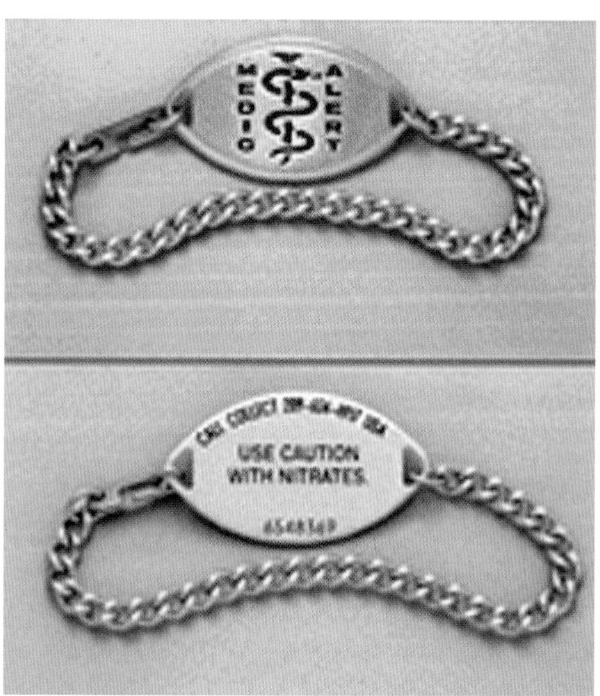

Figure 18-11. Medical alert bracelet provides vital medical information about the patient.

remains, "I'm allergic to Novocain." This response, received from a patient who has been managed properly in the past after an adverse reaction, indicates that the patient was sensitive to ester local anesthetics but not necessarily to amide local anesthetics. However, the answers usually are too general and vague for any conclusions to be drawn.[77]

QUESTION: What amount of drug was administered?

This question seeks to determine whether there was a definite dose–response relationship, as might occur with an overdose reaction. The problem is that patients rarely know these details and can provide little or no assistance. The doctor who was involved in the prior episode(s) may be of greater assistance.

QUESTION: Did the anesthetic solution contain a vasoconstrictor or preservative?

The presence of a vasoconstrictor might lead to the thought of an overdose reaction (relative or absolute) to this component of the solution. A preservative, such as methylparaben (if a multidose vial was used) or sodium bisulfite (if the solution contained a vasoconstrictor), in the solution might lead to the belief that an allergic reaction did occur to the preservative, not to the local anesthetic. Unfortunately, however, most patients are unable to furnish this information. Today, methylparaben is found only in multidose vials of local anesthetics (and most other drugs). Bisulfites are found in all dental local anesthetic cartridges containing a vasopressor.

QUESTION: Were you taking any other drugs or medications at the time of the reaction?

This question seeks to determine the possibility of a drug–drug interaction or a side effect of another drugs being responsible for the reported adverse response. Reidenburg and Lowenthal, reporting in 1968 on adverse nondrug reactions, demonstrated that "adverse" effects and side effects, which so often are blamed on medications, occur with considerable regularity in persons who have received no drugs or medications for weeks.[78] In other words, many so-called adverse drug reactions may be nothing more than a coincidental event: the person is becoming overly tired, irritable, nauseated, or dizzy for reasons unrelated to drugs. Unfortunately, however, it seems that whenever such symptoms develop in a patient taking a medication, the drug is immediately thought to be responsible, with the label "allergy" often applied.

QUESTION: Can you provide the name and address of the doctor (dentist, physician, or hospital) who was treating you at the time of the incident?

If possible, it is usually valuable to speak to the person who managed the previous episode. In most instances, this person is able to locate patient records and describe in detail what transpired. If it is not possible to locate or contact the doctor, the patient's primary care physician should be consulted. Direct discussion with the patient and the doctor can provide a wealth of information that the knowledgeable dentist can use to determine more precisely the nature of the previous reaction.

QUESTIONS FOR THE PATIENT WITH AN ALLEGED ALLERGY TO LOCAL ANESTHETIC

1. **Describe your reaction.**
   Itching, hives, rash, feeling faint, dizziness, lightheadedness, perspiration, shaking, palpitation
2. **How was your reaction treated?**
   Epinephrine, histamine blocker, corticosteroid, oxygen, spirits of ammonia ("smelling salts"), no treatment necessary
3. **What position were you in at the time of the reaction?**
   Supine, upright, partially reclined
4. **What is the name, address, and telephone number of the doctor in whose office this reaction occurred?**

Consultation and Allergy Testing. Consultation should be considered if any doubt remains as to the cause of the reaction after the dialogue history. Referral to a doctor who will test for allergy to local anesthetics is recommended.

Although no form of allergy testing is 100% reliable, skin testing is the primary mode of assessing a patient for local anesthetic allergy. Intracutaneous injections are among the most reliable means available, because they are 100 times more sensitive than cutaneous testing, and involve depositing 0.1 mL of test solution into the patient's forearm.[2,76,79-82] In all such instances, the local anesthetic solutions should contain neither vasoconstrictor nor preservative. Methylparaben, if evaluated, should be tested separately.[83]

The protocol for intracutaneous testing for local anesthetic allergy used at the Ostrow School of Dentistry of U.S.C. for the past 35 years involves the administration of 0.1 mL of each of the following: 0.9% sodium chloride, 1% or 2% lidocaine, 3% mepivacaine, and 4% prilocaine, without methylparaben, bisulfites, or vasopressors. After successful completion of this phase of testing, 0.9 mL of one of the previously noted local anesthetic solutions that produced no reaction is injected intraorally via supraperiosteal infiltration atraumatically (but without topical anesthesia) above a maxillary right or left premolar or anterior tooth. This is called an *intraoral challenge test,* and it frequently provokes the "allergic" reaction: fainting, sweating, and palpitations.

After performing more than 210 local anesthetic allergy testing procedures, the author has encountered four allergic responses to the paraben preservative (before 1984, the protocol included testing for parabens) and none to the amide local anesthetic itself. Numerous psychogenic responses (syncope, hyperventilation, palpitations) have been observed during intracutaneous or intraoral testing phases.

Such testing may be carried out by any person who is knowledgeable about the procedure and is fully prepared to manage whatever adverse reactions may develop. It must be remembered that skin testing is not without risk. Severe immediate allergic reactions may be precipitated by as little as 0.1 mL of drug in a sensitized patient. Emergency drugs, equipment, and trained personnel always must be available whenever allergy testing is performed.

Intracutaneous allergy testing should be carried out only after an intensive dialogue history in which the evaluator has become convinced that the prior reaction to the local anesthetic was not allergy. The testing procedure is used to confirm this fact for the patient. The intraoral challenge test was added to the protocol when several patients with negative responses to intracutaneous testing stated, "But the dentist will give me a larger amount in the mouth." It was intended to provide the patient with the psychological support needed to receive intraoral local anesthetic injections safely.

Informed consent is obtained before allergy testing. This consent includes, among other possible complications, acute allergy (anaphylaxis), cardiac arrest, and death.

A continuous intravenous infusion is started before all allergy testing procedures are performed, and emergency drugs and equipment are readily available throughout the testing.

Dental Management in the Presence of Alleged Local Anesthetic Allergy

When doubt persists concerning a history of allergy to local anesthetics, do not administer these drugs to the patient. Assume that allergy exists. Do not use local anesthetics, including topical anesthetics, unless and until allergy has been absolutely disproved – to the patient's satisfaction.

Elective Dental Care. Dental treatment requiring local anesthesia (topical or injectable) should be postponed until a thorough evaluation of the patient's "allergy" is completed. Dental care not requiring local anesthesia may be completed during this time.

Emergency Dental Care. Pain or oral infection presents a more difficult situation in the "I am allergic to Novocain" patient. Commonly, this patient is new to the dental office, requiring tooth extraction, pulpal extirpation, or incision and drainage (I&D) of an abscess, with an unremarkable medical history except for the alleged "allergy to Novocain." If, after dialogue history, the "allergy" appears to have been a psychogenic reaction but some doubt remains, consider one of several courses of action.

Emergency Protocol No. 1. The most practical approach to this patient is to provide no treatment of an invasive nature. Arrange an appointment for immediate consultation and allergy testing. Do not carry out any dental care requiring the use of injectable or topical local anesthetics. For incision and drainage of an abscess, inhalation sedation with nitrous oxide and oxygen might be an acceptable alternative.

Acute pain may be managed with oral analgesics, infection with oral antibiotics. These constitute only temporary measures. After complete evaluation of the "allergy," definitive dental care may proceed.

Emergency Protocol No. 2. Use general anesthesia in place of local anesthesia for management of a dental emergency. When properly used, general anesthesia is a highly effective and relatively safe alternative. Its lack of availability is a major problem in most dental practices.

When general anesthesia is used, be careful to avoid local anesthetics in these procedures:

1. Topical application (via spray) to the pharynx and tracheal mucosa immediately before intubation.
2. Infiltration of the skin with local anesthetic before venipuncture to decrease discomfort.

General anesthesia, administered in the dental office or in a hospital operating theater, is a viable short-term alternative to local anesthetic administration in managing the "allergic" patient, provided adequate facilities and well-trained personnel are available.

Emergency Protocol No. 3. Histamine blockers used as local anesthetics should be considered if general anesthesia is not available, and if it is deemed necessary to intervene physically in the dental emergency. Most injectable histamine blockers have local anesthetic properties. Diphenhydramine hydrochloride in a 1% solution with 1:100,000 epinephrine provides pulpal anesthesia for up to 30 minutes.[84] Although the quality of soft and hard tissue anesthesia attained with diphenhydramine, lidocaine, or prilocaine is equivalent, an undesirable side effect frequently noted during injection of diphenhydramine is a burning or stinging sensation, which limits the use of this agent for most patients to emergency procedures only.[85-87] Nitrous oxide and oxygen used along with diphenhydramine minimize patient discomfort while increasing the pain reaction threshold. Another (possibly positive) side effect of diphenhydramine and many histamine blockers is CNS depression (sedation, drowsiness), which may prove somewhat beneficial during treatment but mandates that a responsible adult guardian be available to take the patient home after treatment.

Management of the Patient With Confirmed Allergy. Management of the dental patient with a confirmed allergy to local anesthetics varies according to the nature of the allergy. If the allergy is limited to ester anesthetics, an amide anesthetic may be used (provided it does not contain a paraben preservative, which is closely related to the esters). No dental local anesthetic cartridge manufactured in the United States since January 1984 contains methylparaben.

If, in the exceedingly unlikely case, a documented allergy to an amide local anesthetic exists, other amide local anesthetics may be employed because cross-allergenicity between amide locals does not occur.[66]

If allergy does truly exist to an ester local anesthetic (a much more likely situation), dental treatment may be safely completed via one of the following:

1. Administration of an amide local anesthetic.
2. Use of histamine blockers as local anesthetics.
3. General anesthesia.
4. Alternative techniques of pain control:
   a. Hypnosis
   b. Acupuncture

On occasion, it is reported that a patient is "allergic to all 'caine' drugs." Such a report should provoke close scrutiny by the dentist, and the method by which this conclusion was reached should be re-examined.

All too often, patients are mislabeled as "allergic to local anesthetics." Such patients ultimately must have dental treatment carried out in a hospital setting, usually under general anesthesia, when a proper evaluation might have saved the patient time and money and decreased the risk of dental care.[60,77]

Clinical Manifestations

Table 18-9 lists the various forms of allergic reactions. It is also possible to classify allergic reactions by the time elapsing between contact with the antigen (allergen) and onset of clinical manifestations of allergy. Immediate reactions develop within seconds to hours of exposure. (They include types I, II, and III in Table 18-9.) With delayed reactions, clinical manifestations develop hours to days after antigenic exposure (type IV).

Immediate reactions, particularly type I, anaphylaxis, are significant. Organs and tissues involved in immediate allergic reactions include the skin, cardiovascular system, respiratory system, and gastrointestinal system. Generalized (systemic) anaphylaxis involves all these systems. Type I reactions may involve only one system, in which case they are referred to as *localized allergy.* Examples of localized anaphylaxis and their "targets" include bronchospasm (respiratory system) and urticaria (skin).

Time of Onset of Symptoms

The time elapsing between a patient's exposure to the antigen and the development of clinical signs and symptoms is important. In general, the more rapidly signs and symptoms develop following antigenic exposure, the more intense the reaction is likely to be.[88] Conversely, the more time between exposure and onset, the less intense the reaction. Cases have been reported of systemic anaphylaxis arising many hours after exposure.[89]

The rate of progression of signs and symptoms once they appear is also significant. Situations in which signs and symptoms rapidly increase in intensity are likely to be more life threatening than those progressing slowly or not at all once they appear.

Signs and Symptoms

Dermatologic Reactions. The most common allergic drug reaction associated with local anesthetic administration consists of urticaria and angioedema. Urticaria is associated with wheals, which are smooth, elevated patches of skin. Intense itching (pruritus) frequently is present. Angioedema is localized swelling in response to an allergen. Skin color and temperature usually are normal (unless urticaria or erythema is present). Pain and itching are uncommon. Angioedema most frequently involves the face, hands, feet, and genitalia, but it can also involve the lips, tongue, pharynx, and larynx. It is more common following application of topical anesthetics to oral mucous membranes. Within 30 to 60 minutes, the tissue in contact with the allergen appears swollen.

Allergic skin reactions, if the sole manifestation of an allergic response, normally are not life threatening; however, those that occur rapidly after drug administration may be the first indication of a more generalized reaction to follow.

Respiratory Reactions. Clinical signs and symptoms of allergy may be solely related to the respiratory tract, or respiratory tract involvement may occur along with other systemic responses.

Signs and symptoms of bronchospasm, the classic respiratory allergic response, include the following:

- Respiratory distress
- Dyspnea
- Wheezing
- Erythema
- Cyanosis
- Diaphoresis
- Tachycardia
- Increased anxiety
- Use of accessory muscles of respiration

Laryngeal edema, an extension of angioneurotic edema to the larynx, is a swelling of the soft tissues surrounding the vocal apparatus with subsequent obstruction of the airway. Little or no exchange of air from the lungs is possible. Laryngeal edema represents the effects of allergy on the upper airway, whereas bronchospasm represents the effects on the lower airway (smaller bronchioles). Laryngeal edema is a life-threatening emergency.

Generalized Anaphylaxis. The most dramatic and acutely life-threatening allergic reaction is generalized anaphylaxis. Clinical death can occur within a few minutes. Generalized anaphylaxis can develop after administration of an antigen by any route but is more common after parenteral administration (injection). Time of response is variable, but the reaction typically develops rapidly, reaching maximum intensity within 5 to 30 minutes. It is extremely unlikely that this reaction will ever be noted after administration of amide local anesthetics.

Signs and symptoms of generalized anaphylaxis, listed according to their typical progression, follow:

- Skin reactions
- Smooth muscle spasm of the gastrointestinal (cramping) and genitourinary tracts and of respiratory smooth muscle (bronchospasm)
- Respiratory distress
- Cardiovascular collapse

In fatal anaphylaxis, respiratory and cardiovascular disturbances predominate and are evident early in the reaction. The typical reaction progression is shown in Box 18-7.

In rapidly developing reactions, all signs and symptoms may occur within a very short time with considerable overlap. In particularly severe reactions, respiratory and cardiovascular signs and symptoms may be the only ones present. The reaction or any part of it can last from minutes to a day or longer.[88,90]

With prompt and appropriate treatment, the entire reaction may be terminated rapidly. However, hypotension and laryngeal edema may persist for hours to days despite intensive therapy. Death, which may occur at any time during the reaction, usually is secondary to upper airway obstruction produced by laryngeal edema.[91]

BOX 18-7 Typical Reaction Progression of Generalized Anaphylaxis

1. Early phase: skin reactions
   a. Patient complains of feeling sick
   b. Intense itching (pruritus)
   c. Flushing (erythema)
   d. Giant hives (urticaria) over the face and upper chest
   e. Nausea and possibly vomiting
   f. Conjunctivitis
   g. Vasomotor rhinitis (inflammation of mucous membranes in the nose, marked by increased mucous secretion)
   h. Pilomotor erection (feeling of hair standing on end)
2. Associated with skin responses are various gastrointestinal or genitourinary disturbances related to smooth muscle spasm
   a. Severe abdominal cramps
   b. Nausea and vomiting
   c. Diarrhea
   d. Fecal and urinary incontinence
3. Respiratory symptoms usually develop next
   a. Substernal tightness or pain in chest
   b. Cough may develop
   c. Wheezing (bronchospasm)
   d. Dyspnea
   e. If the condition is severe, cyanosis of the mucous membranes and nail beds
   f. Possible laryngeal edema
4. The cardiovascular system is next to be involved
   a. Pallor
   b. Lightheadedness
   c. Palpitations
   d. Tachycardia
   e. Hypotension
   f. Cardiac dysrhythmias
   g. Unconsciousness
   h. Cardiac arrest

Management

Skin Reactions. Management is predicated on the rate at which the reaction appears after antigenic challenge.

Delayed Skin Reactions. Signs and symptoms developing 60 minutes or longer after exposure usually do not progress and are not considered life threatening. Examples include a localized mild skin and mucous membrane reaction after application of topical anesthetic. In most instances, the patient already may have left the dental office and is calling back later describing these signs and symptoms, or the patient may still be in the dental office at the conclusion of his or her treatment.

Basic management follows the usual **P→A→B→C→D** algorithm used in management of all medical emergencies.

P→A→B→C. Position the conscious patient comfortably. A, B, and C are assessed as adequate (patient is conscious and talking).

D (definitive care):

1. Oral histamine blocker: 50 mg diphenhydramine or 10 mg chlorpheniramine; a prescription for diphenhydramine, 50 mg capsules, one q6h for 3 to 4 days should be given to the patient.
2. If still in the dental office, the patient should remain in the office under observation for 1 hour before discharge to ensure that the reaction does not progress.
3. Obtain medical consultation, if necessary, to determine the cause of the reaction. A complete list of all drugs and chemicals administered to or taken by the patient should be compiled for use by the allergy consultant.
4. If drowsiness occurs after oral histamine blocker administration, the patient should not be permitted to leave the dental office unescorted.

Immediate Skin Reactions. Signs and symptoms of allergy developing within 60 minutes require more vigorous management. Examples include conjunctivitis, rhinitis, urticaria, pruritus, and erythema.

P→A→B→C. Position the conscious patient comfortably. A, B, and C are assessed as adequate (patient is conscious and talking).

D (definitive care):

1. Administer parenteral (IM, IV) histamine blocker: 50 mg diphenhydramine (25 mg if less than 30 kg [66 lb]) or 10 mg chlorpheniramine (5 mg if less than 30 kg [66 lb]).
2. Monitor and record vital signs (blood pressure, heart rate and rhythm, respiratory rate) every 5 minutes for 1 hour.

3. Observe the patient a minimum of 60 minutes for evidence of recurrence. Discharge in the custody of a responsible adult if any parenteral drugs have been given.
4. Prescribe an oral histamine blocker for 3 days.
5. Fully evaluate the patient's reaction before further dental care is provided.
6. If, at any time during this period, uncertainty exists as to the condition of the patient, activate EMS (9-1-1).

Respiratory Reactions

Bronchospasm.

P→A→B→C. Position the conscious patient comfortably. Most persons experiencing respiratory distress prefer to be seated upright to varying degrees. A, B, and C are assessed. Airway is patent, although patient is exhibiting respiratory distress. C is assessed as adequate.

D (definitive care):

1. Terminate treatment (if started).
2. Administer oxygen via full face mask, nasal hood, or nasal cannula at a flow of 5 to 6 liters/min.
3. Administer epinephrine IM in the vastus lateralis muscle (0.3 mg if >30 kg; 0.15 mg if <30 kg) or another appropriate bronchodilator via metered dose inhaler (MDI) (albuterol) (Fig. 18-12). Dose may be repeated every 5 to 10 minutes until recovery or help (EMS) arrives on the scene to take over management.
4. Activate EMS (9-1-1). If alone with victim, it is important to administer epinephrine *before* activating EMS.
5. On recovery (bronchospasm resolves), administer histamine blocker to minimize risk of relapse (50 mg IM diphenhydramine [25 mg if <30 kg] or 10 mg IM chlorpheniramine [5 mg if <30 kg]).
6. EMS will evaluate the patient's status and will determine whether transport to the hospital emergency department for observation or additional treatment is warranted.

Laryngeal Edema. Laryngeal edema may be present when movement of air through the patient's nose and mouth cannot be heard or felt in the presence of spontaneous respiratory movements, or when it is impossible to carry out artificial ventilation in the presence of a patent airway (tongue not causing obstruction). Partial obstruction of the larynx produces stridor (a characteristic high-pitched crowing sound), in contrast to the wheezing associated with bronchospasm. A partial obstruction may gradually or rapidly progress to total obstruction accompanied by the ominous "sound" of silence (in the presence of spontaneous respiratory movements). The patient rapidly loses consciousness from lack of oxygen.

P→A→B→C. Position the unconscious patient supine. A, B, and C are assessed. If airway is maintained and the victim's chest is making spontaneous respiratory movements but no air is being exchanged, immediate and aggressive treatment is mandatory to save the victim's life.

D (definitive care):

1. Epinephrine. Administer 0.3 mg (if >30 kg) (0.15 mg if <30 kg) epinephrine IM in the vastus lateralis muscle. Epinephrine may be administered every 5 to 10 minutes as needed until recovery, or until help (9-1-1) arrives on the scene to take over management.
2. Following administration of epinephrine, activate EMS. Summon emergency medical assistance and administer oxygen.
3. Maintain the airway. If only partially obstructed, epinephrine may halt the progress of the edema through its vasoconstrictive actions.
4. Additional drug management: histamine blocker IM or IV (50 mg diphenhydramine or 10 mg chlorpheniramine), corticosteroid IM or IV (100 mg hydrocortisone sodium succinate to inhibit and decrease edema and capillary dilation).
5. Perform cricothyrotomy. If the preceding steps have failed to secure a patent airway, an emergency procedure to create an airway is critical for survival. Figures 18-13 and 18-14 both illustrate the anatomy of the region and the technique. Once established, the airway must be maintained, oxygen administered, and artificial ventilation used as needed. Monitor the patient's vital signs. The patient definitely will require hospitalization following transfer from the dental office by paramedical personnel.

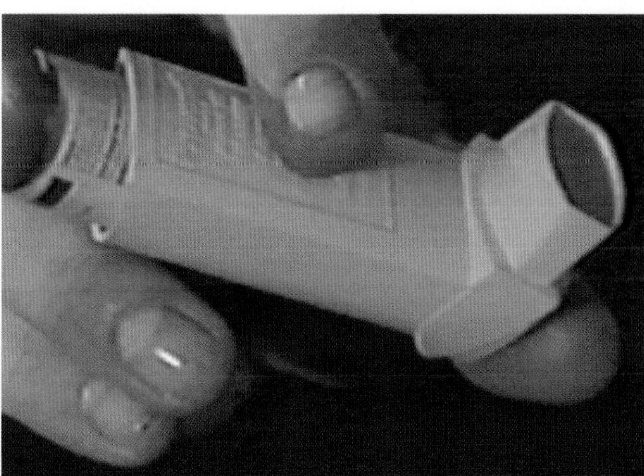

Figure 18-12. Bronchodilator inhaler (albuterol).

Generalized Anaphylaxis. Generalized anaphylaxis is highly unlikely to develop in response to local anesthetic administration. Its management is included here, however, for completeness. The most common causes of death from anaphylaxis are parenterally administered penicillin and stinging insects (the Hymenoptera: wasps, hornets, yellow jackets, and bees).

Signs of Allergy Present. When signs and symptoms of allergy (e.g., urticaria, erythema, pruritus, wheezing) are present, they should signal an immediate diagnosis of allergy. The patient usually is unconscious.

P→A→B→C. Position the unconscious patient supine. A, B, and C are assessed and performed as indicated (Fig. 18-15). If conscious, position the patient comfortably.

D (definitive care):

1. Administer epinephrine. The doctor should have previously called for the office emergency team. Epinephrine from the emergency kit (0.3 mL of 1 : 1000 for >30 kg, 0.15 mL for <30 kg, and 0.075 mL for <15 kg) is administered IM as quickly as possible, or IV (but only if available in a 1 : 10,000 solution). Because of the immediate need for epinephrine in this situation, a preloaded syringe of epinephrine is recommended for the emergency kit (Fig. 18-16). Epinephrine is the only injectable drug the author recommends that should be kept in a preloaded delivery system so as to prevent confusion when looking for it in this near-panic situation.

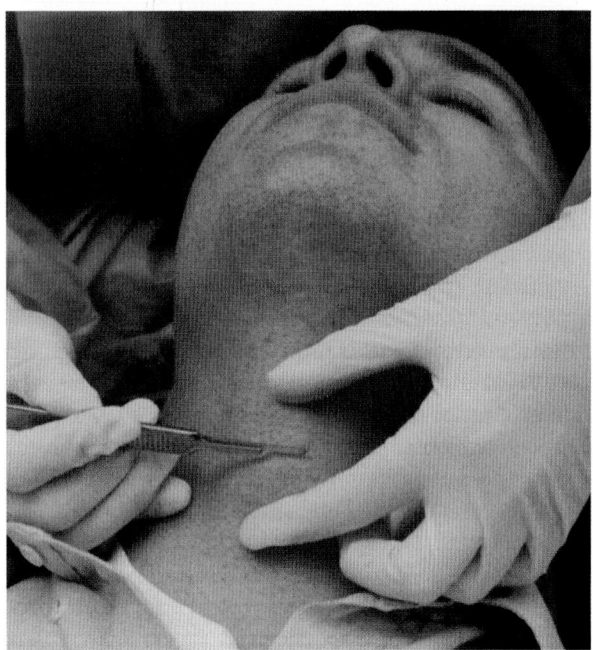

Figure 18-13. With fingers placed on the thyroid and cricoid cartilages, a horizontal incision is made through the cricothyroid membrane to gain access to the trachea.

2. Summon medical assistance (9-1-1). As soon as a severe allergic reaction is considered a possibility, emergency medical care should be summoned. If alone with the victim, it is important to administer the epinephrine first, then activate EMS.
3. Should the clinical picture fail to improve or continue to deteriorate (increased severity of symptoms) within 5 to 10 minutes of the initial epinephrine dose, a second dose is administered. Subsequent doses may be administered as needed every 5 to 10 minutes. *There is no absolute contraindication to epinephrine administration in anaphylaxis.*[88]
4. Administer oxygen.
5. Monitor vital signs. The patient's cardiovascular and respiratory status must be monitored continuously. Blood pressure and heart rate (at the carotid artery) should be recorded at least every 5 minutes, with chest compression started if no palpable pulse (cardiac arrest) is detected.
   During this acute, life-threatening phase of what is obviously an anaphylactic reaction, management consists of epinephrine administration (q5-10min), basic life support (as needed), administration of oxygen, and continual monitoring (and recording) of vital signs. Until improvement in the patient's clinical status is noted, no additional drug therapy is indicated.
6. Additional drug therapy. Additional drug therapy may be started once clinical improvement (increased blood pressure, decreased bronchospasm) is noted. This includes administration of a histamine blocker and a corticosteroid (both drugs IM or, if available, IV). They function to prevent a recurrence of signs and symptoms, obviating the need for continued

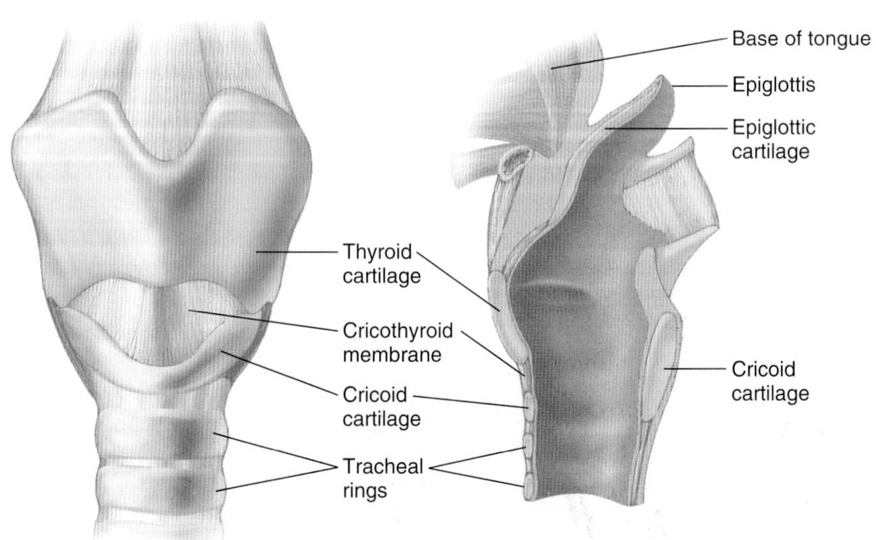

Figure 18-14. Anatomy of the cricothyrotomy site.

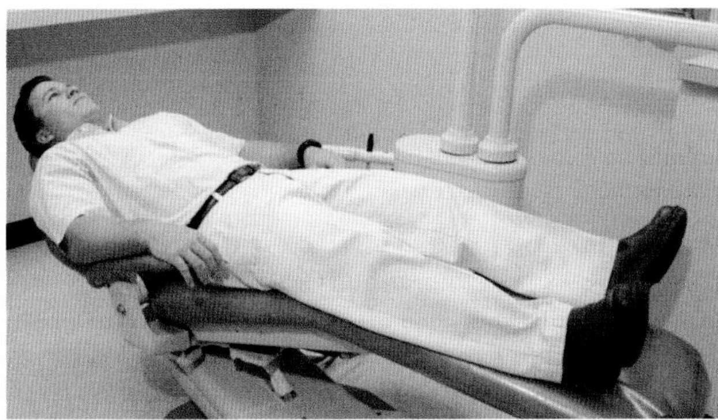

Figure 18-15. Positioning for basic life support.

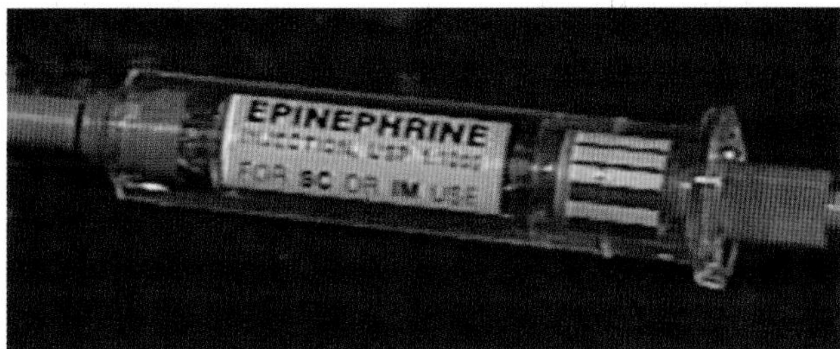

Figure 18-16. Syringe preloaded with 1 : 1000 epinephrine.

administration of epinephrine. They are not administered during the acute phase of the reaction because they are too slow in onset and they do not do enough immediate good to justify their use at this time. Epinephrine and oxygen are the only drugs that should be administered during the acute phase of the anaphylactic reaction.

No Signs of Allergy Present. If a patient receiving a local anesthetic injection loses consciousness and no signs of allergy are present, the differential diagnosis includes psychogenic reaction (vasodepressor syncope), cardiac arrest, overdose reaction, and allergic reaction involving only the cardiovascular system, among other possibilities.

P→A→B→C. Position the unconscious patient supine (see Fig. 18-15).

1. Terminate treatment, if started.
2. Position the patient. Management of this situation, which might prove to result from any of a number of causes (see earlier), requires immediate placement of the patient in the supine position with the legs elevated slightly. Low blood pressure (in the brain) is, far and away, the leading cause of unconsciousness in humans, and the supine position (with feet elevated) increases blood flow to the brain.
3. Provide basic life support, as indicated (Fig. 18-17). A, B, and C are assessed and performed as indicated. Victims of vasodepressor syncope or postural hypotension rapidly recover consciousness once properly positioned with a patent airway maintained. Patients who do not recover at this juncture should continue to have the elements of basic life support applied (breathing, circulation) as needed.

D (definitive care):

1. Summon EMS. If consciousness does not return rapidly after institution of the steps of basic life support, EMS should be sought immediately.
2. Administer oxygen.
3. Monitor vital signs. Blood pressure, heart rate and rhythm, and respirations should be monitored and recorded, at least every 5 minutes, with the elements of basic life support started at any time necessary.
4. Provide additional management. On arrival, emergency medical personnel will seek to make a diagnosis of the cause of the loss of consciousness. If this is possible, appropriate drug therapy will be instituted and the patient stabilized and then transferred to a local hospital emergency department.

In the absence of definitive signs and symptoms of allergy, such as edema, urticaria, or bronchospasm, epinephrine and other allergy drug therapy (e.g., histamine blockers, corticosteroids) are not indicated. Any of a number of other situations may be the cause of the unconsciousness, for example, drug overdose, hypoglycemia, cerebrovascular accident, acute adrenal insufficiency, or cardiopulmonary arrest. Continued basic life support until medical assistance arrives is the most prudent course of action in this situation.

SUMMARY

Systemic complications associated with local anesthetic drug administration and techniques are frequently preventable. Following is a summary of those procedures recommended to minimize their occurrence:

1. Preliminary medical evaluation should be completed before administration of any local anesthetic.
2. Anxiety, fear, and apprehension should be recognized and managed before administration of a local anesthetic.
3. All dental injections should be administered with the patient supine or semi-supine. Patients should not receive local anesthetic injections in the upright position unless special conditions (e.g., severe cardiorespiratory disease) dictate.
4. Topical anesthetic should be applied before all injections for a minimum of 1 minute.
5. The weakest effective concentration of local anesthetic solution should be injected at the minimum volume compatible with successful pain control.
6. The anesthetic solution selected should be appropriate for the dental treatment contemplated (duration of action).
7. Vasoconstrictors should be included in all local anesthetics unless specifically contraindicated by the desired duration of action (e.g., short duration procedure) or the patient's physical status (e.g., ASA 4 as a result of cardiovascular disease).

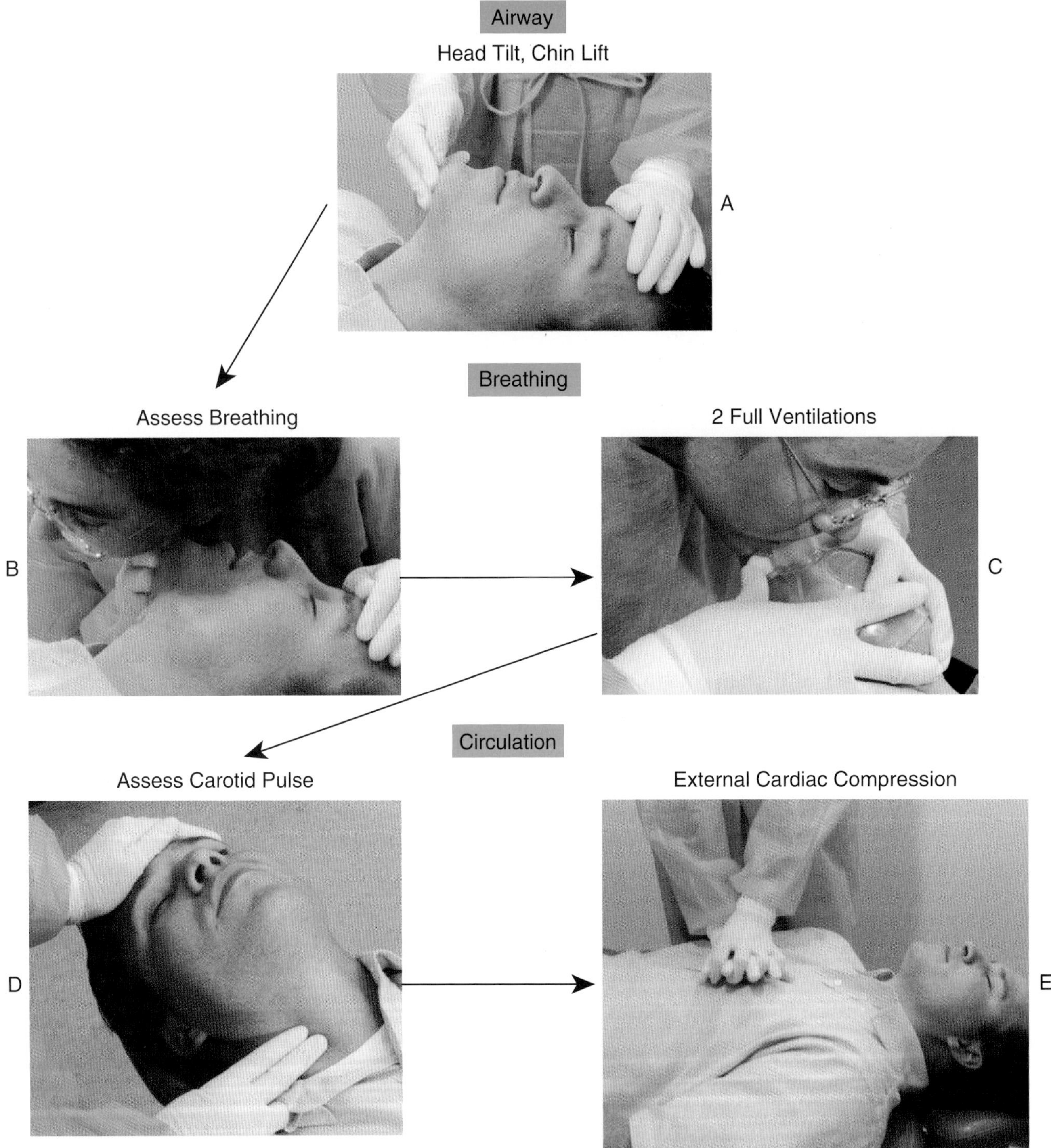

Figure 18-17. Summary of basic life support. **A,** Airway—head tilt, chin lift. **B,** Assess breathing. **C,** Two full ventilations. **D,** Assess carotid pulse. **E,** External chest compression—15 compressions: 2 ventilations.

8. Needles should be disposable, sharp, rigid, capable of reliable aspiration, and of adequate length for the contemplated injection techniques.
9. Aspirating syringes must always be used for all injections.
10. Aspiration should be carried out in at least two planes before injection.
11. Injection should be made slowly, over a minimum of 60 seconds if 1.8 mL of local anesthetic is deposited.
12. Observe the patient both during and after local anesthetic administration for signs and symptoms of undesirable reaction. Never give an injection and leave the patient alone while doing other procedures.

References

1. Pallasch TJ: Pharmacology for dental students and practitioners, Philadelphia, 1980, Lea & Febiger.
2. Speca SJ, Boynes SG, Cuddy MA: Allergic reactions to local anesthetic formulations, Dent Clin North Am 54:655–664, 2010.
3. Finder RL, Moore PA: Adverse drug reactions to local anesthesia, Dent Clin North Am 46:747–757, 2002.
4. Vinckier F: Local anesthesia in children, Rev Belge Medec Dent 55:61–71, 2000.
5. Malamed SF: Morbidity, mortality and local anesthesia, Prim Dent Care 6:11–15, 1999.
6. Meechan J: How to avoid local anaesthetic toxicity, Br Dent J 184:334–335, 1998.
7. Meechan J, Rood JP: Adverse effects of dental local anaesthesia, Dent Update 24:315–318, 1997.
8. Davis MJ, Vogel LD: Local anesthetic safety in pediatric patients, N Y State Dent J 62:32–35, 1996.
9. Prince BS, Goetz CM, Rihn TL, et al: Drug-related emergency department visits and hospital admissions, Am J Hosp Pharm 49:1696–1700, 1992.
10. Kishikawa K, Namiki A, Miyashita K, et al: Effects of famotidine and cimetidine on plasma levels of epidurally administered lignocaine, Anaesthesia 45:719–721, 1990.
11. Shibasaki S, Kawamata Y, Ueno F, et al: Effects of cimetidine on lidocaine distribution in rats, J Pharmacobiodynam 11:785–793, 1988.
12. Dailey PA, Hughes SC, Rosen MA, et al: Effect of cimetidine and ranitidine on lidocaine concentrations during epidural anesthesia for cesarean section, Anesthesiology 69:1013–1017, 1988.
13. de Jong RH: Bupivacaine preserves newborns' muscle tone, JAMA 237:53–54, 1977.
14. Steen PA, Michenfelder JD: Neurotoxicity of anesthetics, Anesthesiology 50:437–453, 1979.
15. Hazma J: Effect of epidural anesthesia on the fetus and the neonate, Cah Anesthesiol 42:265–273, 1994.
16. Shammas FV, Dickstein K: Clinical pharmacokinetics in heart failure: an updated review, Clin Pharmacokinet 15:94–113, 1988.
17. Hammermeister KE: Adverse hemodynamic effects of antiarrhythmic drugs in congestive heart failure, Circulation 81:1151–1153, 1990.
18. Pedersen NA, Jensen FS: Clinical importance of plasma cholinesterase for the anesthetist, Ann Acad Med Singapore 23(Suppl 6):120–124, 1994.
19. Barcelos KC, Furtado DP, Ramacciato JC, et al: Effect of PaCO2 and PaO2 on lidocaine and articaine toxicity, Anesth Prog 57:104–108, 2010.
20. Malagodi MH, Munson ES, Embro MJ: Relation of etidocaine and bupivacaine toxicity to rate of infusion in rhesus monkeys, Br J Anaesth 49:121–125, 1977.
21. Hersh EV, Helpin ML, Evans OB: Local anesthetic mortality: report of a case, ASDC J Dent Child 58:489–491, 1991.
22. Moore PA: Preventing local anesthetic toxicity, J Am Dent Assoc 123:60–64, 1992.
23. Yagiela JA: Local anesthetics. In Dionne RA, Phero JC, Becker DE, editors: Management of pain and anxiety in the dental office, ed 2, Philadelphia, 2002, WB Saunders.
24. Kaplan EL, editor: Cardiovascular disease in dental practice, Dallas, Tex, 1986, American Heart Association.
25. Adriani J, Campbell D: Fatalities following topical application of local anesthetics to mucous membrane, J Am Med Assoc 162:1527, 1956.
26. Wilburn-Goo D, Lloyd LM: When patients become cyanotic: acquired methemoglobinemia, J Am Dent Assoc 130:826–831, 1999.
27. Moos DD, Cuddeford JD: Methemoglobinemia and benzocaine, Gastroenterol Nurs 30:342–345, 2007.
28. Trapp L, Will J: Acquired methemoglobinemia revisited, Dent Clin North Am 54:665–675, 2010.
29. Smith M, Wolfram W, Rose R: Toxicity: seizures in an infant caused by (or related to) oral viscous lidocaine use, J Emerg Med 10:587–590, 1992.
30. Hess GP, Walson PD: Seizures secondary to oral viscous lidocaine, Ann Emerg Med 17:725–727, 1988.
31. Garrettson LK, McGee EB: Rapid onset of seizures following aspiration of viscous lidocaine, J Pediatr 30:413–422, 1992.
32. Rothstein P, Dornbusch J, Shaywitz BA: Prolonged seizures associated with the use of viscous lidocaine, J Pediatr 101:461–463, 1982.
33. Bartlett SZ: Clinical observations on the effects of injections of local anesthetics preceded by aspiration, Oral Surg Oral Med Oral Pathol 33:520, 1972.
34. Aldrete JA, Narang R, Sada T, et al: Reverse carotid blood flow: a possible explanation for some reactions to local anesthetics, J Am Dent Assoc 94:1142–1145, 1977.
35. Malamed SF: Allergic and toxic reactions to local anesthetics, Dent Today 22:114-121, 2003.
36. Tavares M, Goodson JM, Studen-Pavlovich D, et al, Local Anesthesia Reversal Group: Reversal of soft tissue anesthesia with phentolamine mesylate in pediatric patients, J Am Dent Assoc 139:1095–1104, 2008.
37. Moore PA, Hersh EV, Papas AS, et al: Pharmacokinetics of lidocaine with epinephrine following local anesthesia reversal with phentolamine mesylate, Anesth Prog 55:40–48, 2008.
38. Cheatham BD, Primosch RE, Courts FJ: A survey of local anesthetic usage in pediatric patients by Florida dentists, J Dent Child 59:401–407, 1992.
39. Malamed SF: Report of a case, unpublished data, 2002.
40. Munson ES, Tucker WK, Ausinsch B, et al: Etidocaine, bupivacaine, and lidocaine seizure thresholds in monkeys, Anesthesiology 42:471–478, 1975.
41. Rey E, Radvanyi-Bouvet MF, Bodiou C, et al: Intravenous lidocaine in the treatment of convulsions in the neonatal period: monitoring plasma levels, Ther Drug Monit 12:316–320, 1990.
42. Aggarwal P, Wali JP: Lidocaine in refractory status epilepticus: a forgotten drug in the emergency department, Am J Emerg Med 11:243–244, 1993.
43. Pascual J, Ciudad J, Berciano J: Role of lidocaine (lignocaine) in managing status epilepticus, J Neurol Neurosurg Psychiatr 55:49–51, 1992.
44. Jaffe AS: The use of antiarrhythmics in advanced cardiac life support, Ann Emerg Med 22:307–316, 1993.
45. Bruelle P, de La Coussaye JE, Eledjam JJ: Convulsions and cardiac arrest after epidural anesthesia: prevention and treatment, Cah Anesthesiol 42:241–246, 1994.
46. de La Coussaye JE, Eledjam JJ, Brugada J, et al: Cardiotoxicity of local anesthetics, Cah Anesthesiol 41:589–598, 1993.
47. Bachmann MB, Biscoping J, Schurg R, et al: Pharmacokinetics and pharmacodynamics of local anesthetics, Anaesthesiol Reanim 16:359–373, 1991.

48. Ryan CA, Robertson M, Coe JY: Seizures due to lidocaine toxicity in a child during cardiac catheterization, Pediatr Cardiol 14:116–118, 1993.
49. Rivera R, Segnini M, Baltodano A, et al: Midazolam in the treatment of status epilepticus in children, Crit Care Med 21:991–994, 1993.
50. Bertz RJ, Howrie DL: Diazepam by continuous intravenous infusion for status epilepticus in anticonvulsant hypersensitivity syndrome, Ann Pharmacother 27:298–301, 1993.
51. Lahat E, Aladjem M, Eshel G, et al: Midazolam in treatment of epileptic seizures, Pediatr Neurol 8:215–216, 1992.
52. Wroblewski BA, Joseph AB: Intramuscular midazolam for treatment of acute seizures or behavioral episodes in patients with brain injuries, J Neurol Neurosurg Psychiatr 55:328–329, 1992.
53. Hanley DF Jr, Pozo M: Treatment of status epilepticus with midazolam in the critical care setting, Int J Clin Pract 54:30–35, 2000.
54. Feldman HS, Arthur GR, Pitkanen M, et al: Treatment of acute systemic toxicity after the rapid intravenous injection of ropivacaine and bupivacaine in the conscious dog, Anaesth Analg 73:373–384, 1991.
55. Daublander M: The role of the vasoconstrictor. Paper presented at: 3M ESPE Expert Conference, Munich, Germany, April 2011.
56. Kellam SA, Smith JR, Scheffel SJ: Epinephrine absorption from commercial gingival retraction cords in clinical patients, J Prosthet Dent 68:761–765, 1992.
57. ADA/PDR: Ada guide to dental therapeutics, ed 5, Chicago, 2009, The American Dental Association.
58. Gomes ER, Demoly P: Epidemiology of hypersensitivity drug reactions, Curr Opin Allergy Clin Immunol 5:309–316, 2005.
59. Brown DT, Beamish D, Wildsmith JA: Allergic reaction to an amide local anaesthetic, Br J Anaesth 53:435–437, 1981.
60. Aldrete JA, O'Higgins JW: Evaluation of patients with history of allergy to local anesthetic drugs, South Med J 64:1118–1121, 1971.
61. Boren E, Teuber SS, Nguwa SM, et al: A critical review of local anesthetic sensitivity, Clin Rev Allergy Immunol 32:119–128, 2007.
62. Jackson D, Chen AH, Bennett CR: Identifying true lidocaine allergy, J Am Dent Assoc 125:1362–1366, 1994.
63. Doyle KA, Goepferd SJ: An allergy to local anesthetics? The consequences of a misdiagnosis, ASDC J Dent Child 56:103–106, 1989.
64. Thyssen JP, Menne T, Elberling J, et al: Hypersensitivity to local anaesthetics—update and proposal of evaluation algorithm, Contact Dermatitis 59:69–78, 2008.
65. Harboe T, Guttormsen AB, Aarebrot S, et al: Suspected allergy to local anaesthetics: follow-up in 135 cases, Acta Anaesthesiol Scand 54:536–542, 2010.
66. Haas DA: An update on local anesthetics in dentistry, J Can Dent Assoc 68:546–551, 2002.
67. Schwartz HJ, Sher TH: Bisulfite sensitivity manifesting as allergy to local dental anesthesia, J Allergy Clin Immunol 75:525–527, 1985.
68. Seng GF, Gay BJ: Dangers of sulfites in dental local anesthetic solutions: warnings and recommendations, J Am Dent Assoc 113:769–770, 1986.
69. Perusse R, Goulet JP, Turcotte JY: Sulfites, asthma and vasoconstrictors, Can Dent Assoc J 55:55–56, 1989.
70. Shojaie AR, Haas DA: Local anesthetic cartridges and latex allergy: a literature review, J Can Dent Assoc 68:622–626, 2002.
71. Perusse R, Goulet JP, Turcotte JY: Contraindications to vasoconstrictors in dentistry. Part II. Hyperthyroidism, diabetes, sulfite sensitivity, cortico-dependent asthma, and pheochromocytoma, Oral Surg Oral Med Oral Pathol 74:687–691, 1992.
72. Bruze M, Gruvberger B, Thulin I: PABA, benzocaine, and other PABA esters in sunscreens and after-sun products, Photodermatol Photoimmunol Photomed 7:106–108, 1990.
73. Boyce JA, Assa'ad A, Burks AW, et al: Guidelines for the diagnosis and management of food allergy in the United States: report of the NIAID-Sponsored Expert Panel, J Allergy Clin Immunol 126(Suppl 6):S1–S58, 2010.
74. Malamed SF: Medical emergencies in the dental office, ed 6, St Louis, 2007, Mosby.
75. Peter R: Sudden unconsciousness during local anesthesia, Anesth Pain Control Dent 2:140–142, 1993.
76. Chandler MJ, Grammer LC, Patterson R: Provocative challenge with local anesthetics in patients with a prior history of reaction, J Allergy Clin Immunol 79:883–886, 1987.
77. Orr DL II: It's not Novocain, it's not an allergy, and it's not an emergency! Nev Dent Assoc J 11:3–6, 2009.
78. Riedenburg MM, Lowenthal DT: Adverse nondrug reaction, N Engl J Med 279:678–679, 1968.
79. Hodgson TA, Shirlaw PJ, Challacombe SJ: Skin testing after anaphylactoid reactions to dental local anesthetics: a comparison with controls, Oral Surg Oral Med Oral Pathol 75:706–711, 1993.
80. Rozicka T, Gerstmeier M, Przybilla B, et al: Allergy to local anesthetics: comparison of patch test with prick and intradermal test results, J Am Acad Dermatol 16:1202–1208, 1987.
81. Eggleston ST, Lush LW: Understanding allergic reactions to local anesthetics, Ann Pharmacother 30:851–857, 1996.
82. Canfield DW, Gage TW: A guideline to local anesthetic allergy testing, Anesth Prog 34:157–163, 1987.
83. Swanson JG: An answer for a questionable allergy to local anesthetics, Ann Emerg Med 17:554, 1988.
84. Malamed SF: The use of diphenhydramine HCl as a local anesthetic in dentistry, Anesth Prog 20:76–82, 1973.
85. Ernst AA, Anand P, Nick T, et al: Lidocaine versus diphenhydramine for anesthesia in the repair of minor lacerations, J Trauma 34:354–357, 1993.
86. Uckan S, Guler N, Sumer M, et al: Local anesthetic efficacy for oral surgery: comparison of diphenhydramine and prilocaine, Oral Surg Oral Med Oral Pathol Oral Radiol Endod 86:26–30,1998.
87. Willett J, Reader A, Drum M, et al: The anesthetic efficacy of diphenhydramine and the combination diphenhydramine/lidocaine for the inferior alveolar nerve block, J Endod 34:1446–1450, 2008.
88. Lieberman P, Kemp SF, Oppenheimer J, et al. The Diagnosis and Management of Anaphylaxis: An Updated Practice Parameter, Allerg Clin Immunol 115(3):S483-S523, 2005
89. Oh VM: Treatment of allergic adverse drug reactions, Singapore Med J 30:290–293, 1989.
90. Adkinson NF Jr, Busse WW, Bochner BS, et al: Middleton's allergy: principles and practice, ed 7, St Louis, 2009, Mosby.
91. Stafford CT: Life-threatening allergic reactions: anticipating and preparing are the best defenses, Postgrad Med 86:235–242, 245, 1989.

CHAPTER 19

Legal Considerations

There exist several legal theories by means of which plaintiffs may proceed against defendant health professionals.

For instance, contract law has provided a basis for suits in which a health professional is accused of guaranteeing a result related to treatment such as promising that administration of local anesthesia and any subsequent procedure will be pain free. When the result does not meet the plaintiff's personal satisfaction, remedy may be sought in court. Because the contract in this example was based on the patient's subjective opinion, the defendant doctor must prove that the patient never felt pain—an extremely difficult assignment. Plaintiff suits based in contract law against health providers are relatively rare.

Recent history has seen a disturbing and dramatic increase in the number of suits filed under criminal law theories by government prosecutors in areas such as alleged fraudulent activity on the part of the health care provider and for plaintiff morbidity or mortality. Historically, prosecutors criminally attacking health providers must be able to prove that a criminal mind *(mens rea)* exists and that society has been injured. The current trend is to rewrite the law to not require proof of mens rea (such as in the Patient Protection and Affordable Care Act or "Obamacare") to negate any real analyses of intent. This change bodes ill for health professionals and others in that they now have the burden of proof that requires defendants to prove their innocence, rather than requiring prosecutors to prove guilt. This singularly significant change in criminal law is exacerbated by the fact that the forum for such controversies may be a regulatory agency, rather than a courtroom with its attendant Constitutional safeguards.

However, the legal theory covering most health professional lawsuit activity is that of the tort. A *tort* is a private civil wrong not dependent on a contract. The tort may or may not lead to further prosecution under criminal or other legal theories, such as trespass to the person. Classically, a viable suit in tort requires perfection of four essential elements: duty, a breach of that specific duty, proximate cause leading to damage, and damage related to the specific breach of duty. A health professional may successfully defend a suit in tort by proving that no duty existed, that no breach of duty occurred, that the health professional's conduct was not the cause of damage, or that no damage exists. In addition, the elements must be logically linked. For instance, if a doctor negligently administers a drug that the patient is historically allergic to and the patient contemporaneously develops agoraphobia, the doctor would not be liable for the agoraphobia.

DUTY

Briefly, the health professional owes a duty to the patient if the health professional's conduct created a foreseeable risk to the patient. Generally, a duty is created when a patient and a health professional personally interact for health care purposes. Face-to-face interaction at the practitioner's place of practice most likely would fulfill the requirement of a created duty; interaction over the telephone, Internet, etc., may not be as clear-cut regarding establishment of duty.

Breach of Duty

A *breach of duty* occurs when the health care professional fails to act as a reasonable health care provider, and this in medical or dental malpractice cases is proved to the jury by comparison of the defendant's conduct with the reasonable conduct of a similarly situated health professional. Testimony for this aspect of a suit for malpractice is developed by expert witnesses. Exceptions to the rule requiring experts are cases in which damage results after no consent was given or obtained for an elective procedure, and cases in which the defendant's conduct is obviously erroneous and speaks for itself *(res ipsa loquitur)*, such as wrong-sided surgery. In addition, some complications are defined as malpractice per se by statute, such as unintentionally leaving a foreign body in a patient after a procedure.

STANDARD OF CARE

Experts testifying as to alleged breach of duty are arguing about *standard of care* issues. It is often mistakenly assumed that the standard of the practitioner's community is the one by which he will be judged. Today, the community standard is the national standard. If specialists are reasonably accessible to the patient, the standard will be the national standard for specialists, whether or not the practitioner is a specialist. The standard of care may also be illustrated by the professional literature. Health care professionals are expected to be aware of current issues in the literature, such as previously unreported complications with local anesthetics. Often articles will proffer preventative suggestions and will review treatment options.

Simply because an accepted writing recommends conduct other than that which the health care provider used is not necessarily indicative of a breach of duty. For instance, specific drug use other than that recommended by the generic *Physicians' Desk Reference* (PDR) is commonplace and legally acceptable as long as the health care provider can articulate a reasonable purpose for his conduct. Part of this reasoning may likely include a benefit/risk analysis of various treatment options for a specific patient.

In addition, there is no single standard of care treatment plan for a given situation. Several viable treatment plans may exist and all may be within the standard of care, such as the option of choosing different local anesthetic formulations for a procedure.

Finally, ultimately, the standard of care may be determined by the jury itself after it weighs expert opinion, the professional literature, opinions of professional societies or boards, and so forth.

PROXIMATE CAUSE

Proximate cause is the summation of actual cause and legal cause. Actual cause exists if a chain of events factually flows from the defendant's conduct to the plaintiff's injury. Legal cause is present if actual cause exists, and if the plaintiff's attorney can prove that the harm sustained was foreseeable or was not highly extraordinary in hindsight.

DAMAGE

Damage is the element of the cause of action that usually is most easy to identify because it is most often manifested physically. Simply because damage is present does not mean that malpractice has been committed, but damage must be present to fulfill all elements of the tort.

The nation has seen a dramatic rise not only in tort-based malpractice lawsuits over the past several years, but also in regulatory activity (Obamacare alone will result in the creation of at least 159 new regulatory agencies), both or which result in the predictable sequelae of increased costs and decreased access to doctors for patients. Trauma centers have closed, doctors are actively and passively (i.e., by limiting their practice or opting for early retirement) leaving lawsuit-friendly communities or states, and patient consumers now are starting to feel directly the loss of health professional availability and other consequences of a litigation system that has never been busier.

The administration of local anesthesia is a procedure that is not immune to the liability crisis. Although extremely safe, given estimates that more than 300,000,000 dental local anesthetic administration procedures are performed annually in the United States, at times the administration of local anesthesia will result in unintended damage to the patient. If the elements of duty, breach of duty, and proximate cause accompany that damage, malpractice may have been committed. However, complications most often occur with no fault on the part of the local anesthetic administrator. In these situations, most complications are still foreseeable, and because they are predictable, the reasonable practitioner needs to be aware of optimal immediate and long-term treatment for the complications of local anesthetic administration.

The purpose of this chapter is not to describe in great detail the prevention or treatment of various local anesthetic complications, but to simply mention foreseeable complications and comment on the standard of care with regard to appropriate prevention and treatment. Obviously, some complications are common and others are rare, and frequency is an issue that would be considered in legal evaluation of a case. In any case, the health professional who is administering potent local anesthetics by definition tells the public that it can trust in that professional while in his or her care. When pretreatment questions arise, it is the health professional's duty to investigate controversial or unknown areas to minimize risk and maximize the benefits of his or her therapeutic decisions. When foreseen or unforeseen complications arise, the health professional must be able to act in a reasonable manner to address these untoward events.

Adequate legal response to a local anesthetic complication or emergency is often equivalent to adequate dental or medical response. However, when damage persists, plaintiff attorneys will argue that the dental or medical response was not an adequate legal response and will seek damages. The fact that the treatment rendered by the practitioner may be recognized by most of the profession as optimal may not convince a jury when the plaintiff can find an expert who offers an opposite opinion. However, damage alone will not prove malpractice. The tort can be successfully defended by showing no duty, no breach of duty, or no proximate cause. In many cases, no matter what the complication discussed in this chapter, these legal defenses are the same in theory and are applicable across the board, although the dental/medical responses are more specific to the specific situation.

If one is uncomfortable with any of the various situations mentioned in this chapter, further individual research in that area may be warranted.

In addition to the civil, or tort, remedies available to the plaintiff patient, a health care practitioner may have to defend conduct in other forums. Depending on the disposition of the plaintiff and his or her representative, the conduct of the health practitioner may be predictably evaluated not only civilly, but perhaps criminally, or via other governmental agencies such as licensing boards, better business bureaus, and so forth. Although theoretically, the arguments presented by competing sides in these varying forums are the same no matter what the forum, very real differences are involved. In particular, the penalties and the burden of proof are significantly different.

If the case is taken to a state agency, typically the board that issued the health professional's license, the rules of evidence are not onerous as far as admission by the plaintiff. Essentially, the regulatory agency can accept any evidence it deems relevant, including hearsay, which means the defendant may not have the right of facing an accuser. The burden of proof, which typically rests with the moving party or plaintiff, may even be arbitrarily assigned to the defendant by the agency. The reason why the rules of evidence are so liberal in state agency forums is because the issuance of an agency professional license may be deemed a privilege and not a right. The significance of proper representation and preparation if one is called before a regulatory agency cannot be understated when one considers the very real possibility of loss of a license and subsequent loss of ability to practice.

If one is summoned to a civil forum, the rules of evidence and the burden of proof are more strictly defined. Rules of evidence are subject to state and federal guidelines, although this is an area that is not black and white, and attorneys frequently are required to argue zealously for or against admission of evidence. In a civil forum, the burden of proof generally remains with the plaintiff, and the plaintiff is required to prove his or her allegations by a preponderance of evidence. Expressed mathematically, a preponderance is anything over 50%. This essentially means that anything that even slightly tips the scales in favor of the plaintiff in the jury's opinion signifies that the plaintiff has met the burden and thus may prevail.

In criminal cases, which again may be initiated for exactly the same conduct that may place the defendant in other forums, the burden of proof rests squarely with the prosecution (i.e., the state or federal government). In addition, the burden is met only by proof that is beyond a reasonable doubt, not simply a preponderance of evidence. Although the definition of *reasonable doubt* is open to argument, reasonable doubt is a more difficult standard to meet than is found in agency or civil forums.

CONSENT

The consent process is an essential part of patient treatment for health care professionals. Essentially, consent involves explaining to the patient the advantages and disadvantages of differing treatment options, including the benefits and risks of no treatment at all. Often treatment planning will result in several viable options that may be recommended by the doctor. The patient makes an informed decision as to which option is most preferable to that patient, and treatment can begin.

Consent is essential because many of the procedures that doctors perform would be considered illegal in other settings, for instance, an incision developed by a doctor during surgery versus an equivalent traumatic wound placed in a criminal battery.

Consent may be verbal or written, but when a controversy presents at a later date, a written consent is extremely beneficial (Fig. 19-1). In fact, because many times consent is required to fulfill the standard of care for a procedure, lack of written consent may reduce the fact finding to a "he said/she said" scenario. This circumstance may greatly diminish the plaintiff's burden of proving the allegations and may even shift the burden of proof to the defendant.

When the mentally challenged or children younger than the age of majority are treated, consent from a legal guardian is necessary for elective procedures. Whenever restraint is planned or anticipated, consent is warranted.

Consent obtained before one procedure is performed may not be assumed for the same procedure at a different time, or for a different procedure at the same time. In addition, consent obtained for one health care provider to treat may not be transferable to another health care provider, such as a partner doctor or an employee dental hygienist or registered nurse.

Consent is not necessary at times. When a patient is treated in an emergency setting (e.g., a spontaneously or traumatically unconscious patient), consent is implied. However, when possible, consent may be obtained from a legal guardian. The possibility of obtaining consent from a guardian before an emergency procedure is performed is time dependent. In an urgent situation, time may be available to discuss treatment options with a guardian. However, during a more emergent situation, taking time to discuss treatment options may actually compromise the patient.

Generally, emergency aid rendered in nondental or nonmedical settings does not require consent secondary to Good Samaritan statutes, which apply to "rescues." However, a source of liability even when one is being a Good Samaritan is reckless conduct. Reckless conduct in a rescue situation often involves leaving the victim in a situation that is worse than when the rescuer found the victim. An example of such conduct is seen when a rescuer offers to transport a victim to a hospital for necessary treatment and then abandons the victim farther from a hospital than where the victim was initially found.

The patient who offers to sign a waiver to convince a practitioner to provide treatment, for instance, will not likely be held to that waiver if malpractice is suspected and then is adjudicated to exist; it is a recognized principle that a patient may not consent to malpractice because such consent goes against public policy.

With regards to local anesthetic administration, is consent necessary?

Consent is required for any procedure that poses a foreseeable risk to the patient. If the administration of local anesthetic could foreseeably result in damage to the patient, consent should be considered.

INFORMED CONSENT

I hereby request that ______________________ provide treatment for me for the following condition: ____.
I have been afforded the time and opportunity to discuss this proposed treatment, the alternatives, and risks with ______________________, and I understand:

1. The means of treatment will be: ______________________
____

2. The alternative means of treatment are: ______________________
____

3. The advantages of proposed treatment over alternative treatment are:
____
____

4. That all treatments including the one proposed have some risks. The risks of importance involved in my treatment have been explained to me, and they are: ______________________
____

5. The risks of nontreatment are: ______________________
____

____
Signature of Patient

____
Date

____
Signature of Witness

____
Signature of Healthcare Practitioner

Figure 19-1. Sample informed consent form.

Further, some patients prefer to not be given any local anesthesia, even for significant operative procedures, thus rendering the administration of local anesthesia for dentistry optional and not necessarily required. It cannot be assumed that local anesthesia is automatically part of most dental procedures. If a patient is forced to have a local anesthetic without consent, technically a battery has occurred.

At times, local anesthetic administration is all that is necessary for certain diagnostic or therapeutic procedures such as differential diagnosis or treatment of atypical facial pain syndromes, thus establishing the administration of local anesthesia as both diagnostic and therapeutic in and of itself.

Finally, local anesthetic administration involves injecting or otherwise administering potent pharmaceutical agents. These agents or the means used to administer them may inadvertently damage a patient. Any health professional conduct that may reasonably be expected to predictably result in damage requires consent.

HEALTH INSURANCE PORTABILITY AND ACCOUNTABILITY ACT OF 1996

The Health Insurance Portability and Accountability Act (HIPAA) of 1996 was signed into law by former President Bill Clinton on August 21, 1996. Conclusive regulations were issued on August 17, 2000, to be instated by October 16, 2002. HIPAA requires that the transactions of all patient health care information be formatted in a standardized electronic style. In addition to protecting the privacy and security of patient information, HIPAA includes legislation on the formation of medical savings accounts, the authorization of a fraud and abuse control program, the easy transport of health insurance coverage, and the simplification of administrative terms and conditions.

HIPAA encompasses three primary areas, and its privacy requirements can be broken down into three types: privacy standards, patients' rights, and administrative requirements.

Privacy Standards

A central concern of HIPAA is the careful use and disclosure of protected health information (PHI), which generally is electronically controlled health information that is able to be distinguished individually. PHI also refers to verbal communication, although the HIPAA Privacy Rule is not intended to hinder necessary verbal communication. The U.S. Department of Health and Human Services (USDHHS) does not require restructuring, such as soundproofing, architectural changes, and so forth, but some caution is necessary when health information is exchanged by conversation.

An Acknowledgment of Receipt Notice of Privacy Practices, which allows patient information to be used or divulged for treatment, payment, or health care operations (TPO), should be procured from each patient. A detailed and time-sensitive authorization also can be issued; this allows the dentist to release information in special circumstances other than TPOs. A written consent is also an option. Dentists can disclose PHI without acknowledgment, consent, or authorization in very special situations, for example, perceived child abuse, public health supervision, fraud investigation, or law enforcement with valid permission (e.g., a warrant). When divulging PHI, a dentist must try to disclose only the minimum necessary information, to help safeguard the patient's information as much as possible.

Dental professionals must adhere to HIPAA standards because health care providers (as well as health care clearinghouses and health care plans) who convey electronically formatted health information via an outside billing service or merchant are considered covered entities. Covered entities may be dealt serious civil and criminal penalties for violation of HIPAA legislation. Failure to comply with HIPAA privacy requirements may result in civil penalties of up to \$100 per offense with an annual maximum of \$25,000 for repeated failure to comply with the same requirement. Criminal penalties resulting from illegal mishandling of private health information can range from \$50,000 and/or 1 year in prison to \$250,000 and/or 10 years in prison.

Patients' Rights

HIPAA allows patients, authorized representatives, and parents of minors, as well as minors, to become more aware of the health information privacy to which they are entitled. These rights include, but are not limited to, the right to view and copy their health information, the right to dispute alleged breaches of policies and regulations, and the right to request alternative forms of communicating with their dentist. If any health information is released for any reason other than TPO, the patient is entitled to an account of the transaction. Therefore dentists must keep accurate records of such information and provide them when necessary.

The HIPAA Privacy Rule indicates that the parents of a minor have access to their child's health information. This privilege may be overruled, for example, in cases in which child abuse is suspected, or when the parent consents to a term of confidentiality between the dentist and the minor. Parents' rights to access their child's PHI also may be restricted in situations in which a legal entity, such as a court, intervenes, and when the law does not require a parent's consent. To obtain a full list of patients' rights provided by HIPAA, a copy of the law should be acquired and well understood.

Administrative Requirements

Complying with HIPAA legislation may seem like a chore, but it does not need to be so. It is recommended that health care professionals become appropriately familiar with the law, organize the requirements into simpler tasks, begin compliance early, and document their progress in compliance. An important first step is to evaluate current information and practices of the dental office.

Dentists should write a privacy policy for their office—a document for their patients that details the office's practices concerning PHI. The American Dental Association (ADA) HIPAA Privacy Kit includes forms that the dentist can use to customize his or her privacy policy. It is useful to try to understand the role of health care information for patients and the ways in which they deal with this information while visiting the dental office. Staff should be trained and familiar with the terms of HIPAA and the office's privacy policy and related forms. HIPAA requires a designated privacy officer—a person in the practice who is responsible for applying the new policies in the office, fielding complaints, and making choices involving the minimum necessary requirements. Another person in the role of contact person will process complaints.

A *Notice of Privacy Practices*—a document that details the patient's rights and the dental office's obligations concerning PHI—also must be drawn up. Furthermore, any role of a third party with access to PHI must be clearly documented. This third party is known as a *business associate* (BA) and is defined as any entity who, on behalf of the health care provider, takes part in any activity that involves

BUSINESS ASSOCIATE CONTRACT

This contract between the office of Dr. ______________________________
(the *entity*) and ______________________________ (the *business associate*) discloses the conditions to satisfactorily ensure compliance with the Privacy Rule of the Health Insurance Portability and Accountability Act (HIPAA).

During the contract period the business associate must observe the following responsibilities with respect to protected health information:

1. A business associate must limit requests for protected health information on behalf of the covered entity to that which is reasonably necessary to accomplish the intended purpose, a covered entity is permitted to reasonably rely on such requests from a business associate of another covered entity as the minimum necessary.

2. Make information available including information held by business associate as necessary to determine compliance by the covered entity.

3. Fulfill an individual's rights to access and amend his or her protected health information contained in a designated record set, including information held by a business associate, if appropriate, and receive an accounting of disclosures by a business associate.

4. Mitigate, to the extent practicable, any harmful effect that is known to the covered entity of an impermissible use or disclosure of protected health information by its business associate.

5. A business associate cannot use protected health information for his or her own purposes. This includes, but is not limited to, selling protected health information to third parties for the third party's own marketing activities, without authorization.

6. The covered entity is required to ensure, in whatever reasonable manner deemed effective by the covered entity, the appropriate cooperation by his or her business associate in meeting these requirements.

7. If the covered entity discovers a material breach of violation of the contract by the business associate, it will take reasonable steps to cure the breach or end the contract with the business associate. If termination is not feasible the covered entity will report the problem to the Department of Health and Human Services Office for Civil Rights.

Figure 19-2. Sample business associate contract for compliance with the privacy rule of the Health Insurance Portability and Accountability Act.

exposure of PHI. The HIPAA Privacy Kit provides a copy of the USDHHS "Business Associate Contract Terms"; this document provides a concrete format for detailing BA interactions (Fig. 19-2).

The main HIPAA privacy compliance date, including all staff training, was April 14, 2003, although many covered entities who submitted a request and a compliance plan by October 15, 2002, were granted 1-year extensions. Local branches of the ADA may be contacted for details. It is recommended that dentists prepare their offices ahead of time for all deadlines, including preparation of privacy policies and forms, business associate contracts, and employee training sessions (Fig. 19-3).

For a comprehensive discussion of all terms and requirements, a complete list of HIPAA policies and procedures, and a full collection of HIPAA privacy forms, the ADA should be contacted for an HIPAA Privacy Kit. The relevant ADA Website is www.ada.org/goto/hipaa. Other Websites that may contain useful information about HIPAA include the following:

- USDHHS Office of Civil Rights: www.hhs.gov/ocr/hipaa
- Work Group on Electronic Data Interchange: www.wedi.org/SNIP
- Phoenix Health: www.hipaadvisory.com
- USDHHS Office of the Assistant Secretary for Planning and Evaluation: http://aspe.os.dhhs.gov/admnsimp/

OFFICE STAFF TRAINING REGISTRY

I hereby certify that the following employees of the below named dental office have received the office policy regarding the Health Insurance Portability and Accountability Act (HIPAA) Privacy Rule.

Privacy Officer____________________ Date__________

Dental Office ____________________

Address____________________

____

City ____________________ State__________

I understand the office privacy policy and procedures needed to protect the private health information of patients and will access only information that is reasonably needed to carry out my duties.

Name	Date

Figure 19-3. Sample staff training registry to be signed by all employees to verify receipt of the office policy to comply with the privacy rule of the Health Insurance Portability and Accountability Act.

THIRD PARTIES

When any untoward reaction occurs, including during local anesthetic administration, the complication will be treated more ideally by a responsive team trained to handle such events, rather than by the local anesthetic administrator alone.

Along with providing additional trained hands, third parties are witnesses and can testify to events leading up to, during, and after the event in question, and may prove invaluable in describing an event such as a psychogenic patient phenomenon.

OVERDOSE

The term *local anesthesia* actually describes the desired effect of such a drug, not what actually occurs physiologically. Administration of a local anesthetic may or may not produce the desired depression of area nerve function, but it will definitely produce systemic effects. One must be prepared to articulate systemic considerations with regard to injection of these "local" agents.

Dosages of local anesthetic drugs administered to patients are most properly given and recorded in milligrams, not in milliliters, carpules, cartridges, cc's, and so forth. The most standard limiting factor in the administration of certain doses of local anesthetics to a patient is the patient's weight. Other factors that need to be considered include medical history, particularly cardiovascular disease, and previous demonstration of sensitivity to normal dosing. The presence of acute or chronic infection and concomitant administration of other oral, parenteral, or inhaled agents may alter the textbook recommendations for local anesthetic dosages. The reasonable practitioner needs to be able to readily determine the proper dosage levels to be administered to patients before the time of administration. At times, one local anesthetic formulation may be significantly more advantageous than another. The minimal amount of local anesthetic, and of vasoconstrictor contained therein if applicable, needed to achieve operative anesthesia should be used. An inability to properly dose most patients leads to provision of health care below the standard of care.

Overdose may occur without health professional error, as in a previously undiagnosed hypersensitive patient, or in a patient who gives an incomplete medical history. Intravascular injection can occur even with judicious negative aspiration through an appropriate needle and following slow injection and may result in overdose.

Generally, the initial presentation of overdose is physiologic excitement, which is followed by depression. Depending on the timing of the diagnosis of overdose, the treatment protocol will vary. Rapid accurate evaluation is very beneficial as opposed to a delayed diagnosis, and speaks favorably for the responsible health care provider. It is much more desirable to treat syncope secondary to overdose rather than cardiac arrest, which may follow inadequately treated syncope and respiratory arrest.

Adding to the diagnostic challenge is the fact that often more than one chemical is present within the local anesthetic solution that may cause overdose (e.g., lidocaine and epinephrine). The operator must be cognizant of the latency and duration of different components of the local anesthetic solution.

However, no matter the particular manifestation or whether fault is or is not included in the origin of any situation of overdose, the reasonable practitioner needs to be prepared to effectively handle the overdose. An inability to reasonably treat complications that are foreseeable, such as overdose, is a breach of duty.

If an overdose occurs, results can range from no damage whatsoever to death, and often depend on the preparedness of the health practitioner for this foreseeable emergency.

ALLERGY

Related to overdose, but not a dose-dependent manifestation of local anesthetic administration, allergic reactions are foreseeable, although relatively rare, particularly for severe allergic responses such as anaphylaxis.

An accurate medical history is mandatory in minimizing the occurrence of allergy. Patients, in part because doctors do not take the time to explain the difference between allergy, overdose, and sensitivity, often list any adverse drug reaction as an "allergy." Inaccurate reporting of drug-related allergy by patients is not rare. In fact, more than half of patient-reported allergies are not allergies at all, but some other reaction that may not have even been drug related.

The duty of the health professional when administering local anesthetics includes avoiding known allergenic substances, including the local anesthetic in particular and any chemical additions to the local anesthetic solution. If an allergic reaction occurs, whether fault is present or not, the health care provider must be able to treat the drug-related allergy in a reasonable manner. Reasonable treatment may be the difference between resultant transient rhinorrhea versus death.

INSTRUMENTS

Syringe

A compromised syringe may still be usable in administering a local anesthetic. But if, for instance, the syringe cannot be controlled in a normal manner (e.g., secondary to an ill-fitting thumb ring), any damage resulting from such lack of control would be foreseeable and a breach of duty. A properly prepared and functioning syringe is mandatory for safe local anesthetic administration. Factors to be aware of in evaluating a syringe include all components of the syringe from the thumb ring, to the slide assembly, to the harpoon, to the threads that engage the needle, and so forth.

Local Anesthetic Cartridge

Originally, cartridges were much different than they are now. Problems that have been identified through the years include the fact that chemicals can leach from or into the solution within the cartridge, and that the contents are subject to extremes of heat or cold or prolonged shelf life. Cartridges are now coated with a protective film, thus helping to prevent any shattered glass effect from cartridge fracture, which can occur even with normal injection pressures.

Local Anesthetic Needle

Disposable needles have been the norm for decades; although they avoid many problems formerly manifest with reusable needles, malfunction can still occur. Needle breakage can occur with or without fault from the operator. Absent intentional bending and hubbing of the needle into loose mucosa, underlying muscle, and bone, needles still occasionally break for other reasons, as when a patient grabs the operator's hand during an injection. Also, latent manufacturing defects will occasionally be noted during routine inspection of the needle before local anesthetic administration. In addition to needle barbs, the author has discarded preoperatively inspected needles with defects such as those seen in needles with patency in the needle shaft; needles that were partially or totally occluded; needles loose within the plastic hub; and needles with plastic hubs that did not effectively engage the metal threads of the syringe.

A needle-related complication is a plastic barb that is occasionally present when one separates the plastic casings of the needle preparatory to threading the needle hub onto the syringe. Such a barb may be present at the point where the heat sear secures the two casings together. Those who prepare the needle/syringe delivery system need to be aware of this barb not only when separating the casings, but also when recovering then needle after use.

Once again, broken needle instrument damage is foreseeable, as are other instrument failures. The prudent operator will be prepared to deal with this complication and will prevent further morbidity by means such as using a throat pack, not hubbing the needle, and having a prepared assistant who can pass a hemostat to the operator in a fashion that does not require the operator to take his eyes from the field. If a needle is lost in tissue, protocols have been established for retrieval of such foreign bodies, and if the operator is not comfortable with these procedures, an expeditious referral should be considered.

Contamination of the local anesthetic solution or delivery system (i.e., the needle) will likely produce complications, and thus should be assiduously avoided. It would be reasonable to expect a practitioner to be able to intelligently describe in some detail, if called upon to do so, the methods used to minimize any potential contamination. Limiting contamination has the added benefit of not compromising the health of the practitioner or any member of his team.

Any damage resulting from an unorthodox use of the syringe, needle, or cartridge may lead to open argument that a breach of the standard of care and thus breach of duty had occurred.

ALTERNATIVE DELIVERY SYSTEMS/TECHNIQUES

At times practitioners may elect to use alternative delivery systems or techniques, such as periodontal ligament, intraosseous, or extraoral injections via specialized armamentaria. The standard of care, which includes the reasoning that a practitioner will, all things considered, choose the best treatment for his or her patient, certainly includes these alternate local anesthetic delivery systems or techniques.

As with any other routine or less than routine clinical treatment plan, the practitioner should be able to intelligently articulate reasoning for the decision. This is mandatory not only if a disgruntled patient seeks legal recourse, but also for nonlitigious patients who simply want to know why they have "never seen that before."

Although promotional materials from a drug or equipment manufacturer may be helpful to the clinician in identifying advantages of new drugs or equipment, it is incumbent upon the health professional to make an independent and reasonable effort to identify potential disadvantages of new modalities.

LOCAL REACTIONS TO LOCAL ANESTHETIC ADMINISTRATION

Topical or injected local anesthetics can cause reactions ranging from erythema to tissue sloughing in local areas secondary to several factors, including multiple needle penetrations, hydraulic pressure within the tissues, or a direct tissue reaction to the local anesthetic. Topical anesthetics in particular generally are more toxic to tissues than injected solutions, and dosages must be carefully administered. For instance, the practice of letting the patient self-administer prescription strength topical at home could certainly be criticized if an adverse reaction occurs.

Local tissue reactions may be immediate or delayed by hours or days; thus it is mandatory in this situation, as it is in others, for the patient to have access to a professional familiar with such issues, even during off hours. Simply letting patients fend for themselves or advising them to go to the emergency room may not be the best option in providing optimal care.

Finally, one should be able to reasonably justify the use of topical anesthetics for intraoral injection purposes because some authors have opined that these relatively toxic agents are not objectively effective.

LIP CHEWING

Local tissue maceration secondary to lip chewing most often occurs in children status post an inferior alveolar nerve or other trigeminal nerve third division injection. Tissue maceration may also be seen in patients whose mental status has been compromised by sedatives, general anesthetics, central nervous system trauma, or during development. A prudent practitioner will advise any patient who may be prone to such an injury, and that patient's guardian, to be aware of the complication. If this complication is not prevented, it must be properly treated when diagnosed.

SUBCUTANEOUS EMPHYSEMA

Emphysema or air embolism can occur when air is introduced into tissue spaces. This complication usually is seen after incisions have been made through skin or mucosa, but it can also occur via needle tracts, particularly when gas-propelled pressure sprays, pneumatic handpieces, and so forth, are used near the needle tract. The sequelae of air embolism usually are fairly benign, although disconcerting to the patient. An unrecognized and progressive embolism can be life threatening. When a progressive embolism is diagnosed, the practitioner will not be criticized for summoning paramedics and for accompanying the patient to the hospital.

VASCULAR PENETRATION

Even with the most careful technique, excessive bleeding can occur when vessels are partially torn by needles. The fact that aspirating syringes are used reveals that placing needles into soft tissues is indeed a blind procedure. At times, the goal of an injection is intravenous or intra-arterial injection. This is not typically the case with the use of local anesthetics for pain control, and a positive aspiration necessitates that additional measures be taken for a safe injection. The prepared health professional should be able to articulate exactly what the goal of administration of a local anesthetic is, and how that is technically accomplished. For instance, why was a particular anesthetic and needle chosen? What structures might be encountered by the needle during administration of a block? In addition, what measures are taken if a structure is inadvertently compromised by a needle? Even with optimal preparation, vascular compromise can result in tumescence, ecchymosis, or overt hemorrhage that may need to be addressed. These conditions can be magnified by bleeding dyscrasia. The medical history may reveal certain prescriptions that may alter bleeding time; this may indicate the need for preoperative hematologic consultation.

NEURAL PENETRATION

Just as a rich complex of vessels is present in the head and neck area, so it is with nerves. Neural anatomy can vary considerably from the norm, and penetration of a nerve by a needle can occur on rare occasions, even in the most careful and practiced hands. Permanent changes in neural function can result from a single needle-stick; although this complication does not necessarily imply a deviation from the standard of care, the practitioner must be prepared to treat the complication as optimally as possible.

Lingual nerve injury is an event that has been zealously contested in the courts in recent years. Typically, rare instances of loss or change in lingual nerve function have occurred during mandibular third molar surgery. Plaintiff experts readily opine that but for negligence (i.e., malpractice), this injury will not occur, period. In these experts' opinions, lingual nerves are damaged only secondary to unintentional manipulation with a surgical blade, periosteal elevator, burr, and so forth, when the operator is working in an anatomic area that should have been avoided. In spite of the fact that defense experts routinely counter these plaintiff opinions, occasionally juries will rule for the plaintiff, and lingual nerve awards have exceeded $1,000,000.

Although lingual nerve injury occasionally occurs secondary to unintentional contact with surgical blades, periosteal elevators, burrs, and so forth, when an operator unintentionally directly encounters an unintended anatomic structure, it is more likely that the injury results secondary to other means. For instance, lingual nerve anatomy has been shown to be widely variant from the average position lingual to the lingual plate in the third molar area. Lingual nerve position has been shown to vary from within unattached mucosal tissue low on the lingual aspect of the lingual plate, to firmly adherent within lingual periosteum high on the lingual plate, to within soft tissues over the buccal cusps of impacted third molars.

Permanent lingual nerve injury also occurs in the absence of third molar surgery and secondary to needle penetration during inferior alveolar/lingual nerve blocks. Lingual nerve injury can result from pressure placed on the nerve during operative procedures (e.g., with lingual retractors).

A higher incidence of lingual nerve injury has been noted with certain local anesthetic solution formulations over others. The practitioner whose patient develops paresthesia after routine use of, for instance, 4% local anesthetic solution instead of 2% solution must be prepared to explain such decisions as why solutions that are twice as toxic as others and generally are equally effective may have been habitually used. Obviously, the suggestion here is that no treatment should be rote; rather, treatment should be planned on a patient-by-patient basis after a thoughtful risk/benefit analysis has been performed.

Finally, lingual nerve injury can occur when no health care professional treatment whatsoever is provided. Paresthesia can occur with mastication, and a presenting chief complaint of anesthesia can occur spontaneously. Both of these conditions may be rectified by dealing with the pathology associated with the change in function, such as by removing impacted third molars or freeing the lingual nerve from an injury-susceptible position within the periosteum.

However, no matter what the cause, the prudent operator will be prepared to address neural injury effectively when it occurs.

CHEMICAL NERVE INJURY

It is not surprising that potent chemicals such as local anesthetics occasionally will compromise nerve function to a greater degree than they are designed to do. Local anesthetics, after all, are specifically formulated in an effort to alter nerve function, albeit reversibly. Just as systemic toxicity varies from local anesthetic to local anesthetic, so limited nerve/local toxicity at times may alter nerve function in a way that is not typically seen. Deposition of local anesthetic solutions directly on a nerve trunk or too near a nerve trunk in a susceptible patient may result in long-term or permanent paresthesia. Local anesthetic toxicity generally increases as potency increases. In addition, nontargeted nerves in the head and neck may be affected by local anesthetic deposition, as when transient amaurosis occurs after maxillary or mandibular nerve block when the optic nerve is affected. One should not be particularly surprised at the various neural manifestations of these potent agents given that toxic overdose is actually a compromise of higher neural functions. Anyone who chooses to utilize agents designed to relieve pain directly on or near nerve tissue must be prepared for even the rare complications seen. Adequate treatment may range from reassuring a patient who has transient amaurosis to treating or referring for treatment a patient with permanent anesthesia resulting from an adverse chemical compromise of the nerve caused by the local anesthetic solution or other agents.

LOCAL ANESTHETIC DRUG INTERACTIONS

Use of other local or systemic agents certainly will predictably affect and alter the latency, effect, duration, and overall metabolism of local anesthetics. Modern polypharmacy only complicates the situation. However, the health care professional must be aware of specific well-known drug interactions, in addition to the pharmacology of common drug classes. Oral contraceptives, β-blockers, calcium channel blockers, angiotensin-converting enzyme (ACE) inhibitors, other cardiovascular prescriptions such as antihypertensives and anticoagulants, thyroid medications, antihistamines, antibiotics, anabolic steroids or corticosteroids, psychogenic medications, and various street drugs may be considered common to the routine dental population.

Drugs interact with various receptor sites; drug therapy is based on potentiation or inhibition of normal physiologic responses to stimuli. Ideally, with local anesthetic, no unwanted systemic reactions occur, and local nerve tissues are reversibly inhibited for a relatively brief time, after which the tissues regain full function. Concomitant use of other agents can change the usually predictable course of a local anesthetic and vice versa.

For instance, the commonly used β-blocker propranolol has been shown to create a chemically induced decrease in liver function, specifically, hepatic blood flow, which can decrease lidocaine metabolism by as much as 40%. Long-term alcohol use induces enzymes dramatically. Methemoglobinemia has been reported to result from use of topical local anesthetics and over-the-counter Anbesol©.

Therapeutic areas of special concern arise in patients who are obviously ill, who report significant medical history, who report significant drug use (whether prescribed, over-the-counter, or herbal), and who are at extremes of age. The incidence of adverse local anesthetic drug interaction increases with patients who report risk factors, particularly cardiovascular risk factors, as opposed to the general population. Before the time of treatment, clinicians should acquire the knowledge needed to optimally treat such patients with increased potential for adverse drug reactions.

PSYCHOGENIC REACTIONS

At times the practitioner may have to deal with psychogenic reactions that may be mild or can be severe. For instance, the initial manifestation of a toxic overdose, whether noted or not, is excitement. Excitement may also occur secondary to nothing other than stress resulting from a situation in which the patient is not comfortable. Excitement may be manifested, for instance, by controlled or uncontrolled agitation, disorientation, hallucination, or somnolence.

Such reactions may be potentiated by pharmaceuticals administered acutely by the health professional, or by authorized or unauthorized agents taken by the patient before an appointment. The incidence of such reactions is increased with increased utilization of pharmaceuticals, particularly those that may affect the central nervous system, such as local anesthetics. These reactions can occur in children, adolescents, adults, or the aged.

Psychogenic reactions are often frustrating to diagnose and treat. It may be difficult to determine whether the reaction is occurring secondary to an administered drug, including local anesthesia, or as the result of other causes.

Treatment may require restraint if the patient is in danger of inflicting harm upon himself or herself, as might be seen in an epileptic seizure. Fortunately, most of these reactions are short term (i.e., often lasting only moments). However, occasionally, they may occur regularly over long periods of time. Some, such as hysterical conversion manifest by unresponsiveness, may require hospitalization.

Although many practitioners may diagnose such an event, prudence requires that one be aware of the cause and treatment of such reactions. Even when psychogenic reactions are handled appropriately, patients may assume that the health care professional "did something wrong" and may seek the advice of an attorney.

Eroticism

A singularly troublesome psychogenic reaction to potent agents is observed in which the patient reacts with sexual affections that may or may not be recalled at a later time. Historically, such reactions were fairly common during administration of cocaine solutions. Generally speaking, these reactions appear to be rare and usually are of relatively short duration. However, as with other psychogenic or hysterical phenomena, rapid diagnosis and treatment is optimal.

Although concomitant use of agents such as nitrous oxide or administration of minor tranquilizers may be of general benefit during administration of local anesthesia, these and many other agents have been reported to produce erotic hallucinations or behaviors in patients so predisposed.

In the case of eroticism, the practitioner who has administered local or other agents without a neutral third party present when such reactions occur will have more difficulty exonerating conduct than the practitioner who had witnesses to the reaction. In addition, with regard to eroticism, it has historically been more optimal to have witnesses of the same sex as the patient.

Occasionally, a patient may request to speak with or be treated privately by the health practitioner. Absent unusual circumstances, such as treating a close relative, practitioners may want to consider avoidance of situations such as treating an emergency patient alone after hours, or even speaking to a patient behind closed doors.

POSTPROCEDURE EVALUATION

Any time that potent agents are utilized, an evaluation of the patient is necessary. This evaluation consists of at least a preoperative assessment, continuous examination during treatment when the drugs utilized are at peak effect, and a postoperative appraisal.

Although most adverse reactions to local anesthetics occur rapidly, delayed sequelae are possible. Just as patients who have been administered agents by intravenous, inhalation, oral, or other routes are evaluated post procedure, so too should patients who have been administered local anesthetics. Any question about a less than optimal recovery from local anesthesia should be addressed before the patient is released from direct care.

For instance, it is widely accepted that patients may drive after administration of local anesthesia for dental purposes. Occasionally, a postprocedure concern that may arise secondary to local anesthesia and/or other procedures may dictate that a patient who was not accompanied may need to obtain assistance before leaving the place of treatment. Patients whose employment requires higher than normal mental or physical performance may be cautioned about the potential effects of local anesthetic administration. As an example, U.S. Air Force and U.S. Navy pilots are restricted from flying for 24 hours status post local anesthetic administration.

Some practitioners routinely call each patient after release and several hours after treatment has been terminated to ensure that recovery is uneventful. Such calls are usually welcomed by patients as a sign that their health care provider is truly concerned about his or her welfare. Occasionally, the practitioner's call may enable one to address a developing concern or an objective complication early on.

RESPONDEAT SUPERIOR

Respondeat superior ("let the superior reply"), or vicarious liability, is the legal doctrine that holds an employer responsible for an employee's conduct during the course of employment. The common law principle that all have a duty to conduct themselves so as to not harm another thus also applies to employees assigned tasks by an employer. Respondeat superior is justified in part by the assumption that the employer has the right to direct the actions of employees. For the health professional, responsibility may be shared by clerical staff, surgical or other assistants, dental hygienists, laboratory technicians, and so forth. At times vicarious liability will be applied between employer doctors and employee doctors if the employee doctors are agents of the employer doctor within a practice.

Respondeat superior does not relieve the employee of responsibility for employee conduct; it simply enables a plaintiff to litigate against the employer.

An employer is not responsible for employee conduct that is not related to employment. What type of employee conduct is related to the job is an arguable proposition, as are most legal issues. For instance, the question of whether an employer is responsible for employee conduct outside the normal workplace is open to a case-by-case evaluation. Conduct during trips to and from the workplace may or may not be related to employment. For example, an employer probably would not be responsible for employee conduct when the employee is driving home from the place of employment. However, if the employer asked the employee to perform a task on the way home, responsibility for that employee conduct may attach. An employer generally is not responsible for statute violation or criminal conduct by employees.

An employer may not be responsible for an independent contractor. One test used to evaluate the relationship between an employer and another is to discern whether the employer has the authority to direct how a task is done, as opposed to simply requesting that a task be completed. For instance, a dentist may request that a plumber make repairs, but likely will not direct how the repairs are to be accomplished, so the plumber would likely be independent. The same dentist will request that a dental hygienist perform hygiene duties, but the dentist may choose to instruct how the duties will be performed, thus rendering the hygienist less independent.

With regard to the administration of local anesthesia, dentists and dental hygienists routinely accomplish this task. Generally speaking, and subject ultimately to state statutes, although a dental hygienist may be an independent contractor according to many elemental definitions, the dental hygienist generally is not an independent contractor with regard to the provision of health care services. This includes the administration of local anesthetics. Thus, the employee dentist may be adjudicated responsible for any negligent conduct that causes damage to a patient during the course of hygiene treatment.

With regard to the degree of supervision, one must consult the state statutes. Often verbiage such as "direct" or "indirect" supervision is used, and understanding the definitions of these or other terms is paramount for both supervising and supervised health care providers.

STATUTE VIOLATION

Violation of a state or federal statute usually leads to an assumption of negligence if statute-related damage to a patient occurs. In other words, the burden of proof now shifts to the defendant to prove that the statute violation was not such that it caused any damage claimed.

Two basic types of statutes exist: malum in se and malum prohibitum. Malum in se (bad in fact) statutes restrict behavior that in and of itself is recognized as harmful, such as driving while inebriated. Malum prohibitum (defined as bad) conduct in and of itself may not be criminal, reckless, wanton, etc., but is regulated simply to, for instance, promote social order. Driving at certain speeds is an example of a malum prohibitum statute. The difference between legally driving at 15 mph in a school zone and driving at 16 mph in a school zone is not the result of a criminal mind but is a social regulatory decision.

For instance, if one is speeding while driving, several sequelae may result when that statute violation is recognized. First, the speeder may simply be warned to stop speeding. Second, the speeder may be issued a citation and may have to appear in court, argue innocence, pay a fine if found guilty, attend traffic school, etc. Third, if the speeder's conduct causes damage to others, additional civil or criminal sanctions may apply. Fourth, the situation may be compounded civilly or criminally if multiple statute violations are present, such as speeding and driving recklessly or driving while intoxicated.

Occasionally, statute violation is commendable. For instance, a driver may swerve to the "wrong" side of the centerline to avoid a child who suddenly runs into the street from between parked cars. At times, speeding may be considered a heroic act, such as when a driver is transporting a patient to a hospital during an emergency. However, even if the speeder has felt that he is contributing to the public welfare somehow, the statute violation is still subject to review.

For health professionals, for instance, administration of local anesthetic without a current health professional license or Drug Enforcement Agency (DEA) certification is likely a violation of statute. If the type of harm sustained by the patient is the type that would have been prevented by obeying the statute, additional liability may attach to the defendant.

Conversely, an example of a beneficial statute violation occurred when a licensee did not fulfill mandatory basic CPR (cardiopulmonary resuscitation) certification, but chose to complete ACLS (advanced cardiac life support) certification instead. When admonished by the state board that a violation of statute had occurred, potentially putting the public at greater risk, the licensee pointed out to the regulatory board that ACLS certification is actually more beneficial to the public than CPR. The licensing board then changed the statute to allow CPR or ACLS certification as a requirement to maintain a license.

Generally, employers are not responsible for statute violations of employees. An exception to this guideline is seen in the health professions. When employees engage in the practice of dentistry or medicine, even without the knowledge or approval of the employer, both that employee and the employer may be held liable for damage. Employer sanctions may be magnified, such as loss of one's professional license, if an employee practices dentistry or medicine with employer knowledge.

Finally, at times some types of specific conduct are defined statutorily as malpractice per se. For instance, unintentionally leaving a foreign body in a patient after a procedure may be deemed malpractice per se. In these types of cases, theoretically simply the plaintiff's demonstration of the foreign body, via radiograph, a secondary procedure to remove the foreign body, etc., may be all that is required to establish malpractice.

IF MALPRACTICE EXISTS

Although attorneys and doctors do not always agree on when all the elements of malpractice are present, occasionally the health professional may feel that he or she has made a mistake that has damaged a patient. As can be easily and successfully argued, simply the fact that a patient has damage, even significant damage, does not fulfill all requirements of the tort of malpractice.

If, however, the practitioner determines that a duty existed, the duty was breached, and breach was the proximate cause of damage, it is likely that malpractice has occurred. In this instance, the health professional is likely ethically, if not yet legally, responsible for making the patient "whole." If the damage is minimal (e.g., transient ecchymoses), nominal recompense, perhaps even a judicious apology, may be all that is required. If, however, the damage is significant, significant recompense may be required.

Certainly, any significant damage whatsoever from malpractice requires that the health professional contact his liability carrier as soon as possible. The same holds true, even if damage is not evident, when the health care professional receives notice of patient dissatisfaction, often in the form of a request for records. The liability insurance carrier's representative will help evaluate the situation and will provide valuable insight from a significant experience pool. In all likelihood, the carrier will be more successful in negotiating a settlement to any case that is controversial as far as damages. The practitioner should be very cautious about undertaking any such negotiations without his carrier's input. Such unauthorized negotiations, or similar conduct, such as not informing the carrier about a potential complaint in a timely fashion, may even cause liability coverage to become the practitioner's sole responsibility. At times, if the practitioner and the patient still have a good working relationship, the carrier will allow the practitioner to negotiate a reasonable settlement. This course of action is advantageous in that the patient receives immediate financial aid that may be necessary for additional expenses or time off from work. In addition, the plaintiff patient will not be required to overcome the assumption that the health care provider acted reasonably and to prove malpractice, which may be very difficult.

No matter whether the damage is secondary to negligence, the practitioner must try to treat the patient optimally. It is hoped that the patient will not independently seek treatment elsewhere because this course of action may simply prolong recovery and aggravate future legal considerations. One near universal finding in filed and served malpractice actions is criticism, usually unwarranted, by a nontreating health professional. If, on the other hand, referral would be beneficial, the practitioner should facilitate that referral for the patient and not just send the patient out to fend alone. After a referral is made, continued care as needed for the patient is advisable if possible.

Once legal action has been initiated, it may be wise to refuse further treatment for the patient because the patient has now effectively expressed the opinion that the practitioner's conduct was below the level of the standard of care and has resulted in damage. It is an unfortunate circumstance when a plaintiff patient realizes that the perceived malpractice did not exist and is unable to continue care with the health professional most familiar with the intricacies of that patient's individual circumstances.

Many patients shortsightedly and unintentionally limit their health care options by pursuing malpractice actions. Most malpractice cases take years to resolve and involve great expense for both the defendant and the plaintiff. Ultimately, a vast majority of alleged malpractice claims result in adjudication in favor of the defendant doctor. No matter who prevails in a malpractice claim, for both the defendant and the plaintiff the victory is often Pyrrhic when the temporal, social, and economic costs are factored in.

CONCLUSION

The administration of local anesthetics may undergo change with time secondary to new drugs, new instrumentation, and new knowledge bases. The law is even more subject to variation, often with each session of a legislative body or secondary to a significant court case. For instance, the philosophy of detailed versus general informed consent has undergone several permutations over the years. The decision of one court in a contractual, criminal, or civil tort proceeding may be appealed by the losing party and eventually reversed by another court secondary to a new fact pattern or simply as the result of re-evaluation of the same fact pattern under different legal formulae.

However, one thing that never changes is that reasonable and responsible health care practitioners will continue to be informed as to the current standard of care and will attempt to optimize their decision making and treatment planning for patients on an individual basis after a realistic risk versus benefit analysis. The opinions printed in this chapter and in this text are meant as guidelines and may be subject to modification on an individual patient treatment basis by knowledgeable practitioners and informed patients.

Selected Bibliography

Arroliga ME, Wagner W, Bobek MB, et al: A pilot study of penicillin skin testing in patients with a history of penicillin allergy admitted to a medical ICU, Chest 118:1106–1108, 2000.

Associated Press: Jury acquits Pasadena dentist of 60 child endangering charges. March 5, 2002.

Bax NDS, Tucker GT, Lennard MS, et al: The impairment of lignocaine clearance by propranolol: major contribution from enzyme inhibition, Br J Clin Pharm 19:597–603, 1985.

Burkhart CG, Burkhart KM, Burkhart AK: The Physicians' Desk Reference should not be held as a legal standard of medical care, Arch Pediatr Adolesc Med 152:609–610, 1998.

Cohen JS: Adverse drug effects, compliance, and initial doses of antihypertensive drugs recommended by the Joint National Committee vs the Physicians' Desk Reference, Arch Intern Med 161:880–885, 2001.

Cohen JS: Dose discrepancies between the Physicians' Desk Reference and the medical literature, and their possible role in the high incidence of dose-related adverse drug events, Arch Intern Med 161:957–964, 2001.

College C, Feigal R, Wandera A, et al: Bilateral versus unilateral mandibular block anesthesia in a pediatric population, Pediatr Dent 22:453–457, 2000.

Covino BG, Vassallo HG: Local anesthetics mechanisms of action and clinical use, New York, 1976, Grune & Stratton.

Daublander M, Muller R, Lipp MD: The incidence of complications associated with local anesthesia in dentistry, Anesth Prog 44:132–141, 1997.

Dyer C: Junior doctor is cleared of manslaughter after feeding tube error, BMJ 325:414, 2003.

Evans IL, Sayers MS, Gibbons AJ, et al: Can warfarin be continued during dental extraction? Results of a randomized controlled trial, Br J Oral Maxillofac Surg 40:248–252, 2002.

Faria MA: Vandals at the gates of medicine, Macon, Ga, 1994, Hacienda Publishing.

Fischer G, Reithmuller RH: Local anesthesia in dentistry, ed 2, Philadelphia, 1914, Lea & Febiger.

Gill CJ, Orr DL: A double-blind crossover comparison of topical anesthetics, J Am Dent Assoc 98:213–214, 1979.

Gilman CS, Veser FH, Randall D: Methemoglobinemia from a topical oral anesthetic, Acad Emerg Med 4:1011–1013, 1997.

Goldenberg AS: Transient diplopia as a result of block injections: mandibular and posterior superior alveolar, N Y State Dent J 63:29–31, 1997.

Kern S: Saying I'm sorry may make you sorry, N V Dent Assoc J 12:18–19, Winter 2010–2011.

Lang MS, Waite PD: Bilateral lingual nerve injury after laryngoscopy for intubation, J Oral Maxillofac Surg 59:1497–1498, 2001.

Lee TH: By the way, doctor…My hair has been thinning out for the past decade or so, but since my doctor started me on Lipitor (atorvastatin) a few months ago for high cholesterol, I swear it's been falling out much faster. My doctor discounts the possibility, but I looked in the Physicians' Desk Reference (PDR) and alopecia is listed under "adverse reactions." What do you think? Harv Health Lett 25:8, 2000.

Lustig JP, Zusman SP: Immediate complications of local anesthetic administered to 1,007 consecutive patients, J Am Dent Assoc 130:496–499, 1999.

Lydiatt DD: Litigation and the lingual nerve, J Oral Maxillofac Surg 61:197–199, 2003.

Malamed SF: Handbook of local anesthesia, ed 4, St Louis, 1997, Mosby.

Malamed SF, Gagnon S, Leblanc D: Efficacy of articaine: a new amide local anesthetic, J Am Dent Assoc 131:635–642, 2000.

Meechan JG: Intra-oral topical anaesthetics: a review, J Dent 28:3–14, 2000.

Meechan JG, Cole B, Welbury RR: The influence of two different dental local anaesthetic solutions on the haemodynamic responses of children undergoing restorative dentistry: a randomised, single-blind, split-mouth study, Br Dent J 190:502–504, 2001.

Meyer FU: Complications of local dental anesthesia and anatomical causes, Anat Anz 181:105–106, 1999.

Moore PA: Adverse drug interactions in dental practice: interactions associated with local anesthetics, sedatives, and anxiolytics. Part IV of a series, J Am Dent Assoc 130:541–554, 1999.

Mullen WH, Anderson IB, Kim SY, et al: Incorrect overdose management advice in the Physicians' Desk Reference, Ann Emerg Med 29:255–261, 1997.

Olson WK: The litigation explosion, what happened when America unleashed the lawsuit, New York, 1991, Penguin Books.

Orr DL: Airway, airway, airway, N V Dent Assoc J 9:4–6, 2008.

Orr DL: The broken needle: report of case, J Am Dent Assoc 107:603–604, 1983.

Orr DL: Conversion part I, Pract Rev Oral Maxillofac Surg 8(7), 1994 (audiocassette).

Orr DL: Conversion part II, Pract Rev Oral Maxillofac Surg 8(8), 1994 (audiocassette).
Orr DL: Conversion phenomenon following general anesthesia, J Oral Maxillofac Surg 43:817–819, 1985.
Orr DL: Intraseptal anesthesia, Compend Cont Educ Dent 8:312, 1987.
Orr DL: Is there a duty to rescue? N V Dent Assoc J 12:14–15, 2010.
Orr DL: It's not Novocain, it's not an allergy, and it's not an emergency! N V Dent Assoc J 11:3, 2009.
Orr DL: Medical malpractice, Pract Rev Oral Maxillofac Surg 3(4), 1988 (audiocassette).
Orr DL: Paresthesia of the second division of the trigeminal nerve secondary to endodontic manipulation with N2, J Headache 27:21–22, 1987.
Orr DL: Paresthesia of the trigeminal nerve secondary to endodontic manipulation with N2, J Headache 25:334–336, 1985.
Orr DL: PDL injections, J Am Dent Assoc 114:578, 1987.
Orr DL: Pericardial and subcutaneous air after maxillary surgery, Anesth Analg 66:921, 1987.
Orr DL: A plea for collegiality, J Oral Maxillofac Surg 64:1086–1092, 2006.
Orr DL: Protection of the lingual nerve, Br J Oral Maxillofac Surg 36:158, 1998.
Orr DL: Reduction of ketamine induced emergence phenomena, J Oral Maxillofac Surg 41:1, 1983.
Orr DL: Responsibility for dental emergencies, N V Dent Assoc J 10:34, 2008.
Orr DL, Curtis W: Frequency of provision of informed consent for the administration of local anesthesia in dentistry, J Am Dent Assoc 136:1568–1571, 2005.
Orr DL, Park JH: Another eye protection option, Anesth Analg 112:739–740, 2011.
Orr TM, Orr DL: Methemoglobinemia secondary to over the counter Anbesol, OOOOE. October 2010.
Penarrocha-Diago M, Sanchis-Bielsa JM: Opthalmologic complications after intraoral local anesthesia with articaine, Oral Surg Oral Med Oral Pathol Oral Radiol Endod 90:21–24, 2009.
Pogrel MA, Schmidt BL, Sambajon V, et al: Lingual nerve damage due to inferior alveolar nerve blocks: a possible explanation, J Am Dent Assoc 134:195–199, 2003.
Pogrel MA, Thamby S: Permanent nerve involvement resulting from inferior alveolar nerve blocks, J Am Dent Assoc 131:901–907, 2000.
Rawson RD, Orr DL: A scientific approach to pain control, 2000, University Press.
Rawson RD, Orr DL: Vascular penetration following intraligamental injection, J Oral Maxillofac Surg 43:600–604, 1985.
Rosenberg M, Orr DL, Starley E, et al: Student-to-student local anesthesia injections in dental education: moral, ethical, and legal issues, J Dent Educ 75:127–132, 2009.
Sawyer RJ, von Schroeder H: Temporary bilateral blindness after acute lidocaine toxicity, Anesth Analg 95:224–226, 2002.
Webber B, Orlansky H, Lipton C, et al: Complications of an intra-arterial injection from an inferior alveolar nerve block, J Am Dent Assoc 132:1702–1704, 2001.
Wilkie GJ: Temporary uniocular blindness and opthalmoplegia associated with a mandibular block injection: a case report, Aust Dent J 45:131–133, 2000.
Younessi OJ, Punnia-Moorthy A: Cardiovascular effects of bupivacaine and the role of this agent in preemptive dental analgesia, Anesth Prog 46:56–62, 1999.

CHAPTER 20

Future Trends in Pain Control

Although local anesthesia remains the backbone of pain control in dentistry, research continues in both medicine and dentistry with the goal of improving all areas of the local anesthetic experience, from that of the administrator to that of the patient. Much of this research has focused on improvements in the area of local anesthesia—safer needles and syringes; more successful techniques of regional nerve block, such as the anterior middle superior alveolar (AMSA) and palatal anterior superior alveolar (P-ASA) (see Chapter 13); and newer drugs, such as articaine HCl. These advances have been discussed in some depth in previous editions of this text and in preceding chapters of this 6th edition: intraosseous anesthesia (see Chapter 15); self-aspirating, pressure, and safety syringes and computer-controlled local anesthetic delivery (C-CLAD) systems (see Chapter 5); and articaine HCl (see Chapter 4). These drugs, devices, and techniques are now a part of the mainstream of pain control in the United States and elsewhere.

Some of the items discussed in previous editions have not progressed into the dental mainstream: the local anesthetics centbucridine and ropivacaine; the ultra-long-acting local anesthetics tetrodotoxin (TTX) and saxitoxin (STX); the topical anesthetic EMLA (eutectic mixture of local anesthetics); and the technique of electronic dental anesthesia (EDA). The reader who is interested in these items is referred to the 5th edition of this textbook.[1]

Since publication of the 5th edition in 2004, the dental profession in the United States has witnessed the introduction of products and devices that enable the doctor to dramatically decrease the onset time of pulpal anesthesia (the local anesthetic "on" switch), and significantly reduce the duration of the residual soft tissue anesthesia associated with intraoral injections of local anesthetics containing vasopressors (the local anesthetic "off" switch). In addition, recent research appears to demonstrate the usefulness of the infiltration of articaine HCl in providing pulpal anesthesia in the adult mandible.

Increasing the pH of a local anesthetic solution (i.e., buffering) toward a more physiologic pH, although not new in medicine or dentistry, had never been shown to provide consistently reliable clinical results (e.g., shorter onset time, more comfortable injection). Recent changes in the formulation of the buffering solution and in its delivery have greatly increased the effectiveness of this technique.

Residual soft tissue anesthesia—anesthesia of the lips, tongue, chin, or face—oftentimes lasting 5 hours or longer after injection of a vasopressor-containing local anesthetic, is usually unneeded and may, on occasion, present as a potential inconvenience or problem for the patient. Administration of a vasodilating drug into the site of previous local anesthetic administration increases vascular perfusion, allowing the local anesthetic drug to be removed from the site of injection more rapidly, thereby decreasing the duration of residual soft tissue anesthesia.

The inability of the traditional (Halsted approach) inferior alveolar nerve block (IANB) to provide consistently reliable pulpal anesthesia has been a vexing problem for all dentists. The lack of reliable, easy to visualize landmarks and extreme variations in patient anatomy have led to exceedingly high failure rates with this vitally important dental nerve block. Infiltration anesthesia, a mainstay in maxillary anesthesia, did not demonstrate significant clinical success when lidocaine, mepivacaine, and prilocaine were employed by mandibular infiltration in adult patients. However, recent clinical trials of mandibular infiltration with articaine have shown promise.

A current area of clinical research that has demonstrated early promise is the use of intranasally (IN) administered local anesthesia as a means of providing pulpal anesthesia to maxillary teeth without the need for injection (i.e., no needle). Phase II clinical trials comparing IN local anesthetic versus injected local anesthetic have demonstrated significant clinical success in providing pulpal anesthesia bilaterally from the second premolar to the second premolar.

Computer-controlled local anesthetic delivery (C-CLAD) has been included in this chapter on future developments since 1997. Today, C-CLAD has moved into mainstream dentistry. Recent research in this area is reviewed in this chapter.

BUFFERED LOCAL ANESTHETICS (THE LOCAL ANESTHETIC "ON" SWITCH)

With the introduction of the first amide local anesthetic (LA), lidocaine HCl, in 1948, providing profound anesthesia of long duration became almost a certainty. Other amides introduced since 1948 include mepivacaine HCl, prilocaine HCl, bupivacaine HCl, etidocaine HCl, and articaine HCl (the latter is considered an amide, although technically it is a hybrid drug, possessing both amide- and ester-type characteristics).

Onset of pulpal anesthesia commonly occurs within 5 to 10 minutes and persists for approximately 60 minutes with articaine HCl, lidocaine HCl, mepivacaine HCl, and prilocaine HCl formulations containing a vasopressor (epinephrine or levonordefrin).

Local anesthetics work. They represent the safest and most effective drugs in medicine for the prevention and management of pain. If deposited in close proximity to a nerve, they will block nerve conduction. However, as good as they are, LAs are not perfect:

- LAs containing a vasopressor sting on injection.
- LAs are associated with a degree of postinjection tissue injury.
- LAs have relatively slow onset.
- LAs do not work as reliably in the presence of infection and inflammation.

These drawbacks can be addressed by buffering the anesthetic solution to a more physiologic pH, which:

- Eliminates the sting on injection
- Reduces tissue injury and postinjection soreness
- Reduces latency
- Introduces the independent anesthetic effect of carbon dioxide
- Introduces the catalytic effect of carbon dioxide

Reducing Stinging and Postinjection Tissue Injury

The burning and stinging of acidic injections represent one of the most common complaints in dentistry. LAs containing a vasopressor have a pH of approximately 3.5; "plain" solutions have a pH of approximately 5.9. LA injections that contain epinephrine typically have a very low pH; therefore, a more significant degree of soft tissue injury may be produced by the injection, leading to increased postinjection soreness.

Chemistry and Anesthetic Latency

To achieve anesthesia, two things must happen: (1) the LA must be deposited in close proximity to a nerve, and (2) the LA must diffuse across the nerve membrane to the interior of the nerve, where it blocks sodium channels. The first requirement is met through the injection technique. However, without modification of the solution, the ability of the anesthetic to cross the nerve membrane is dependent on biochemical processes that are out of the practitioner's control.

Two ionic forms of the LA exist in equilibrium within the anesthetic cartridge: RN (the uncharged, de-ionized, "active" free base form of the drug, which is lipid soluble) and RNH^+ (the "charged" or ionized cationic form, which is not lipid soluble). Only the lipid-soluble de-ionized form can cross the nerve membrane. This is described more completely in Chapter 1.

The equilibrium between de-ionized RN and ionized RNH^+ is illustrated as follows:

$$RN + H^+ \longleftrightarrow RNH^+$$

The relative amounts of de-ionized and ionized forms of LA in a dental cartridge are dependent on the pH of the solution, in accordance with the Henderson-Hasselbalch equation. For instance, at a pH of 3.5, 99.996% of lidocaine HCl exists in the non–lipid-soluble ionized (RNH^+) form, and only 0.004% is present in the lipid-soluble de-ionized (RN) form. Only the lipid-soluble RN form can cross the nerve membrane. Once within the nerve, the RN picks up an H^+ with the resultant RNH^+ entering an Na^+ channel to block nerve conduction. Only after the body buffers the injected anesthetic solution to a pH closer to the physiologic range (7.35 to 7.45) will enough of the anesthetic enter into the nerve to effectively block nerve conduction. The time that this transformation requires is a key factor in anesthetic latency (e.g., 5 to 10 minute onset for most vasopressor-containing local anesthetic solutions).

Local Anesthesia in the Presence of Infection

Infection represents an additional factor in anesthetic effectiveness. (See Chapter 16 for a more complete description of the effects of infection on LAs and potential solutions to the problem of less effective pain control.) Lower tissue pH at the site of infection makes it extremely difficult for the typical LA injection to provide adequate pulpal anesthesia. Infected tissue is more acidic, making it more difficult for the RN conversion to occur.

Buffering Local Anesthetic Immediately Before Injection

Increasing the pH of a cartridge of lidocaine HCl with epinephrine immediately before administering the injection significantly increases the amount of the active anesthetic form (RN) available: for example, raising the pH of lidocaine HCl from 3.5 to 7.4 produces a 6000-fold increase. This "anesthetic buffering" process results in several clinical advantages, including (1) greater patient comfort during injection; (2) more rapid onset of anesthesia; and (3) decreased postinjection tissue injury. The percentage of RN ions available in local anesthetic solutions at various pH values is shown in Table 20-1.

Introducing Carbon Dioxide via the Buffering Process

When sodium bicarbonate ($NaHCO_3$) solution is mixed with an LA, it interacts with the hydrochloric acid in the LA to create water and carbon dioxide (CO_2). The CO_2 begins

TABLE 20-1
Percentage of RN Ions Present in LA Solution at Various pH Values

pH	Lidocaine pKa 7.9	Articaine pKa 7.8	Mepivacaine pKa 7.6	Bupivacaine pKa 8.1
7.4 (body pH)	24.03	28.47	38.69	16.63
6.5 (plain)	3.83	4.77	7.36	2.45
3.5 (with epi)	0.004	0.005	0.008	0.003

to diffuse out of solution immediately and continues to do so even after the solution has been injected. Catchlove concluded that CO_2 in combination with lidocaine HCl potentiates the action of lidocaine HCl by (1) providing a direct depressant effect of CO_2 on the axon, (2) concentrating the local anesthetic inside the nerve trunk through ion trapping, and (3) changing the charge of the local anesthetic inside the nerve axon.[2] Condouris and Shakalis demonstrated that CO_2 possesses an independent anesthetic effect and caused a sevenfold potentiation in anesthetic action.[3]

Buffering Local Anesthetic in Medicine

Buffering is well known and accepted in medicine where injections of local anesthetic into the skin are considerably more uncomfortable than intraoral injections. Buffering is used frequently in ophthalmology,[4] ear nose and throat,[5] and dermatology.[6] Prefilled cartridges of LA are not used in medicine, so preparation of a buffered solution is relatively simple: the physician adds a volume of $NaHCO_3$ to the local anesthetic solution just before injection. The ratio of LA to bicarbonate in published studies has varied significantly, from 2:1 (LA-to-bicarbonate) to 3:1, 5:1, 6:1, 10:1, 30:1, and 33:1, as have their results, from "no positive effect" to "excellent results" to "the formation of a precipitate" within the solution. From these and other studies, it appears that an LA-to-bicarbonate ratio of between 5:1 and 10:1 provides the greatest opportunity of achieving a more comfortable and more rapid-acting local anesthetic injection.

Buffering Local Anesthetic in Dentistry

The "problem" (as related to buffering) in dentistry is the prefilled local anesthetic cartridge. Because the addition of $NaHCO_3$ must occur within minutes of injection, it is not possible for the local anesthetic manufacturer to produce buffered LA cartridges. Until recently, dentists who attempted to buffer LAs would do so by expelling a volume of LA from the cartridge and replacing it with an equal volume of $NaHCO_3$. This means of buffering led to inconsistent results.[7]

A recently introduced product (February 2011) provides a means of consistently buffering dental cartridges of LA to a pH ranging between 7.35 and 7.5 (Figs. 20-1 and 20-2).

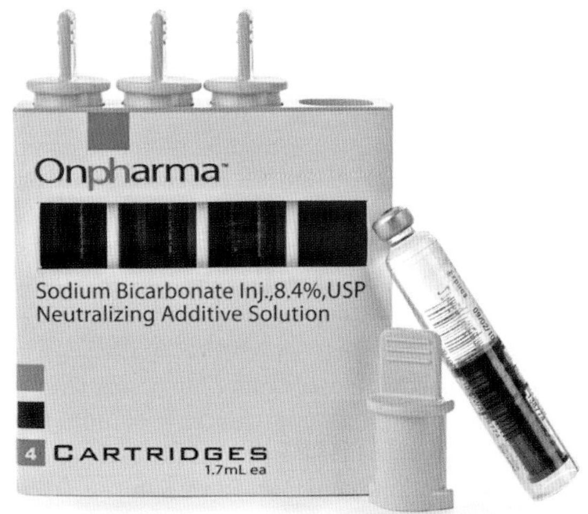

Figure 20-1. Sodium bicarbonate cartridges for buffering local anesthetic solution. (Photo courtesy Onpharma Inc., Los Gatos, Calif.)

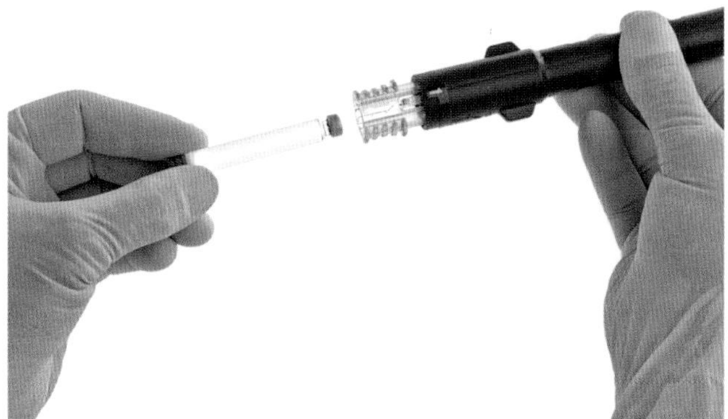

Figure 20-2. Dental local anesthetic cartridge inserted into mixing pen. (Photo courtesy Onpharma Inc., Los Gatos, Calif.)

A prospective, randomized, double-blind, crossover trial (N = 20) compared "standard" LA with epinephrine versus LA with epinephrine buffered toward physiologic pH using sodium bicarbonate.[8] Patients served as their own controls, receiving inferior alveolar nerve blocks, once with a standard cartridge of lidocaine 2% with epinephrine 1:100,000 (pH ≈3.5), the other time with the same solution buffered with sodium bicarbonate (pH ≈7.4), on two visits separated by at least 2 weeks. The study assessed (1) comfort of injection and (2) speed of onset of pulpal anesthesia.

Seventy-two percent of subjects rated the buffered LA injection as more comfortable than the unbuffered injection, 17% rated them the same, and 11% rated the unbuffered LA as more comfortable (P =.003). When a visual analog scale (VAS) was used to rate pain from "0" (felt nothing) to "10" (worst pain imaginable), 44% of injections with buffered LA were reported to be painless (VAS = 0) versus 6% of injections with traditional LA (P =.004).[8]

The study also assessed the onset of pulpal anesthesia. Average time to pulpal anesthesia (as determined by electrical pulp testing) was 7 minutes 29 seconds for standard LA and 1 minute 51 seconds for buffered LA (P <.05). Eighty percent of buffered subjects obtained pulpal anesthesia within 2 minutes.[8]

At this time (January 2012), clinical trials are under way to determine whether buffered local anesthetic solution provides a more profound level of pulpal anesthesia, as seems likely given that approximately 6000 times the RN ionic form of local anesthetic is available to penetrate the nerve membrane.

Developments Since the 5th Edition. Previous editions of this book referenced studies in both medicine and dentistry in which $NaHCO_3$ or hyaluronidase was added to local anesthetic cartridges with extremely variable results.[9] The introduction of a stabilized form of $NaHCO_3$ along with use of a delivery device makes addition of $NaHCO_3$ to the dental cartridge with removal of a like volume of LA from the cartridge an easy to accomplish chairside procedure.

PHENTOLAMINE MESYLATE (THE LOCAL ANESTHETIC "OFF" SWITCH)

The local anesthetic armamentarium today consists of drugs that provide a range of durations of pain control, from short-acting drugs (≈30 minutes of pulpal anesthesia) to long-acting drugs that provide pulpal anesthesia up to 7 hours and soft tissue anesthesia up to 12 hours.[10] Short-duration drugs provide pulpal anesthesia for approximately 30 minutes and include mepivacaine HCl 3% and prilocaine HCl 4%. The long-duration category consists of bupivacaine HCl 0.5% with epinephrine 1:200,000, providing pulpal anesthesia for up to 7 hours (commonly from 90 to 180 minutes) with soft tissue anesthesia for up to 12 hours. It is interesting to note that bupivacaine HCl is a long-acting anesthetic only when administered by nerve block (e.g., inferior alveolar nerve block). It is not nearly as long acting when administered by supraperiosteal (infiltration) injection.

Because the usual length of dental treatment is approximately 44 minutes, the short-duration anesthetics fail to meet the pain control needs of many patients.[11] The intermediate-duration category is used most often. With inclusion of a vasopressor (epinephrine or levonordefrin [in North America]), the drugs in this group provide pulpal anesthesia of approximately 60 minutes' duration. Intermediate-duration drugs include articaine HCl 4% with epinephrine 1:100,000 and 1:200,000; lidocaine HCl 2% with epinephrine 1:50,000 and 1:100,000; mepivacaine HCl 2% with levonordefrin 1:20,000; and prilocaine HCl 4% with epinephrine 1:200,000.

It is pulpal anesthesia that allows a tooth to be treated painlessly. Anesthesia of associated soft tissues (STA) occurs hand-in-hand with pulpal anesthesia. Although necessary for many treatments such as curettage, periodontal surgery, extractions, implants, and subgingival tooth preparation, to be completed painlessly, the duration of STA is considerably longer than that of pulpal anesthesia, averaging 3 to 5 hours in the intermediate-duration group of LAs.

In the mandible, where anesthesia in the adult is usually limited to nerve blocks (inferior alveolar, Gow-Gates), large areas of soft tissue anesthesia develop along with the desired pulpal anesthesia. The anterior two thirds of the tongue, the lower lip, and the cheek are left without sensation for many hours following completion of dental treatment.

Techniques such as periodontal ligament (PDL) injection (also known as intraligamentary injection [ILI][12] and intraosseous [IO] injection)[13] provide localized areas of pulpal anesthesia with a minimum of associated soft tissue anesthesia. Anesthesia of the tongue or lip is essentially nonexistent following these injections.

Residual Soft Tissue Anesthesia

Although a long duration of residual STA may be desirable following some dental procedures such as surgery (oral surgical, periodontal, and endodontic), most operative dental care requires profound anesthesia (pulpal) during the relatively brief treatment period while the patient is in the dental chair. Once the traumatic part of the treatment is completed, continued anesthesia of the tissues, hard or soft, is no longer needed. However, the need for effective intraoperative pain control normally mandates the use of a vasoconstrictor-containing local anesthetic.[14] Patients commonly are discharged from the dental office with residual numbness to their lips and tongue, which typically persists for an additional 3 to 5 hours.[15]

Residual STA presents as an inconvenience or embarrassment to the patient, who is unable to function normally for many hours after leaving the dental appointment. In a survey by Rafique and associates[16] of patients receiving intraoral local anesthesia, the authors stated that several aspects of the post–local anesthetic experience were disliked by patients, including three major areas—functional, sensory, and perceptual.

Functionally, patients disliked their diminished ability to speak (lisping), to smile (asymmetric), or to drink (liquid runs from the mouth), and their inability to control drooling while still numb. Sensorially, lack of sensation was described as quite discomforting, and the perception that their body was distorted (e.g., swollen lips) was equally unpleasant. For many patients, these sequelae become a significant detriment to their quality of life, making it difficult for them to return to their usual activities for hours after treatment. When the dental appointment concludes at a time approaching a meal—either lunch or dinner—the patient must consider whether to eat while numb or postpone dining until residual STA resolves.

Although not normally a significant problem, residual STA occasionally may lead to self-inflicted injury in any patient. Self-inflicted injury to soft tissues, most commonly the lip or tongue, is more apt to be noted in younger children and in mentally disabled adult and pediatric patients[17,18] (Fig. 20-3).

A study of pediatric patients by College and colleagues[17] revealed that a significant percentage of inferior alveolar nerve blocks were associated with inadvertent biting of the

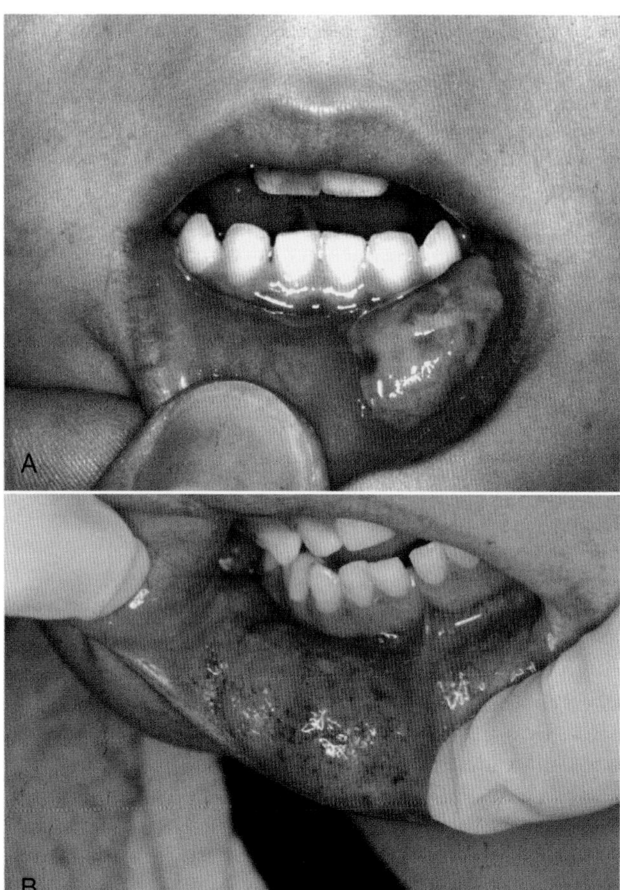

Figure 20-3. Self-inflicted soft tissue injury of lips.

TABLE 20-2
Percentage of Patients, by Age, With Self-Inflicted Soft Tissue Injury Following IANB

Age, yr	% With Soft Tissue Trauma
<4	18
4-7	16
8-11	13
12+	7

Data from College C, Feigal R, Wandera A, et al: Bilateral versus unilateral mandibular block anesthesia in a pediatric population, Pediatr Dent 22:453–457, 2000.
IANB, Inferior alveolar nerve block.

lips. By age group, the frequency of trauma to the lips was as follows: 18% (<4 yr), 16% (4 to 7 yr), 13% (8 to 11 yr), and 7% (>12 yr) (Table 20-2). This can be explained by the fact that the younger patient will test (by biting) his or her un-numb lip—which hurts—and then will test the still numb side—which doesn't hurt. Although the adult normally would not proceed beyond this point, the younger child may "play" with this "feeling" and continue to bite ever harder and harder, not realizing the damage that is being inflicted. Mentally handicapped adults are just as likely to incur self-inflicted soft tissue injury. Another group—geriatric patients with dementia—presents a risk of soft tissue injury following LA injection equal to or greater than that of children and mentally challenged adults.

HOW LOCAL ANESTHETICS WORK—AN OVERVIEW

When a local anesthetic is deposited close to a nerve, it diffuses into the nerve. When the dental drill stimulates a tooth distal to this site (the area that is "numb"), a nerve impulse is propagated. However, this impulse travels only so far as the area of the nerve where the LA has been deposited. The nerve impulse then dies out, never reaching the patient's brain. As long as enough LA stays in the nerve, the painful nerve impulse does not reach the brain. This defines the duration of anesthesia produced by the LA drug.

Local anesthetics "stop working" when the volume of LA within the nerve is greater than the volume of LA outside the nerve. The process of diffusion reverses, and the drug begins to leave the nerve and move into the soft tissues surrounding it. Individual nerve fibers are gradually unblocked, causing the patient to tell the doctor that he or she is "starting to feel it again."

As the drug exits the nerve, it is absorbed into capillaries that carry LA molecules away from the injection site via the venous circulation. The greater the volume of blood flowing through the area where the LA was deposited, the more rapidly this diffusion out of the nerve occurs. This explains why "plain" LAs have a shorter duration of both soft tissue and pulpal anesthesia than those containing a vasopressor. Local anesthetics inherently are vasodilators. Injection of a plain LA increases vascular perfusion at the injection site, allowing entry of a lesser volume of LA into the nerve and more rapid diffusion of the drug back out of the nerve. As a group, plain LAs provide a shorter duration with less profound anesthesia than is provided by anesthetics containing a vasopressor.

The addition of epinephrine or levonordefrin to LA diminishes blood flow into the site of LA deposition. This permits a greater volume of LA to diffuse into the nerve and, because less blood flows through the region, allows LA to remain within the nerve in a higher concentration for a longer time, thus providing a longer duration of more profound anesthesia.

Decreasing the Duration of Residual STA

Increasing the flow of blood through the site in which LA was injected facilitates more rapid diffusion of LA from the nerve into the cardiovascular system, thus decreasing the length of residual STA. Any technique that causes vasodilation can produce this effect.

In the 1980s, the technique known as TENS (transcutaneous electrical nerve stimulation) was successful in shortening the duration of residual STA. TENS is commonly used in sports medicine and in rehabilitation from soft tissue injury.[19] Electrodes are placed on the site of injury, and a low-frequency electrical current is delivered to the area (Fig. 20-4). Application of this low-frequency (2.5 Hz) electrical current to an area that has been recently injured is beneficial for the patient in two ways: (1) it acts to increase tissue perfusion produced by capillary and arteriolar dilation, and (2) it simultaneously stimulates the contraction of skeletal muscle. The net effect of these two processes is a pumping action in the area of application of the current. Therapeutically, a 1 hour treatment given at a low frequency helps to decrease edema (skeletal muscle–stimulating effect), and increased perfusion and skeletal muscle stimulation act to "cleanse" the area of tissue injury breakdown products.[19] With electrodes placed intraorally around the site where local anesthetic is injected, it was possible to shorten the duration of STA. This technique was short-lived because it was difficult to position the electrodes intraorally and to have them adhere firmly to the moist intraoral mucous membranes.

Another approach to the question of how to minimize residual STA consists of injection of a vasodilating drug into the area of prior local anesthetic administration. In theory, this should hasten the redistribution of LA from the nerve into the cardiovascular system (CVS), thereby decreasing the duration of residual STA.

Phentolamine Mesylate

Phentolamine is an α-adrenergic receptor antagonist approved for use by the U.S. Food and Drug Administration (FDA) in 1952 (Fig. 20-5). Approved uses of phentolamine currently include (1) diagnosis of pheochromocytoma, (2) treatment of hypertension in pheochromocytoma,[20,21] and (3) prevention of tissue necrosis after norepinephrine extravasation.[22,23] An early use of injectable phentolamine involved the management of impotence (erectile dysfunction).[24]

Phentolamine is a short-acting, competitive antagonist at peripheral α-adrenergic receptors. It antagonizes both α_1 and α_2 receptors, thus blocking the actions of the circulating catecholamines epinephrine and norepinephrine. Phentolamine also stimulates β-adrenergic receptors in the heart and lungs.

The clinical effects of phentolamine include peripheral vasodilation and tachycardia. Vasodilation results from both direct relaxation of vascular smooth muscle and α blockade. The drug produces positive inotropic and chronotropic effects, leading to an increase in cardiac output. In smaller doses, the positive inotropic effect can predominate and raise blood pressure; in larger doses, peripheral vasodilation can mask the inotropic effect and lower blood pressure. These actions make phentolamine useful in treating hypertension caused by increased circulating levels of epinephrine and norepinephrine, as occurs in pheochromocytoma.

The effects of phentolamine in treating impotence are mediated by α-adrenergic blockade in penile blood vessels. Actions of the drug cause relaxation of the trabecular cavernous smooth muscles and dilation of the penile arteries; this increases arterial blood flow into the corpus cavernosa and subsequently causes an erection.[24] Phentolamine is administered IV or IM but can be injected subcutaneously to prevent local tissue necrosis when vasoconstrictor drugs extravasate.[23] The pharmacokinetics of phentolamine is largely unknown; 10% of a parenteral dose is excreted in the urine unchanged.

Availability. Phentolamine is available as a 5 mg/mL solution for parenteral administration.

Phentolamine Mesylate for Reversal of Residual STA

Clinical Trials—Adults and Adolescents. An injectable form of phentolamine mesylate (PM) has been formulated to terminate the numbing sensation associated with local anesthesia when it is no longer required. The product, which is available under the proprietary name OraVerse (Septodont Inc. Lancaster, Pa), contains 0.4 mg PM (0.235 mg/mL) packaged in a 1.7 mL dental cartridge[22] (Fig. 20-6). In May 2008, the FDA approved phentolamine mesylate, which was

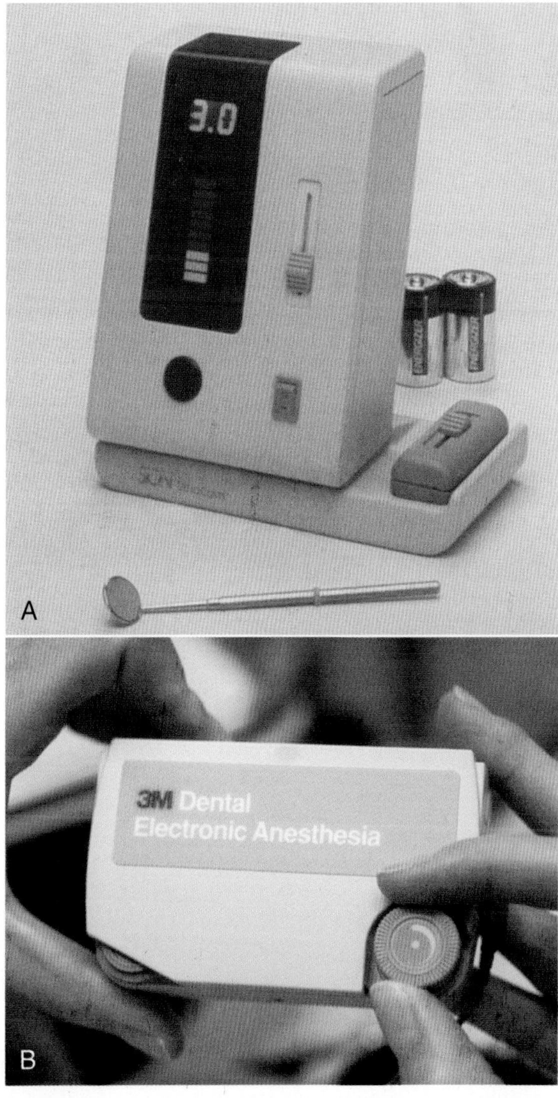

Figure 20-4. A and B, Electronic dental anesthesia (EDA) unit, circa 1980.

Continued

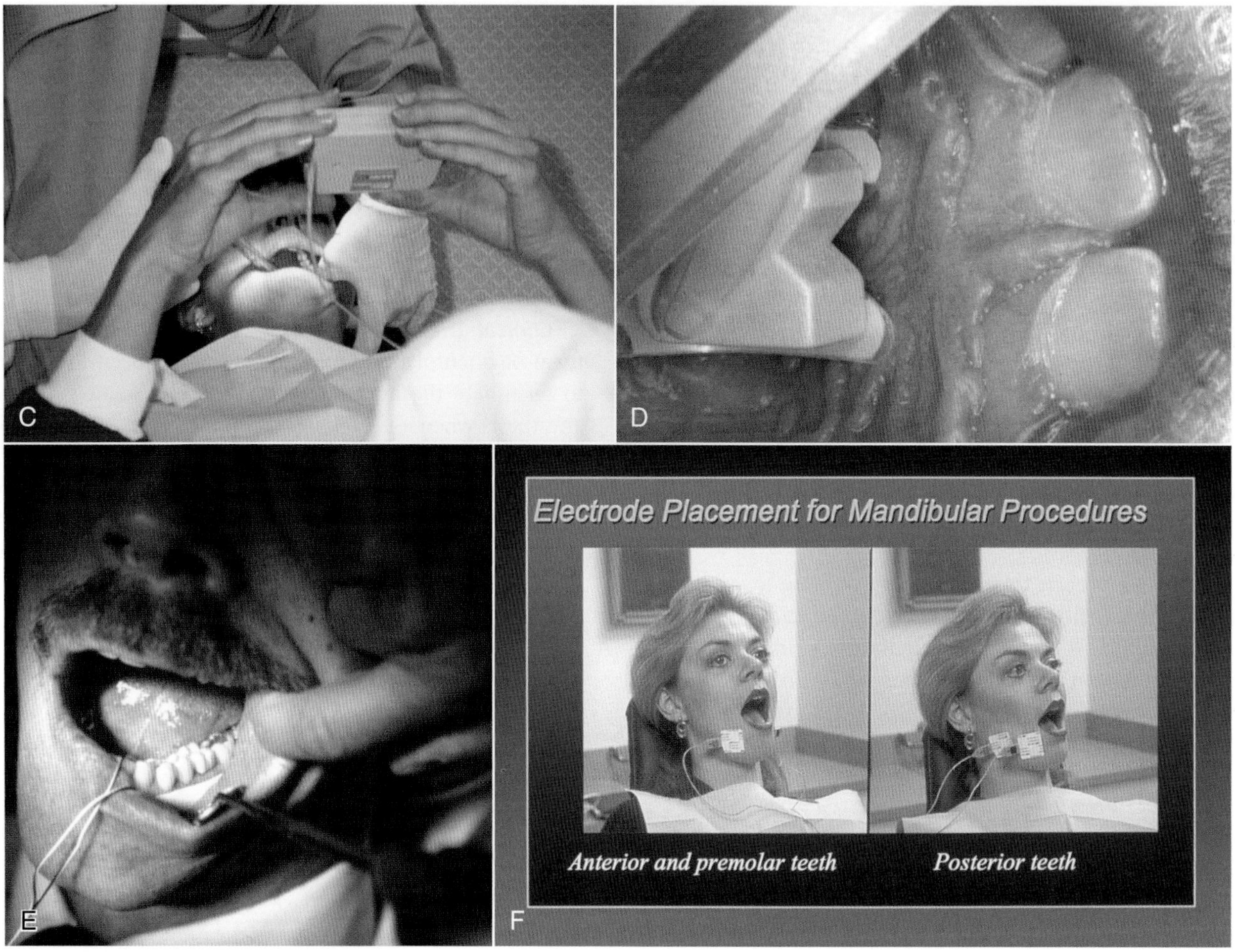

Figure 20-4, cont'd. C and D, Intraoral use of transcutaneous electrical nerve stimulation (TENS) for comfortable administration of local anesthesia and (E and F) for treatment without the need for local anesthesia.

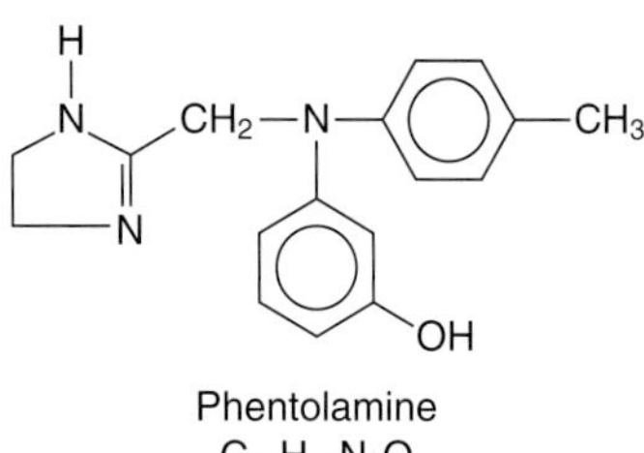

Figure 20-5. Chemical formula of phentolamine.

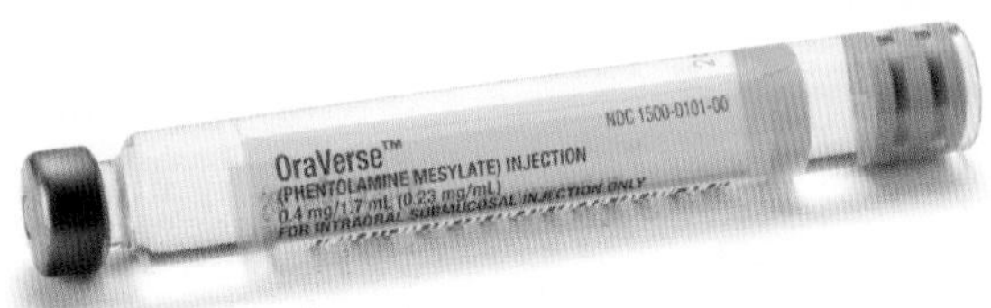

Figure 20-6. Phentolamine mesylate (OraVerse) cartridge. (Photo courtesy Septodont, Lancaster, Pa.)

marketed in February 2009.[25] The dental formulation of phentolamine is approximately $\frac{1}{30}$ the concentration used in medicine (0.17 mg/mL vs. 5.0 mg/mL).

Before receiving FDA approval, PM went through a series of clinical trials to demonstrate its safety and efficacy for this new therapeutic indication. Two Phase III, double-blind, randomized, multicenter, controlled studies were conducted.[26] One trial studied the safety and efficacy of PM in reversing mandibular STA; the second trial studied the safety and efficacy of PM in reversing maxillary STA. A pediatric Phase II, double-blinded, randomized, multicenter, controlled study was conducted in dental patients, aged 4 to 11 years, who had received 2% lidocaine with 1:100,000 epinephrine.[27]

In Phase III trials for this new indication for PM, patients received a local anesthetic containing a vasoconstrictor on one side of the mouth before a restorative or periodontal maintenance procedure was begun. The primary endpoint was elapsed time to the return of normal lip sensation as measured by patient-reported responses to lip palpation. Secondary endpoints included patients' perceptions of altered function, sensation, and appearance, and functional deficits in smiling, speaking, drinking, and drooling, as

STAR QUESTIONNAIRE

	Not at all	A little bit	Some what	Qutie a bit	Very much
I feel like my lip, tongue or cheek is swollen	0	1	2	3	4
I am uncomfortable with how my lip, tongue or cheek feels	0	1	2	3	4
I am concerned about biting my lip, tongue or cheek	0	1	2	3	4
I have trouble drinking form a glass or cup	0	1	2	3	4
I have trouble eating	0	1	2	3	4
I have trouble speaking clearly	0	1	2	3	4
I have trouble smiling	0	1	2	3	4
I am concerned about drooling	0	1	2	3	4
I am concerned about how long my numbness will last	0	1	2	3	4
I am concerned about my ability to speak at work or home	0	1	2	3	4
I am concerned about the way my mouth might look to others	0	1	2	3	4
The numbness I feel now would cause me to avoid social activities	0	1	2	3	4

Figure 20-7. Soft Tissue Anesthesia Recovery (STAR) Questionnaire.

assessed by both the patient and an observer blinded to the treatment.[26-29] To determine the impact of functional deficits, a patient-reported outcomes questionnaire (Soft Tissue Anesthesia Recovery [STAR]) was developed (Fig. 20-7). In the mandibular study, the time to recovery of tongue sensation was also a secondary endpoint. The dental procedure had to be completed within 60 minutes of the LA injection, and the patient's lip had to still be numb at that time, or he or she was excluded from the study. All 244 patients randomized in the mandibular study reported lip anesthesia at 1 hour; only 194 reported that their tongue was still numb at this time. The maxillary study enrolled 240 patients.

Patients were randomized to receive one of four local anesthetics: 2% lidocaine + epinephrine 1:100,000; 2% mepivacaine + levonordefrin 1:20,000; 4% articaine + epinephrine 1:100,000; or 4% prilocaine + epinephrine 1:200,000. Drugs were randomized using a 6:1:1:1 ratio based on usage patterns in the United States.

At the conclusion of treatment, the patient received either PM or a control injection. The patient and all investigators were blinded to the treatment assigned. The study drug was administered at the same site, and in the case of PM, the same number of cartridges (one or two) was used as in the previous LA injection(s). The control was a sham injection in which the plastic needle cap attached to the dental syringe containing an empty cartridge was pushed against, but did not penetrate, intraoral soft tissue at the site of the previous LA injection. This sham allowed for a blinded comparison of injection site pain. After receiving PM or the sham injection, all patients were observed for 5 hours for collection of efficacy and safety data, and were monitored for up to 48 hours.

The 5 hour observation and testing period was a primary determinant of the lower age limit (4 years) for patients. It was believed (correctly, it turned out) that younger patients would be unable to cooperate fully with the assessments (see later) required over the 5 hour period of observation.

Lip and Tongue Palpation. All patients were trained in assessing the numbness of their lip. Those in the mandibular protocol were also trained to tap their tongue. The procedure involved light tapping of these soft tissues with the index or middle finger. Research assistants instructed patients that during the study, they would rate the injected side as feeling normal, tingling, or numb, and that they may tap the non-injected side as a comparison. Assessments were made every 5 minutes.

STAR Questionnaire. The STAR questionnaire measures quality of life (see Fig. 20-7). It was developed specifically for these studies to quantify a patient's perceived clinical benefit derived from reversing soft tissue anesthesia.

Functional Assessment Battery (FAB). The FAB included measurements of smiling, speaking, and drooling, and drinking 3 ounces of water at various time points during the study.[28] Each functional assessment was rated as normal or abnormal by a research assistant and by the patient.

Heft-Parker Visual Analog Scale (H-P VAS). The H-P VAS is a 170 mm visual analog scale that contains the following verbal descriptors: none, faint, weak, mild, moderate, strong, intense, and maximum possible.[29] Patients were asked to place a mark on the line that corresponded to their current assessment of pain at the injection site and at the procedural site.

Efficacy of Phentolamine Mesylate: Adolescents and Adults.[26] In the maxillary trial, the median time to recovery of normal sensation in the upper lip was 50 minutes for PM patients and 132.5 minutes for sham patients, for a reduction in upper lip anesthesia of 82.5 minutes (P <.0001).

In the mandibular trial, the median time to recovery of normal sensation in the lower lip was 70 minutes for PM patients and 155 minutes for sham patients, for a reduction in lower lip anesthesia of 85 minutes (P <.0001).

Within 30 minutes of PM administration, 26.7% of maxillary patients reported return of normal lip sensation as compared with 1.7% in the control group. At 1 hour, 59.2% had normal upper lip sensation versus 11.7% for sham. At 90 minutes, these figures were 75% and 25%, respectively. Upper lip anesthesia persisted beyond 2 hours

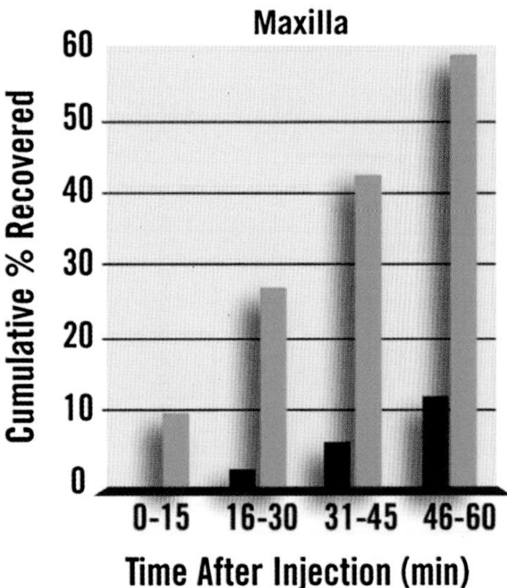

Figure 20-8. Percentage of Patients Reporting Return of Normal Upper Lip Sensation Following Administration of Phentolamine Mesylate *(green)* or Sham Injection *(blue)*.

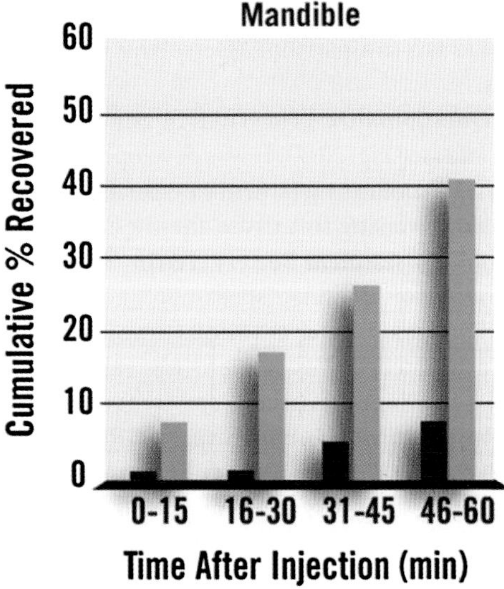

Figure 20-9. Percentage of Patients Reporting Return of Normal Lower Lip Sensation Following Administration of Phentolamine Mesylate *(green)* or Sham Injection *(blue)*.

in 54.2% of sham patients versus 11.6% of PM patients (Fig. 20-8).

In the mandible, within 30 minutes of PM administration, 17.2% of patients reported normal lower lip sensation as compared with 0.8% in the control group. At 1 hour, 41% had normal lower lip sensation versus 7.4% for sham. At 90 minutes, these figures were 70.5% and 13.1%, respectively. Lower lip anesthesia persisted beyond 2 hours in 70.5% of sham patients versus 18.9% of PM patients (Fig. 20-9).

The median time to return of normal sensation to the tongue was 60 minutes for PM and 125 minutes for sham-treated patients—a statistically significant (P <.0001) difference of 65 minutes.

Safety of Phentolamine Mesylate: Adolescents and Adults.[26] The overall frequency and the nature of adverse events (AEs) reported in the maxillary and mandibular studies appeared similar in nature and frequency. In the maxillary study, a total of 38 patients reported 50 AEs: 32 AEs in 22 patients in the PM group, and 18 AEs in 16 patients in the sham group. In the mandibular study, a total of 63 patients reported 77 AEs: 44 AEs in 34 patients in the PM group, and 33 AEs in 29 patients in the sham group. None of the AEs in either study were serious or rated severe, and no patient was discontinued from the study because of an AE.

Dental patients were administered a dose of 0.2, 0.4, or 0.8 mg of PM. Adverse reactions in which the frequency was greater than or equal to 3% in any PM dose group and was equal to or exceeded that of the control group include diarrhea, facial swelling, increased blood pressure/hypertension, injection site reactions, jaw pain, oral pain, paresthesia, pruritus, tenderness, upper abdominal pain, and vomiting. Most adverse reactions were mild and resolved within 48 hours.[30]

Safety and Efficacy of Phentolamine Mesylate: Children.[31] In a Phase II, double-blind, randomized, multicenter (N = 11), controlled study, pediatric patients between the ages of 4 and 11 years received 2% lidocaine + epinephrine 1:100,000 and either PM or sham injection. One hundred fifty-two patients were enrolled and completed the study. A total of 96 patients were included in the PM group and 56 in the sham injection group. Patients received ½ cartridge of local anesthetic if they weighed more than 15 kg but less than 30 kg, and ½ or a full cartridge if they weighed 30 kg or more. Median time to normal lip sensation was evaluated in patients 6 to 11 years of age who were trainable for lip palpation procedures (see earlier). The reduction in median time to normal lip sensation for PM patients (n = 60) was 60 minutes compared with 135 minutes in the sham group (n = 43), representing a reduction in residual STA of 75 minutes (55.6%) for both maxillary and mandibular. Within 1 hour following administration of PM, 61% of patients reported normal lip sensation, but only 21% of patients in the sham injection group reported normal lip sensation. This finding was statistically significant (P <.0001).

Among the 152 patients, 35 (23%) reported 37 adverse events with similar frequencies in the PM (20.8%) and sham (26.8%) groups. No deaths or other serious AEs were reported, and all patients completed the study. All but 3 AEs were mild or moderate in severity. One patient in the PM group and 2 in the sham group reported severe AEs: post–dental procedure pain (PM, sham) and injection site pain (sham). All AEs were transient and resolved within the study period.

Clinical Indications for Reversal of Local Anesthesia. Administration of phentolamine mesylate should be a treatment option whenever prolonged STA presents a potential risk (soft tissue injury) or will negatively impact the patient's

BOX 20-1 Candidates for Phentolamine Reversal

Conservative dentistry
Nonsurgical periodontics
Pediatric dentistry
Medically compromised patients (e.g., type 1 diabetic patient)
Geriatric patients
Special needs patients
Post mandibular implants

lifestyle (e.g., inability to speak or eat). Box 20-1 lists potential candidates for reversal of STA.

Situations that do not usually represent indications for STA reversal involve postsurgical patients in whom prolonged STA is welcomed as a means of preventing breakthrough pain. Further, following local anesthetic administration via the PDL, also known as ILI or IO injection, the extremely localized area of STA associated with these injections precludes the use of PM.

Clinical Use of Phentolamine Mesylate in Dentistry. Phentolamine mesylate is indicated for the reversal of soft tissue anesthesia (i.e., anesthesia of the lip and tongue) and associated functional deficits resulting from intraoral submucosal injection of a local anesthetic containing a vasoconstrictor. Phentolamine mesylate is not recommended for use in children younger than 6 years of age or weighing less than 15 kg (33 lb).[30]

The recommended dose of phentolamine mesylate is based on the number of cartridges of LA + vasoconstrictor administered. It is administered in an equal volumes, up to a maximum of two cartridges. Phentolamine mesylate is administered at the same location(s) and by the same technique(s) (nerve block or infiltration) used earlier for LA administration.[30]

Adverse reactions associated with the administration of PM were discussed earlier (safety and adverse reaction discussion). Other potential complications include trismus and paresthesia, both of which are related to the act of injection rather than to the drug itself.

Summary

Phentolamine mesylate (OraVerse) enables the dentist or the dental hygienist (in states or provinces where permitted) to significantly decrease the duration of residual soft tissue anesthesia in patients in whom such numbness may prove to be potentially injurious (children, geriatric patients, and special needs patients) or a negative influence on their quality of life (speaking, eating, negative body image). (*Note:* As of October 24, 2011, dental hygienists are permitted to administer phentolamine mesylate in the following states: Alaska, Arkansas, California, Hawaii, Idaho, Iowa, Louisiana, Montana, Nevada, New York, North Dakota, Oklahoma, Rhode Island, Tennessee, Utah, and Wisconsin.) Additionally, phentolamine mesylate may be administered following placement of a mandibular implant to aid in the rapid determination of implant impingement on the inferior alveolar nerve.[32]

Developments Since the 5th Edition. Local anesthetic reversal with phentolamine mesylate was not yet a consideration when the 5th edition of this textbook was published in 2004.

ARTICAINE HCL BY BUCCAL INFILTRATION IN THE ADULT MANDIBLE

Providing effective pain control is one of the most important aspects of dental care. Indeed, patients rate a dentist "who does not hurt" and one who can "give painless injections" as meeting the second and first most important criteria used in evaluating dentists.[33] Unfortunately, the ability to obtain consistently profound anesthesia for dental procedures in the mandible has proved extremely elusive. This is even more of a problem when infected teeth are involved, primarily mandibular molars. Anesthesia of maxillary teeth on the other hand, although on occasion difficult to achieve, is rarely an insurmountable problem. Reasons for this include the fact that the cortical plate of bone overlying maxillary teeth is normally thin, thus allowing the local anesthetic drug to diffuse when administered by supraperiosteal injection (infiltration). Additionally, relatively simple nerve blocks, such as posterior superior alveolar (PSA), middle superior alveolar (MSA), anterior superior alveolar (ASA; infraorbital), and anterior middle superior alveolar (AMSA),[34] are available as alternatives to infiltration.

It is commonly stated that the significantly higher failure rate for mandibular anesthesia is related to the thickness of the cortical plate of bone in the adult mandible. Indeed it is generally acknowledged that mandibular infiltration *is* successful when the patient has a full primary dentition.[35,36] Once a mixed dentition develops, it is a general rule of teaching that the mandibular cortical plate of bone has thickened to the degree that infiltration might not be effective, leading to the recommendation that "mandibular block" techniques should now be employed.[37]

A second difficulty with the traditional Halsted approach to the inferior alveolar nerve (i.e., IANB, or "mandibular block") is an absence of consistent landmarks. Multiple authors have described numerous approaches to this oftentimes elusive nerve.[38-40] Indeed, reported failure rates for the IANB are commonly quite high, ranging from 31% and 41% in mandibular second and first molars to 42%, 38%, and 46% in second and first premolars and canines, respectively,[9] and 81% in lateral incisors.[41]

Not only is the inferior alveolar nerve elusive, but studies using ultrasound[42] and radiographs[43,44] to accurately locate the inferior alveolar neurovascular bundle or the mandibular foramen have revealed that accurate needle location did not guarantee successful pain control.[45] The central core theory best explains this problem.[46,47] Nerves on the outside of the nerve bundle supply the molar teeth, and nerves on the inside (core fibers) supply the incisor teeth. Therefore the local anesthetic solution deposited near the inferior alveolar nerve may diffuse and block the outermost fibers but not those located more centrally, leading to incomplete mandibular anesthesia.

The difficulty in achieving mandibular anesthesia has, over the years, led to the development of alternative techniques to the traditional (Halsted approach) inferior alveolar nerve block. These have included the Gow-Gates mandibular nerve block,[48] the Akinosi-Vazirani closed-mouth nerve block,[49] the PDL (intraligamentary) injection,[50] intraosseous anesthesia,[51] and, most recently, buffered local anesthetics.[52] Although all maintain some advantages over the traditional Halsted approach, none is without its own faults and contraindications.

The ability to provide localized areas of anesthesia by infiltration injection without the need for nerve block injections has a number of benefits. Meechan[53] has enumerated them as follows: (1) technically simple, (2) more comfortable for patients, (3) can provide hemostasis when needed, (4) in many cases obviates the presence of collateral innervation, (5) avoids the risk of potential damage to nerve trunks, (6) lesser risk of intravascular injection, (7) safer in patients with clotting disorders, (8) reduces risk of needle-stick injury, and (9) preinjection application of topical anesthetic masks needle penetration discomfort.

Mandibular Infiltration

Attempts at mandibular infiltration have been made in the past. In a 1976 study of 331 subjects receiving IANB with lidocaine HCl 2% with epinephrine 1:80,000, 23.7% had unsuccessful anesthesia.[54] Supplemental infiltration of 1.0 mL of the same drug on the buccal aspect of the mandible proved successful in 70 of the 79 subjects. Of the remaining 9, 7 were successfully anesthetized following additional infiltration of 1.0 mL on the lingual aspect of the mandible.

Yonchak and associates investigated infiltration on incisors and reported 45% success following labial infiltration (lidocaine 2% with 1:100,000 epinephrine) and 50% with lingual infiltrations of the same solution for lateral incisors, and 63% and 47% for central incisors on labial and lingual infiltration.[55]

Meechan and Ledvinka found similar success rates (50%) on central incisor teeth following labial or lingual infiltration of 1.0 mL of lidocaine 2% with 1:80,000 epinephrine.[56]

In 1990 Haas and colleagues compared mandibular buccal infiltrations for canines with prilocaine HCl versus articaine HCl and found no significant differences.[57] Success rates were 50% for prilocaine and 65% for articaine (both 4% with epinephrine 1:200,000). A second study noted a 63% success rate on mandibular second molars with articaine, and 53% with prilocaine (both 4% with epinephrine 1:200,000).[58]

Recent Findings—Mandibular Infiltration With Articaine HCl. Since the introduction of articaine HCl 4% with epinephrine 1:100,000 in the United States in June 2000, numerous anecdotal reports have been received from doctors claiming that they no longer needed to administer the IANB to work in the adult mandible painlessly. They claimed that mandibular infiltration with articaine HCl was uniformly successful. These claims were initially met with skepticism. Over the past 5 years, four well-designed clinical trials have compared infiltration in the adult mandible of articaine HCl 4% with epinephrine 1:100,000 versus lidocaine 2% with epinephrine 1:100,000 or 1:80,000.

Kanaa MD, Whitworth JM, Corbett IP, et al: Articaine and lidocaine mandibular buccal infiltration anesthesia: a prospective randomized double-blind cross-over study, J Endod 32:296–298, 2006.[59]

Robertson D, Nusstein J, Reader A, et al: The anesthetic efficacy of articaine in buccal infiltration of mandibular posterior teeth, J Am Dent Assoc 138:1104–1112, 2007.[60]

These first two papers assessed the effectiveness of articaine buccal infiltration administered in lieu of an IANB.

Haase A, Reader A, Nusstein J, et al: Comparing anesthetic efficacy of articaine versus lidocaine as a supplemental buccal infiltration of the mandibular first molar after an inferior alveolar nerve block, J Am Dent Assoc 139:1228–1235, 2008.[61]

Kanaa MD, Whitworth JM, Corbett IP, et al: Articaine buccal infiltration enhances the effectiveness of lidocaine inferior alveolar nerve block, Int Endod J 42:238–246, 2009.[41]

These two papers studied the effectiveness of an articaine buccal infiltration as a supplement to the IANB.

These clinically important clinical trials are summarized in the following section.

Kanaa MD, Whitworth JM, Corbett IP, et al: Articaine and lidocaine mandibular buccal infiltration anesthesia: a prospective randomized double-blind cross-over study, J Endod 32:296–298, 2006.[59]

Design. Infiltrations were administered to 31 subjects in the buccal fold adjacent to the mandibular first molar. A dose of 1.8 mL was administered at a rate of 0.9 mL per 15 seconds. The order of drug administration was randomized, with the second injection administered at least 1 week after the first. The same investigator administered all injections. Electrical pulp testing (EPT) was used to determine pulpal sensitivity. Baseline readings were obtained, and EPT was repeated once every 2 minutes after injection for 30 minutes. If no response (to maximal EPT stimulation of 80 μA) occurred, the number of episodes of no response at maximal stimulation was recorded. The criterion for successful anesthesia was no volunteer response to maximal stimulation on two or more consecutive episodes of testing. (This had been established as the criterion for success in many previous clinical trials.)

Results. The total number of episodes of no sensation on maximal stimulation in first molars over the period of the trial (32 minutes) was greater for articaine (236 episodes) than for lidocaine (129) ($P < .001$). Twenty (64.5%) subjects experienced anesthetic success following articaine, whereas 12 (38.7%) did so with lidocaine ($P < .08$). The design of the trial allowed for a maximal possible duration of anesthesia of 28 minutes. Six subjects receiving articaine achieved 28 minutes of anesthesia compared with 2 given lidocaine.

Discussion. The difference between articaine and lidocaine was most obvious toward the end of the study period. The percentage of patients showing no response at maximal stimulation was reduced at all reference points after 22 minutes with lidocaine. With articaine, however, the greatest percentage of nonresponders was noted at the end of the trial (32 minutes).

Conclusion. Overall, 4% articaine with epinephrine was more effective than 2% lidocaine with epinephrine in producing pulpal anesthesia in lower molars following buccal infiltration.

Robertson D, Nusstein J, Reader A, et al: The anesthetic efficacy of articaine in buccal infiltration of mandibular posterior teeth, J Am Dent Assoc 138:1104–1112, 2007.[60]

Design. A total of 60 blinded subjects randomly received buccal infiltration injections of 1.8 mL of 2% lidocaine with epinephrine 1:100,000 and 4% articaine with epinephrine 1:100,000 in two separate appointments at least 1 week apart. Each subject served as his/her own control. Sixty infiltrations were administered on the right side, and 60 on the left side. For the second infiltration in each subject, the investigator used the same side randomly chosen for the first infiltration. The teeth chosen for evaluation were the first and second molars and the first and second premolars. The same investigator administered all injections. Before injections were administered, baseline values were determined on the experimental teeth with EPT. A single infiltration was administered buccal to the first mandibular molar, bisecting the approximate location of the mesial and distal roots. The 1.8 mL was deposited over a period of 1 minute. One minute after injection, the first and second molars were pulp tested. At 2 minutes, the premolars were tested. At 3 minutes, the control canine (contralateral side) was tested. This testing cycle was repeated every 3 minutes for 60 minutes. Complete absence of sensation to maximal EPT stimulation on two or more consecutive readings was the criterion for successful anesthesia. The onset of anesthesia was defined as the time at which the first of two consecutive no responses to EPT of 80 occurred.

Results. Articaine was significantly better than lidocaine in achieving pulpal anesthesia in each of the four teeth ($P < .0001$ for all four teeth). Table 20-3 summarizes these findings.

The onset of successful anesthesia was significantly faster for articaine than for lidocaine for all four teeth tested (Table 20-4).

Discussion. The exact mechanism of the increased efficacy of articaine is not known. One theory relates to the 4% concentration of articaine versus the 2% lidocaine solution. However, Potocnik and coworkers found that 4% and 2% articaine formulations were superior to 2% lidocaine in blocking nerve conduction.[62] A second theory is that the thiophene ring of articaine enables it to diffuse more effectively than the benzene ring found in other local anesthetics.

Regarding onset of anesthesia, previous studies of lidocaine following IANB found onset times ranging from 8

TABLE 20-3
Success Rate in Achieving Pulpal Anesthesia-Articaine versus Lidocaine

Tooth	Articaine, % Success*	Lidocaine, % Success*
Second molar	75	45
First molar	87	57
Second premolar	92	67
First premolar	86	61

Modified from Robertson D, Nusstein J, Reader A, et al: The anesthetic efficacy of articaine in buccal infiltration of mandibular posterior teeth, J Am Dent Assoc 138:1104–1112, 2007.
*$P < .0001$ for all four teeth.

TABLE 20-4
Onset Time (Minutes) of Pulpal Anesthesia-Articaine versus Lidocaine

Tooth	Articaine Onset (Min) ± Standard Deviation	Lidocaine Onset (Min) ± Standard Deviation	*P* Value
Second molar	4.6 ± 4.0	11.1 ± 9.5	.0001
First molar	4.2 ± 3.1	7.7 ± 4.3	.0002
Second premolar	4.3 ± 2.3	6.9 ± 6.6	.0014
First premolar	4.7 ± 2.4	6.3 ± 3.1	.0137

Modified from Robertson D, Nusstein J, Reader A, et al: The anesthetic efficacy of articaine in buccal infiltration of mandibular posterior teeth, J Am Dent Assoc 138:1104–1112, 2007.

to 11 minutes for the first molar, and from 8 to 12 minutes for the first premolar.[63-68] Articaine provided a more rapid onset of pulpal anesthesia for all tested teeth than for IANB. However, pulpal anesthesia declined steadily over the 60 minute test period. Therefore, if profound pulpal anesthesia is required for 60 minutes, buccal infiltration of 4% articaine with epinephrine 1:100,000 will not provide the duration needed because of declining pulpal anesthesia.

Conclusion. Buccal infiltration of the first mandibular molar with 1.8 mL of 4% articaine with epinephrine 1:100,000 is significantly better than a similar infiltration of 2% lidocaine with epinephrine 1:100,000 in achieving pulpal anesthesia in mandibular posterior teeth. Clinicians should keep in mind that pulpal anesthesia will likely decline slowly over 60 minutes.

Haase A, Reader A, Nusstein J, et al: Comparing anesthetic efficacy of articaine versus lidocaine as a supplemental buccal infiltration of the mandibular first molar after an inferior alveolar nerve block, J Am Dent Assoc 139:1228–1235, 2008.[61]

Design. Seventy-three subjects participated in a prospective, randomized, double-blind, crossover study comparing the degree of pulpal anesthesia achieved by means of mandibular buccal infiltration of two anesthetic solutions: 4% articaine with epinephrine 1:100,000 and 2% lidocaine with epinephrine 1:100,000, following an IANB with 4% articaine with epinephrine 1:100,000. Subjects served as their own controls. The side chosen for the first infiltration was used again for the second infiltration. Injections were administered at least 1 week apart. The same investigator administered all injections. An EPT was used to test the first molar for anesthesia in 3 minute cycles for 60 minutes. The IANB was administered over 60 seconds. Fifteen minutes after completion of the IANB, the infiltration was administered buccal to the first mandibular molar, bisecting the approximate location of the mesial and distal roots. The 1.8 mL was deposited over a period of 1 minute. Sixteen minutes after completion of the IANB (1 minute following the infiltration), EPT testing of the first molar was performed. At 3 minutes, the contralateral canine was tested. This cycle was repeated every 3 minutes for 60 minutes. Anesthesia was considered successful when two consecutive EPT readings of 80 were obtained within 10 minutes of the IANB and infiltration injection, and the 80 reading was maintained continuously through the 60th minute.

Results. The articaine formulation was significantly better than the lidocaine formulation with regard to anesthetic success: 88% versus 71% for lidocaine ($P < .01$), with anesthesia developing within 10 minutes after IANB and buccal infiltration, sustaining the 80 reading on the EPT continuously for the 60 minute testing period.

Discussion. Anesthetic success was significantly better with the 4% articaine formulation than with the 2% lidocaine formulation. Both anesthetic formulations demonstrated a gradual increase in pulpal anesthesia. This is likely a result of the effect of the infiltrations' overcoming failure or the slow onset of anesthesia following IANB. Therefore, for a maximum effect with the 4% articaine infiltration, a waiting time is required before onset of pulpal anesthesia is achieved. It may be prudent to wait for signs of lip numbness before administering the infiltration. Without an effective IANB, buccal infiltration of articaine alone has a relatively short duration (see previous two citations). A fairly high percentage of patients receiving the articaine infiltration maintained pulpal anesthesia through the 50th minute. Articaine infiltration demonstrated a decline in the incidence of pulpal anesthesia after the 52nd minute. Because most dental procedures require less than 50 minutes for completion, this injection protocol should prove successful for most dental treatments. The 2% lidocaine demonstrated a decline after the 60th minute.

Conclusion. Buccal infiltration of the first molar with a cartridge of 4% articaine with epinephrine 1:100,000 resulted in a significantly higher success rate (88%) than was attained with buccal infiltration of a cartridge of 2% lidocaine with epinephrine 1:100,000 (71%) after IANB with 4% articaine with epinephrine 1:100,000.

Kanaa MD, Whitworth JM, Corbett IP, et al: Articaine buccal infiltration enhances the effectiveness of lidocaine inferior alveolar nerve block, Int Endod J 42:238–246, 2009.[41]

Design. The goal of this study was to compare mandibular tooth anesthesia following lidocaine IANB with and without supplementary articaine buccal infiltration. In this prospective, randomized, double-blind, crossover study, 36 subjects received two IANB injections with 2.2 mL lidocaine 2% with epinephrine 1:80,000 over two visits. At one visit, infiltration of 2.2 mL of articaine 4% with epinephrine 1:100,000 was administered in the mucobuccal fold opposite the mandibular first molar. At the other visit, a dummy injection was performed. At least 1 week separated the two visits. Pulpal anesthesia of the first molar, the first premolar, and the lateral incisor teeth was assessed with an EPT every 2 minutes for the first 10 minutes, and then at 5 minute intervals for 45 minutes post injection. Successful anesthesia was the absence of sensation on two or more consecutive maximal EPT stimulations. The number of episodes of no response to maximal EPT stimulation was recorded. The onset of pulpal anesthesia was considered the first episode of no response to maximal stimulation (two consecutive readings), whereas the duration of anesthesia was taken as the time from the first of at least two consecutive maximal readings with no response until the onset of more than two responses at less than maximal stimulation, or the end of the 45 minute test period, whichever was sooner.

Results. IANB with supplemental articaine infiltration produced greater success than IANB alone in first molars (33 vs. 20 subjects, respectively; $P < .001$), premolars (32 vs. 24;

TABLE 20-5
Articaine Buccal Infiltration Enhances the Effectiveness of Lidocaine Inferior Alveolar Nerve Block

	First Molar	First Premolar	Lateral Incisor
Success IANB + dummy	55.6%	66.7%	19.4%
Success IANB + infiltration	91.7% (*P* <.001)	88.9% (*P* =.021)	77.8% (*P* <.001)
Onset (mean) IANB + dummy (minutes)	6.8	8.9	10.9
Onset (mean) IANB + infiltration (minutes)	4.5 (*P* <.06)	4.2 (*P* <.002)	6.9 (*P* =.40)
Duration of pulpal anesthesia (mean) IANB + dummy (minutes)	29.0	31.3	29.1
Duration of pulpal anesthesia (mean) IANB + infiltration (minutes)	38.8 (*P* <.001)	37.8 (*P* =.013)	30.0 (*P* =.90)

Modified from Kanaa MD, Whitworth JM, Corbett IP, et al: Articaine buccal infiltration enhances the effectiveness of lidocaine inferior alveolar nerve block, Int Endod J 42:238–246, 2009.

P =.021), and lateral incisors (28 vs. 7; *P* <.001). Additionally, IANB with articaine supplemental infiltration produced significantly more episodes of no response than IANB alone for first molars (339 cases vs. 162, respectively; *P* <.001), premolars (333 cases vs. 197; *P* <.001), and lateral incisors (227 cases vs. 63; *P* <.001) (Table 20-5).

Discussion. Onset of pulpal anesthesia In this study, the anesthetic effect for mandibular first molars peaked 25 minutes post injection with the dummy injection versus 6 minutes following articaine infiltration. For first premolars, peak anesthetic effect occurred at 30 minutes post injection versus 8 minutes following articaine infiltration, and for lateral incisors, peak anesthetic effect occurred at 40 minutes post injection versus 20 minutes following articaine infiltration in the first molar region.

Duration of pulpal anesthesia The maximum duration of anesthesia possible in this trial was 43 minutes. Duration of pulpal anesthesia was significantly longer for first molars and first premolars, but not for lateral incisors.

Conclusions. IANB injection supplemented with articaine buccal infiltration was more successful than IANB alone for pulpal anesthesia in mandibular teeth. Articaine infiltration increased the duration of pulpal anesthesia in premolar and molar teeth when given in combination with a lidocaine IANB and produced more rapid onset for premolars.

These four clinical trials clearly demonstrate that articaine by mandibular buccal infiltration in the mucobuccal fold by the first mandibular molar can provide more successful anesthesia of longer duration to mandibular teeth when administered alone or as a supplement to IANB.

One thing to consider is that in each of these trials, buccal infiltration of articaine was administered adjacent to the first mandibular molar. The trials demonstrated the effectiveness of articaine in improving pulpal anesthesia success rates in molars and premolars. However, success rates and duration of anesthesia were not improved as significantly in lateral incisors (i.e., teeth at a distance from the site of local anesthetic deposition).

In 2002, Meechan and Ledvinka studied the effects of infiltrating 1.0 mL of 2% lidocaine with 1:80,000 epinephrine buccally or lingually to the mandibular central incisor.[56] A success rate of 50% was achieved with the buccal or the lingual injection site. However, when the injection dose was split (0.5 mL per site) between buccal *and* lingual, the success rate increased to a statistically significant 92%.

Jaber and colleagues used a split dose (0.9 mL per site) of 2% lidocaine with 1:100,000 epinephrine to confirm this finding.[69] For buccal infiltration of 1.8 mL alone, successful anesthesia of the central incisor was 77%, and it was 97% for the split buccal/lingual dose. Investigators also compared articaine 4% with epinephrine 1:100,000 versus lidocaine 2% with epinephrine 1:100,000 as an anesthetic for infiltration in the anterior mandible and found that articaine was superior to lidocaine in obtaining pulpal anesthesia of the central incisor when infiltrated adjacent to the tooth buccally alone (94%) or in split buccal/lingual injections (97%).

The increased success rate for infiltration in the adult mandibular incisor region is thought to be due to the fact that the cortical plate of bone, both buccal and lingual, is thin and might provide little resistance to infiltration.

Developments Since the 5th Edition. Although anecdotal reports and several studies had hinted at the efficacy of articaine in providing pulpal anesthesia following administration via mandibular infiltration in adults, it had not received serious consideration at the time the 5th edition of this textbook was published in 2004.

Summary and Conclusions

Failure rates for profound pulpal anesthesia following traditional IANB on non–pulpally involved teeth are quite high. This has led to the development of several alternative techniques, including the Gow-Gates mandibular nerve block, the Akinosi-Vazirani closed-mouth mandibular nerve block, periodontal ligament injection, and intraosseous anesthesia. The introduction of the articaine HCl has spurred interest in the use of this local anesthetic by infiltration in the adult mandible.

Initial studies in which articaine was infiltrated in the buccal fold adjacent to the first mandibular molar showed significantly greater success rates compared with lidocaine 2% infiltration (all with epinephrine). Additional studies using articaine mandibular infiltration (by the first molar) as a supplement to IANB (with lidocaine or articaine) revealed the same significant increases. In each of these studies, a full cartridge of local anesthetic (1.8 mL or 2.2 mL) was administered. Future studies are called for to determine the minimal volume of LA solution needed to produce the best clinical result. At this time, the recommendation is to administer a full cartridge of articaine 4% with epinephrine 1:100,000 (or 1:200,000) in the mucobuccal fold adjacent to the mandibular first molar when treating molars or premolars in the adult mandible.

When mandibular incisors are treated, the recommendation is to administer a split dose of articaine, 0.9 mL in the buccal fold adjacent to the tooth being treated and 0.9 mL on the lingual aspect of the same tooth. Splitting of the LA dose is *not* effective in the mandibular molar region.

The articaine mandibular infiltration injection can be repeated later in the dental procedure if pulpal anesthesia begins to wane and the patient starts to become sensitive.

An EPT can be used effectively to assess pulpal anesthesia before invasive dental treatment is started.[60] Studies have demonstrated that absence of patient response to an 80 reading was an assurance of pulpal anesthesia in vital asymptomatic teeth.[70,71] Two consecutive EPT readings at maximal output (80 μA) 2 or 3 minutes apart is almost always indicative of profound anesthesia. Certosimo and Archer reported that patients who had EPT readings of less than 80 experienced pain during operative procedures in asymptomatic teeth.[71]

INTRANASAL LOCAL ANESTHESIA

Absorption of drugs through the nasal mucosa to achieve a systemic effect has a long and varied history. The nares are extremely vascular, so most drugs instilled into them will be absorbed rapidly and distributed systemically (Fig. 20-10). "Snorting a line" of cocaine is an example of illicit use of this route of drug administration. Critical care medicine has used intranasal (IN) drug administration of the central nervous system (CNS)-depressant drug midazolam in the management of status epilepticus in young children.[72-74] Lahat and associates compared IN midazolam (0.2 mg/kg) versus intravenous (IV) diazepam (0.3 mg/kg) in 47 children aged 6 months to 5 years.[72] Twenty-three of 26 seizures were terminated with IN midazolam—24 of 26 with IV diazepam. The speed at which seizures were terminated was considerably faster with IN midazolam (5.5 minutes) than with IV diazepam (8.0 minutes).

Pediatric dentistry has utilized IN sedation dating as far back as the early 1990s.[75-78] The dosage of midazolam most often cited as most effective and safe is 0.2 mg/kg—the same dose employed in critical care medicine for termination of seizures.

Intranasal instillation of local anesthetics has been employed in medicine primarily in the realm of ear nose and throat (ENT) procedures.[79,80] Tetracaine, an ester-type local anesthetic, is commonly used to provide a numbing effect before surgical manipulations in the nose. Many patients receiving IN tetracaine have commented on how their upper teeth felt numb, sparking interest in a possible dental application of IN local anesthetic. For dental application, the vasoconstrictor oxymetazoline was added to the tetracaine to enhance effectiveness. Oxymetazoline is the active ingredient in the nasal decongestant spray, Afrin.

In a Phase II double-blind, randomized clinical trial, Ciancio and colleagues compared IN tetracaine with oxymetazoline versus injectable lidocaine 2% with 1:100,000 epinephrine in providing pulpal anesthesia bilaterally in the maxilla from first molar to first molar (teeth #3 through #14)[81] (Fig. 20-11). Success was defined as the ability to accomplish the dental procedure without the need for rescue medication (injectable local anesthetic) (Fig. 20-12). The tetracaine nasal spray group had a success rate of 88% (22 of 25) versus 93% (14 of 15) in the lidocaine injection group. In the IN group, all failures to achieve adequate pulpal anesthesia occurred on first molars (#3 or #14). Teeth #4 through #13 had 100% success.[81]

Phase III clinical trials have just begun as this text is being written (October 2011).

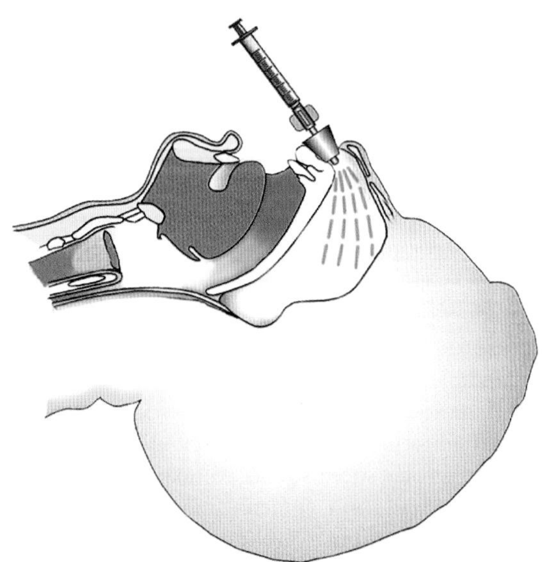

Figure 20-10. Intranasal instillation of local anesthesia.

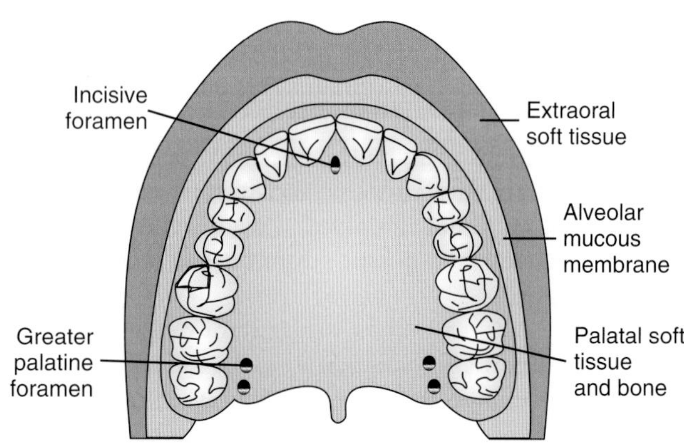

Figure 20-11. Diagram of extent of intranasal local anesthesia.

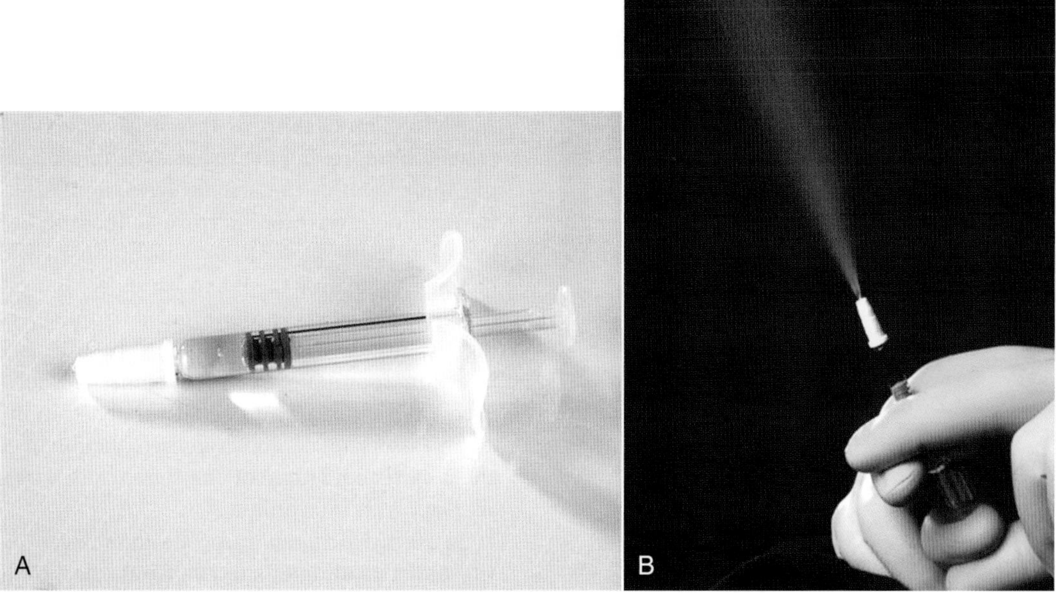

Figure 20-12. Intranasal local anesthesia device. (Photos courtesy St. Renatus, LLC, Ft Collins, Colo.)

Developments Since the 5th Edition. Intranasal local anesthetic administration was not yet a consideration when the 5th edition of this textbook was published in 2004.

COMPUTER-CONTROLLED LOCAL ANESTHETIC DELIVERY (C-CLAD)

During the late 1880s, physicians Sigmund Freud, Carl Koller, and William Halsted were pursuing a common area of clinical research: the development of the drug benzoylmethyl ecognine, more commonly known today as cocaine, for medicinal use and for application as the first local anesthetic.[82]

Although Freud and Koller were the first to notice the anesthetic effects of cocaine, it was Halsted who introduced cocaine as a local anesthetic in dentistry.[83] Using a hypodermic syringe, Halsted demonstrated that interstitial injection of aqueous cocaine resulted in an effective nerve block of the inferior alveolar nerve, and that a small amount of anesthetic solution injected into the trunk of a sensory and motor nerve resulted in blockage of sensory and motor function from the terminal nerve branches. This discovery represented the starting point for local pain control in both dentistry and medicine as we know it today.

This pioneering event relied on the required knowledge of bringing together three separate elements: a drug, a drug delivery instrument, and an anatomic technique. Each of these components had the potential to influence the success or failure of achieving the desired result. The drug delivery instrument commonly known as the hypodermic syringe as used by Halsted was a simple hand-driven mechanical instrument developed in 1853 by the French general surgeon Charles Gabriel Pravas.[84] It consisted of a hollow-bore needle connected to a fluid-containing chamber with a sealed plunger. Remarkably, the basic design, mechanics, and manual operation of the Pravaz syringe, invented more than 150 years ago, were virtually identical to those of medical and dental syringes in current use.

What have we learned over the past century about local anesthetic delivery systems? What do clinical data reveal about their common use today? Aside from the noted obvious benefit in providing a convenient means of delivery of a liquid drug, we know (numerous dental studies and consumer surveys have documented this) that the dental syringe predictably invokes fear and anxiety in our patients.[85-87] The term *trypanophobia* (needle phobia) is the extreme and irrational fear of medical and dental procedures involving injection. It is estimated that nearly one in five adults are dental phobics who will avoid, cancel, or fail to appear for required dental treatment because of their fear of the dental injection.[88,89]

In 1997, a new local anesthetic delivery system was introduced.[90] Originally called The Wand (later renamed The CompuDent/Wand; Milestone Scientific, Inc., Livingston, NJ), it represented the first computer-controlled local anesthetic delivery (C-CLAD) system (Fig. 20-13). Within but a few years, C-CLAD technology had helped to redefine our perception and, even more important, the perception of our patients, as to how local anesthesia can and could be achieved.[91]

C-CLAD devices provide clinicians with the ability to precisely control the rate of delivery of the local anesthetic solution.[92] In addition, C-CLAD introduced the concept of using a disposable handpiece weighing less than 10 g, allowing the clinician to hold it in a pen-like fashion, greatly increasing tactile control and improving dexterity during injection[90] (Fig. 20-14). C-CLAD devices represent a significant advancement for subcutaneous injections and have

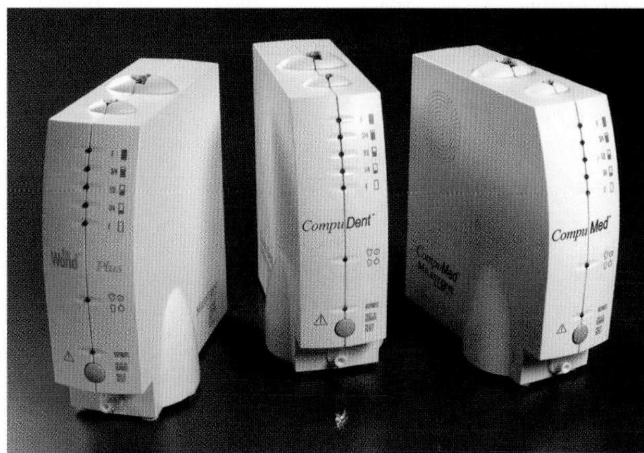

Figure 20-13. Early computer-controlled local anesthetic delivery (C-CLAD) devices (1997-2005). (Photo courtesy Milestone Scientific, Livingstone, NJ.)

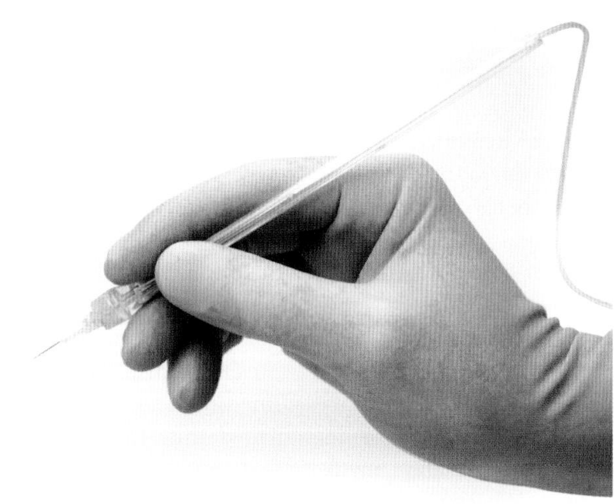

Figure 20-14. Lightweight handpiece for computer-controlled local anesthetic delivery (C-CLAD). (Photo courtesy Milestone Scientific, Livingstone, NJ.)

markedly improved outcomes and experiences for millions of patients over the past decade, helping to mitigate the "fear factor" that has become so closely linked to the dental visit.[93-97]

As a result of this new technology, several new injection techniques were introduced. The first was the anterior middle superior alveolar (AMSA) nerve block (NB), described in 1997 by Friedman and Hochman.[96] The AMSA NB achieves maxillary anesthesia of multiple maxillary teeth from a single palatal injection site without the undesired collateral anesthesia to the lip and face. (The AMSA injection is described in Chapter 13.) Subsequently, Friedman and Hochman introduced a technique that they named the palatal-approach anterior superior alveolar (P-ASA) nerve block, in which dental and soft tissue anesthesia of the central and lateral incisors is achieved by a single palatal injection.[97] This appears to be the first dental injection that allows practitioners to anesthetize multiple maxillary teeth across the midline during administration of a local anesthetic. (The P-ASA injection is described in Chapter 13.)

A third innovation of this new delivery instrument is related to improving the success rate of the IANB by reducing and/or eliminating needle deflection.[98] The IANB injection technique was modified to include use of the bi-rotational insertion technique (BRIT), which is used with the Wand handpiece. Holding the Wand handpiece in a pen-like grasp, the clinician can easily rotate it while simultaneously advancing the needle in a forward direction. This bi-rotational insertion technique has been clinically shown to reduce needle deflection during deep tissue penetration.[98,99] Aboushala and associates demonstrated a reduction in missed IANBs and a more rapid onset of anesthesia caused by the increased accuracy of this technique.[99]

In 2001, Hochman and colleagues advanced the science and understanding of subcutaneous injection fluid dynamics by identifying a predictable method for measuring the precise value of fluid exit-pressure in situ (at the tip of the needle) during drug administration.[100] This led to the next significant improvement in C-CLAD technology—the development of an instrument for medical and dental injections capable of controlling all variables of a subcutaneous injection event. This instrument was initially named the CompuFlo (Milestone Scientific).

The CompuFlo technology consists of a C-CLAD device that precisely regulates fluid pressure at the needle tip while a subcutaneous injection or aspiration is performed. The instrument provides the clinician with continuous real-time audible and visual feedback during the injection. The core technology includes a series of mathematical algorithms that function in concert with pressure transducers, allowing instantaneous real-time measurement of fluid exit-pressure at the tip of the needle. This approach to fluid injection dynamics is called *dynamic pressure-sensing (DPS) technology,* which was developed for the delivery and aspiration of medicaments.[101] DPS provides visual and audible in-tissue pressure feedback that helps to (1) identify tissue types for the health care provider; (2) show when certain types of tissue have been penetrated; and (3) ensure that injection of drugs occurs at the precise targeted location. Ghelber and coworkers were the first to publish clinical data related to a medical application for this innovative technology.[102] CompuFlo was clinically tested among several human pilot studies involving administration of epidural injections and succeeded in identifying false-positives of anesthesia.[103,104] Epidural administration is just one of the many medical and extra-medical applications identified for this sophisticated C-CLAD instrument.

In 2007, CompuFlo technology was applied in dentistry to address an important challenge: performing more predictable single-tooth anesthesia (e.g., the PDL injection). With the decreasing trend of generalized dental caries and the increasing trend toward site-specific treatment of an individual tooth, the use of nerve block anesthesia has

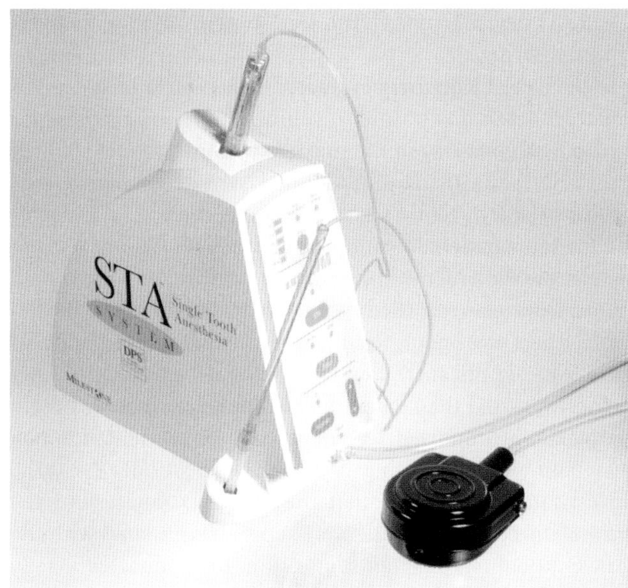

Figure 20-15. STA-Single Tooth Anesthesia computer-controlled local anesthetic delivery (C-CLAD) device incorporates dynamic pressure sensing (DPS) to aid in locating the precise site for periodontal ligament (PDL) injection. (Photo courtesy Milestone Scientific, Livingstone, NJ.)

become less necessary. Coupled with the unpredictable nature of the IANB, these trends have caused clinicians to look for a more predictable alternative.[105-107] To address these findings, the development of a new technology that uses a safer, more predictable approach to performing the PDL injection was pursued.[108,109] The STA-Single Tooth Anesthesia system allows dentists to perform a dental injection with real-time feedback, indicating when the needle tip is in the correct location when a dental injection is performed[108] (Fig. 20-15).The system incorporates the safety of using dynamic pressure-sensing technology, allowing low-pressure administration of local anesthetic drugs. This same technology allows the easy administration of any traditional injection that may be performed with a manual syringe, in addition to newer dental injections that were developed using C-CLAD instruments (e.g., AMSA, P-ASA, STA-Intraligamentary [PDL] injections).

Over the past decade, numerous clinical trials have been conducted to evaluate the validity and use of this new drug delivery technology for dentistry.[110-113] The largest cohort of studies has been related to pain-disruptive behavior in the pediatric dental population.[114-121] Two recent publications from Ashkenazi and associates have confirmed several consistent findings, including a measurable reduction in pain-disruptive behavior in children receiving a C-CLAD injection[122] and the clinical effectiveness of the PDL injection as a primary injection in primary teeth.[123]

Ashkenazi and colleagues reported on a study population of 193 children, aged 2 to 13 years, after treating 159 mandibular molars and 48 maxillary molars.[123] They reported success rates of 97% mandibular molars and 96% maxillary molars for restorative dentistry treatment when C-CLAD technology was used as the primary dental injection technique. Ashkenazi concluded that pain-disruptive behavior was consistently reported as "relatively nonstressful" for patients, and that a change in the behavior management mode was not required. In essence, dental local anesthesia using low-pressure intrasulcular PDL injection was nondisruptive to these patients. The study concluded that using a C-CLAD device resulted in higher success rates for single-tooth anesthesia, in addition to general absence of pain-disruptive behavior in the pediatric dental patient.

In 2010, Ashkenazi and coworkers published the results of a long-term, controlled clinical study evaluating developmental effects on unerupted permanent teeth following use of a regulated low-pressure PDL injection performed with the STA-System instrument.[123] The study population consisted of 78 children (aged 4.1 to 12.8 years) who received STA-Intraligamentary (PDL) injections to 166 primary molar teeth.[123] A structured form was designed to include information regarding age at treatment, gender, type of treated tooth, tooth location, type of dental treatment, and type of developmental disturbance(s) present in associated permanent tooth. For each patient, teeth that received conventional dental anesthesia or teeth that were not anesthetized previously served as intrapatient controls. Upon reviewing data collected between 1999 and 2007, Ashkenazi and associates concluded that performing the PDL injection with the use of a low-pressure C-CLAD injection instrument, specifically, the STA-System with dynamic pressure sensing, did not produce damage to the underlying developing permanent tooth bud.[123]

This finding is important because it represents a new perspective on the PDL injection technique, which contrasts with the long-held position of Brannstrom and colleagues, whose previously published data demonstrated that a PDL injection performed on primary teeth using a hand-controlled high-pressure syringe (e.g., traditional syringe) resulted in developmental disturbances of the underlying tooth bud and had influenced a generation of practitioners.[124] Ashkenazi's findings conclusively demonstrated that use of a precisely regulated low-pressure C-CLAD instrument to perform the PDL injection on primary teeth produced a different outcome based on fluid-pressure differences known between the manual hand-driven syringe and a C-CLAD instrument.[123]

One can conclude upon reviewing the dental literature that a consensus has been reached over the past 10 years supporting the use of a C-CLAD system to perform dental local anesthesia in the pediatric patient and in the adult patient population. The collective data support the clinical rationale, with the consistent finding of a marked and measurable reduction in pain-disrupted behavior compared with the standard syringe. The following groups have published data supporting this position: Versloot and associates,[125] Ram and Kassirer,[126] Palm and colleagues,[127] Oztas and coworkers,[128] Gibson and associates,[129] and Allen and colleagues.[130]

Versloot, Veerkamp, and Hoogstraten compared the behavioral reactions of 125 children, aged 4 to 11 years, who received dental local anesthesia with a traditional syringe compared with a C-CLAD instrument.[125] The occurrence of muscle tension, crying, verbal protest, movement, and resistance was scored on the Venham Distress Scale by two independent observers at 15 second intervals. Parents completed the Dental Subscale of the children's Fear Survey Schedule. Results demonstrated a measurable reduction in overall behavior reactions and patient anxiety when C-CLAD injections were used as compared with the standard syringe. The C-CLAD system demonstrated its greatest effect on low-anxiety children by producing the most positive reaction, making the C-CLAD system useful in treatment of the pediatric patient.

Ram and Kassirer compared the reactions of 138 children, 24 to 38 months old, who received dental local anesthesia of the maxillary incisors by comparing a C-CLAD system with a conventional syringe.[126] PDL and P-ASA injection techniques using a C-CLAD instrument were compared with conventional supraperiosteal buccal infiltration performed with a traditional syringe. Behavior reactions related to crying, facial expression, and eye squeeze were independently scored for each injection. Results demonstrated that children receiving the C-CLAD instrument injection displayed better overall behavior than those given supraperiosteal buccal infiltration injection performed with a traditional syringe. The authors concluded that the C-CLAD instrument provided a benefit in treatment of the pediatric patient and recommended its use in this population.

Palm, Kirkegaard, and Poulsen studied the perception of pain and the onset of anesthesia following IANB administered with a C-CLAD device and a traditional dental anesthesia syringe.[127] A split-mouth design was used, with each patient serving as his or her own control. Thirty-three patients between the ages of 7 and 18 years were included. All patients were blindfolded, and a sound from the C-CLAD instrument was heard during each injection. Pain ratings were scored on a 10 point Visual Analog Pain-Perception Scale. Results showed that the C-CLAD instrument produced significantly lower pain ratings than were produced by the traditional syringe. Time to onset of anesthesia was similar in this study. Researchers concluded that using a C-CLAD instrument is more effective in reducing subjective pain perception compared with a traditional syringe when IANB is performed.

Oztas, Tezer, Bodur, and Dogan studied 25 children, aged 6 to 10 years, with each child serving as his or her own control.[128] Contralateral primary mandibular molars were treated in two separate visits with random use of the C-CLAD device or traditional syringe injection. Pain perception levels for each injection were assessed with the Eland Color Scale. Results of this study show that an overwhelming number of patients preferred the PDL injection performed with the C-CLAD device over IANB injection performed with a traditional syringe.

Jalevik and Klingberg evaluated 20 adolescents in need of bilateral surgical exposure of canines and/or extractions for orthodontic reasons in the maxilla.[120] Conventional infiltration anesthesia using a traditional syringe was compared with a palatal injection performed using the C-CLAD device on the same patient. A randomized study design was used to determine the order of injection, and scoring of patient pain perceptions was recorded using a visual analog scale immediately post treatment. Results indicate that the sensation of pain was significantly lower ($P < .01$) when the C-CLAD device was used than when the traditional syringe was used; patients who reported fear of injection experienced much less pain when receiving a C-CLAD injection ($P < .001$). Investigators concluded that the C-CLAD device and the palatal injection technique were superior compared with the conventional syringe and injection technique, especially among those who reported fear of injections.

Gibson and associates published results from 62 patients between the ages of 5 and 13 years who required dental local anesthesia.[129] Patients were randomly assigned a C-CLAD device or a traditional syringe injection. Pain ratings were recorded, and subjects rated their satisfaction with treatment. Investigators found that C-CLAD injections resulted in significantly fewer disruptive behaviors during initial moments of the injection. Nearly twice as many children receiving a traditional palatal injection were disruptive compared with those receiving a C-CLAD device injection. Disruptive behaviors included significantly increased intervals of crying and disruptive body movements. In addition, five times more patients receiving a traditional palatal injection required restraint compared with patients anesthetized with the C-CLAD device. Gibson and colleagues concluded by stating, "the C-CLAD instrument injection offers a valuable means of reducing the disruptive behavior of children during injections."[129]

Allen and coworkers studied 40 preschool patients between 2 and 5 years of age.[116] The purpose of the investigation was to evaluate the efficacy of a C-CLAD injection in reducing pain behavior in the preschool-aged child when compared with a traditional syringe. A C-CLAD palatal injection technique was compared with traditional syringe infiltration. Results demonstrated the largest difference related to the need for patient restraint, with only 3% of C-CLAD patients requiring restraint compared with 34% of the intervals for traditional syringe injections. Allen and associates concluded that preschool-aged children anesthetized with the C-CLAD device demonstrated significantly fewer disruptive behaviors when compared with those given a traditional injection regimen. Additionally, even with control applied for the increased duration of the injection, the slower rate of anesthetic delivery of the C-CLAD did appear to reliably reduce pain-related behavior in children. These young children were significantly less likely to cry or to move in a disruptive manner. The authors stated, "most impressively the results showed that none of the preschool-aged children exposed to the C-CLAD instrument required restraint during the initial interval, while nearly half of the children receiving a traditional injection required some type of immediate restraint. These results are important because they demonstrate that the C-CLAD instrument can significantly reduce disruptive behavior in a population of young children who are traditionally more difficult to manage. Reducing disruptive behavior in preschool-aged children is important not only because it creates a more positive experience for the child, but it also creates a more positive experience for the practitioner."[116]

Asarch and associates conducted a study of 57 patients between 5 and 13 years of age to evaluate pain-disruptive behavior and each subject's subjective pain perception when a traditional syringe injection was compared with the C-CLAD system injection.[114] IANB injection and palatal and buccal infiltration were the only injections administered, with each subject receiving a single injection. Authors stated the method of use for the C-CLAD device as follows: "A slow rate of administration was used prior to needle insertion. Upon evidence of negative aspiration, the fast-rate of administration was used." Pain perceptions were rated using a 10 point visual analog scale; pain behavior was evaluated by an external examiner, and subjects rated their overall satisfaction. Results of this study show no significant differences between the C-CLAD device and the traditional syringe. However, two subsequent studies published by three of Asarch's coauthors[116,129] found that Asarch's study design and methods were suspect and called into question whether injection methods and failure to identify specific injection sites were shortcomings in that study. Subsequently, two published studies were consistent with the findings of other research groups presenting on this topic (i.e., a reduction in pain-disruptive behavior and the ability to reduce fear during a dental injection).[116,129]

Consistent findings in the dental literature support the use of a C-CLAD device, reporting a significant reduction in general pain perception; a measurable reduction in disruptive pain behavior; and a substantial reduction in the need for restraint in the management of pediatric patients requiring dental local anesthesia.

Most recently, Ferrari and coworkers published data from 60 adult patients receiving a PDL injection and compared the STA-System device versus two other manual syringes: a high-pressure PDL syringe (Ligmaject, IMA Associates, Bloomington, Ind) and a traditional dental syringe.[130] EPT was performed on all tested teeth at regular intervals to determine success or failure, and the different instruments and techniques used were compared. In addition to pulp testing, patient subjective pain responses were recorded after treatment. Ferrari reported that the STA-System had 100% success in achieving pulpal anesthesia; in addition, rapid onset of anesthesia was observed. The PDL injection was used as the primary injection for restorative dental care in mandibular teeth in this study. All patients receiving the PDL injection with the STA device reported subjective pain responses of "minimal or no pain." In contrast, those receiving injections with one of the other two instruments (high-pressure mechanical syringe or conventional syringe) were found to have generally higher pain scores throughout the testing period and required repeated attempts to achieve a successful outcome. Researchers concluded that the STA-System device resulted in more predictable, more reliable, and more comfortable anesthesia than the high-pressure mechanical syringe and/or the conventional dental syringe.[130]

The STA-System device and its predecessors—The Wand, CompuDent, and the Midwest Comfort Control Syringe—(Dentsply Professional 901 West Oakton Street, Des Plaines, IL 60018) represent a material improvement over the traditional (antiquated) 150-year-old hand-driven manual dental syringe. C-CLAD devices have been shown to enable the dental practitioner to administer a more comfortable and less anxiety-provoking injection. The STA-System instrument adds to those previous advances by introducing dynamic pressure-sensing (DPS) technology that provides continuous real-time injection feedback and identification of specific patient tissues and has been shown to enhance the predictability of the PDL injection[130,131] (Fig. 20-16). This is accomplished while adverse tissue reactions are minimized, resulting in a safer, more positive patient and operator experience during administration of dental local anesthetics.[123]

Dental local anesthesia delivery has been changed with the introduction of C-CLAD devices. It can be expected that current and future C-CLAD devices will continue to permit clinicians to perform dental injections more

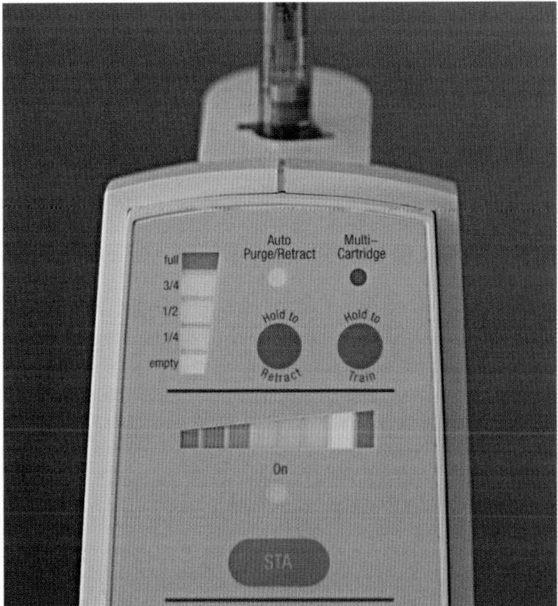

Figure 20-16. Dynamic pressure-sensing (DPS) technology that provides continuous real-time injection feedback and identification of specific patient tissues has been shown to enhance the predictability of the periodontal ligament (PDL) injection. (Photo courtesy Milestone Scientific, Livingstone, NJ.)

successfully and painlessly than in the past. No longer are primary advances in dental local anesthesia concentrated in the areas of pharmacology and pharmacokinetics. Instead, dentistry has entered an era in which advances in local anesthesia are being made by altering the fluid dynamics and physical means by which these drugs are administered to patients. Fifteen years has passed since the first C-CLAD device was introduced into dentistry (The Wand, 1997). It is understood by many in this field that future advances in dental pain control will be derived by improving the drug delivery system, in addition to the drugs used for dental local anesthesia.

Developments Since the 5th Edition. C-CLAD has been a part of this "Future Considerations" chapter ever since the late 1990s. At the present time (January 2012), it is safe to say with confidence that the concept of C-CLAD works (in enabling the LA administrator to provide essentially painless injections to patients). The numbers of dentists and physicians using C-CLAD are growing rapidly.

References

1. Malamed SF: Future considerations. In Handbook of local anesthesia, ed 5, St Louis, 2004, CV Mosby.
2. Catchlove RFH: The influence of CO_2 and pH on local anesthetic action, J Pharmacol Exp Ther 181:298–309, 1972.
3. Condouris GA, Shakalis A: Potentiation of the nerve-depressant effect of local anaesthetics by carbon dioxide, Nature 204:57–58, 1964.
4. Metzinger SE, Rigby PL, Bailey DJ, et al: Local anesthesia in blepharoplasty: a new look? South Med J 87:225–227, 1994.
5. Metzinger SE, Bailey DJ, Boyce RG, et al: Local anesthesia in rhinoplasty: a new twist? Ear Nose Throat J 71:405–406, 1992.
6. Stewart JH, Chinn SE, Cole GW, et al: Neutralized lidocaine with epinephrine for local anesthesia, part II, J Derm Surg Oncol 16:842–845, 1990.
7. Whitcomb M, Drum M, Reader A, et al: A prospective, randomized, double-blind study of the anesthetic efficacy of sodium bicarbonate buffered 2% lidocaine with 1:100,000 epinephrine in inferior alveolar nerve blocks, Anesth Prog 57:59–66, 2010.
8. Malamed SF, Hersh E, Poorsattar S, Falkel M. Reduction of local anesthetic injection pain using an automated dental anesthetic cartridge buffering system: A randomized, double-blind, crossover study, J Amer Dent Assoc October 2011.
9. Courtiss EH, Ransil BJ, Russo J: The effects of hyaluronidase on local anesthesia: a prospective, randomized, controlled, double-blind study, Plast Reconstr Surg 95:876–883, 1995.
10. Malamed SF, Yagiela JA: Pain control in dentistry, ADA News, September 15, 2007 (supplement).
11. American Dental Association: 2006 survey of dental practice—characteristics of dentists in private practice and their patients, Chicago, 2007, American Dental Association.
12. Malamed SF: The periodontal ligament (PDL) injection: an alternative to inferior alveolar nerve block, Oral Surg 53:117–121, 1982.
13. Kleber CH: Intraosseous anesthesia: implications, instrumentation and techniques, J Am Dent Assoc 134:487–491, 2003.
14. Yagiela JA: Local anesthetics. In Yagiela JA, Dowd FJ, Neidle EA, editors: Pharmacology and therapeutics for dentistry, ed 5, St Louis, 2004, CV Mosby, pp 251–270.
15. Hersh EV, Hermann DG, Lamp CJ, et al: Assessing the duration of mandibular soft tissue anesthesia, J Am Dent Assoc 126:1531–1536, 1995.
16. Rafique S, Fiske J, Banerjee A: Clinical trial of an air-abrasion/chemomechanical operative procedure for restorative treatment of dental patients, Caries Res 37:360–364, 2003.
17. College C, Feigal R, Wandera A, et al: Bilateral versus unilateral mandibular block anesthesia in a pediatric population, Pediatr Dent 22:453–457, 2000.
18. Tavares M, Goodson JM, Studen-Pavlovich D, et al: Reversal of soft tissue local anesthesia with phentolamine mesylate in pediatric patients, J Am Dent Assoc 139:1095–1104, 2008.
19. Smith MJ, Hutchins RC, Hehenberger D: Transcutaneous neural stimulation use in postoperative knee rehabilitation, Am J Sports Med 11:75–82, 1983.
20. Tuncel M, Ram VC: Hypertensive emergencies: etiology and management, Am J Cardiovasc Drugs 3:21–31, 2003.
21. Rhoney D, Peacock WF: Intravenous therapy for hypertensive emergencies, part 2, Am J Health-Syst Pharm 66:1448–1457, 2009.
22. Phentolamine, MD Consult, St Louis, September 3, 2010, CV Mosby, accessed June 26, 2011.
23. Simons FE, Lieberman RL, Read EJ Jr, et al: Hazards of unintentional injection of epinephrine from autoinjectors: a systematic review, Ann Allergy Asthma Immunol 102:282–287, 2009.
24. Zentgraf M, Ludwig G, Ziegler M: How safe is the treatment of impotence with intracavernous autoinjection? Eur Urol 16:165–171, 1989.
25. U.S. Food and Drug Administration (FDA): New dental anesthetic reversal agent receives FDA approval. May 12, 2008.
26. Hersh E, Moore P, Papas A, et al: Reversal of soft tissue local anesthesia with phentolamine mesylate in adolescents and adults, J Am Dent Assoc 139:1080–1093, 2008.
27. Tavares M, Goodson JM, Studen-Pavlovich D, et al: Reversal of soft tissue local anesthesia with phentolamine mesylate in pediatric patients, J Am Dent Assoc 139:1095–1104, 2008.
28. DePippo KL, Holas MA, Reding MJ: Validation of the 3-oz water swallow test for aspiration following stroke, Arch Neurol 49:1259–1261, 1991.
29. Heft M, Parker S: An experimental basis for revising the graphic rating scale for pain, Pain 19:153–161, 1984.
30. OraVerse prescribing information, San Diego, 2009, Novalar Pharmaceuticals.
31. Tavares M, Goodson JM, Studen-Pavlovich D, et al: Reversal of soft tissue local anesthesia with phentolamine mesylate in pediatric patients, J Am Dent Assoc 139:1095–1104, 2008.
32. Froum SJ, Froum SH, Malamed SF: The use of phentolamine mesylate to evaluate mandibular nerve damage following implant placement. Compendium 31:520, 522–528, 2010.
33. De St Georges J: How dentists are judged by patients, Dent Today 23:96, 98–99, 2004.
34. Friedman MJ, Hochman MN: The AMSA injection: a new concept for local anesthesia of maxillary teeth using a computer-controlled injection system, Quintessence Int 29:297–303, 1998.
35. Oulis CJ, Vadiakis GP, Vasilopoulou A: The effectiveness of mandibular infiltration compared to mandibular block

anesthesia in treating primary molars in children, Pediatr Dent 18:301–305, 1996.

36. Sharaf AA: Evaluation of mandibular infiltration versus block anesthesia in pediatric dentistry, J Dent Child 64:276–281, 1997.
37. Malamed SF: Local anesthetic considerations in dental specialties. In Malamed SF, editor: Handbook of local anesthesia, ed 5, St Louis, 2004, CV Mosby.
38. Bennett CR: Techniques of regional anesthesia and analgesia. In Bennett CR, editor: Monheim's local anesthesia and pain control in dental practice, ed 7, St Louis, 1984, CV Mosby.
39. Evers H, Haegerstam G: Anaesthesia of the lower jaw. In Evers H, Haegerstam G, editors: Introduction to dental local anaesthesia, Fribourg, Switzerland, 1990, Mediglobe SA.
40. Trieger N: New approaches to local anesthesia. In Pain control, ed 2, St Louis, 1994, CV Mosby.
41. Kanaa MD, Whitworth JM, Corbett IP, et al: Articaine buccal infiltration enhances the effectiveness of lidocaine inferior alveolar nerve block, Int Endod J 42:238–246, 2009.
42. Hannan L, Reader A, Nist R, et al: The use of ultrasound for guiding needle placement for inferior alveolar nerve blocks, Oral Surg Oral Med Oral Pathol Oral Radiol Endod 87:658–665, 1999.
43. Berns JM, Sadove MS: Mandibular block injection: a method of study using an injected radiopaque material, J Am Dent Assoc 65:736–745, 1962.
44. Galbreath JC: Tracing the course of the mandibular block injection, Oral Surg Oral Med Oral Pathol 30:571–582, 1970.
45. Reader A, American Association of Endodontists: Taking the pain out of restorative dentistry and endodontics: current thoughts and treatment options to help patients achieve profound anesthesia, Endodontics: Colleagues for Excellence. Winter 2009.
46. DeJong RH: Local anesthetics, St Louis, 1994, CV Mosby, pp 110–111.
47. Strichartz G: Molecular mechanisms of nerve block by local anesthetics, Anesthesiology 45:421–444, 1976.
48. Gow-Gates GA: Mandibular conduction anesthesia: a new technique using extraoral landmarks, Oral Surg Oral Med Oral Pathol 36:321–328, 1973.
49. Akinosi JO: A new approach to the mandibular nerve block, Br J Oral Surg 15:83–87, 1977.
50. Malamed SF: The periodontal ligament (PDL) injection—an alternative to inferior alveolar nerve block, Oral Surg 53:117–121, 1982.
51. Coggins R, Reader A, Nist R, et al: Anesthetic efficacy of the intraosseous injection in maxillary and mandibular teeth, Oral Surg Oral Med Oral Pathol 81:634–641, 1996.
52. Hanna MN, Elhassan A, Veloso PM, et al: Efficacy of bicarbonate in decreasing pain on intradermal injection of local anesthetics: a meta analysis, Reg Anesth Pain Med 34:122–125, 2009.
53. Meechan JG: Infiltration anesthesia in the mandible, Dent Clin N Am 54:621–629, 2010.
54. Rood JP: The analgesia and innervation of mandibular teeth, Br Dent J 140:237–239, 1976.
55. Yonchak T, Reader A, Beck M, et al: Anesthetic efficacy of infiltrations in mandibular anterior teeth, Anesth Prog 48:55–60, 2001.
56. Meechan JG, Ledvinka JI: Pulpal anaesthesia for mandibular central incisor teeth: a comparison of infiltration and intraligamentary injections, Int Endod J 35:629–634, 2002.
57. Haas DA, Harper DG, Saso MA, et al: Comparison of articaine and prilocaine anesthesia by infiltration in maxillary and mandibular arches, Anesth Prog 37:230–237, 1990.
58. Haas DA, Harper DG, Saso MA, et al: Lack of differential effect by Ultracaine (articaine) and Citanest (prilocaine) in infiltration anaesthesia, J Can Dent Assoc 57:217–223, 1991.
59. Kanaa MD, Whitworth JM, Corbett IP, et al: Articaine and lidocaine mandibular buccal infiltration anesthesia: a prospective randomized double-blind cross-over study, J Endod 32:296–298, 2006.
60. Robertson D, Nusstein J, Reader A, et al: The anesthetic efficacy of articaine in buccal infiltration of mandibular posterior teeth, J Am Dent Assoc 138:1104–1112, 2007.
61. Haase A, Reader A, Nusstein J, et al: Comparing anesthetic efficacy of articaine versus lidocaine as a supplemental buccal infiltration of the mandibular first molar after an inferior alveolar nerve block, J Am Dent Assoc 139:1228–1235, 2008.
62. Potocnik I, Tomsic M, Sketelj J, et al: Articaine is more effective than lidocaine or mepivacaine in rat sensory nerve conduction block in vitro, J Dent Res 85:162–166, 2006.
63. Vreeland DL, Reader A, Beck M, et al: An evaluation of volumes and concentrations of lidocaine in human inferior alveolar nerve block, J Endod 15:6–12, 1989.
64. Hinkley SA, Reader A, Beck M, et al: An evaluation of 4 percent prilocaine with 1:200,000 epinephrine and 2% mepivacaine with 1:20,000 levonordefrin compared with 2% lidocaine with 1:100,000 epinephrine for inferior alveolar nerve block, Anesth Prog 38:84–89, 1991.
65. Chaney MA, Kerby R, Reader A, et al: An evaluation of lidocaine hydrocarbonate compared with lidocaine hydrochloride for inferior alveolar nerve block, Anesth Prog 38:212–216, 1991.
66. McClean C, Reader A, Beck M, et al: An evaluation of 4% prilocaine and 3% mepivacaine compared with 2% lidocaine (1:100,000 epinephrine) for inferior alveolar nerve block, J Endod 19:146–150, 1993.
67. Ridenour S, Reader A, Beck M, et al: Anesthetic efficacy of a combination of hyaluronidase and lidocaine with epinephrine in inferior alveolar nerve blocks, Anesth Prog 48:9–15, 2001.
68. Steinkruger G, Nusstein J, Reader A, et al: The significance of needle bevel orientation in achieving a successful inferior alveolar nerve block, J Am Dent Assoc 137:1685–1691, 2006.
69. Jaber A, Whitworth JM, Corbett IP, et al: The efficacy of infiltration anesthesia for adult mandibular incisors: a randomized double-blind cross-over trial comparing articaine and lidocaine buccal and buccal plus lingual infiltrations, Br Dent J 209:E16, 2010.
70. Dreven LJ, Reader A, Beck M, et al: An evaluation of the electric pulp tester as a measure of analgesia in human vital teeth, J Endod 13:233–238, 1987.
71. Certosimo AJ, Archer RD: A clinical evaluation of the electric pulp tester as an indicator of local anesthesia, Oper Dent 21:25–30, 1996.
72. Lahat E, Goldman M, Barr J, et al: Comparison of intranasal midazolam with intravenous diazepam for treating febrile seizures in children: prospective randomised study, BMJ 321:83–86, 2000.
73. Owen R, Castle N: Intranasal midazolam, Emerg Med J 26:217–218, 2009.

74. Holsti M, Sill BL, Firth SD, et al: Prehospital intranasal midazolam for the treatment of pediatric seizures, Pediatr Emerg Care 23:148–153, 2007.
75. Fukota O, Braham RL, Yanase H, et al: The sedative effect of intranasal midazolam administration in the dental treatment of patients with mental disabilities. Part 1. The effect of a 0.2 mg/kg dose, J Clin Pediatr Dent 17:231–237, 1993.
76. Fuks AB, Kaufman E, Ram D, et al: Assessment of two doses of intranasal midazolam for sedation of young pediatric dental patients, Pediatr Dent 16:301–305, 1994.
77. Dallman JA, Ignelzi MA Jr, Briskie DM: Comparing the safety, efficacy and recovery of intranasal midazolam vs. oral chloral hydrate and promethazine, Pediatr Dent 23:424–430, 2001.
78. Lam C, Udin RD, Malamed SF, et al: Midazolam premedication in children: a pilot study comparing intramuscular and intranasal administration, Anesth Prog 52:56–61, 2005.
79. Chadha NK, Repanos C, Carswell AJ: Local anaesthesia for manipulation of nasal fractures: systematic review, J Laryngol Otol 123:830–836, 2009.
80. Jones TM, Nandapalan V: Manipulation of the fractured nose: a comparison of local infiltration anaesthesia and topical local anaesthesia, Clin Otolaryngol Allied Sci 24:443–446, 1999.
81. Ciancio S, Ayoub F, Pantera E, et al: Nasal spray for anesthesia of maxillary teeth. Poster presentation at International Association for Dental Research (IADR) General Session, July 14–17, 2010, Barcelona, Spain.
82. Liljestrand G: The historical development of local anesthesia, vol I, International encyclopedia of pharmacology and therapeutics: local anesthetics, New York, 1965, Pergamon Press, pp 546–549.
83. Hoffmann-Axtheim W: History of dentistry, Chicago, 1981, Quintessence.
84. Dobbs EC: A chronological history of local anesthesia in dentistry, J Oral Ther Pharmacol 1:546–549, 1965.
85. Milgrom P, Weinstein B, Kleinknect R: Treating fearful dental patients, Reston, Va, 1985, Reston Publishing.
86. Naini FB, Mellow AC, Getz T: Treatment of dental fears: pharmacology or psychology, Dental Update 26:270–276, 1999.
87. Dionne R, Phero J, Becker D: Management of pain and anxiety in the dental office, Philadelphia, 1985, Saunders.
88. Agras S, Sylvester D, Oliveau D: The epidemiology of common fears and phobia, Compr Psychiatry 10:151–156, 1979.
89. Kleinknecht RA, McGlynn FD, Thorndike RM, et al: Factor analysis of the dental fear survey with cross validation, J Am Dent Assoc 108:59–61, 1984.
90. Hochman MN, Chiarello D, Hochman CB, et al: Computerized local anesthetic delivery vs. traditional syringe technique: subjective pain response, N Y Dent J 63:24–29, 1997.
91. Clinical Research Associates: Local anesthesia, automated delivery, Clin Res Associates Newsltr 22:1–2, 1999.
92. Friedman MJ, Hochman MN: 21st century computerized injection for local pain control, Compend Contin Educ Dent 18:995–1003, 1997.
93. Murphy D: Ergonomics and the dental care worker, Washington, DC, 1998, American Public Health Association.
94. Yesilyurt C, Bulut G, Tasdemir T: Pain perception during inferior alveolar injection administered with the Wand or conventional syringe, Br Dent J 205:E10, discussion 258–259, 2008.
95. Krochak M, Friedman N: Using a precision-metered injection system to minimize dental injection anxiety, Compend Contin Educ Dent 19:137–148, 1998.
96. Friedman MJ, Hochman MN: The AMSA injection: a new concept for local anesthesia of maxillary teeth using a computer-controlled injection system, Quintessence Int 29:297–303, 1998.
97. Friedman MJ, Hochman MN: P-ASA block injection: a new palatal technique to anesthetize maxillary anterior teeth, J Esthet Dent 11:63–71, 1999.
98. Hochman MN, Friedman MJ: In vitro study of needle deflection: a linear insertion technique versus a bidirectional rotation insertion technique, Quintessence Int 31:33–39, 2000.
99. Aboushala A, Kugel G, Efthimiadis N, et al: Efficacy of a computer-controlled injection system of local anesthesia in vivo, IADR Abstract, 2000. Abstract #2775.
100. Hochman MN, inventor: Pressure/force computer controlled drug delivery system and the like, 2001, U.S. Patent #6,200,289.
101. Hochman MN, inventor: Computer controlled drug delivery system with dynamic pressure sensing, 2006, U.S. Patent #7,618,409.
102. Ghelber O, Gebhard R, Vora S, et al: Utilization of the CompuFlo in determining the pressure of the epidural space: a pilot study, Anesth Analg 100:S-189, 2005.
103. Ghelber O, Gebhard R, Szmuk P, et al: Identification of the epidural space—a pilot study of a new technique, Anesth Analg 100:S-255, 2005.
104. Ghelber O, Gebhard RE, Vora S, et al: Identification of the epidural space using pressure measurement with the CompuFlo injection pump—a pilot study, Reg Anesth Pain Med 33:346–352, 2008.
105. Kaufman E, Weinstein P, Milgrom P: Difficulties in achieving local anesthesia, J Am Dent Assoc 108:205–208, 1984.
106. Roda RS, Blanton PL: The anatomy of local anesthesia, Quintessence Int 25:27–38, 1994.
107. Meechan JG: Intraligamentary anaesthesia, J Dent 20:325–332, 1992.
108. Hochman MN: Single-tooth anesthesia: pressure sensing technology provides innovative advancement in the field of dental local anesthesia, Compendium 28:186–193, 2007.
109. Hochman MN, inventor: Drug infusion device with tissue identification using pressure sensing. 2008, U.S. Patent #7,449,008.
110. Nicholson JW, Berry TG, Summitt JB, et al: Pain perception and utility: a comparison of the syringe and computerized local injection techniques, Gen Dent 49:167–173, 2001.
111. Fukayama H: Research for improving local anesthesia method in dentistry, Kokubyo Gakkai Zasshi 77:169–175, 2010.
112. Rosenberg E: A computer-controlled anesthetic delivery system in a periodontal practice: patient satisfaction and acceptance, J Esthet Restor Dent 13:25–32, 2001.
113. Kudo M, Ohke H, Katagiri K, et al: The shape of local anesthetic injection syringes with less discomfort and anxiety: evaluation of discomfort and anxiety caused by various types of local anesthetic injection syringes in high level trait-anxiety people, J Japan Dent Soc Anesthesiol 29:173–178, 2001.
114. Asarch T, Allen K, Petersen B, et al: Efficacy of a computerized local anesthesia device in pediatric dentistry, Pediatr Dent 21:421–424, 1999.
115. Gibson RS, Allen K, Hutfless S, Beiraghi S: The Wand vs. traditional injection: a comparison of pain related behaviors, Pediatr Dent 22:458–462, 2000.

116. Allen KD, Kotil D, Larzelere RE, et al: Comparison of a computerized anesthesia device with a traditional syringe in preschool children, Pediatr Dent 24:315–320, 2002.
117. Palm AM, Kirkegaard U, Paulsen S: The Wand versus traditional injection for mandibular nerve block in children and adolescents: perceived pain and time of onset, Pediatr Dent 26:481–484, 2004.
118. Oztas N, Ulusu T, Bodur H, et al: The Wand in pulp therapy: an alternative to inferior alveolar nerve block, Quintessence Int 36:559–564, 2005.
119. Versloot J, Veerkamp JSJ, Hoogstraten J: Computerized anesthesia delivery system vs. traditional syringe: comparing pain and pain-related behavior in children, Eur J Oral Sci 113:448–493, 2005.
120. Jalevik B, Klingberg G: Sensation of pain when using computerized injection technique, the Wand, IADR Pan Federation, September 13–16, 2006. Dublin, Ireland. Abstract # 0070.
121. Ram D, Kassirer J: Assessment of a palatal approach-anterior superior alveolar (P-ASA) nerve block with the Wand in paediatric dental patients, Intern J Paediatr Dent 16:348–351, 2006.
122. Ashkenazi M, Blumer S, Eli I: Effective of computerized delivery of intrasulcular anesthetic in primary molars, J Am Dent Assoc 136:1418–1425, 2005.
123. Ashkenazi M, Blumer S, Eli I: Effect of computerized delivery intraligamental injection in primary molars on their corresponding permanent tooth buds, Intern J Paediatr Dent 20:270–275, 2010.
124. Brannstrom M, Nordenvall KJ, Hedstrom KG: Periodontal tissue changes after intraligamentary anesthesia, J Dent Child 49:417–423, 1982.
125. Versloot J, Veerkamp JSJ, Hoogstraten J: Computerized anesthesia delivery system vs. traditional syringe: comparing pain and pain-related behavior in children, Eur J Oral Sci 113:448–493, 2005.
126. Ram D, Kassirer J: Assessment of a palatal approach-anterior superior alveolar (P-ASA) nerve block with the Wand in paediatric dental patients, Intern J Paediatr Dent 16:348–351, 2006.
127. Palm AM, Kirkegaard U, Paulsen S: The Wand versus traditional injection for mandibular nerve block in children and adolescents: perceived pain and time of onset, Pediatr Dent 26:481–484, 2004.
128. Oztas N, Ulusu T, Bodur H, et al: The Wand in pulp therapy: an alternative to inferior alveolar nerve block, Quintessence Int 36:559–564, 2005.
129. Gibson RS, Allen K, Hutfless S, et al: The Wand vs. traditional injection: a comparison of pain related behaviors, Pediatr Dent 22:458–462, 2000.
130. Ferrari M, Cagidiaco MC, Vichi A, et al: Efficacy of the computer-controlled injection system STA, the Ligamaject, and the dental syringe for intraligamentary anesthesia in restorative patients, Intern Dent SA 11:4–12, 2010.
131. Hochman MN, Friedman MF, Williams WP, et al: Interstitial pressure associated with dental injections: a clinical study, Quintessence Int 37:469–476, 2006.

CHAPTER 21

Questions

LOCAL ANESTHETICS

QUESTION: Why is it said that intravascular administration of local anesthetics is dangerous when physicians frequently administer intravenous (IV) lidocaine to correct serious cardiac dysrhythmias?

Intravenous administration of local anesthetics is potentially hazardous at all times and in all patients. However, IV local anesthetics, such as lidocaine and procainamide, do have an important place in the management of pre-fatal ventricular dysrhythmias, such as premature ventricular contractions and ventricular tachycardia. Several factors, including weighing the risk versus the benefit, must be considered whenever local anesthetics are to be administered "safely" intravenously.

1. *The patient's physical status.* Patients receiving IV lidocaine or other antidysrhythmic drugs have potentially life-threatening cardiac dysrhythmias. The myocardium is highly irritable (usually secondary to ischemia), which is often the primary cause of the dysrhythmia. Local anesthetics are myocardial depressants. By depressing the myocardium, lidocaine decreases the incidence of dysrhythmias. However, patients with normal cardiac rhythms receiving IV local anesthetics will also have their myocardium depressed; their cardiac function may be impaired by the local anesthetic in this circumstance.
2. *The form of lidocaine used.* Lidocaine for IV use in the management of ventricular dysrhythmias, so-called cardiac lidocaine, is prepared in single-use ampules or prefilled syringes. These ampules and syringes contain only lidocaine and sodium chloride. The typical dental cartridge of lidocaine contains lidocaine, distilled water, vasopressor, sodium bisulfite, and sodium chloride. IV injection of these ingredients, in and of itself, might precipitate unwanted cardiovascular responses rather than terminate them.
3. *The rate of injection.* Lidocaine for antidysrhythmic use is titrated slowly into the cardiovascular system to achieve a therapeutic blood level in the myocardium. The accepted therapeutic blood level is 1.8 to 5 μg/mL. To achieve this, lidocaine is administered IV slowly and is titrated until ventricular dysrhythmias on the electrocardiogram (ECG) are eliminated—typically, a total dose of between 1.0 and 1.5 mg/kg. In the typical dental practice, a 1.8 mL cartridge of lidocaine (36 mg) is deposited in 15 seconds or less. The rate at which the drug is administered intravenously has a significant bearing on its peak blood level. Overly rapid IV administration results in lidocaine blood levels that quickly enter into the overdose range, whereas a more slowly administered dose results in blood levels well within the therapeutic range for terminating dysrhythmias.[1-6]
4. *Risk versus benefit.* An overdose reaction is always a possibility whenever IV lidocaine is administered. Even under controlled conditions in a hospital, adverse reactions related to overly high blood levels do develop.[1-6] The risk of administering local anesthetics intravenously always must be weighed against the potential benefit to be gained from their use. For high-risk patients with a specific life-threatening dysrhythmia, the benefit clearly outweighs the risk. For dental patients seeking relief from intraoral pain, IV local anesthetic administration confers no benefit yet adds many risks.

QUESTION: What should I do when a patient claims to be allergic to a local anesthetic?

Believe the patient! Do not use any form of local anesthetic (especially topical anesthetic preparations) on this patient until you are able to definitively determine whether a true, documented, reproducible allergy exists. Seek to determine what actually happened to the patient to prompt such a claim and how his or her "reaction" was managed. (A detailed discussion of this problem is found in Chapter 18.)

QUESTION: Are any local anesthetics safer than others? Some appear to be implicated more than others in adverse reactions.

No. When used properly, all currently available local anesthetic formulations are extremely safe and effective. "Used properly" is the key phrase. Aspiration before injection (to minimize the risk of intravascular administration) and slow administration of the drug are vital. A medical history and physical evaluation, to determine potential contraindications to specific local anesthetics or additives, must be completed before their use. Maximum dosage of a drug should be determined for a given patient and not exceeded. Charts for the most commonly used local anesthetics are found in Chapters 4 and 18. The figures cited are maximum recommended doses (MRDs). The stated MRD should be decreased in patients with certain medical complications and in older individuals. Most systemic reactions to local anesthetics are entirely preventable. Overdose reactions that have led to death or significant morbidity frequently result from the administration of too large a dose to a younger, lighter-weight, well-behaved patient requiring multiple quadrants of dental care, or, less commonly, after "accidental" IV administration. Psychogenic reactions, by far the most common adverse response to the administration of a local anesthetic, may be virtually eliminated through enhanced rapport with the patient, use of an atraumatic injection technique (see Chapter 11), placement of the patient in a supine position during injection, and ample doses of empathy.

QUESTION: Do some local anesthetics have a greater risk of producing nerve damage (e.g., paresthesia)?

Discussion in dental circles continues regarding 4% local anesthetic formulations and the reported incidence of paresthesia. Such concern started in 1995 with the publication of a paper by Haas and Lennon,[7] which stated the incidence of paresthesia following all local anesthetic solutions with 1:785,000. For 0.5%, 2%, and 3% local anesthetic, the calculated risk was 1:1,125,000, and for 4% local anesthetics, it was 1:485,000. A subsequent retrospective study from Denmark provided similar results.[8] Neither publication presents scientific documentation that 4% solutions are the cause of the paresthesia. Hillerup reported that 79% of the cases of paresthesia involved the lingual nerve, and 21% the inferior alveolar.[8] Malamed, responding to Hillerup's paper, suggested that the likely cause of lingual nerve damage associated with inferior alveolar nerve block administration is direct needle trauma to the lingual nerve, which lies directly in the path of needle insertion.[9] In response to the Hillerup paper, the Pharmacovigilance Committee of the European Union initiated an inquiry into these allegations. Its report, released on October 20, 2006, concluded, "Regarding articaine, the conclusion is that the safety profile of the drug has not significantly evolved since its initial launch (1998). Thus, no medical evidence exists to prohibit the use of articaine according to the current guidelines listed in the summary of product characteristics."[10] The Committee further reported, "All local anaesthetics may cause nerve damage (they are neurotoxic in nature). Nerve injuries may result from several incidents: mechanical trauma due to needle insertion, direct toxicity from the drug, and neural ischaemia." Their concluding statement read as follows: "There is no need for new experimental studies or clinical trials."

Another possible "etiology" of these reports, especially as related to articaine HCl, is a phenomenon in epidemiology known as the *Weber effect,* after Dr. J.C.P. Weber.[11] The Weber effect states that the number of reported adverse reactions to a drug rises until about the middle to the end of the second year of marketing; it peaks and then steadily declines, despite steadily increasing prescribing rates. The validity of the Weber effect has been demonstrated in many studies of adverse drug reactions.[12,13]

In 2007, Pogrel reported on 57 nonsurgical dental patients whom he evaluated for post–dental care paresthesia over a 3-year period.[14] He commented in the introduction to the paper, "We were aware of the discussion in dental circles as to the use of articaine for inferior alveolar nerve blocks, and are aware of recommendations suggesting that it not be used for IANBs. This was the predominant reason for submitting this paper at this time." Lidocaine was responsible for 35% of the cases of paresthesia, articaine and prilocaine each 29.8%. However, at the time the paper was published (2007), lidocaine had approximately a 54% share of the U.S. local anesthetic market, giving it a risk of paresthesia below that which would be calculated if all drugs were equally neurotoxic. The lidocaine ratio was 0.64. Prilocaine, with a 6% market share, had a ratio of 4.96—the highest of any of the local anesthetics in use in the United States, and articaine, at the time possessing a 25% market share, had a ratio of 1.19.[14] Pogrel concluded, "Therefore, using our previous assumption that approximately half of all local anesthetic used is for inferior alveolar nerve blocks, then on the figures we have generated from our clinic we do not see disproportionate nerve involvement from articaine."[14]

In 2010, Garisto and associates published a report on the occurrence of paresthesia in the United States.[15] Although again demonstrating that 4% solutions had a higher reported rate of paresthesia, their reported incidences for all local anesthetics were quite astounding: the overall incidence of reported paresthesia was 1 in 13,800,970 injections. For mepivacaine, the incidence was 1:623,112,900, and for lidocaine, 1:181,076,673. For articaine and prilocaine, investigators reported 1:4,159,848 and 1:2,070,678, respectively. This author might report, for the sake of comparison, that the risk of being struck by lightning in the United States on an annual basis is 1:750,000.[16]

A meta-analysis comparing articaine HCl with lidocaine (lignocaine) HCl reported that articaine is more likely than lidocaine to achieve anesthetic success in the posterior first molar area, and that there is no difference in postinjection adverse events.[17] A 2011 review of the articaine literature (116 papers reviewed) concluded, "although there may be controversy regarding its safety and advantages in comparison to other local anaesthetics, there is no conclusive evidence demonstrating neurotoxicity or significantly superior anaesthetic properties of articaine for dental procedures."[18]

QUESTION: How do I select an appropriate local anesthetic for a given patient and procedure?

Two factors are particularly important:

1. The duration of pain control necessary to complete the procedure and the possible need for posttreatment pain control (e.g., after surgical procedures). Box 4-1 lists currently available local anesthetic formulations by their approximate duration of action—both soft tissue and pulpal anesthesia.
2. The patient's physical status (e.g., American Society of Anesthesiologists [ASA] classification), hypersensitivity, methemoglobinemia, or sulfur allergy, which may preclude the use of some drugs.

For most patients, the duration of desired pain control is the ultimate deciding factor in local anesthetic selection, because usually there are no contraindications to the administration of any particular agent.

QUESTION: What local anesthetics should be available in my office?

It is suggested that a number of local anesthetics be available at all times. The nature of the dental practice will dictate the number and types of local anesthetics needed. In a typical dental practice, selection of a local anesthetic formulation is based on the desired duration of pulpal anesthesia, for example, less than 30 minutes, approximately 60 minutes, in excess of 90 minutes. One local anesthetic preparation from each group, as necessitated by the nature of the doctor's practice, should be available. For example, the pediatric dentist has little need or desire for long-acting local anesthetics such as bupivacaine, whereas the oral and maxillofacial surgeon may have little need for shorter-acting drugs such as mepivacaine plain, but a greater need for bupivacaine. Remember that not all patients have similar local anesthetic requirements, and the same patient may require a different local anesthetic for a dental procedure of a different duration. Amide local anesthetics are preferred to esters because of their decreased incidence of allergy.

QUESTION: Do topical anesthetics really work?

Absolutely, if the topical anesthetic preparation is applied to mucous membrane for an adequate length of time.[19] The American Dental Association recommends a 1 minute application.[20] The Food and Drug Administration recommends application for a minimum of 1 minute. Gill and Orr recommend application for 2 to 3 minutes.[21] Topical anesthetics containing benzocaine are not absorbed from their site of application into the cardiovascular system. Therefore risk of overdose is minimal when benzocaine-containing topical anesthetic preparations are used. Because of the rapid absorption of some topically applied local anesthetics such as lidocaine, it is recommended that their use be restricted to the following situations:

1. Locally, at the site of needle puncture before injection.
2. For scaling or curettage, over not more than one quadrant at a time.

Pressurized sprays of topical anesthetics cannot be recommended unless they release a metered dose of the drug, not a steady uncontrolled dose. Sterilization of the spray nozzle must be possible if a spray is used. Many pressurized topical anesthetic sprays are available in metered form with disposable spray nozzles.

EMLA (eutectic mixture of local anesthetics), a combination of lidocaine and prilocaine, designed to provide cutaneous anesthesia before venipuncture, has been employed in dentistry with some degree of success.[22,23]

VASOCONSTRICTORS

QUESTION: Are there any contraindications to the use of vasopressors in dental patients?

Yes. Use of local anesthetics with vasopressors should be avoided or kept to an absolute minimum in the following cases[24-26]:

1. Patients with blood pressure in excess of 200 mm Hg systolic or 115 mm Hg diastolic.
2. Patients with uncontrolled hyperthyroidism.
3. Patients with severe cardiovascular disease.
   a. Less than 6 months after myocardial infarction
   b. Less than 6 months after cerebrovascular accident
   c. Daily episodes of angina pectoris or unstable (preinfarction) angina
   d. Cardiac dysrhythmias despite appropriate therapy
   e. Post coronary artery bypass surgery, less than 6 months
4. Patients who are undergoing general anesthesia with halogenated agents.
5. Patients receiving nonspecific β-blockers, monoamine oxidase inhibitors, or tricyclic antidepressants.

Patients in categories 1 to 3a through 3d are classified as ASA 4 risks and normally are not considered candidates for elective or emergency dental treatment in the office. (Refer to Chapter 3 for a more detailed discussion; also see the next question.)

QUESTION: Often medical consultants recommend against inclusion of a vasopressor in a local anesthetic for a cardiovascular risk patient. Why? And what can I do to achieve effective pain control?

As indicated, there are several instances in which it is prudent to avoid the use of vasopressors in local anesthetics. Most of these situations (e.g., severely elevated, untreated high blood pressure; severe cardiovascular disease) also represent absolute contraindications to elective dental care because of greater potential risk to the patient. If a dental patient with cardiovascular disease is deemed treatable (ASA 2 or 3), then local anesthetics for pain control are indicated. The patient's physician often states that, although local anesthetics can be used, epinephrine should be avoided.

QUESTION: When should epinephrine be avoided?

One of the few valid reasons for avoiding epinephrine is the patient with cardiac rhythm abnormalities that are unresponsive to medical therapy. The presence of dysrhythmias (especially ventricular) usually indicates an irritable or ischemic myocardium. Epinephrine, exogenous or endogenous, further increases myocardial sensitivity, thereby predisposing this patient to a greater frequency of dysrhythmias or to more significant types of dysrhythmias, such as ventricular tachycardia or ventricular fibrillation. In these patients, epinephrine-containing local anesthetics should be avoided, if at all possible. However, many cardiologists today do not even consider the ischemic myocardium a valid reason for excluding vasoconstrictors from local anesthetics, provided the dose of epinephrine administered is minimal and intravascular administration is avoided.

It is my recommendation that with a patient who is deemed able to tolerate the stresses involved in the planned dental treatment, a vasoconstrictor should be included in the local anesthetic if there is a reason for its inclusion (e.g., depth or duration of anesthesia, need for hemostasis). As Bennett has stated, "the greater the medical risk of a patient, the more important effective control of pain and anxiety becomes."[27]

QUESTION: Why do many physicians still recommend against the use of epinephrine (and other vasopressors) in cardiovascular risk patients?

Most physicians never, or at best rarely, use epinephrine in their practice. The only physicians who do so on a regular basis are anesthesiologists, emergency medicine specialists, and surgeons. As used in medicine, epinephrine is almost always used in emergency situations. At those times, the dose is considerably higher than that used in dentistry. The average emergency dose of intramuscular (IM) or IV epinephrine (used in a 1:1000 or 1:10,000 concentration) for anaphylaxis or cardiac arrest is 0.3 to 1 mg, whereas one dental cartridge with 1:100,000 epinephrine contains only 0.018 mg.

Therefore it is understandable that many physicians, lacking an intimate knowledge of the practice of dentistry, think of epinephrine in terms of the doses used in emergency medicine and not in the much more dilute forms used for anesthesia in dentistry.

An example follows. In a hospital situation, a patient with a serious cardiovascular problem (ASA 4) who requires a surgical procedure (e.g., emergency appendectomy) may be considered too great a risk for general anesthesia. Many anesthesiologists opt to use a regional local anesthetic (spinal) block with an intravenous antianxiety agent (diazepam or midazolam) for sedation in place of general anesthesia. The local anesthetic usually contains a vasopressor such as epinephrine in a 1:100,000 or 1:200,000 concentration, added primarily to decrease the rate at which the local anesthetic is absorbed into the cardiovascular system, but also to minimize bleeding and prolong the duration of clinical action.

QUESTION: Why is the use of vasopressors in local anesthetics recommended for cardiac risk patients?

Pain is stressful to the body. During stress, endogenous catecholamines (e.g., epinephrine, norepinephrine) are released from their storage sites into the cardiovascular system at a level approximately 40 times greater than the resting level. (Refer to Chapter 3 for a review of the pharmacology of this group of drugs.)

Release of epinephrine and norepinephrine into the blood increases the cardiovascular workload; thus the myocardial oxygen requirement increases. In patients with compromised (partially occluded) coronary arteries, this greater myocardial oxygen requirement may not be met; ischemia may develop subsequently and may lead to dysrhythmias, anginal pain (if ischemia is transient), or myocardial infarction (if prolonged). Increased cardiac workload may also lead to acute exacerbation of heart failure (acute pulmonary edema). Elevated catecholamine levels can produce a dramatic increase in blood pressure; this can precipitate another life-threatening situation (e.g., a hemorrhagic stroke [cerebrovascular accident {CVA}, "brain attack"]).

Therefore the goal is to minimize endogenous catecholamine release during dental therapy. The stress reduction protocol is designed to accomplish this. A local anesthetic without vasopressor provides pulpal anesthesia of shorter duration than the same drug with a vasopressor. Profound pain control of adequate duration is less likely to be achieved when a vasopressor is excluded from a local anesthetic solution. If the patient experiences pain during treatment, an exaggerated stress response is observed.

With proper use (aspiration and slow injection) of a local anesthetic with minimum concentration of exogenous vasopressor (e.g., 1:100,000, 1:200,000), pain control of longer duration is virtually guaranteed, and the exaggerated stress response is avoided. Levels of catecholamine in the blood are elevated when exogenous epinephrine is administered, but these levels usually are not clinically significant.

An often repeated and essentially true statement is that the cardiovascularly impaired patient is more at risk from endogenously released catecholamines than from exogenous epinephrine administered in a proper manner.

QUESTION: Can I administer a local anesthetic with a vasopressor even if a physician has advised against it?

Yes. A medical consultation is a request for advice from you to a person with more knowledge of the matter being discussed. You are not obligated to heed this advice if you feel it may be inaccurate. If doubt persists in your mind concerning the proper treatment protocol following this initial consultation, additional opinions should be sought, preferably from a specialist in the "area" of concern, such as a cardiologist, an anesthesiologist, or a dental expert in local anesthesia. Of course, for some patients, exogenous catecholamines may prove too great a risk; in these cases, "plain" local anesthetic solutions should be administered.

It must always be remembered that the primary responsibility for the care and well-being of a patient rests solely in the hands of the person who performs the treatment, not the one who gives advice.

An incident concerning a medical consultation is worth relating. A periodontal graduate student was planning four quadrants of osseous surgery on a patient whose medical history was within normal limits, except for a torticollis for which she was receiving imipramine, a tricyclic antidepressant. A written consultation was sent to the patient's physician requesting that the patient be taken off the imipramine before the surgical procedure was performed. The response was that the patient could not be taken off the drug, because it had taken longer than a year to get her medical condition stabilized. Moreover, it was recommended that epinephrine be avoided during this patient's surgery. It was decided to contact the physician directly to discuss the matter and to attempt to explain the importance of epinephrine during the surgical procedure. In the ensuing conversation, it was agreed that epinephrine could be used, but in a limited dose, and that the patient was to be monitored (vital signs) throughout the procedure. The surgery was carried off without incident.

The lesson to be learned from this episode is that the wording of the original consult was too constricting, or indeed might have been construed as threatening, to the physician. Whenever possible, direct contact and discussion with both parties explaining their needs should be obtained, because this is more likely to lead to a satisfactory compromise and to better and safer patient management.

QUESTION: If epinephrine is used in cardiac risk patients, is there a maximum dose?

Yes. Bennett recommends, and others agree, that the maximum dose of epinephrine in a cardiac risk patient should be 0.04 mg.[27] This equates to roughly the following:

- One cartridge of 1:50,000 epinephrine
- Two cartridges of 1:100,000 epinephrine
- Four cartridges of 1:200,000 epinephrine

I do not recommend the use of 1:50,000 epinephrine for pain control purposes. (Further information on dental management of the cardiovascular risk patient is available.[28-30])

QUESTION: What about epinephrine-containing gingival retraction cord?

Racemic epinephrine gingival retraction cord should never be used for cardiovascular risk patients, and it is my opinion that it should not be used for any patient. Gingival retraction cord contains 8% racemic epinephrine. Half of this is the levorotatory form, which provides a concentration of active epinephrine of 4% (or 40 mg/mL). This is 40 times the concentration used in the management of anaphylaxis or cardiac arrest. Absorption of epinephrine through mucous membrane into the cardiovascular system normally is rapid but is even more so with active bleeding, such as that occurring after subgingival tooth preparation. Levels of epinephrine in the blood rise rapidly, leading to cardiovascular manifestations of epinephrine overdose (p. 325).

This increase in cardiovascular activity may prove to be life threatening in patients with preexisting clinically evident or subclinical cardiovascular disease.

QUESTION: If I elect not to use a vasopressor for a patient, which local anesthetics are clinically useful?

The clinically available local anesthetics are listed by their duration of action in Box 4-1. Mepivacaine 3% (via nerve block) can provide up to 40 minutes of pulpal anesthesia for the average patient, whereas prilocaine 4% (via nerve block) can provide up to 60 minutes.

SYRINGES

QUESTION: What type of syringe is recommended?

Although a wide variety of syringes are available, two factors have primary importance in their selection:

1. A syringe must be capable of aspiration. Never use a syringe that does not permit aspiration.
2. A syringe must be sterilizable, unless it is disposable.

In addition, with the introduction of so-called safety syringes, it is my recommendation that every consideration be given to the use of a syringe that is designed to minimize the risk of accidental needle-stick after injection is completed. Although the unit cost of the disposable safety syringe increases office expenses, the decreased liability faced by the doctor in needle-stick injuries should more than cover this consideration. Although in theory, safety syringes are mandatory, the lack of effective devices in the American dental market has severely limited implementation in clinical practice. Traditional dental syringes continue to represent the standard of care.

QUESTION: Do computer-controlled local anesthetic delivery systems (C-CLADs) work well enough to justify their purchase?

Yes. In most instances, C-CLADs enable the patient to receive effective local anesthesia in an entirely pain-free manner. Response from dentists using C-CLADs varies from those who are extremely ecstatic to those who do not feel they are worth the expense. Most responses are favorable. In my experience, C-CLADs make it easier to more comfortably deliver those injections that are "difficult" to administer painlessly.

These include all palatal injections and periodontal ligament (PDL) techniques.

NEEDLES

QUESTION: What gauge and length of needles are recommended for injection?

Selection of a needle depends on several factors, foremost among which are the aspiration potential of the injection and the estimated depth of soft tissue penetration:

1. A long dental needle is recommended for inferior alveolar, Gow-Gates mandibular, Vazirani-Akinosi mandibular, ASA (infraorbital), and maxillary nerve blocks in adults.
2. A short needle is recommended for posterior superior alveolar, mental, and incisive nerve blocks; maxillary infiltration (supraperiosteal injection); palatal nerve blocks and infiltration; and periodontal ligament and intraseptal injections.

In earlier editions, I specified the gauge of the needle for each injection. A 25-gauge needle was recommended for the techniques in number 1 (above), a 27-gauge needle for those in number 2 (above). These remain my recommendations today.

If only two needles were to be available in my dental office, I would opt for a 25-gauge long and a 27-gauge short. I have absolutely no need or desire to ever use a 30-gauge needle for an intraoral injection. However, this is not the case in dentistry in the United States. Information received from needle manufacturers indicates that the most commonly purchased needles in dentistry in the United States are the 27-gauge long and the 30-gauge short.

I do not recommend a 30-gauge short, but it may be used for local infiltration to produce hemostasis. The major problem, in this author's opinion, is the increased risk of needle breakage and retention within soft tissues if it is used for an injection technique that mandates use of a long dental needle. The problem of broken needles is reviewed in Chapter 17.

CARTRIDGES

QUESTION: Why do you (the author) call this a cartridge when everyone else calls it a carpule?

Carpule is a proprietary name for the glass cartridge. The name is trademarked by the Cook-Waite Corporation (now Kodak).

QUESTION: Can glass cartridges be autoclaved?

No. Autoclaving of glass cartridges destroys their seals. The heat of autoclaving also degrades the heat-labile vasopressor.

QUESTION: Should local anesthetic cartridges be stored in alcohol or cold sterilizing solution?

No. Alcohol or cold sterilizing solution diffuses into the cartridge. Injection of these into tissues may produce burning, irritation, or paresthesia. (The care and handling of local anesthetic cartridges are discussed in Chapter 7.)

QUESTION: Are cartridge warmers effective in making local anesthetic solutions more comfortable on injection?

No. Most cartridge warmers make the local anesthetic solution too warm, leading to increased discomfort on injection, and possible destruction of the heat-sensitive vasopressor. Cartridges of local anesthetic solution stored at room temperature produce no discomfort to patients and are greatly preferred.

QUESTION: Why do some patients complain of a burning sensation when a local anesthetic is injected?

Because of its pH, any local anesthetic may cause a slight burning sensation during the initial injection. The pH of a plain solution is in the range of 5.5 to 6.0, and that of a vasopressor-containing solution is in the mid-3 to mid-4 range. Other causes include an overly warm solution, the presence of alcohol or cold sterilizing solution within the cartridge, or a solution with a vasopressor at or near its expiration date.

The recent introduction of a simple system of buffering local anesthetic cartridges immediately before injection, raising the pH to a body-compatible 7.35 to 7.5, enables the delivery of more comfortable local anesthetic to patients. Local anesthetic buffering is discussed in Chapter 20.

QUESTION: What causes local anesthetic solution to run down the outside of the needle into a patient's mouth?

Improper preparation of the armamentarium is to blame for this. (See Chapter 9.) The recommended sequence for preparation (using a metal syringe and a disposable needle) is as follows:

1. Place the cartridge in the syringe.
2. Embed the aspirating harpoon with finger pressure only. (No tapping or hitting of the plunger is necessary.)
3. Place the needle on the syringe.

This sequence provides a perfectly centric perforation of the rubber diaphragm by the needle, with a tight seal formed around the needle. No leakage of anesthetic occurs.

When the needle is placed onto the syringe first, followed by the cartridge, it is possible for the perforation of the diaphragm to be ovoid, not round. The ovoid perforation does not seal itself as well around the metal needle, leading to leakage of anesthetic around this area as the anesthetic drug is injected.

QUESTION: What causes cartridges to break during injection?

1. Damage during shipping. Visually check cartridges before use.
2. Using excessive force to engage the aspirating harpoon in the rubber stopper. Proper preparation of the needle, cartridge, and syringe (see previous question) precludes breakage caused by excessive force. When the needle is placed onto the syringe before the cartridge, it is necessary to "hit" the plunger to embed the harpoon into the rubber stopper. This may cause a cartridge to shatter.
3. Attempting to force a cartridge with an extruded plunger into the syringe.
4. Using a syringe with a bent aspirating harpoon.
5. Bent needle with an occluded lumen. Always expel a small volume of anesthetic from the syringe before inserting the needle into the patient's tissues to ensure patency of the needle.

TECHNIQUES OF REGIONAL ANESTHESIA IN DENTISTRY

QUESTION: What should always be done before local anesthetic administration in a patient?

Review of the patient's medical history questionnaire (visually or verbally) and a physical examination, including vital signs and visual inspection, are recommended when a patient is seen for the first time or after a long absence from the office. This identifies possible contraindications to the use of local anesthetics or vasopressors and in general determines a patient's ability to tolerate physically and psychologically the stresses of dental care without undue risk.

QUESTION: What are medical contraindications to the use of local anesthetics and vasopressors?

These are discussed in Chapter 4 and in excellent review articles by Perusse, Goulet, and Turcotte.[24-26]

QUESTION: Should a patient be advised that a local anesthetic injection will hurt before the injection is started?

No. Local anesthetic injections need not hurt. Careful adherence to the atraumatic injection protocol described in Chapter 11 can make virtually all injections, including palatal, painless.

QUESTION: Is any specific chair position best for administration of local anesthetics?

Yes, absolutely! Because the most commonly observed adverse reactions to local anesthetics are psychogenic (e.g., syncope), the position of choice during intraoral injections is one in which the patient's chest (heart) and head are parallel to the floor with the feet slightly elevated. Presyncopal episodes may still occur (pallor, lightheadedness), but actual loss of consciousness is extremely unlikely to develop with the patient in this position.

After completion of several mandibular injections (inferior alveolar, Gow-Gates mandibular, and Vazirani-Akinosi mandibular nerve blocks), it is suggested that the patient be returned to a comfortable, more upright position during the ensuing 5 to 10 minutes. This change in patient position appears to help speed the onset of mandibular block anesthesia.

QUESTION: Why do you (the author) recommend regional block anesthesia in the maxilla instead of infiltration (supraperiosteal) anesthesia?

Regional block anesthesia in the maxilla is preferred to infiltration whenever more than two teeth are to be treated. Its advantages include the following:
1. Fewer penetrations of tissue, thus less likelihood of postinjection problems.
2. Smaller volume of local anesthetic (e.g., than for multiple infiltrations of the same area), thereby decreasing the risk of systemic reactions such as overdose.
3. Clinically adequate anesthesia more likely when infiltration is ineffective because of the presence of infection.

QUESTION: Do palatal injections always hurt?

No. Careful adherence to the protocol for atraumatic injections can do much to minimize any discomfort associated with palatal anesthesia. In addition, the following are important:
1. Topical anesthesia.
2. Pressure anesthesia.
3. Control of the needle.
4. Slow deposition of solution.
5. Positive attitude of the administrator.

An area of considerable interest among practicing dentists is palatal anesthesia and how to increase patient comfort. Over the years, I have received many devices designed by dentists in an attempt to minimize or eliminate pain during palatal injections, and I have been told of many techniques. These include using vibrating wands, letting the needle trace along the palate for a second or two so patients know it is coming and it is not a "shock" to them, and avoiding the use of palatal injections unless they are absolutely necessary.

The clinical introduction of C-CLADs (see the preceding and Chapter 5) permits the delivery of local anesthetic injections in any area of the oral cavity in a pain-free manner in most situations.

Research into the use of intranasally administered local anesthetics has shown promising results. Pulpal anesthesia bilaterally from second premolar to second premolar was achieved in a Phase II clinical trial.[31]

QUESTION: Why do I miss inferior alveolar nerve blocks more often than any other injection?

Of all nerve blocks in dentistry and, with few exceptions, in medicine too, the inferior alveolar is the most elusive of consistent success. A success rate, bilaterally, of 85% or greater indicates that one's technique is basically correct. However, many factors can, and do, affect this rate of success:

1. *Anatomic variation.* It is well known that if any one aspect of human anatomy is consistent, it is its inconsistency. Strict adherence to injection technique does not always produce adequate inferior alveolar anesthesia.
2. *Technical error.* The most common technical error observed with the inferior alveolar nerve block is insertion of the needle too low on the medial side of the ramus (below the mandibular foramen, where the inferior alveolar nerve enters onto the mandibular canal). A second common technical error is insertion of the needle too far anteriorly (laterally) on the medial side of the ramus (thus contacting bone quite soon after penetration).
3. *Accessory innervation.* When isolated regions of mandibular teeth remain sensitive when all other areas are insensitive, the possibility of accessory innervation should be considered. The technique used in eliminating this problem (which usually is produced by the mylohyoid nerve) is described in Chapter 14.

In September 2011, a supplement to the *Journal of the American Dental Association,* titled *Is the Mandibular Block Passé?* was published.[32-35] It concluded that although the time had not yet arrived to bid farewell to the traditional inferior alveolar nerve block, sufficient alternative techniques are available to enable the doctor to provide successful pain control in the mandible in virtually all treatment situations: Gow-Gates, Akinosi-Vazirani, and incisive (mental) nerve blocks; intraosseous and periodontal ligament injections; and the use of mandibular infiltration anesthesia in adults. These techniques are discussed in Chapters 14, 15, and 20.

QUESTION: Why do I have a much higher failure rate with inferior alveolar nerve block on one side than on the other?

Because of significantly different operator positions during administration of the inferior alveolar nerve block on contralateral sides of the mouth, it is not uncommon for some doctors to encounter significant differences in their success rates. The inferior alveolar is the only intraoral nerve block for which significant differences in success rates are noted on opposite sides of the mouth. Although basic protocols are the same on the right and left sides, the view of the target area as seen by the administrator, the angle of needle entry, and other factors may be responsible for an increased failure rate on one side. The solution to this problem is to critically evaluate one's technique on the less successful side and to seek to correct it without interfering with success on the opposite side. Patience is often necessary.

QUESTION: How can I achieve adequate pain control when gaining access in pulpally involved teeth?

The recommended sequence of injection techniques for pulpally involved teeth follows:

1. Local infiltration, if possible and not contraindicated.
2. Regional nerve block.
3. PDL injection, if not contraindicated by the presence of infection.
4. Intraosseous injection.
5. Intraseptal injection.
6. Intrapulpal injection.
7. Psychosedation, if pain control techniques have proved unsuccessful in completely blocking pain impulses from reaching brain.
8. Prayer…when nothing else works! However, with the introduction of intraosseous anesthesia, this step is rarely, if ever, needed.

The recent (2011) introduction of a method by which local anesthetic cartridges can be consistently buffered to a pH of between 7.35 and 7.5 brings with it the expectation that, along with increased comfort during injection and more rapid onset of anesthesia, the depth of anesthesia will be greater because more of the lipid-soluble RN ionic form of the local anesthetic molecule is available to diffuse through the lipid-rich nerve membrane.[36] Research projects in this area have been undertaken. Buffered local anesthetics are discussed in Chapter 20.

For all teeth in the mouth, with the probable exception of mandibular molars, clinically adequate pain control for pulpal extirpation can be obtained with local infiltration or nerve block injection. Difficulties arise most often in the mandibular molars. A working knowledge of alternative mandibular anesthesia techniques, such as the Gow-Gates mandibular block or the Vazirani-Akinosi mandibular block,[33] increases the likelihood of obtaining anesthesia. In addition, the use of intraosseous anesthesia greatly increases success rates in mandibular molars.[34]

Mandibular premolars and anterior teeth can be anesthetized adequately for pulpal extirpation with the incisive nerve block.

QUESTION: What special concerns are involved with local anesthesia in pediatric dentistry?

Pain control generally is easier to achieve in pediatric dentistry. However, two concerns should always be considered:

1. *Increased potential for overdose* exists because (most) children are smaller and weigh less than adults. Use milligram-per-weight formulas to minimize doses in children.

2. *Prolonged anesthesia* can lead to traumatization of the lips and tongue, unless shorter-duration drugs are used, and both patient and parent are warned of this possible complication.

A third concern relates to injection technique and the appropriate needle to be used in specific techniques. A long dental needle is recommended for the injections described in this book for which a considerable thickness of soft tissue is to be penetrated. The rationale for this is the rule of thumb that "a needle should not be inserted into tissue all the way to its hub, unless it is absolutely necessary for the success of that injection." If it is possible for an injection technique to be administered in a child with a short (≈20 mm length) needle within the parameters of this rule, then use of this needle is warranted. Psychologically, however, the sight of a long needle is more traumatic than the sight of a short needle (in point of fact, needles and syringes should always be kept out of a patient's line of sight, if possible).

QUESTION: What is the recommended method of achieving hemostasis in surgical areas?

The recommended technique is local infiltration of a vasopressor-containing anesthetic into the region of the surgery. Only small volumes are necessary for this purpose. Epinephrine in a concentration of 1:100,000 is recommended (although 1:50,000 also may be used).

References

1. Radowicka A, Kochmanski M, Zochowski RJ: Rare case of asystolic cardiac arrest after administration of xylocaine, Kardiol Pol 24:237–242, 1981.
2. Applebaum D, Halperin E: Asystole following a conventional therapeutic dose of lidocaine, Am J Emerg Med 4:143–145, 1986.
3. Mishima S, Kasai K, Yamamoto M, et al: Cardiac arrest due to lidocaine, Masui 38:1365–1368, 1989.
4. Gilbert TB: Cardiac arrest from inadvertent overdose of lidocaine hydrochloride through an arterial pressure line flush apparatus, Anesth Analg 93:1534–1536, 2001.
5. Doumiri M, Moussaoui A, Maazouzi W: Cardiac arrest after gargling and oral ingestion of 5% lidocaine, Can J Anaesth 55:882–883, 2008.
6. Yang JJ, Shen J, Xu J: Cardiac asystole after nasal infiltration of lidocaine with epinephrine in a transsphenoidal hypophysectomy patient with hypertrophic cardiomyopathy, J Neurosurg Anesthesiol 22:81–82, 2010.
7. Haas DA, Lennon D: A 21 year retrospective study of reports of paresthesia following local anesthetic administration, J Can Dent Assoc 61:319–320, 343–326, 329–330, 1995.
8. Hillerup S, Jensen R: Nerve injury caused by mandibular block analgesia, Int J Oral Maxillofac Surg 35:437–443, 2006.
9. Malamed SF: Nerve injury caused by mandibular block analgesia. Letter to the Editor, Int J Oral Maxillofac Surg 35:876–877, 2006.
10. Pharmacovigilance Committee of the European Union: Adverse effects from local anaesthetics used in relation with dental care with a special focus on anaesthetics containing articaine, Case number 3200-1367, October 20, 2006.
11. Weber JCP: Epidemiology of adverse reactions to nonsteroidal anti-inflammatory drugs. In Rainsford KD, Velo GP, editors: Advances in inflammatory research, vol 6, New York, 1984, Raven Press, pp 1–7.
12. Hartnell NR, Wilson JP: Replication of the Weber effect using postmarketing adverse event reports voluntarily submitted to the United States Food and Drug Administration, Pharmacotherapy 24:743–749, 2004.
13. Wallensteim EJ, Fife D: Temporal patterns of NSAID spontaneous adverse event reports: the Weber effect revisited, Drug Saf 24:233–237, 2001.
14. Pogrel MA: Permanent nerve damage from inferior alveolar nerve blocks—an update to include articaine, J Calif Dent Assoc 35:271–273, 2007.
15. Garisto GA, Gaffen AS, Lawrence HP, et al: Occurrence of paresthesia after dental local anesthetic administration in the United States, J Am Dent Assoc 141:836–844, 2010.
16. Available at: www.lightningsafety.noaa.gov. Accessed October 2011.
17. Katyal V: The efficacy and safety of articaine versus lignocaine in dental treatments: a meta-analysis, J Dent 38:307–317, 2010.
18. Yapp KE, Hopcraft MS, Parashos P: Articaine: a review of the literature, Br Dent J 210:323–329, 2011.
19. Meechan JG: Intra-oral topical anaesthetics: a review, J Dent 28:1–14, 2000.
20. American Dental Association Council on Dental Therapeutics: Accepted dental therapeutics, Chicago, 1984, The American Dental Association.
21. Gill CJ, Orr DL: A double blind crossover comparison of topical anesthetics, J Am Dent Assoc 98:213, 1979.
22. Gunter JB: Benefits and risks of local anesthetics in infants and children, Paediatr Drugs 4:649–672, 2002.
23. Bernardi M, Secco F, Benech A: Anesthetic efficacy of a eutectic mixture of lidocaine and prilocaine (EMLA) on the oral mucosa: prospective double-blind study with a placebo, Minerv Somatol 48:39–43, 1999.
24. Perusse R, Goulet JP, Turcotte JY: Contraindications to vasoconstrictors in dentistry: Part I. Cardiovascular diseases, Oral Surg 74:692–697, 1992.
25. Perusse R, Goulet JP, Turcotte JY: Contraindications to vasoconstrictors in dentistry: Part II. Hyperthyroidism, diabetes, sulfite sensitivity, cortico-dependent asthma, and pheochromocytoma, Oral Surg 74:587–691, 1992.
26. Perusse R, Goulet JP, Turcotte JY: Contraindications to vasoconstrictors in dentistry: Part III. Pharmacologic interactions, Oral Surg 74:592–697, 1992.
27. Bennett CR: Monheim's local anesthesia and pain control in dental practice, ed 7, St Louis, 1984, Mosby.
28. Anonymous: Cardiovascular effects of epinephrine in hypertensive dental patients, Evidence Report: Technology Assessment (Summary) 48:1–3, 2002.
29. Silvestre FJ, Verdu MJ, Sanchis JM, et al: Effects of vasoconstrictors in dentistry on systolic and diastolic arterial pressure, Med Oral 6:17–63, 2001.
30. Yagiela JA: Adverse drug interactions in dental practice: interactions associated with vasoconstrictors. Part V of a series, J Am Dent Assoc 130:701–709, 1999.
31. Ciancio S, Ayoub F, Pantera E, et al: Nasal spray for anesthesia of maxillary teeth. Poster presentation at International Association for Dental Research (IADR) General Session, July 14–17, 2010, Barcelona, Spain.

32. Malamed SF. Is the mandibular block passé? J Am Dent Assoc 142(Suppl 9):35–75, 2011.
33. Haas D: Alternative mandibular block techniques: a review of the Gow-Gates mandibular nerve block and Akinos-Vazirani closed-mouth mandibular nerve block techniques, J Am Dent Assoc 142(Suppl 9):8S–12S, 2011.
34. Moore PA, Cuddy MA, Cooke MR, et al: Intraosseous anesthesia techniques: alternatives to mandibular nerve blocks, J Am Dent Assoc 142(Suppl 9):13S–18S, 2011.
35. Meechan JG: Mandibular infiltration anesthesia in adults, J Am Dent Assoc 142(Suppl 9):19S–26S, 2011.
36. Malamed SF: Buffering local anesthetics in dentistry, DSA Pulse 44(1):3, 8-9, 2011.

Index

Note: Page numbers followed by "f" refer to illustrations; page numbers followed by "t" refer to tables; page numbers followed by "b" refer to boxes.

D

I